THE JOURNAL OF

Pathology

A Journal of the Pathological Society of Great Britain and Ireland

1984 Volume 144

A WILEY MEDICAL PUBLICATION
JPTLAS 144(1–4) 1–300 (1984)
ISSN 0022-3417

THE JOURNAL OF

Pathology

Published in association with the
Pathological Society of Great Britain and Ireland

Editor-in-Chief

Professor D. H. Wright
Department of Pathology, University of Southampton, South Laboratory/Pathology Block, Southampton General Hospital, Tremona Road, Southampton SO9 4XY, UK

Editors

Dr A. G. MacIver
Department of Pathology, Southmead General Hospital, Westbury-on-Trym, Bristol BS10 5NB, UK

Professor F. Walker
Department of Pathology, University Medical Buildings, Foresterhill, Aberdeen AB9 2ZD, UK

Aims and Scope

The Journal of Pathology is a journal of the Pathological Society of Great Britain and Ireland. From January 1984, it will incorporate the other affiliated journal, *Diagnostic Histopathology*. The new group of Editors intend that the journal shall reflect the interests of the members of the Society. This will be no easy task since they cover the whole range of experimental and diagnostic histopathology.

High quality papers, written in English and dealing with descriptive histopathology will be welcome. Papers dealing with new techniques and those that elucidate the mechanisms underlying disease processes and histopathological appearance will be particularly encouraged. Single case reports will be accepted only when they are of exceptional interest with important new information and which contain a full, but concise, review of the literature. Good photo-micrographs are of particular value and interest to histopathologists and emphasis will be placed on the quality of the illustrations.

Original articles in the field of experimental pathology, relevant to human disease, will be welcome. Review articles dealing with general and experimental pathology, as well as diagnostic histopathology, will be solicited. Unsolicited reviews will also be accepted if they are clearly written and topical. Editorials, a letter column and reviews of recently published books will form regular features of the Journal. Meetings abstracts of the Pathological Society of Great Britain and Ireland will be published as they become available and the annual CL Oakley Lecture will continue to be included. Symposia proceedings may be published if the Editors consider them appropriate and relevant. The Editors wish to maintain the minimum delay between manuscript submission, decision and publication, and authors are therefore requested to follow the instructions for manuscript preparation as set out in the Notes for Contributors which are printed on the inside back cover.

CONTENTS

Volume, 144 Issue Nos 1–4, 1984

JOURNAL OF PATHOLOGY

Issue No. 1 SEPTEMBER 1984

Editorial Policy i

Original Articles

Functional and Morphologic Studies of the Adrenal Cortex and Kidney in Ovine Toxaemia of Pregnancy, P. A. HILL, J. P. COGHLAN, B. A. SCOGGINS AND G. B. RYAN 1

Ductal Adenoma of the Breast: a Lesion Which Can Mimic Carcinoma, J. G. AZZOPARDI AND R. SALM 15

Cutaneous and Pulmonary Histopathological Response to Platelet Activating Factor (Paf-acether) in the Guinea-Pig, A. DEWAR, C. B. ARCHER, W. PAUL, C. P. PAGE, D. M. MACDONALD AND J. MORLEY 25

Immunohistochemical Localization of Macromolecules of the Basement Membrane and Peritumoral Stroma in Human Laryngeal Carcinomas, Y. CAM, T. CAULET, G. BELLON, G. POULIN, M. LEGROS AND M. PYTLINSKA 35

Ferritin Deposition in the Glomerular Deposits of Focal Glomerular Sclerosis in the Rat, C. MELCION, J. SMITH AND V. CATTELL 45

Short Communication

Pigmented Villonodular Synovitis Associated with Psoriatic Polyarthropathy: an Electron Microscopic and Immunocytochemical Study, J. M. ARCHER-HARVEY, D. W. HENDERSON, J. M. PAPADIMITRIOU AND M. A. M. ROZENBILDS 57

Book Review 69

Announcement 71

Issue No. 2 OCTOBER 1984

Original Articles

Amiodarone Lung Toxicity: A Human and Experimental Study, F. R. COSTA-JUSSÀ, B. CORRIN AND J. M. JACOBS 73

Improved Chimaeric Mouse Model Confirms that Resident Peritoneal Macrophages are Derived Solely from Bone Marrow Precursors, A. R. MURCH, M. D. GROUNDS AND J. M. PAPADIMITRIOU 81

The Cumulative Scanning Electron Microscopic Changes in Baby Mouse Lungs Following Prenatal and Postnatal Exposures to Nicotine, N.-S. WANG, M.-F. CHEN, D. E. SCHRAUFNAGEL AND Y.-T. YAO 89

The Binding of Peroxidase-labelled Lectins to Human Breast Epithelium. II—The Reactivity of Breast Carcinomas to Wheat Germ Agglutinin, R. A. WALKER . . 101

The Binding of Peroxidase-labelled Lectins to Human Breast Epithelium. III—Altered Fucose-binding Patterns of Breast Carcinomas and their Significance, R. A. WALKER 109

Unexpected Inorganic Elements in Oral Lesions: Results of X-ray Energy Spectroscopy (XES) on Particulate Matter in Paraffin Sections, D. A. LEVISON, P. R. CROCKER, G. LEE, N. A. SHEPHERD AND A. P. SMITH 119

Angiofollicular Lymph Node Hyperplasia (Castleman's Disease): An Immunohistochemical and Enzyme-histochemical Study of the Hyaline-vascular Form of Lesion, E. L. JONES, J. CROCKER, J. GREGORY, M. GUIBARRA AND R. C. CURRAN 131

Issue No. 3 NOVEMBER 1984

Original Articles

The Role of Cell Injury and the Continuing Inflammatory Response in the Generation of Silicotic Pulmonary Fibrosis, D. H. BOWDEN AND I. Y. R. ADAMSON . . 149

Histomorphometric Analysis of Sclerotic Bone from Idiopathic Myeloid Metaplasia (Nine Cases), J. M. COINDRE, J. REIFFERS, J. F. GOUSSOT, A. DE MASCAREL AND A. BROUSTET 163

Endocrine Cells in Intestinal Metaplasia of the Stomach, P. MINGAZZINI, F. CARLEI, F. MALCHIODI-ALBEDI, E. LEZOCHE, A. COVOTTA, V. SPERANZA AND J. M. POLAK 171

Persistence of Inert Macromolecules (Imposil) in the Rat Mesangium and Glomerular Functional Disturbance, N. P. GOODE, A. M. DAVISON, G. GOWLAND, S. R. APARICIO AND M. SHIRES 179

Spindle Cell Tumours of the Skin of Debatable Origin. An Immunocytochemical Study, V. EUSEBI, C. CECCARELLI, F. PISCIOLI, M. CRISTOFOLINI AND J. G. AZZOPARDI 189

Alterations in the Biophysical Properties of the Human Endothelial Cell Plasma Membrane Induced by a Chemotactic Tripeptide: Correlation with Enhanced Adherence of Granulocytes, C. J. KIRKPATRICK AND I. MELZNER 201

Endothelial Cell Changes in Acute Hepatitis. A Light and Electron Microscopic Study, K. A. BARDADIN AND P. J. SCHEUER 213

Book Reviews 221

Announcements 222

Issue No. 4 DECEMBER 1984

Editorial

From Where Comes The Osteoclast?, J. C. E. UNDERWOOD 225

Review Article

Reticulum Cells: Characterization and Immune Functions and the Nature of Hodgkin and Reed–Sternberg Cells, E. L. JONES 227

Original Articles

The Application of the Metalophil Method for the Demonstration of Histiocytes, J. A. M. VAN UNNIK 233

Metalophil Histiocytes in Non-Hodgkin's Lymphomas Particularly in Malignant Proliferations of B-Lymphocytes, J. A. M. VAN UNNIK AND R. A. DE WEGER 241

Paranodal Tumour in Breast Cancer: Extranodal Extension Versus Vascular Spread, F. HARTVEIT 253

Ischaemic Changes in Human Mesenteric Lymph Nodes, N. J. MAHY AND J. D. DAVIES 257

Focal Lymphocytic Thyroiditis in Southampton, J. D. MITCHELL, N. KIRKHAM AND D. MACHIN 269

Histogenesis of Adenomatoid Tumour Associated to Pseudofibromatous Periorchitis in an Infant with Hydrocele, M. NISTRAL, R. PANIAGUA, E. FUENTES AND J. REGADERA 275

Cell Surface Characterization of the Human Osteoclast: Phenotypic Relationship to Other Bone Marrow-Derived Cell Types, M. A. HORTON, E. F. RIMMER, D. LEWIS, J. A. S. PRINGLE, K. FULLER AND T. J. CHAMBERS 281

Letter to the Editor

Osteoclasts: Putative, Surrogate and Authentic, J. J. CHAMBERS AND M. A. HORTON 295

Book Reviews 297

Announcement 300

JOURNAL OF PATHOLOGY, VOL. **144**: 1–13 (1984)

FUNCTIONAL AND MORPHOLOGIC STUDIES OF THE ADRENAL CORTEX AND KIDNEY IN OVINE TOXAEMIA OF PREGNANCY

PRUDENCE A. HILL*, J. P. COGHLAN†, B. A. SCOGGINS† AND G. B. RYAN*

**Department of Anatomy and †Howard Florey Institute of Experimental Physiology and Medicine, University of Melbourne, Parkville, Victoria, Australia*

Received 31 March 1983
Accepted 1 September 1983

SUMMARY

Functional and morphologic studies of the adrenal cortex and kidney have been carried out in pregnant sheep with spontaneous or dietary restriction-induced ovine toxaemia. It was found that proteinuria was an inconstant feature and no animal showed glomerular lesions analogous to those found in human preeclampsia; thus ovine toxaemia cannot be regarded as a precise experimental model for human toxaemia of pregnancy. The elevation of blood cortisol levels and the morphologic appearance of the adrenal zona fasciculata found in such animals suggest an adrenal response comparable to that caused by adrenocorticotrophic hormone. In addition, animals with severe disease showed evidence of stimulation of the renin–angiotensin–aldosterone system as reflected by elevated blood renin and aldosterone concentrations and raised renal juxtaglomerular indices. Ultrastructural changes in the adrenal zona glomerulosa and renal juxtaglomerular myoepithelioid cells in toxaemic animals resembled those described in non-pregnant sodium-depleted sheep. The finding of juxtaglomerular peripolar cell mitoses and granule exocytosis, the latter only being previously observed in sodium depleted sheep, together with the ultrastructural changes in the adrenal zona glomerulosa and juxtaglomerular myoepithelioid cells, suggest that sodium depletion may play a role in this disease.

KEY WORDS—Sheep, toxaemia of pregnancy, adrenal glands, juxtaglomerular cells.

INTRODUCTION

Human toxaemia of pregnancy or preeclampsia is a syndrome characterized by hypertension, proteinuria and oedema. In severe cases, it may be associated with convulsions and is then termed eclampsia. Preeclampsia–eclampsia is associated with a unique combination of renal glomerular changes, including endothelial cell swelling, subendothelial and mesangial 'fibrin' deposition and an increase in mesangial matrix and cellularity.[1,2] Most data suggest that preeclampsia is associated with suppression of the renin–angiotensin–aldosterone system as compared with normal pregnancy.[3] There also appears to be a loss of the pregnancy–associated refractoriness to angiotensin II.[4]

There are no recognized spontaneous toxaemia-like states in animals which are completely analogous to human toxaemia of pregnancy. Ovine toxaemia or 'twin lamb disease' is a syndrome which occurs in the latter part of pregnancy in sheep, more commonly in ewes with multiple fetuses, and is characterized by neurological signs, motor weakness, apparent blindness and the development of proteinuria.[5,6] The disease occurs either spontaneously 'in the field' or may be induced by either dietary restriction or a traumatic change in environment.[5,6] The animals show a significant reduction in renal blood flow and glomerular filtration rate[7,8] associated with impaired renal function, dramatically raised plas-

Addressee for reprints: Professor G. B. Ryan, Department of Anatomy, University of Melbourne, Parkville 3052, Victoria, Australia.

0022–3417/84/090001–13$01.30

ma renin activity[6] and elevated plasma cortisol levels.[5] Ovine toxaemia has been advanced as a possible animal model for human preeclampsia. However, unlike the human disease, ovine toxaemia is not associated with hypertension[6,7,9] and there is a decreased pressor response to angiotensin II.[6]

In the present paper, functional and morphologic studies of the adrenal cortex and renal juxtaglomerular apparatus have been performed to define more closely the role of the renin–angiotensin–aldosterone system in ovine toxaemia; additionally, the kidneys have been examined for evidence of glomerular lesions comparable to those in human toxaemia of pregnancy. Sheep with either spontaneous toxaemia or with dietary restriction-induced disease were studied. Special attention was directed towards the adrenal zona glomerulosa (the site of aldosterone production) and zona fasciculata (the site of cortisol production) and, in the juxtaglomerular apparatus, arteriolar myoepithelioid cells and the recently described peripolar cells.[10] The myoepithelioid cells, in the wall of the afferent arteriole, contain granules composed of renin which acts on renin substrate to produce angiotensin I which in turn is converted to angiotensin II by converting enzyme. Apart from its effect in causing contraction of arteriolar smooth muscle, angiotensin triggers aldosterone secretion from adrenal zona glomerulosa cells.[11] Peripolar cells are in an epithelial position, forming a cuff around the origin of the glomerular tuft.[10] They form junctional complexes with podocytic epithelial cells on one side and parietal epithelial cells on the other. One surface is attached to Bowman's capsular basement membrane and the other is directly exposed to the urinary space. They contain multiple secretory-type cytoplasmic granules. Peripolar cells are very prominent in sheep but are also found in a wide range of animal species, including man.[10] The composition of peripolar cell granules is unknown but, in view of their unique potential to be released into the urinary space and thereby added to the glomerular ultrafiltrate, it has been suggested that they contain a factor which affects tubular reabsorptive function.[10] Because release of peripolar cell granules into the urinary space has been detected in sodium-depleted sheep,[12] the morphologic appearance of peripolar cells in ovine toxaemia was of particular interest in view of the elevation in renin levels shared by sodium-depleted and toxaemic sheep.[6]

MATERIALS AND METHODS

Twelve ewes with ovine toxaemia developing in the last third of pregnancy (100–150 days) were examined (Table I).

Spontaneous disease: two Merino-cross ewes with the spontaneous onset of ovine toxaemia occurring 'in the field'.

Induced disease: ten Corriedale ewes in which ovine toxaemia was induced as follows: ewes, greater than 5 years of age and gravida 4 or greater, were mated with young fertile rams and yielded a high incidence of twin lambs; at approximately 40 days of gestation their food intake, particularly its protein content, was reduced by keeping the animals in a paddock that was relatively sparsely stocked with grass, but providing supplementary feeding with barley straw and rice straw.

Within a few hours of the onset of signs of toxaemia, the ewes were transported by truck from the farm over a distance of approximately 20 miles to Melbourne. On arrival in the laboratory, the ewes were assessed clinically and graded from I to III (see below) with Grade III showing the most severe signs of the disease. They were catheterized and a urine sample was tested for protein by the sulphosalicylic acid method[13] and for acetone by Multistix® (Ames). In selected animals (Table I), jugular venous blood samples were taken for the measurement of plasma renin concentration by an antibody capture method;[14,15] and blood aldosterone concentration and blood cortisol concentration by a double isotope derivation dilution procedure.[16] Animals were anaesthetized with thiopentone sodium and killed by exsanguination within 4 h of arrival in the laboratory.

A ventral midline incision was made in the abdominal wall through which the uterus was delivered and opened. The fetus or fetuses were assessed as follows (Table I): single (S) or twins (T); dead (D) or alive (A); and crown rump (CR) measurements for estimation of gestational age.

The left adrenal gland of the ewe was removed and bisected longitudinally. One half of the gland was fixed in buffered formol saline and processed for light microscopy. Paraffin sections, 5 μm thick, were stained with haematoxylin and eosin and projected on to a screen using a Nikon profile projector. A tracing was made of the outline of the gland and the zona glomerulosa–fasciculata junction and, under ×400 light microscopy, mitotic figures were identified and plotted on the tracing. For electron microscopy, 1 mm slices were cut from the other half of the gland and placed immediately in 2·5 per cent glutaraldehyde and 2·0 per cent paraformaldehyde in 0·1 M phosphate buffer, pH 7·4, at room temperature and fixed for 5 h. Radial elongated blocks were cut from each slice, always including the capsule and all zones of the cortex, and rinsed overnight in 5 per cent sucrose in 0·1 M phosphate buffer, pH 7·4. The tissue was then post-fixed in 2 per cent aqueous osmium tetroxide at room temperature, dehydrated through 10 per cent to 100 per cent acetone and embedded in Epon–Araldite. Sections, 0·5 μm thick, were cut from tissue blocks using glass knives on a Huxley ultramicrotome, and then stained with methylene blue and examined by light microscopy to confirm the zonation of the tissue. Blocks were trimmed to include the capsule, zona glomerulosa and superficial zona fasciculata; a diamond knife was used to cut thin sections which were then mounted on copper grids, stained with uranyl acetate and lead citrate and examined with a Siemens 102 electron microscope.

The left kidney of each ewe was also removed, bisected longitudinally and slices of tissue were fixed in either Helly's solution or buffered formol saline and processed for light microscopy. Paraffin sections, 5 μm thick, of Helly's-fixed material were stained with Bowie's stain[17] and of formol saline-fixed material were stained with Lendrum's Martius Scarlet Blue (MSB) stain.[18] For animals with induced disease, using the sections stained by the Bowie's method, the juxtaglomerular granulation index (JGI)[19] was calculated as follows. A representative area in Bowie-stained sections of the kidney was selected so that all zones of the cortex were included. Using an oil immersion objective lens, the area was systematically examined and all glomeruli were counted regardless of whether a vascular pole was included in the plane of section; in addition, all juxtaglomerular units were counted whether or not the glomerulus was included in the plane of section. The juxtaglomerular units were assessed for degree of granulation and graded from + to +++. The total juxtaglomerular units were recorded in categories of +, ++ and +++ and multiplied by the factors 1, 2 and 4, respectively; the sum of the weighted totals was expressed as an index per 100 glomeruli. Two JGI's were performed per animal and the measurements were allocated into groups (see Table II) depending upon the grade of toxaemia. A mean value and standard error were calculated for each group and comparisons of group values with those obtained for the control non-toxaemic pregnant Corriedale sheep (see below) were performed using Student's *t*-test. For statistical analysis, a p value of $<0·05$ was considered significant. A peripolar cell granulation index (PGI) was devised on the same protocol as for the JGI above and was performed on the MSB-stained sections; in such sections, peripolar cell granules stain red.[10] Allocation into groups (see Table II), calculations and statistical analysis were performed as described above for the JGI.

For electron microscopy, 1 mm slices from the left kidney were immediately placed in 2·5 per cent glutaraldehyde and 2·0 per cent paraformaldehyde in 0·1 M phosphate buffer, pH 7·4, and fixed for 5 h. The tissue was rinsed overnight in 5 per cent sucrose in 0·1 M phosphate buffer, pH 7·4, and then post-fixed in 2 per cent aqueous osmium tetroxide, dehydrated and embedded as above. Sections, 0·5 μm thick, were stained with methylene blue and examined by light microscopy to determine the presence of juxtaglomerular regions. Blocks were trimmed to include the appropriate glomerulus and juxtaglomerular region and thin sections were then cut, stained and examined as above with an electron microscope.

The findings in these toxaemic sheep were compared with those in five non-pregnant Corriedale ewes, two pregnant but non-toxaemic Merino-cross ewes with single fetuses at 100–110 days of gestation, and five pregnant but non-toxaemic Corriedale ewes with single fetuses at 100–147 days of gestation. Plasma renin, blood aldosterone and blood cortisol concentrations were estimated as above in three of the pregnant ewes (two Merino-cross, and one Corriedale at 137 days). Morphologic studies of the adrenal zona glomerulosa and renal juxtaglomerular apparatus were performed as above in all control animals.

RESULTS

Clinical assessment

The clinical manifestations were similar in animals with spontaneous and dietary restriction-induced ovine toxaemia. Animals with Grade I disease were listless and unsteady on their feet. Animals with Grade II disease were unable to

Table I—Clinical and biochemical data in sheep with ovine toxaemia

Animal number	Clinical grading (Grade I to III)	Gestational age (days)	Fetus(es) S = single T = twins A = alive D = dead	Urinary protein (mg per cent)	Urinary acetone	Plasma renin concentration (pmol/h · ml)	Blood aldosterone concentration (ng/dl)	Blood cortisol concentration (μg/dl)
Spontaneous disease								
1	I	134	T; A, A	20	3+	17·0	—	—
2	III	134	T; D, D	—	—	27·3	71·0	7·1
Induced disease								
3	I	122	S; A	0	3+	—	—	—
4	I	120	T; A, A	10	3+	—	—	—
5	I	115	T; A, A	0	3+	—	—	—
6	II	129	S; A	50	3+	—	—	—
7	II	130	S; A	—	—	—	—	—
8	II	130	T; A, A	0	3+	—	18·3	4·3
9	III	133	T; D, D	75	0	>33·0	106·0	6·0
10	III	121	T; D, A	5	3+	31·3	17·7	1·5
11	III	121	T; A, A	0	3+	24·3	8·9	4·6
12	III	122	T; A, A	40	3+	—	—	—

— = Not available. 0 = Not detectable.

stand and were in sternal recumbency. Animals with Grade III disease were in lateral recumbency and unable to raise their heads. Apparent blindness was manifest in all grades of the disease, although ophthalmoscopic examination of the eyes of several apparently blind animals revealed no abnormality.

Gestation at the time of onset of the disease varied from 115 to 134 days (Table I). In both ewes with spontaneous disease and in all ewes with Grade III induced disease there were twin fetuses (Table I). In one ewe with Grade III spontaneous disease and in two of the ewes with Grade III induced disease, fetal lambs were dead at the time of sacrifice of the ewe (Table I).

Urine measurement

Proteinuria was a variable finding, ranging from undetectably low levels to the highest level of 75 mg per cent in a ewe with Grade III induced disease (Table I). Acetonuria of moderate to severe degree was a more constant finding but was notably absent from the above ewe with Grade III induced disease and the highest level of proteinuria (Table I).

Biochemical data

Plasma renin concentrations in toxaemic animals were considerably elevated above the normal non-pregnant range (<2·0 pmol/h · ml) and above the levels found in non-toxaemic pregnant sheep (range 4·6–7·3 pmol/h · ml); the highest level of >33·0 pmol/h · ml was recorded in ewe No. 9 with Grade III induced disease, and the lowest level of 17·0 pmol/h · ml was found in the ewe with Grade I spontaneous disease (Table I). Blood aldosterone concentrations in toxaemic animals were also considerably elevated above the normal non-pregnant range (<5·0 ng/dl) and above the levels found in non-toxaemic pregnant sheep (range 0–9·3 ng/dl); the highest levels, 71 and 106 ng/dl, respectively, were found in ewes with Grade III spontaneous disease and Grade III induced disease (Table I). Although the highest blood aldosterone concentration was recorded in the ewe with the highest plasma renin concentration, ewe No. 9, there did not otherwise appear to be a good correlation between the degree of elevation of aldosterone and renin concentrations (Table I).

The blood cortisol concentrations in toxaemic ewes were also elevated above the normal non-pregnant range (0·1–0·8 μg/dl) and above the levels found in non-toxaemic pregnant sheep (range 0·4–1·4 μg/dl); the highest levels of 7·1 and 6·0 μg/dl were recorded in the ewes with the greatest elevations of blood aldosterone concentration (Table I).

Morphology

Adrenal cortex—In normal non-pregnant ewes, mitotic activity was absent throughout the adrenal cortex. Zona glomerulosa cells showed sparse smooth and granular endoplasmic reticulum, compact Golgi profiles, few lipid droplets and numerous oval mitochondria with a dense matrix, lamelliform cristae (Fig. 1) and occasional small, electron dense intramitochondrial inclusion bodies. Zona intermedia cells resembled zona glomerulosa cells except that mitochondria contained both lamelliform and vesicular cristae. Zona fasciculata cells showed prominent smooth endoplasmic reticulum, rare lipid droplets and numerous round mitochondria with closely packed vesicular cristae.

In non-toxaemic sheep in the last third of pregnancy the adrenal cortex showed occasional scattered mitotic figures in the zona glomerulosa. Mitochondrial changes (as described below) affected 40–70 per cent of zona glomerulosa cells, mainly in the mid and superficial regions; no mitochondrial changes were present in intervening zona glomerulosa cells. A minor increase in smooth and granular endoplasmic reticulum was found in some zona glomerulosa cells with altered mitochondria. A moderate increase in cytoplasmic lipid occurred in the deep zona glomerulosa and underlying zona intermedia. No morphologic changes were evident in the superficial zona fasciculata.

The adrenal cortex in toxaemic animals showed striking changes compared with non-toxaemic pregnant sheep.

Mitotic activity

Intense mitotic activity throughout the zona glomerulosa, zona intermedia and superficial zona fasciculata was detected in two animals, each with Grade III signs, one with spontaneous disease (No. 2) and the other with induced disease (No. 9) (Fig. 2). Moderately increased mitotic activity, affecting the zona glomerulosa only, was detected in three animals, all with induced disease, one with Grade I signs (No. 5), one with Grade II signs (No. 8) and one with Grade III signs (No. 10). Occasional mitotic figures in the zona glomerulosa were seen in the remaining animals. Ultrastructurally, mitotic figures were identified in glandular and interstitial cells in animals with intense mitotic activity. In animals with lesser mitotic activity, mitotic figures were identified only in glandular cells.

Mitochondrial changes

In all glands, dividing and non-dividing zona glomerulosa glandular cells contained enlarged, pale, irregularly shaped mitochondria which showed replacement of normal lamelliform cristae by straight 'rod-like' tubular structures, 45–65 nm in diameter, occurring singly or grouped together in parallel arrays or bundles (Figs 3, 4). Bundles of these tubules were commonly found arranged in several directions in the same mitochondria. Intramitochondrial electron dense inclusion bodies were also increased in number (Fig. 5). These mitochondrial changes were uniform, affecting all zona glomerulosa glandular cells, in all glands showing intense or moderate mitotic activity. In glands showing only occasional mitotic figures, the mitochondrial changes were widespread, only occasional scattered zona glomerulosa cells displaying normal mitochondria. Mitochondria in the zona intermedia showed changes resembling those in the zona glomerulosa only in glands with intense or moderate mitotic activity. Similarly, mitochondria in the zona

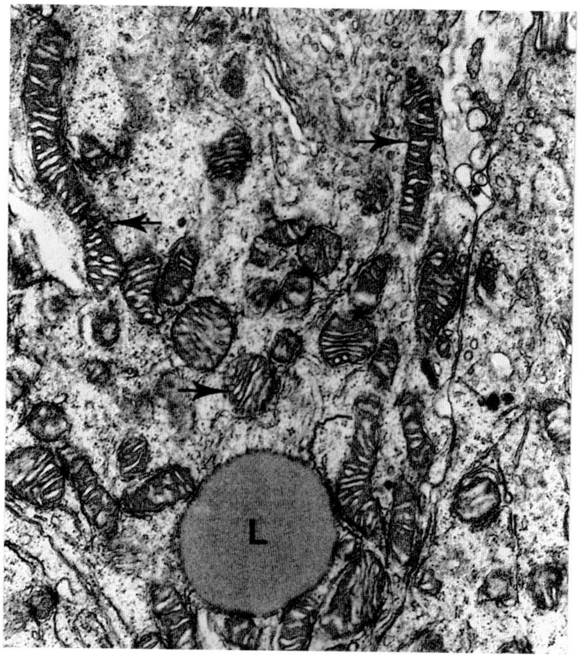

Fig. 1—Mitochondria in adrenal zona glomerulosa cell of non-pregnant ewe showing dense matrix and normal lamelliform cristae (arrows). L, lipid droplet. ×12 750

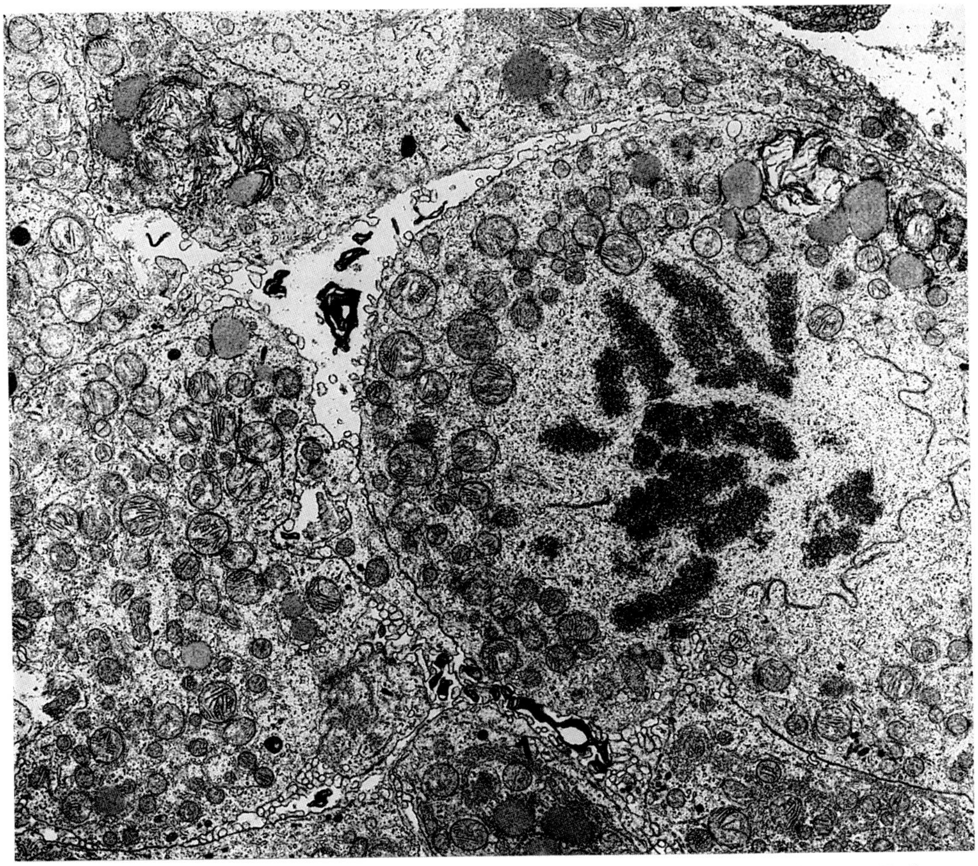

Fig. 2—Adrenal zona glomerulosa of pregnant ewe with induced ovine toxaemia (Grade III disease, sheep No. 9) showing mitotic activity in glandular cell (at right). ×6250

fasciculata were enlarged and showed variation in size and shape only in glands with intense or moderate zona glomerulosa mitotic activity; zona fasciculata mitochondrial cristae remained of normal vesicular type in all animals.

Other changes

As with the mitochondrial changes in the zona glomerulosa, cytologic features associated with increased synthetic activity, i.e. extensive whorls of smooth and granular endoplasmic reticulum and prominent Golgi profiles (Fig. 3), increased and decreased in all zones of the adrenal cortex in direct proportion to the degree of mitotic activity found in the zona glomerulosa. Lipid accumulation (Fig. 5) was prominent in zona glomerulosa and zona intermedia glandular cells in glands showing only occasional mitotic figures, and became less apparent in association with increasing mitotic activity in the zona glomerulosa. The zona fasciculata showed moderate lipid accumulation in all animals. The zona glomerulosa showed extensive interstitial oedema in the animals with intense mitotic activity but not in the other animals.

Kidney—Juxtaglomerular granulation indices (JGI) and peripolar cell granulation indices (PGI) were performed in the ewes with induced toxaemia (Table II). There was a significant ($p<0{\cdot}01$) elevation of the JGI in the group of animals with Grade III disease as compared with the JGI in normal Corriedale ewes in the last third of pregnancy. In animals with Grades I and II disease, the JGI was not significantly different from that of the normal pregnant group. In the groups of animals with Grades I and II disease, the PGI was significantly reduced ($p<0{\cdot}01$ and $<0{\cdot}05$, respectively) as compared with the PGI in normal ewes in the last third of pregnancy, but there was no

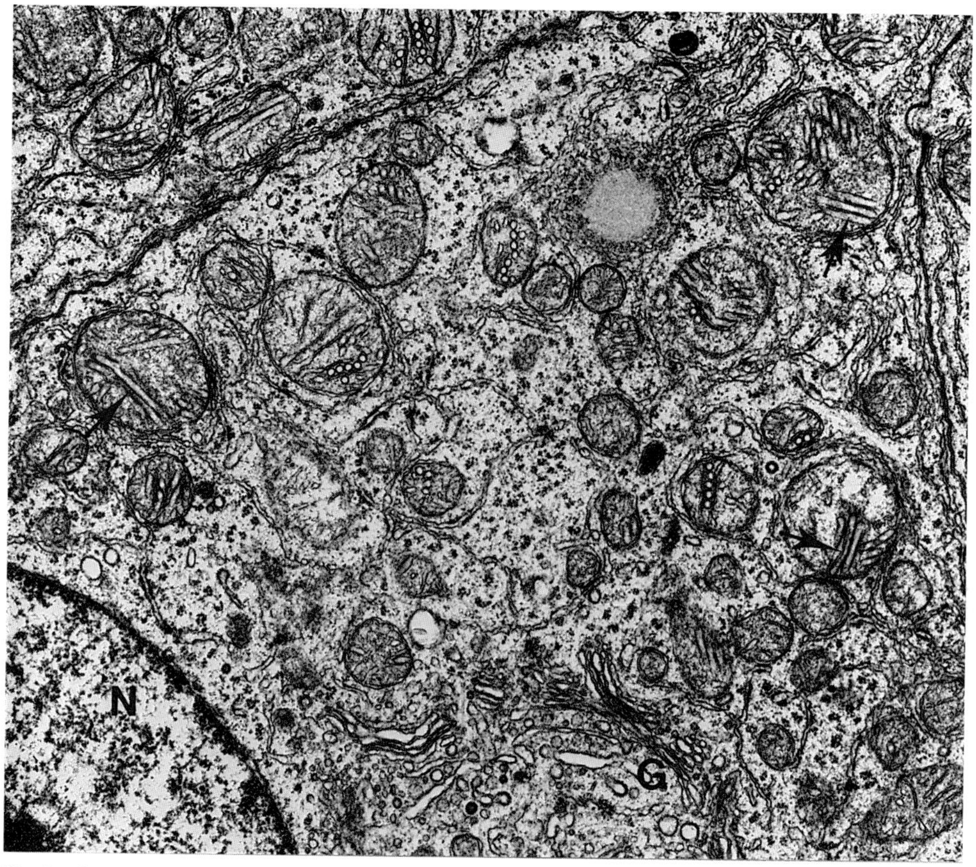

Fig. 3—Cytoplasm of adrenal zona glomerulosa cell of pregnant ewe with induced ovine toxaemia (Grade III disease, sheep No. 9) containing enlarged, pale mitochondria showing replacement of lamelliform cristae by tubular structures (arrows). Note prominent Golgi complex (G). N, nucleus. ×12 500

significant alteration in the PGI in the group with Grade III disease (Table II).

The ultrastructure of the glomerular capillary loops appeared normal (Fig. 6) in all the animals studied except one (No. 10) with Grade III induced disease in which small subendothelial, mesangial and subepithelial deposits were occasionally observed (Fig. 7). In addition, in the same animal there was a moderate increase in mesangial matrix (Fig. 7) but there was no evidence of endothelial cell swelling or epithelial cell abnormalities.

In examining the ultrastructure of the juxtaglomerular region in normal ewes in the last third of pregnancy, there appeared to be a slight increase in granulation of afferent arteriolar myoepithelioid cells compared with non-pregnant ewes; granules were homogeneous in size, shape and density; protogranules were not seen; there was no increase in granular endoplasmic reticulum and Golgi profiles; and there was no sign of exocytosis of granules. In the same animals, juxtaglomerular peripolar cells showed no changes compared with non-pregnant ewes.

There were no distinguishing ultrastructural features in juxtaglomerular arteriolar myoepithelioid cells of animals with Grades I or Grade II toxaemia. However, in the animals with Grade III induced toxaemia there were striking ultrastructural changes in myoepithelioid cells. The cells showed prominent granularity (Fig. 8) and there was considerable heterogeneity of granule density (Fig. 9). Granular endoplasmic reticulum was often dilated and Golgi profiles were prominent (Fig. 9). Protogranules and sacs containing several protogranules were readily apparent. Myoepithelioid cells also contained membrane sacs filled with irregular flocculent material, some of which was

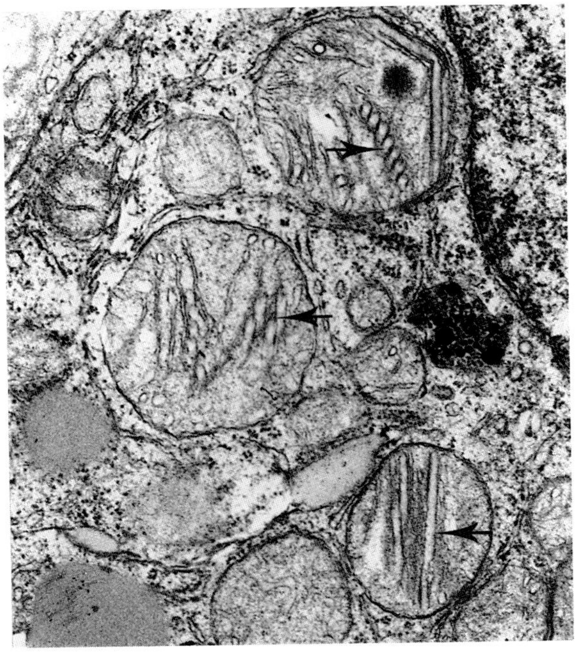

Fig. 4—Detail of adrenal zona glomerulosa cell of pregnant ewe with induced ovine toxaemia (Grade III disease, sheep No. 9) showing bundles of intramitochondrial tubular structures (arrows). ×24 650

Table II—Juxtaglomerular granulation indices (JGI) and peripolar cell granulation indices (PGI) in sheep with induced ovine toxaemia

Animals	JGI	PGI
Normal pregnancy (last third) ($n=5$)	40 ± 5	46 ± 10
Grade I ovine toxaemia ($n=3$)	23 ± 4	5 ± 2
p value	NS	<0·01
Grade II ovine toxaemia ($n=3$)	36 ± 5	15 ± 3
p value	NS	<0·05
Grade III ovine toxaemia ($n=4$)	63 ± 4	21 ± 11
p value	<0·01	NS

Values are mean ± S.E. NS, not significant from normal pregnancy (last third) value.

extruded at the cell periphery and autophagic vacuoles were occasionally seen. Channel-like invaginations of the plasma membrane coming into contact with granules were occasionally detected.

There were no consistent changes in the ultrastructure of juxtaglomerular peripolar cells compared with normal pregnant controls or

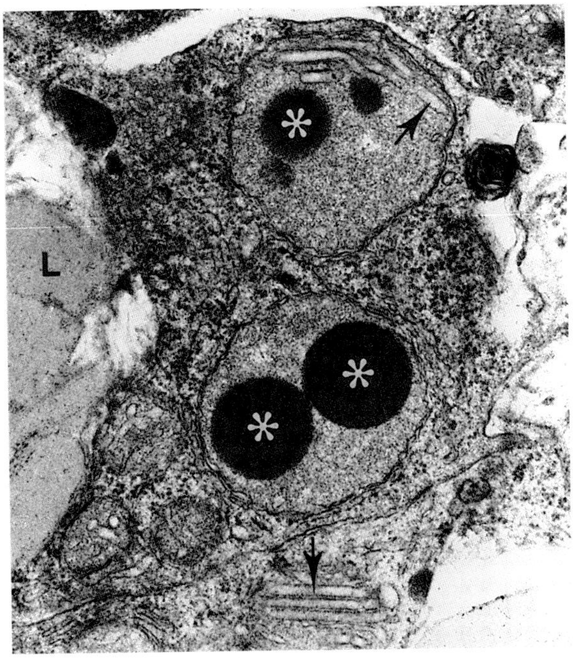

Fig. 5—Detail of adrenal zona glomerulosa cell of pregnant ewe with spontaneous ovine toxaemia (Grade I disease, sheep No. 1) showing prominent intramitochondrial electron dense inclusion bodies (asterisks). Note intramitochondrial tubular structures (arrows). L, lipid droplet. ×24 650

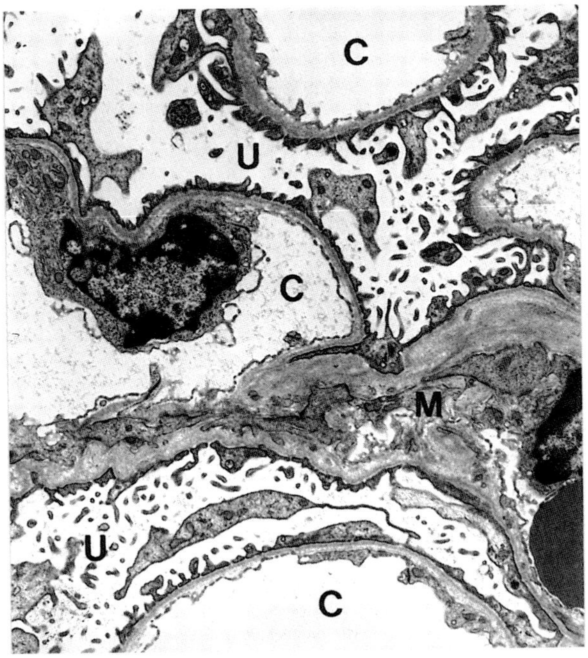

Fig. 6—Portion of renal glomerulus of pregnant ewe with induced ovine toxaemia (Grade III disease, sheep No. 9) showing normal capillary loops (C) and mesangium (M). U, urinary space. All animals except sheep No. 10 (see Fig. 7) showed the same normal glomerular ultrastructure. ×4675

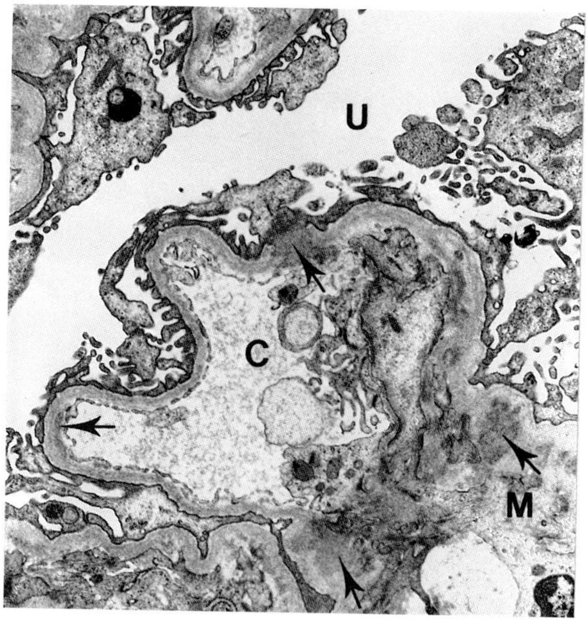

Fig. 7—Portion of renal glomerulus of pregnant ewe with induced ovine toxaemia (Grade III disease, sheep No. 10) showing occasional small deposits (arrows), mainly in moderately expanded mesangial areas (M). C, capillary lumen; U, urinary space. This was the only sheep to show abnormal glomerular ultrastructure. ×5100

between different clinical grades of toxaemia. In one animal (No. 9) with Grade III induced disease, peripolar cells were relatively poorly granulated but showed well developed granular endoplasmic reticulum and Golgi profiles. In contrast, in another animal (No. 10) with Grade III induced disease, peripolar cells were very well granulated, and one example of a peripolar cell in mitosis was observed (Fig. 10). Other peripolar cells showed very prominent microtubules which, in some sections, came into close association with the cell surface. In one animal (No. 8) with Grade II induced disease, evidence of peripolar cell exocytotic activity was detected, granule material

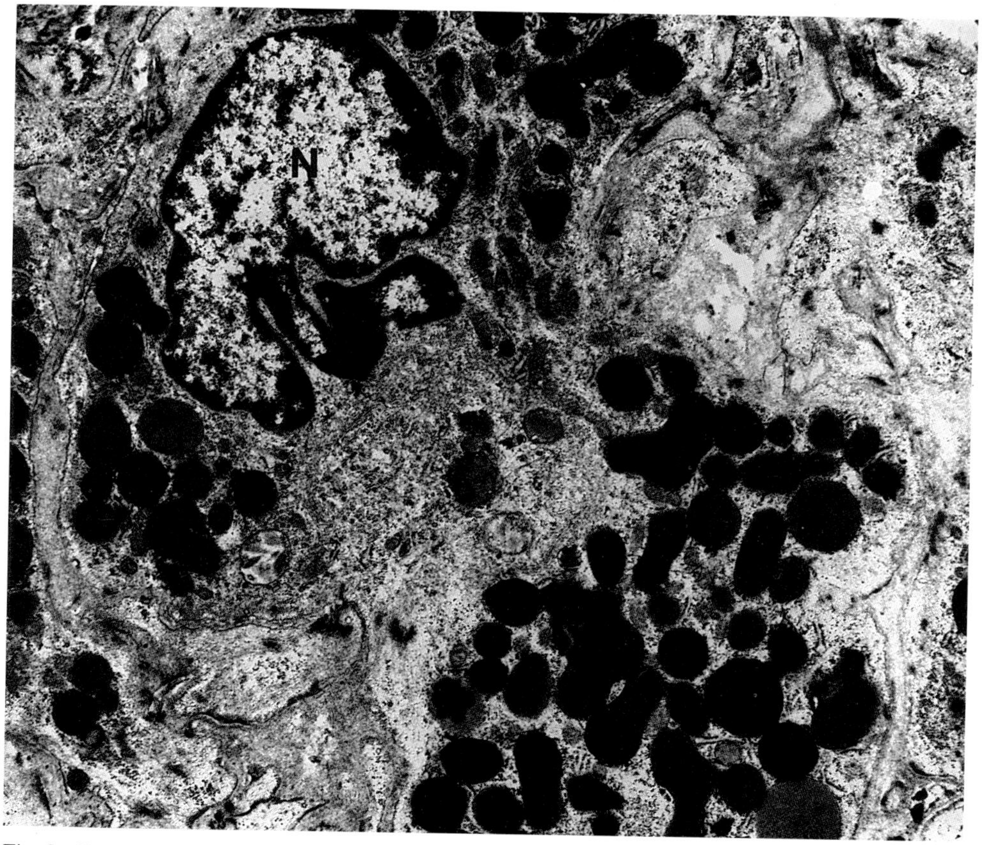

Fig. 8—Renal juxtaglomerular region of pregnant ewe with induced ovine toxaemia (Grade III disease, sheep No. 9) showing large numbers of electron dense cytoplasmic granules in arteriolar myoepithelioid cells. N, nucleus. ×8500

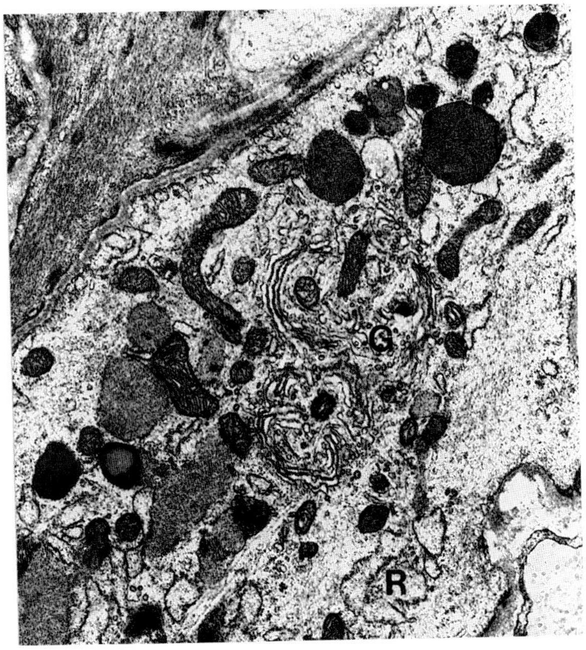

Fig. 9—Detail of juxtaglomerular myoepithelioid cell of pregnant ewe with induced ovine toxaemia (Grade III disease, sheep No. 9) showing heterogeneous cytoplasmic granules, dilated granular endoplasmic reticulum (R) and prominent Golgi complex (G). ×12 750

being observed in the process of release into the urinary space (Fig. 11).

DISCUSSION

In toxaemic pregnant sheep in the present study there were no renal glomerular pathological changes analogous to those found in human preeclampsia. This disagrees with the findings of Ferris *et al.*[6] in sheep with experimentally induced toxaemia, in which they described glomerular endothelial cell swelling, basement membrane reduplication and widespread focal fusion of epithelial foot processes, but accords with the observation of McCausland *et al.*[20] of the absence

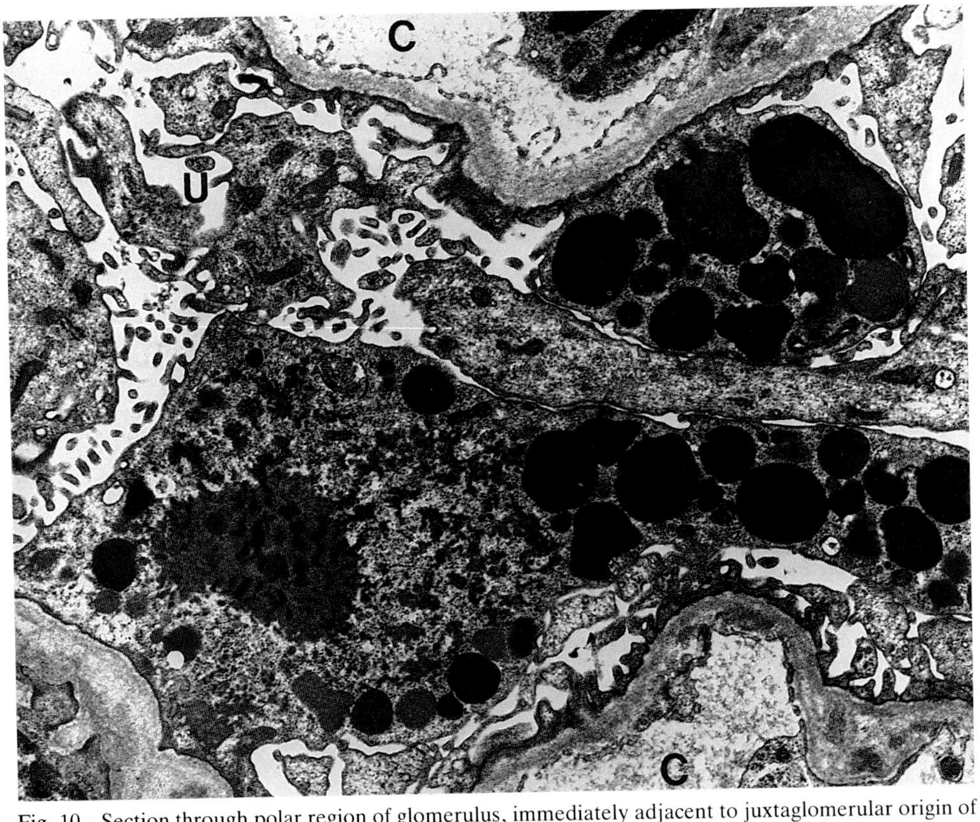

Fig. 10—Section through polar region of glomerulus, immediately adjacent to juxtaglomerular origin of glomerular tuft, in pregnant ewe with induced ovine toxaemia (Grade III disease, sheep No. 10) showing portions of two peripolar epithelial cells which contain multiple electron dense cytoplasmic granules. The lower peripolar cell is in mitosis. C, capillary lumen; U, urinary space. ×13 000

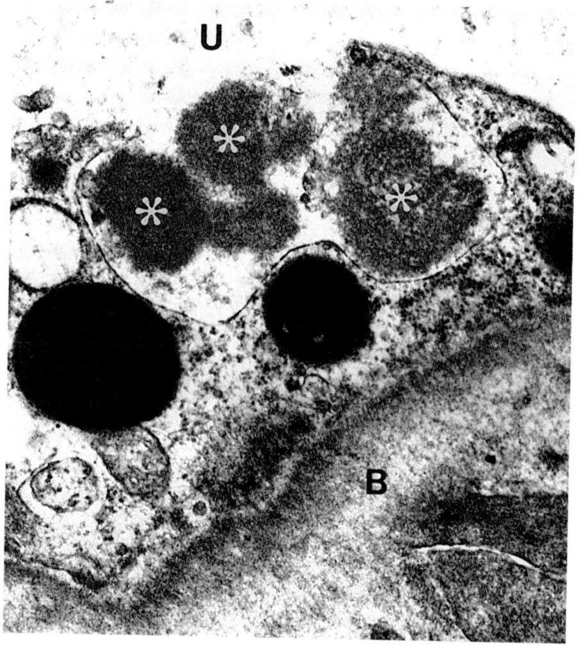

Fig. 11—Detail of juxtaglomerular peripolar cell of pregnant ewe with induced ovine toxaemia (Grade II disease, sheep No. 8) showing evidence of coalescence of granules (asterisks) and their release to the urinary space (U). B, Bowman's capsular basement membrane. ×29 750

of any structural glomerular abnormalities in sheep with spontaneous toxaemia. In the glomeruli of one sheep with Grade III induced disease in the present study there were small subendothelial, mesangial and subepithelial electron dense deposits associated with a moderate increase in mesangial matrix. This appearance is randomly observed in small numbers (less than 5 per cent) of otherwise apparently normal Corriedale ewes in local flocks. The significance of the abnormality is not clear but, with no associated endothelial swelling or fibrin deposition, it did not resemble the characteristic glomerular lesion of human preeclampsia.[1,2]

The inconsistency of the finding of proteinuria in the toxaemic sheep in this study and the failure of its presence to correlate with the severity of the disease also disagrees with the study by Ferris *et al.*[6] in which they reported significant degrees of proteinuria as a constant finding in toxaemic sheep. The mechanisms of proteinuria, when it occurs in toxaemic sheep in the absence of structural changes in the glomerular capillary wall, may relate to alterations in intrarenal haemodynamics, possibly mediated by the very high peripheral plasma renin levels found in the present study and by Ferris *et al.*[6] In favour of this view is the increase in glomerular permeability in rats provoked by renin or angiotensin infusion and attributed to altered intrarenal haemodynamics resulting in an increased filtration fraction.[21]

Hence, two of the features required for a valid experimental model for human preeclampsia, i.e. the characteristic glomerular changes and consistent proteinuria, were not found to be present in this series of animals with ovine toxaemia. In addition, hypertension, another cardinal feature of preeclampsia, does not appear to occur in ovine toxaemia.[6,7,9] In unpublished studies in our laboratory, an increase in blood pressure was not observed in a sheep which developed the clinical signs of Grade I ovine toxaemia after bilateral uterine artery constriction. In contrast, in other species including the dog,[22,23] rabbit,[24] monkey[25] and baboon,[26] uteroplacental ischaemia leads to the development of hypertension, proteinuria and renal glomerular lesions similar to those observed in human preeclampsia.

So what is the nature of ovine toxaemia? The disease was originally considered to result from a metabolic abnormality related to hypoglycaemia and hyperketonaemia but it has since been shown that hypoglycaemia not only bears no relationship to either the presence of toxaemia or the associated neurological signs[6] but also occurs in non-toxaemic starved sheep.[5] Elevated blood cortisol levels are a consistent feature of pregnancy toxaemia in sheep.[27] In the present study, cortisol levels were measured in animals with severe clinical manifestations of the disease and were all found to be elevated above normal; except in one animal, all values reached the range seen in sheep treated with adrenocorticotrophic hormone (ACTH) for 5 days.[28] Reid[27] proposed that elevated blood cortisol levels, as a response to various forms of stress, may inhibit glucose utilization by the tissues and cause the clinical manifestations (particularly the neurological signs) of ovine toxaemia. The more frequent occurrence of the disease in ewes with multiple fetuses may be explained by the high fetal demand for glucose acting as an additional stress factor in already undernourished ewes.[27]

The adrenal gland showed a range of morphologic changes in toxaemic sheep. The ultrastructural appearances in the zona fasciculata suggested significant stimulation of this zone by ACTH.[29] In sheep we have shown previously that ACTH administration for 5 days results in inhibition of aldosterone production associated with severe atrophy of the zona glomerulosa.[30] In the present study, although the toxaemic sheep had appearances in the zona fasciculata consistent with ACTH stimulation, the changes in the zona glomerulosa were more typical of those seen with sodium depletion[31] than with ACTH administration.[30] These zona glomerulosa changes included varying degrees of proliferative activity associated with widespread striking alterations in mitochondria, endoplasmic reticulum and Golgi profiles. In contrast to the ACTH-treated sheep,[30] plasma renin and blood aldosterone concentrations were elevated in toxaemic sheep into the range of values usually found in sodium-depleted sheep.[16,31] It is of interest to speculate that the increased activity of the renin–angiotensin–aldosterone system in these animals played a part in protecting the zona glomerulosa from the atrophic effects of ACTH.[30]

Morphologic studies of the juxtaglomerular regions in sheep with Grade III induced disease showed the highest juxtaglomerular indices and striking ultrastructural changes in myoepithelioid cells. The increase in granularity, the development of protogranules and plasma membrane invaginations are features found in myoepithelioid cells in severely sodium-depleted sheep.[12] In addition, extrusion of membrane sacs at the cell periphery and autophagic vacuoles were observed in the myoepithelioid cells of toxaemic sheep. Trump and Bulger[32] described autophagocytosis as an altered 'steady state' in which the cell may be able to maintain homeostasis but does so at the expense of organelle digestion. De Duve and Wattiaux[33] have suggested that an increase in cellular autophagy is a pathologic response representing a sublethal reaction to injurious stimuli.

The stimulus or stimuli to the increase in renin production in ovine toxaemia are not known but may relate to stress-related increases in sympathetic activity or adrenal medullary catecholamines, each of which is known to directly stimulate renin production.[11] Ferris *et al.*[6] reported a correlation between the degree of elevation of plasma renin concentration in ovine toxaemia and the severity of the disease. The correlation in the present study between the clinical severity of the disease and the plasma renin concentration, juxtaglomerular index and ultrastructural alterations in myoepithelioid cells suggests that the physiological responses to stress may be important factors in provoking the increased renin secretion in ovine toxaemia. However, another important possibility is that the increased activity of the renin–angiotensin–aldosterone system in these animals results from significant sodium depletion.

Examination of peripolar cells revealed a decrease in the granulation index, reflecting a decrease in granule storage, in Grade I with Grade II toxaemia. Of special interest, in one animal with Grade III disease, was the finding of peripolar cell mitotic activity. Other peripolar cells were observed with very prominent, cell surface-associated microtubules, which are known to be important in the process of exocytosis.[29] Exocytosis of peripolar cell granule material was indeed detected in one animal with Grade II disease. Because exocytotic release of granule material from peripolar cells has only been observed previously in sodium-depleted sheep,[12] its finding in sheep with ovine toxaemia accords with the suggestion from the adrenal findings that sodium depletion may play a role in this disease. The detection of peripolar cell mitotic activity in association with changes in the peripolar cell granulation index is supporting evidence that such cells are being subjected to significant stimulation in ovine toxaemia.

ACKNOWLEDGEMENTS

These studies were supported by grants from the National Health and Medical Research Council of Australia and the Australia Wool Corporation. Thc authors thank Mrs Geraldine Cheshire, Mrs Helen Rodgers and Mr Phil Hollis for expert technical assistance.

REFERENCES

1. Pirani CL, Pollak VE, Lannigan R, Folli G. The renal glomerular lesions of pre-eclampsia: electron microscopic studies. *Am J Obstet Gynecol* 1963; **87:** 1047.
2. Sheehan HL. Renal morphology in preeclampsia. *Kidney Int* 1980; **18:** 241.
3. Weir RJ, Brown JJ, Fraser R, Kraszewski A, Lever AF, McIlwaine GM, Morton JJ, Robertson JIS, Tree M. Plasma renin, renin substrate, angiotensin II and aldosterone in hypertensive disease of pregnancy. *Lancet* 1973; **1:** 291.
4. Talledo OE, Chesley LC, Zuspan FP. Renin–angiotensin system in normal and toxemic pregnan-

cies. III: Differential sensitivity to angiotensin II and norepinephrine in toxemia of pregnancy. *Am J Obstet Gynecol* 1968; **100:** 218.
5. Reid RL. The physiopathology of undernourishment in pregnant sheep, with particular reference to pregnancy toxemia. *Adv Vet Sci* 1968; **12:** 163.
6. Ferris TF, Herdson PB, Dunnill MS, Lee MR. Toxaemia of pregnancy in sheep: a clinical, physiological and pathological study. *J Clin Invest* 1969; **48:** 1643.
7. Assali NS, Holm L, Hutchinson DL. Renal haemodynamics, electrolyte excretion and water metabolism in pregnant sheep before and after induction of toxaemia of pregnancy. *Circ Res* 1958; **6:** 468.
8. Kaufman CF, Bergman EN. Renal function studies in normal and toxemic pregnant sheep. *Cornell Vet* 1978; **68:** 124.
9. Parry HB, Taylor WH. Renal function in sheep during normal and toxaemic pregnancies. *J. Physiol* 1956; **131:** 383.
10. Ryan GB, Coghlan JP, Scoggins BA. The granulated peripolar epithelial cell: a potential secretory component of the renal juxtaglomerular complex. *Nature* 1979; **277:** 655.
11. Davis JO, Freeman RH. Mechanisms regulating renin release. *Physiol Rev* 1976; **56:** 1.
12. Hill Prudence A, Coghlan JP, Scoggins BA, Ryan GB. Ultrastructural changes in the sheep renal juxtaglomerular apparatus in response to sodium depletion or loading. *Pathology,* in press.
13. Kingsbury FB, Clark CP, Williams G, Post AL. Rapid determination of albumin in urine. *J Lab Clin Med* 1926; **11:** 981.
14. Poulsen K, Jorgensen J. An easy radioimmunological microassay of renin activity, concentration and substrate in human and animal plasma and tissues based on angiotensin I trapping by antibody. *J. Clin Endocrinol Metab* 1974; **39:** 816.
15. Fei DTW, Graham WF, McDougall JG, Scoggins BA, Coghlan JP. [Des-asp'] angiotensin II in the sheep: blood levels and its effect on plasma renin concentration. *Life Sci* 1980; **27:** 1495.
16. Coghlan JP, Scoggins BA. Measurement of aldosterone in peripheral blood of man and sheep. *J Clin Endocrinol Metab* 1967; **27:** 1470.
17. Bowie DJ. Method for staining pepsinogen granules in gastric glands. *Anat Rec* 1936; **64:** 357.
18. Lendrum AC, Fraser DS, Slidders W, Henderson R. Studies on the character and staining of fibrin. *J Clin Path* 1962; **15:** 401.
19. Hartroft Phyllis M. The juxtaglomerular complex as an endocrine gland. In: Bloodworth JMB, ed. Endocrine Pathology. Baltimore: Williams and Wilkins, 1968: 641.
20. McCausland IP, O'Hara PJ, Herdson PB, Leet NG. Spontaneous toxemia of pregnancy in sheep. A study of renal function and glomerular fine structure. *J Comp Path* 1974; **84:** 375.
21. Hulme B, Pessina AC. Influence of renin and angiotensin II on macromolecular glomerular permeability. In: Giovanetti S, Bonomini V, D'Amico G, eds. Proceedings of the Sixth International Congress of Nephrology. Basel: Karger, 1976; 381.
22. Hodari AA. Chronic uterine ischemia and reversible experimental 'toxemia of pregnancy'. *Am J Obstet Gynecol* 1967; **97:** 597.
23. Abitbol MM, Pirani CL, Ober WB, Driscoll Shirley G, Cohen MW. Production of experimental toxemia in the pregnant dog. *Obstet Gynecol* 1976; **48:** 537.
24. Abitbol MM, Gallo Gloria R, Pirani CL, Ober WB. Production of experimental toxemia in the pregnant rabbit. *Am J Obstet Gynecol* 1976; **124:** 460.
25. Abitbol MM, Ober WB, Gallo Gloria R, Driscoll Shirley G, Pirani CL. Experimental toxemia of pregnancy in the monkey, with a preliminary report on renin and aldosterone. *Am J Path* 1977; **86:** 573.
26. Cavanagh D, Rao PS, Tsai CC, O'Connor TC. Experimental toxemia in the pregnant primate. *Am J Obstet Gynecol* 1977; **128:** 75.
27. Reid RL. Studies on the carbohydrate metabolism of sheep. XI: The role of the adrenals in ovine pregnancy toxaemia. *Aust J Agricult Res* 1960; **11:** 364.
28. Scoggins BA, Coghlan JP, Denton DA, Fan JSK, McDougall JG, Oddie Catherine J, Shulkes AA. Metabolic effects of ACTH in the sheep. *Am J Physiol* 1974; **226:** 198.
29. Nussdorfer GG, Mazzocchi G, Meneghelli V. Cytophysiology of the adrenal zona fasciculata. *Int Rev Cytol* 1978; **55:** 291.
30. McDougall JG, Butkus Aldona, Coghlan JP, Denton DA, Muller J, Oddie Catherine J, Robinson PM, Scoggins BA. Biosynthetic and morphological evidence for inhibition of aldosterone production following administration of ACTH to sheep. *Acta Endocrinol (Copenh)* 1980; **94:** 559.
31. Hill Prudence A, Coghlan JP, Butkus Aldona, Ryan GB. Structural and functional studies of the adrenal zona glomerulosa in sodium-depleted and sodium-loaded sheep. *Cell Tissue Res* 1983; **229:** 515.
32. Trump BF, Bulger RE. Studies of cellular injury in isolated flounder tubule. I: Correlation between morphology and function of control tubules and observations of auto-phagocytosis and mechanical cell damage. *Lab Invest* 1967; **16:** 453.
33. De Duve C, Wattiaux R. Functions of lysosomes. *Annu Rev Physiol* 1966; **28:** 435.

JOURNAL OF PATHOLOGY, VOL. **144**: 15–23 (1984)

DUCTAL ADENOMA OF THE BREAST: A LESION WHICH CAN MIMIC CARCINOMA

J. G. AZZOPARDI AND R. SALM

Department of Histopathology, Royal Postgraduate Medical School, London W12, U.K.

Received 8 March 1984
Accepted 9 April 1984

SUMMARY

Twenty-four cases of a solid benign tumour of breast ducts are described, for which we propose the name 'ductal adenoma'. The lesion consists of a single nodule or multiple nodules involving medium size and small ducts, but not major subareolar ducts. It presents as a palpable lump, and is not associated with a nipple discharge. Clinically, radiologically and macroscopically, it can simulate malignancy because of its occurrence in older age groups, frequent microcalcification and the firmness and irregularity of many lesions. Fibrous sclerosis sometimes results in distortion with apparent invasion of surrounding tissue. It can be mistaken for carcinoma both on frozen and paraffin sections. Differentiation into epithelial and myoepithelial cells is the most reliable criterion in the recognition of this lesion as benign. It has microscopic affinities with ductal papilloma, on the one hand, and with salivary-type adenoma, on the other. Ductal adenoma constitutes the third major type of adenoma in the breast, in addition to the already widely recognized nipple adenoma and tubular adenoma.

KEY WORDS—Breast, ductal adenoma, adenoma of breast.

INTRODUCTION

The purpose of this paper is to draw attention to a hitherto undescribed type of benign breast tumour for which we propose the name of 'ductal adenoma'. After the recognition of the essential features of this distinctive lesion, it soon became apparent that it is not a rare tumour, as one of us (JGA) received many examples in consultation from colleagues who had found the lesions difficult to interpret because of the absence of any description of the entity in the existing literature. Some pathologists regarded them as benign, others were concerned about the possibility of malignancy, but justifiably considered the features sufficiently unusual to require a second opinion. Some cases have been seen in which the patient was subjected to mastectomy on the basis of an erroneous diagnosis of malignancy usually, but by no means always, at frozen section examination. The latter cases have been excluded from this series. The correct identification of the tumour as an innocent lesion is obviously of great practical importance.

0022–3417/84/090015–09$01.00

MATERIALS AND METHODS

We collected 24 examples of this tumour during the past 3 years: three were derived from current material in the files of the department of histopathology, Royal Postgraduate Medical School, 21 were seen in referred material. Paraffin sections were cut at 5 μm and stained with haematoxylin and eosin, Weigert's elastic tissue stain in most cases, and von Kossa and other stains when considered necessary. Step sections were studied in five cases.

CLINICAL FEATURES

All patients were female, with ages ranging from 26 to 73 years, with a mean of 51 years. Nineteen patients were above the age of 40 and only five were younger than 40 years of age. All the patients presented with a palpable breast lump which had been present for periods varying between several weeks or months and several years. One lesion was discovered 7 months after the patient had stopped breast feeding. Significantly, no patient complained of a nipple discharge. All lesions were unilateral.

GROSS PATHOLOGY

Ten tumours were discrete solitary nodules, while in 14 cases there were multiple nodules. The multinodular tumours mostly formed compact aggregates, less frequently the nodules were separated by a distance of up to 1·0 cm and were discontinuous three-dimensionally. The multiple nodules mostly appeared to involve different parts of the same ductal system but, less frequently, adjacent ductal systems may have been affected. In one case as many as 30 more-or-less separate nodules were identifiable in the same area. The lesions varied in size between 0·5 and 3·0 cm in maximum diameter. Individual nodules tended to be small, measuring between 0·25 and 2·2 cm in maximum diameter, with a mean of 0·85 cm.

MICROSCOPIC PATHOLOGY

The tumours present in one of two major ways. Many form an adenomatous nodule which is clearly contained within a ductal lumen (Figs 1, 2). The ductal wall around it is frequently thickened and fibrosed and occasionally it is patchily calcified. Variable amounts of elastic tissue persist in the ductal wall. Occasionally, a nodule of this type is largely sclerosed with glandular structures persisting mainly in the central parts of the lesion. In other lesions a stellate central scar and a crenated outline impart a floral appearance (Fig. 3).

The other adenomatous variant is more complex, with tumour not obviously confined to the ductal lumen, but giving the impression of having outgrown its confines (Fig. 4). In these cases, tumour margins are still fairly well defined and mostly of 'pushing' type, with nodules either abutting directly on adjacent breast tissue or separated from it by a thin fibrous layer.

The detailed microscopical features resemble

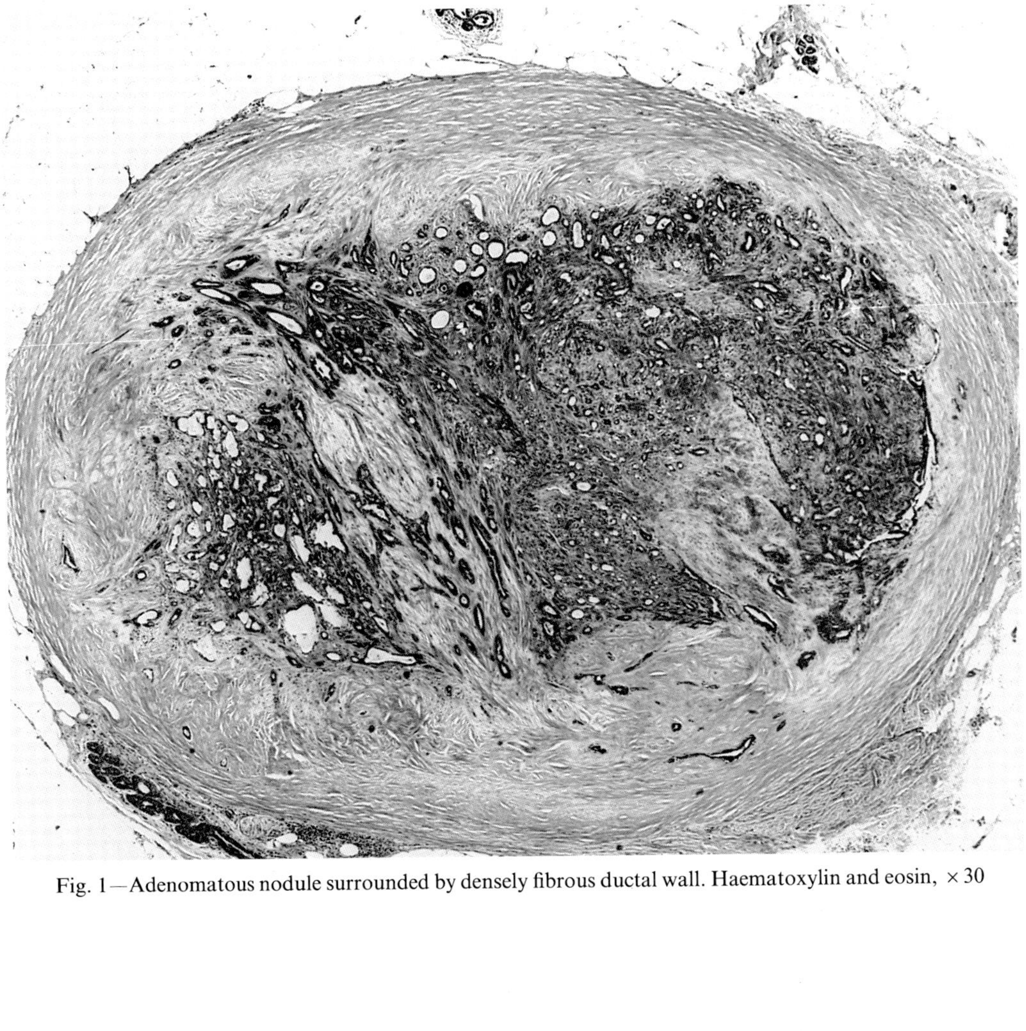

Fig. 1—Adenomatous nodule surrounded by densely fibrous ductal wall. Haematoxylin and eosin, × 30

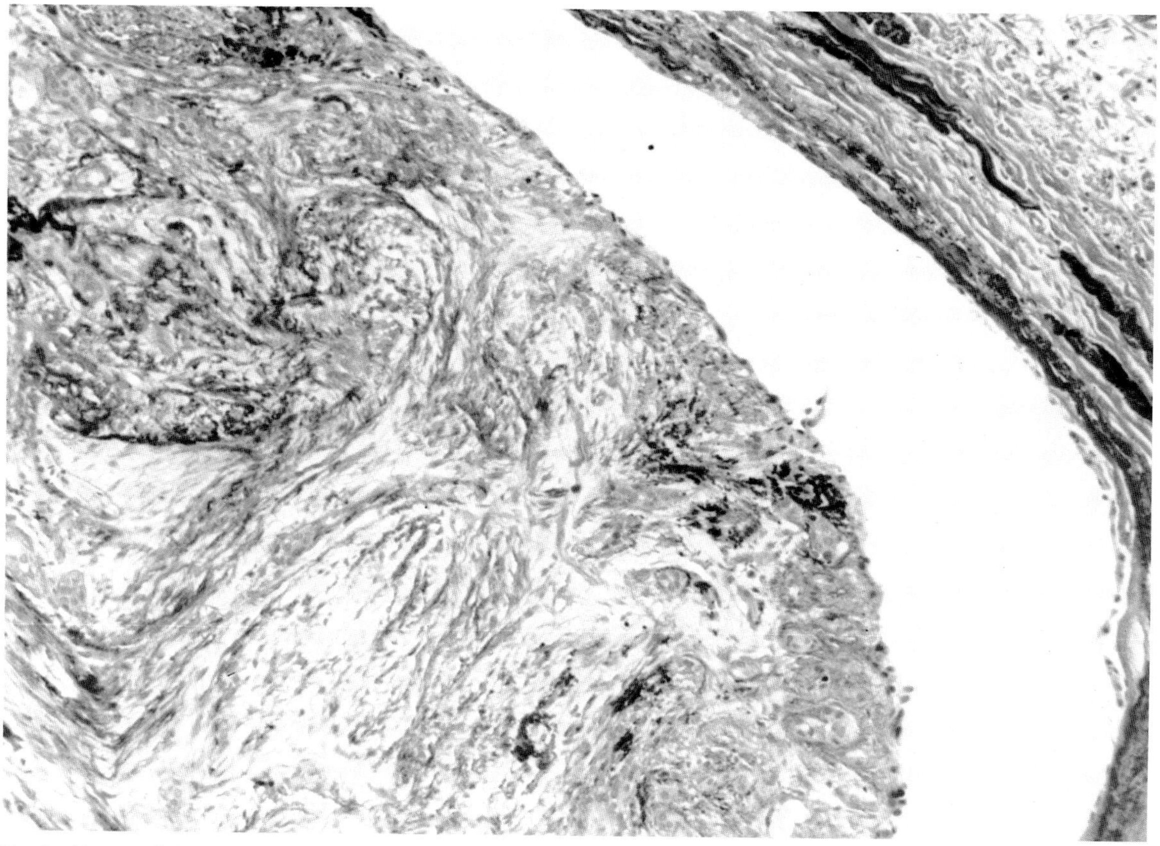

Fig. 2—Tumour lying free in ductal lumen at this level. Elastic tissue of duct wall visible at top right. Weigert elastic stain and Van Gieson, × 150

those seen in ductal papillomas, with the important difference that the lesion is a solid one and is totally devoid of the arborescent and fronded structure of a papilloma (Figs 1–4). The adenomas consist essentially of glandular tubules which are separated either by a modest amount of loose fibrous stroma or occasionally by abundant and dense fibrous tissue (Figs 5, 6). Elastic tissue is often present as coarse and fine fibres between the glandular elements (Fig. 7). This represents newly formed elastic tissue, as opposed to mere pre-existing elastica in the duct wall. The tubules are mostly rounded or ovoid, but some are markedly elongated and rarely even branched (Figs 5, 6).

The glandular tubules are composed of two cell types, epithelial and myoepithelial (Fig. 5). In most tumours, these two cell types can be distinguished easily at least in parts of the lesion, but occasionally the recognition of these distinct cell populations requires closer scrutiny. Epithelial cells vary in shape between cuboidal and columnar, and only more rarely assume a flattened shape. Myoepithelial cells are smaller and low cuboidal to flattened, and sometimes assume a spindled form (Fig 5, 6 and 8). Epithelial cells usually stain deeply with eosin, while the cytoplasm of myoepithelial cells is either clear or palely stained (Figs 5, 8). Apical cytoplasmic snouts on the luminal border of the epithelial component are a striking feature of 15 cases (Fig. 5). Myoepithelial cells occasionally exceed epithelial cells in number, with individual nodules sometimes consisting largely of an overgrowth of spindled myoepithelia (Fig. 8).

Mitotic activity is variable, but it is usually scanty. In 22 cases, mitosis number between zero and four per 20 high power fields. In two otherwise similar tumours, however, there are as many as six to eight mitoses per 20 high power fields. All mitoses seen are of normal appearance.

Apocrine metaplasia is present in 17 tumours, but it is not often a prominent feature (Fig. 8). Calcispherules, mostly situated in glandular lumina, are

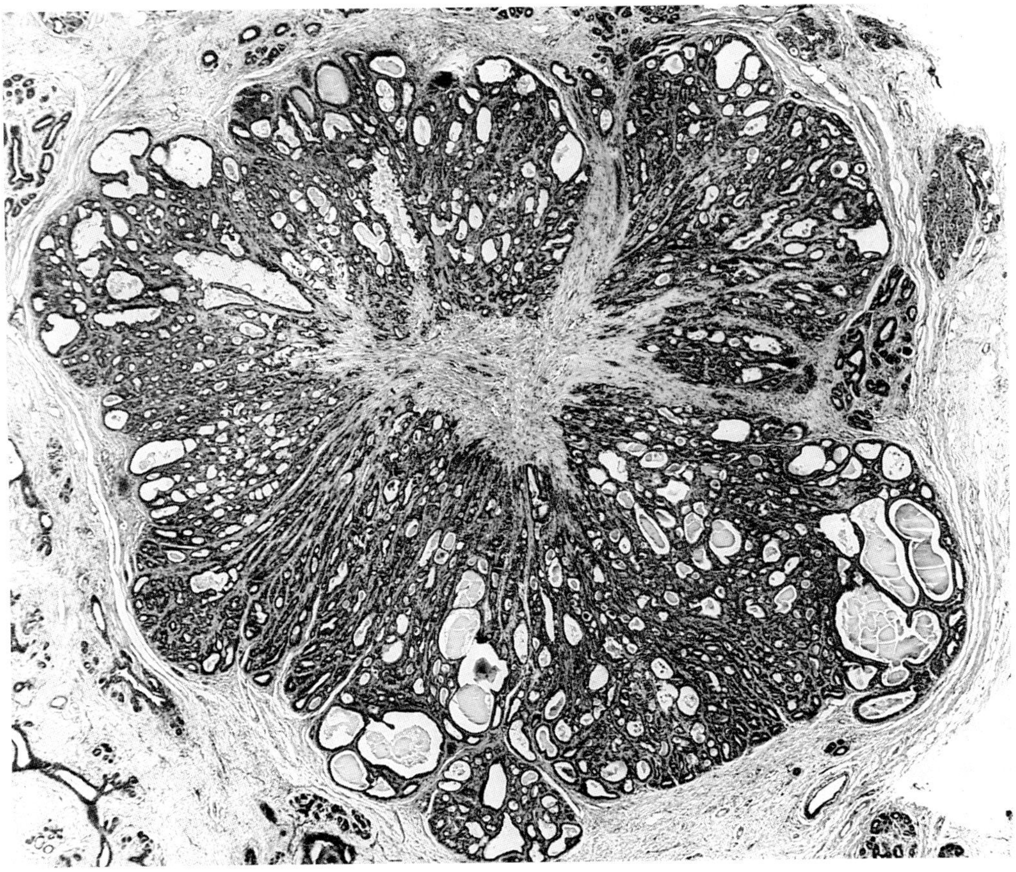

Fig. 3—Crenated outine of ductal adenoma with central scar. HE, × 30

found in nine lesions (Fig. 6). Some lumina contain a homogeneous or granular eosinophilic material, others appear empty.

Other less common and less important features are lipophages, in four cases, and cholesterol granulomas, in two cases: one of the latter was in a lesion which had been needled. A myxoid stromal change is present focally in four adenomas. In none of these cases was there any difficulty in distinguishing this from the myxoid tissue of the salivary-type adenoma. In the latter, the myxoid tissue is an integral part of the neoplasm and not a mere stromal change.

Certain patterns of extension of tumour and the multifocality of some lesions add to the variability and complexity of many of these tumours.

Extension of lesions

One mode of extension is represented by a protrusion of tumour through a breach in the fibrous ductal wall surrounding the bulk of the lesion. This is noted in three of the adenomas. Such extension is comparable with the so-called 'entrapment' of part of a ductal papilloma within the duct wall, an appearance which the unwary can misconstrue as evidence of malignancy.

A second pattern of extension, especially well shown in longitudinal cuts of the ductal system, is an exophytic one into the lumen with the formation of solid intraluminal polypoidal structures which are in continuity with a tumour nidus attached to the ductal wall. This pattern is seen in three tumours.

Multifocality

The apparent multifocality noted macroscopically in 14 cases is confirmed microscopically in 10 cases. Apart from three cases with distinctly separate nodules on gross examination, seven others show tumour foci which are separated from one another

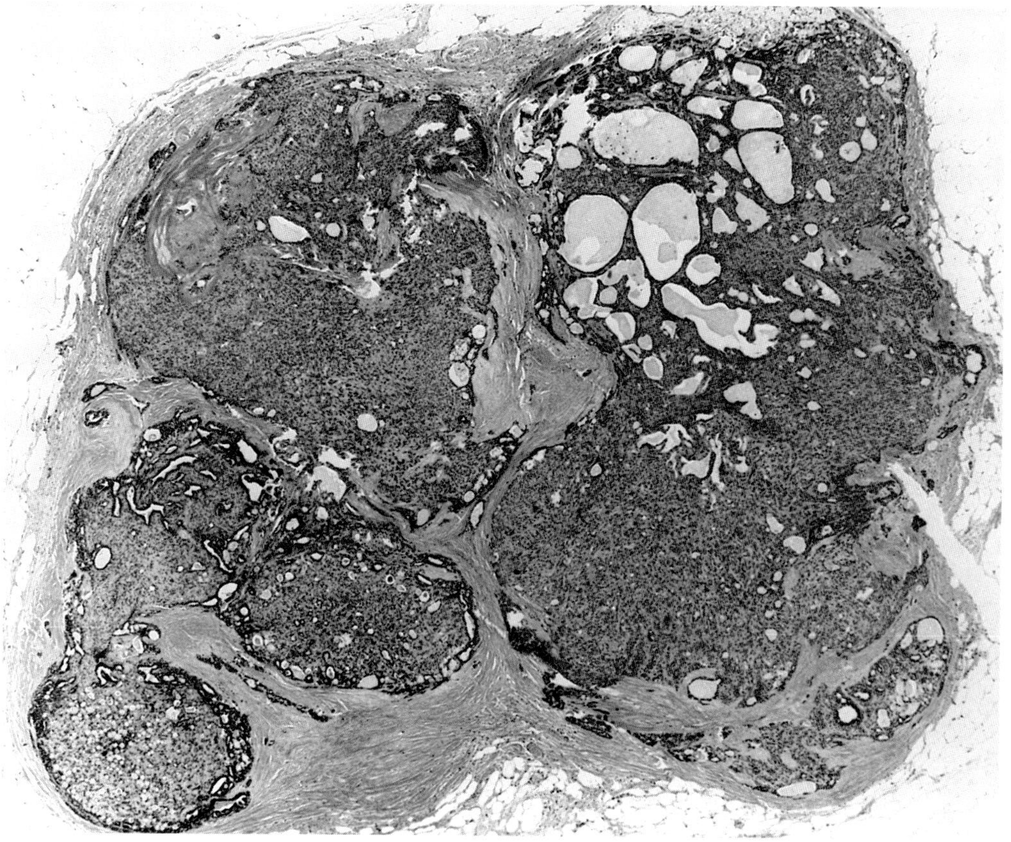

Fig. 4—More complex adenomatous pattern with apparent encroachment on ductal wall. HE, ×30

by way of skip lesions with interposed normal segments of ducts. Such lesions mostly fill the ductal lumina, but occasionally they take the form of an eccentric mural cushion involving only part of the ductal circumference. The genuinely multifocal origin of many of the tumours in the series is further supported by the occasional presence of minute, but otherwise similar, adenomatous foci in the breast tissue surrounding the main lesions (Fig. 9). These minute 'satellite' foci appear to originate in the smallest ductal ramifications, possibly including ductules. The larger lesions involve medium-sized ducts for the most part, but none of our tumours is situated in the largest subareolar ducts, a frequent site of involvement by ductal papillomas.

ASSOCIATED PATHOLOGY

Benign lesions

The ductal adenomas in this series are associated with a wide variety of benign lesions. These include duct ectasia in 12 cases, adenosis and sclerosing adenosis in 11 cases, cystic disease in four cases and benign 'infiltrating epitheliosis'[1] in four cases. In some patients the accompanying benign disease, especially cystic disease and significant degrees of epithelial hyperplasia, was probably mainly responsible for the clinically palpable breast lump. In other patients the ductal adenoma itself was responsible for the clinical presentation with a palpable mass. It was not always possible to determine the relative contributions of the ductal adenoma and of the other pathology to the clinical signs and symptoms.

The high incidence of associated, and presumably coincidental, duct ectasia among these patients is attributed to the high mean age of 51 years in the series as a whole. The frequency of other types of epithelial hyperplasia may partly be due to their frequency in these age groups, but probably also reflects the relative frequency with which different types of epithelial hyperplasia occur together in the same breast other than by chance.

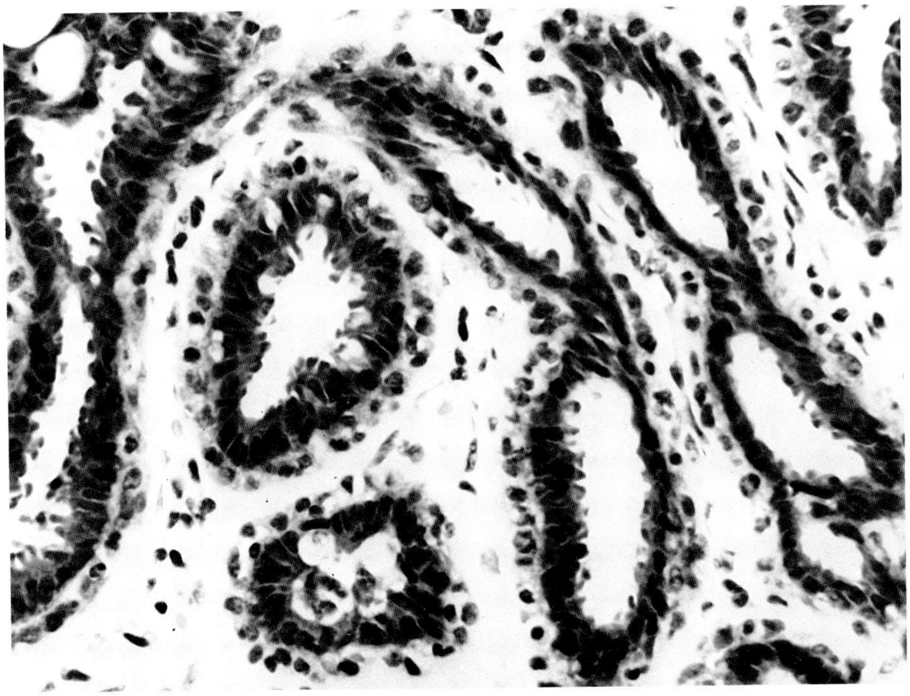

Fig. 5—Typical two-cell-type glandular structure. Note apical snouts. HE, × 340

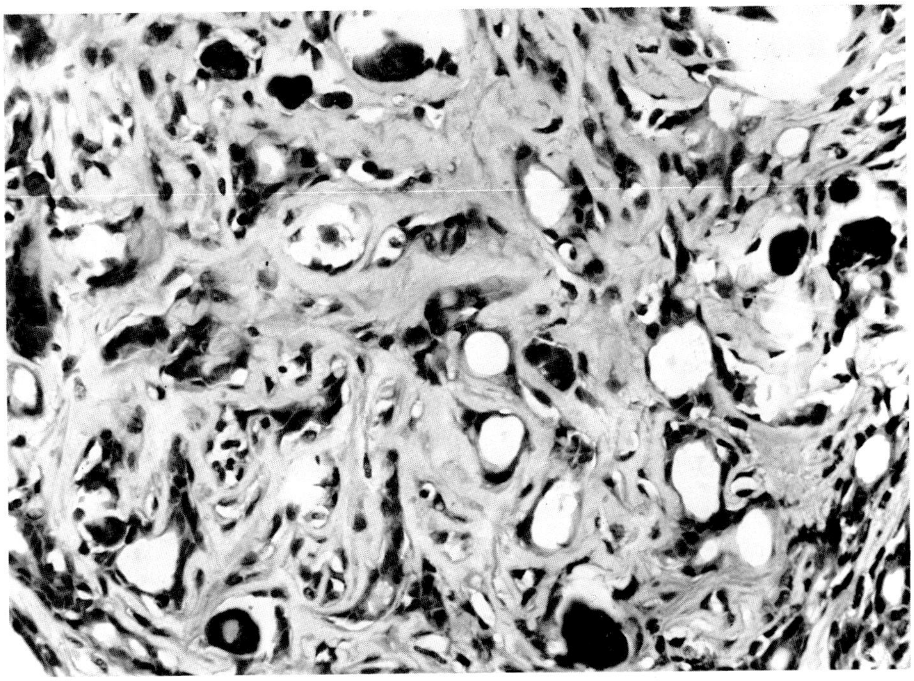

Fig. 6—Unusually fibrous lesion. Densely-stained calcispherites are best seen at bottom and near right edge of illustration. HE, × 340

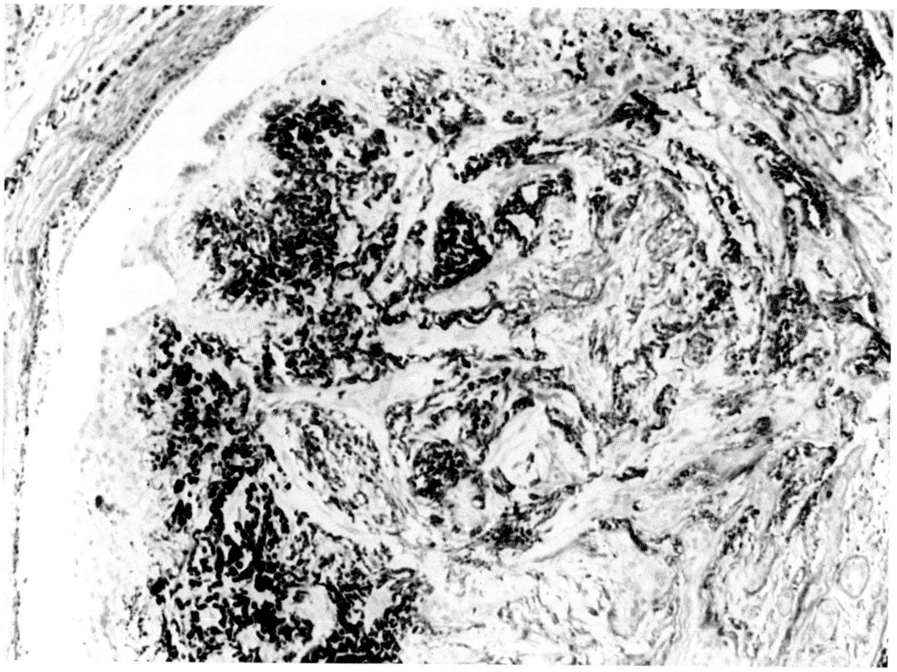

Fig. 7—Abundant elastic fibre between neoplastic glands. A very small amount of elastic tissue persists in duct wall at upper left of illustration. Weigert elastic stain and Van Gieson, ×128

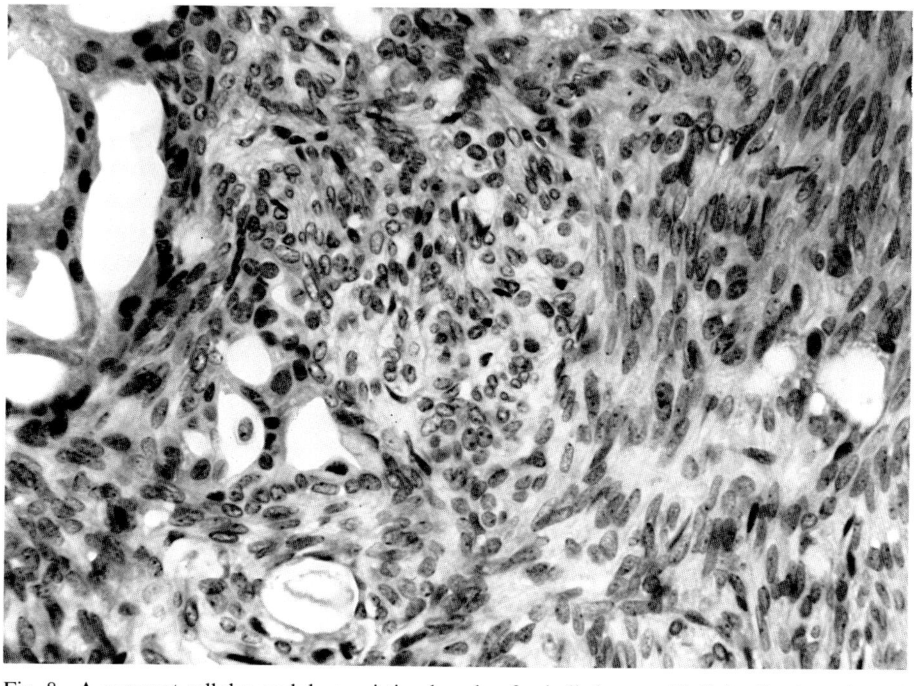

Fig. 8—A compact cellular nodule consisting largely of spindled myoepithelial cells. Apocrine epithelium is visible at upper left. HE, ×340

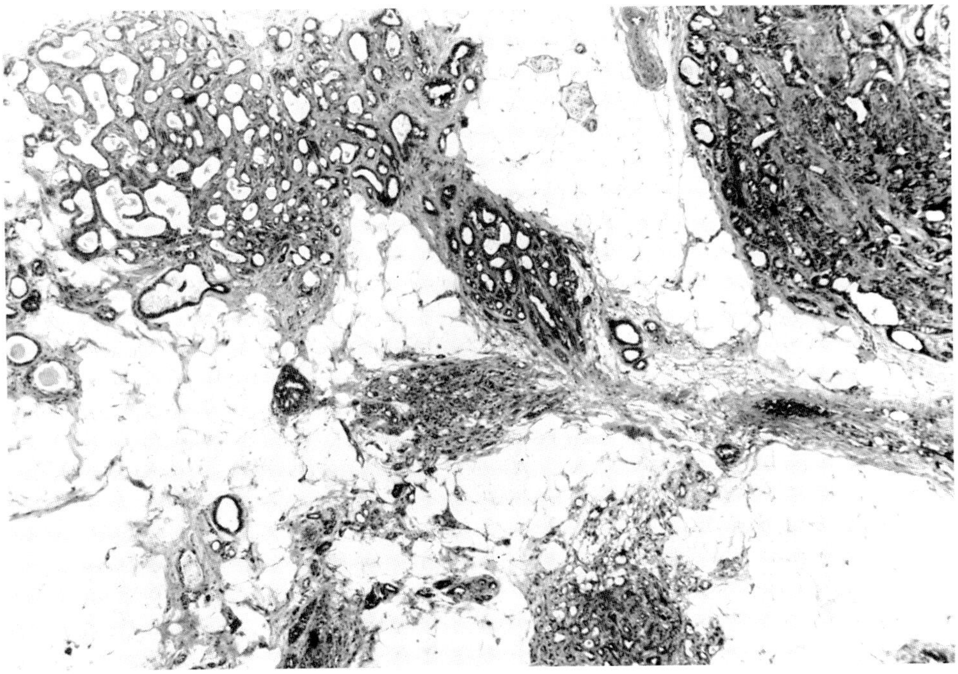

Fig. 9—A part of a large ductal adenoma is visible in the upper right corner. Small similar lesions are present in the adjacent breast tissue. HE, × 36

Malignant lesions

Two patients, aged 56 and 60 years, also have *in situ* malignancy in their biopsy specimens, unrelated topographically to the ductal adenoma. One has a focus of lobular neoplasia, the other has a small focus of ductal carcinoma *in situ*. The latter patient had had a contralateral mastectomy for invasive ductal carcinoma 1 year previously.

DISCUSSION

Ductal adenomas are not uncommon lesions of the female breast. They are benign glandular tumours of ducts which occupy and fill their lumina, distend them and sometimes appear to extend into and perhaps beyond the duct walls. The term 'ductal adenoma' seems an appropriate designation for these lesions. With multiple tumours, 'ductal adenomatosis' is probably more appropriate.

As compared with ductal papilloma, it is noteworthy that none of our 24 cases arose in a major subareolar duct and that no patient presented with a nipple discharge, bloodstained or otherwise. The absence of a discharge presumably reflects the location of ductal adenoma in medium size and small ducts, and the lesser frequency of infarction.

The greatest danger is that this lesion be misinterpreted as a carcinoma, a diagnosis which was seriously entertained in some cases in this series, especially with lesions in the older age groups. A diagnosis of malignancy was made in other cases, but these have been excluded here. The problems of differential diagnosis are clearly formidable.

The histological feature that argues most cogently in favour of a benign lesion is the divergent differentiation into epithelial and myoepithelial cells. This is the single most important feature of this lesion pointing to a benign nature. With the exception of adenoid cystic carcinoma and related tumours, no proliferative epithelial lesion of the breast with clear dual differentiation of this type is malignant. Apocrine metaplasia, when present, provides additional confirmatory evidence. However, it was present in only two-thirds of our cases.

Calcispherules may be confusing to the pathologist, since they are better known in the context of malignant disease. Indeed, in some cases, they had been noted radiologically, and both the clinician and pathologist concerned had been alerted to the possibility of a malignant lesion. It must be stressed that this form of calcification can be found in a variety of benign breast diseases, especially in sclerosing adenosis, other types of adenosis and within the lumina of apocrine cysts. They are occasionally present in ductal papillomas and are even commoner in the lesion under consideration. They are, however, uncommon in epitheliosis or so-called 'papillomatosis' in the sense that the latter term is, regrettably, still used in some centres.

Concentric dense fibrous thickening of the duct wall is not usually a worrisome feature, but the sclerosis observed at times in the interior of some nodules has been a cause for concern.

Tumours with eccentric sclerosis at the periphery, resulting in distortion of the margin and apparent infiltration, generate considerable problems of interpretation. Large lesions, which are often of multiple type, and lesions which appear to breach the ductal confines also give rise to problems in diagnosis: yet even these usually retain an expansile growth pattern and do not closely resemble any known type of breast carcinoma. It is in the presence of a combination of a number of these features that the greatest difficulty of interpretation is experienced. In the final analysis, the criterion which establishes the benign nature of these lesions unequivocally is the identification in them of the two-cell-type structure.

There is an undoubted resemblance between certain ductal adenomas and some salivary-type adenomas of the breast. The classical pleomorphic salivary-type adenoma of breast with myxochondroid tissue and with other features identical to those seen in the common run of pleomorphic adenomas of salivary glands, is an extremely rare lesion.[2] Nevertheless, some ductal adenomas resemble the less pleomorphic varieties of salivary-type adenomas and we suspect that a few have been reported in the literature as such. This occasions no great harm, but it is best to recognize that there is a broader group of ductal adenomas linked, on the one hand, to ductal papillomas and, on the other, to salivary-type adenomas. Indeed there is probably no sharp dividing line since we have seen tumours with a structure which is intermediate between ductual adenomas and salivary-type adenoma.

Since, currently, solitary and multiple ductal papillomas are considered to have different clinicopathological connotations,[1] the solitary and multiple types of ductal adenoma should be separated, at least provisionally, until many more series of cases have been studied. More than one-third of the cases in this series were multifocal, although an element of selection may well have played a part in determining this high incidence. Unlike the 'multiple papilloma syndrome', however, we have not to date seen a case in which multiple ductal adenomas involved a whole segment of breast tissue, nor have we seen bilateral lesions.

It is our hope that the entity 'ductal adenoma', which is distinctive both clinically and pathologically, will become recognized as the third major form of adenoma of the breast: the other two are the nipple adenoma and the tubular adenoma. Study of further series of cases are needed to establish the precise incidence of this lesion, its association with other pathological processes, its malignant potential, if any, and the points of overlap between this lesion, on the one hand, and both ductal papilloma and salivary-type adenoma, on the other. The most important practical reason for its correct identification is to minimize the very real danger of confusion with carcinoma. This applies particularly to the larger and more complex lesions, and especially in the older age groups.

ACKNOWLEDGEMENTS

We are deeply indebted to the following pathologists who referred material included in this study: Dr A. Ahmed, Manchester; Dr A. Casarini, Mantova, Italy; Dr E. F. Gagliano, Brescia, Italy; Dr P. Goddeeris, Louvain, Belgium; Dr W. Guthrie, Dundee; Dr H. C. Ho, Hong Kong; Dr I. P. Hopper, Derby; Dr J. Horwood, Chatham, Ontario; Dr C. J. Hunter-Craig, Haywards Heath; Dr D. Jenkins, Lincoln; Dr C. H. Kelland, Hobart, Tasmania; Dr P. Laidler, Adelaide, Australia; Dr J. W. Magner, Cork; Dr W. R. Parry, Worksop; Dr H. G. Penman, Crawley; Dr J. Rode, London; Dr C. M. D. Ross, Barnstaple; Dr H. M. Ruitenberg, Zwolle, Holland; Dr W. Scarrett, Plymouth; Dr D. Spencer, Jersey; Professor E. C. Sweeney, Dublin. We wish to thank Mr E. G. Hamilton and his staff for technical assistance, Mr W. F. Hinkes for photographic services and Miss J. Flora for typing the manuscript. Professor N. A. Wright offered constructive criticism. One of us (J.G.A.) is suppored by grant SP 1626 of the Cancer Research Campaign.

REFERENCES

1. Azzopardi JG. Problems in breast pathology. In: Bennington JL, ed. Major Problems in Pathology, Vol. 11. London: Saunders, 1979.
2. van der Walt JD, Rohlova B. Pleomorphic adenoma of the human breast. A report of a benign tumour closely mimicking a carcinoma clinically. *Clin Oncol* 1982; **8**: 361–365.

JOURNAL OF PATHOLOGY, VOL. **144**: 25–34 (1984)

CUTANEOUS AND PULMONARY HISTOPATHOLOGICAL RESPONSES TO PLATELET ACTIVATING FACTOR (PAF-ACETHER) IN THE GUINEA-PIG

A. DEWAR

Electron Microscopy Unit, Cardiothoracic Institute, Fulham Road, London SW3 6HP, U.K.

C. B. ARCHER

Department of Dermatology, Guys Hospital, St. Thomas' Street, London SE1 9RT, U.K.

W. PAUL AND C. P. PAGE

Department of Clinical Pharmacology, Cardiothoracic Institute, Fulham Road, London SW3 6HP, U.K.

D. M. MACDONALD

Department of Dermatology, Guys Hospital, St. Thomas' Street, London SE1 9RT, U.K.

AND

J. MORLEY

Department of Clinical Pharmacology, Cardiothoracic Institute, Fulham Road, London SW3 6HP, U.K.

Received 16 January 1984
Accepted 16 April 1984

SUMMARY

The effect of synthetic Paf-acether has been studied in guinea-pig skin, following intradermal injection, and in guinea-pig lung, following intravenous administration. Histopathological responses to Paf-acether were assessed by both light microscopy and electron microscopy. In addition, plasma protein extravasation and platelet accumulation were quantitatively assessed using radiolabelling techniques. Intradermal injection of Paf-acether, but not lyso-Paf, elicited acute increased vascular permeability, accompanied by intravascular accumulation of platelets and neutrophils. There was evidence, 2–8 h after intradermal injection of Paf-acether, of perivascular infiltration with neutrophils. At 24 h there was a mixed cellular infiltrate comprising mononuclear cells in addition to neutrophils. Following systemic administration of Paf-acether, aggregates of platelets in close association with neutrophils were evident within the pulmonary vasculature. Intravenous injection of Paf-acether, but not lyso-Paf, caused intrathoracic accumulation of radiolabelled platelets. These results suggest that Paf-acether has properties consistent with those of a mediator of inflammation.

KEY WORDS—Platelet activating factor, Paf-acether, inflammatory mediator, vascular permeability.

INTRODUCTION

The term platelet activating factor (PAF) was introduced to describe a product released by interaction of antigen with IgE-sensitized rabbit basophils.[1] This active material has now been characterized as 1-*O*-alkyl-2-acetyl-*sn*-glyceryl-3-phosphorylcholine and renamed Paf-acether,[2] or AGEPC.[3] It is now recognized that Paf-acether is generated from ether-linked phospholipids via a two-step pathway, the first being the formation of lyso-PAF, which is biologically inactive, but has

0022–3417/84/090025–10$01.00

similar physiochemical properties to Paf-acether. This is followed by acetylation of lyso-PAF to form biologically active Paf-acether.[4] The availability of synthetic Paf-acether[5] has led to the discovery of biological properties in addition to platelet aggregation and mediator release,[4] and Paf-acether is now considered to be a putative mediator of inflammation as well as of allergy.[6]

The capacity of Paf-acether to elicit inflammatory responses in a number of different species has been recognized by several investigators, both in the skin[7–14] and the lung.[15,16] However, the histological changes accompanying such responses have not been extensively investigated.

The present study has evaluated the histopathological responses in the lung and skin of the guinea-pig following intravenous and intradermal administration of Paf-acether.

MATERIALS AND METHODS

Animals

Male Dunkin Hartley guinea-pigs (450–550 g) were used throughout this study.

Drugs

Paf-acether (obtained from Professor J. J. Godfroid and Dr J. Benveniste, Paris), lyso-PAF (Bachem) and prostaglandin E1 (PGE1; Sigma) were prepared as stock solutions (1 mg/ml) in absolute ethanol and diluted in phosphate buffered saline (PBS, Dulbeccos; Gibco Europe), containing 0·25 per cent bovine serum albumin (BSA, Sigma) immediately prior to use.

Radiolabelling of platelets

Guinea-pig platelets were labelled using ^{111}Indium oxine (^{111}In; Amersham International) as described previously.[17] Briefly, the platelet pellet from citrated arterial blood was washed free of plasma protein, resuspended in Ca^{2+} free Tyrode's solution containing PGE1 (300 ng/ml) (modified Tyrode's) and incubated with 25–50 μCi ^{111}Indium oxine for 2 min at 37°C. Platelets were then centrifuged to remove excess free radioactivity, resuspended in 1 ml modified Tyrode's solution and injected intravenously into anaesthetized recipient animals.

Skin studies

The dorso-lateral skin of animals was shaved at least 2 h prior to the start of experiments. Intradermal injections (each of 0·1 ml) of Paf-acether (0·1–100 ng/site), lyso-Paf (1 μg/site) and PBS-BSA were made at marked sites on the shaved skin of three guinea-pigs which had been injected intravenously with Evans blue dye (0·5 ml, 2·5 per cent in PBS; Sigma). Treatments were allocated to sites according to a balanced Latin square design. The animals were killed 30 min after the intradermal injections, skinned and the inner aspects of the skins were photographed.

Three animals were injected intravenously with Evans blue dye, ^{125}I-human serum albumin (^{125}I-HSA; 1 μCi, Amersham International) and ^{111}In-labelled guinea-pig platelets. These animals were injected intradermally, as above, with Paf-acether, lyso-Paf and PBS-BSA, then killed 30 min later. Blood (5 ml) was collected from each animal and heparinized (10 units/ml). After skinning, discs of skin, wholly including each lesion, were excised with a wad punch (17 mm diameter). Skin discs, whole blood (1 ml) and plasma samples (0·5 ml) were counted in an automatic gamma spectrometer (Nuclear Enterprises). Accumulation of ^{125}I-HSA or ^{111}In-platelets has been expressed as equivalent μl of whole blood [(^{125}I or ^{111}In counts in lesion/^{125}I or ^{111}In counts in 1 ml blood) $\times$ 1000] as described elsewhere.[10]

The time-course of the inflammatory response was established in groups of three animals by injecting Paf-acether (100 ng) or lyso-Paf (100 ng) at various times prior to, or immediately following, intravenous injection of Evans blue dye and ^{125}I-HSA. The animals were killed 30 min after the intravenous injections, bled and skinned. After visual inspection of the injected sites, these were removed and counted as described above.

For histological studies, groups of three animals were injected intravenously with shellac-free colloidal carbon (0·1 ml/100 g; Pelikan, Gunther Wagner). Duplicate sites on the shaved skin were injected with Paf-acether (100 ng), lyso-Paf (100 ng) or PBS–BSA at various times (24, 8, 4, 2, 0 h) prior to injection of the colloidal carbon and the animals were killed 30 min later. Discs of skin, containing the lesions, were removed as described above, fixed in 2·5 per cent glutaraldehyde in cacodylate buffer and embedded in Araldite for light and electron microscopy.

Lung studies

An indwelling 21 gauge cannula (Butterfly-21 INT; Abbott), placed in a foot vein of anaesthetized animals (7 ml/kg of a 25 per cent solution of urethane; Sigma), was used for administration of

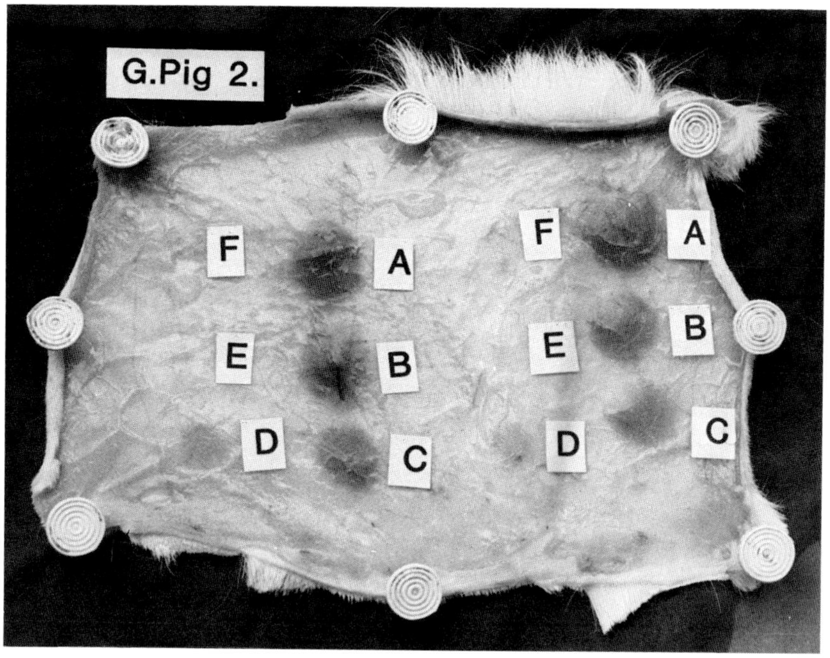

Fig. 1—Photograph of guinea-pig skin showing extravasation of Evans blue dye, 30 min after injection of Paf-acether 0·1, 1, 10, and 100 ng/site (D, C, B, and A respectively), lyso-PAF (1 μg/site) (E) and PBS–BSA (F)

Paf-acether (100 ng/kg) as a 0·3 ml bolus in three animals. After appropriate intervals following administration of Paf-acether, the animals were killed and the lungs removed for fixation by tracheal infusion of 2·5 per cent glutaraldehyde and processed as described for the skin. No other organs or tissues were examined.

To determine the time-course of platelet accumulation, ^{111}In labelled platelets were administered to three anaesthetized guinea-pigs 1 h prior to intravenous injection of lyso-Paf (100 ng/kg) followed 45 min later by Paf-acether (100 ng/kg). The radioactive platelets were monitored using an automated isotopic monitoring system (AIMS 2000; Mumed Ltd.) comprizing a 1 in. crystal scintillation detector (located over the thoracic region) coupled to a gamma spectrometer (Nuclear Enterprises). Counts were logged by a microcomputer (North Star Horizon) controlled by a visual display unit (Lyme 5000). Intrathoracic platelet accumulation was expressed as percentage increase in radioactivity as described elsewhere.[18]

RESULTS

Effects of intradermal administration

Intradermal injection of Paf-acether (0·1–100 ng/site) produced extravasation of Evans blue dye which was dose-related in terms of lesion diameter and intensity (Fig. 1). The lowest dose of 0·1 ng/site produced a lesion which was distinguishable from sites injected with PBS-BSA or lyso-Paf (1 μg/site). These latter sites could not be distinguished from each other (Fig. 1). The dose-related effect of Paf-acether on plasma protein extravasation, and the lack of effect of lyso-Paf, were confirmed in the animals injected with ^{125}I-HSA (Table I). In agreement with our previously published data,[10,11] sig-

Table I—Dose-related effects of Paf-acether and lack of effect of lyso-Paf on plasma protein extravasation (PPE) and platelet accumulation (PA) in guinea-pig skin

Treatment (dose/site)	PPE (μl)*	PA (μl)*
PBS-BSA	18±1	15±3
Paf-acether, 0·1 ng	30±3	15±5
1 ng	99±14	20±2
10 ng	148±19	41±7
100 ng	230±25	111±21
Lyso-Paf, 1 μg	21±5	16±4

*PPE and PA have been expressed as equivalent μl of whole blood [(^{125}I-HSA or ^{111}In counts in skin disc/^{125}I-HSA or ^{111}In counts in 1 ml blood) × 1000]. Values in the table represent mean ± SEM ($n=3$). Animals were killed 30 min after the intradermal injections.

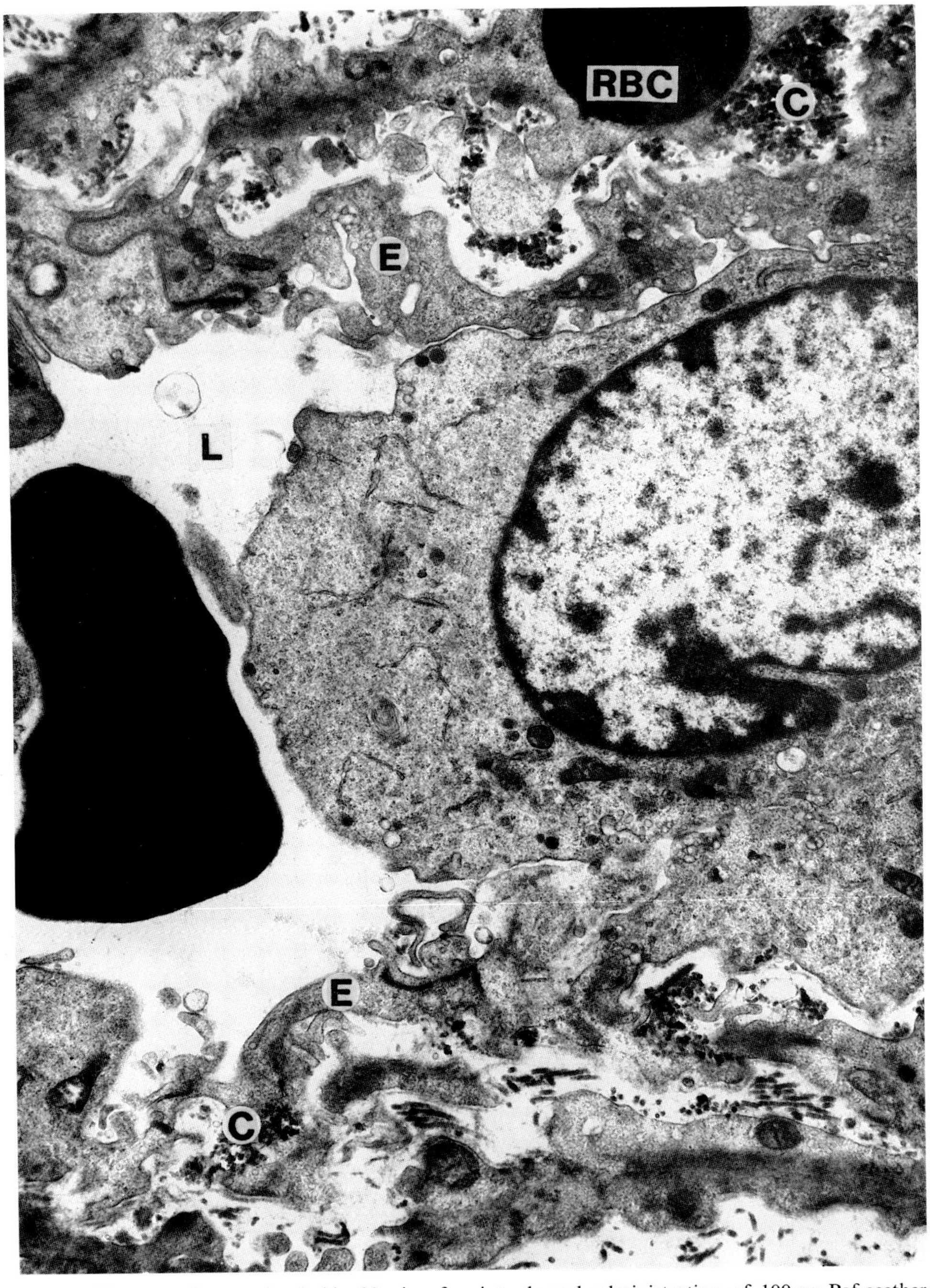

Fig. 2—Electron micrograph of skin 30 min after intradermal administration of 100 ng Paf-ecether illustrating carbon labelling (C) of endothelial cells (E) and extravasated red blood cells (RBC). The vessel lumen is indicated (L). × 10 500

Table II—Time-course of the plasma protein extravasation (PPE) response to Paf-acether (100 ng) in guinea-pig skin

Time (h)*	0·5	1	2	4	24	Control
PPE (μl)	140±11	27±2	9±2	5±1	4±1	8±2

*Time of injection of Paf-acether prior to killing the animals. ^{125}I-HSA was injected intravenously 30 min prior to killing the animals. Results are expressed as equivalent μl of whole blood [(^{125}I-HSA counts in skin sites/^{125}I-HSA counts in 1 ml blood) × 1000]. Values represent mean ± SEM ($n=3$).

nificant accumulation of radiolabelled platelets was evident at sites injected with Paf-acether (10 or 100 ng/site) but not at sites injected with PBS–BSA or lyso-Paf (1 μg/site) (Table I).

In animals injected with Paf-acether (100 ng/site) at various times prior to injection of visual and radioisotopic markers of plasma protein extravasation, leakage of Evans blue dye (results not shown) and accumulation of ^{125}I-HSA occurred only at sites injected within 1 h of killing the animals (Table II). Skin sites injected with lyso-Paf (1 μg/site) showed neither extravasation of Evans blue dye nor accumulation of ^{125}I-HSA at any time (results not shown).

Skin sites excised 30 min after intradermal administration of Paf-acether, showed extensive

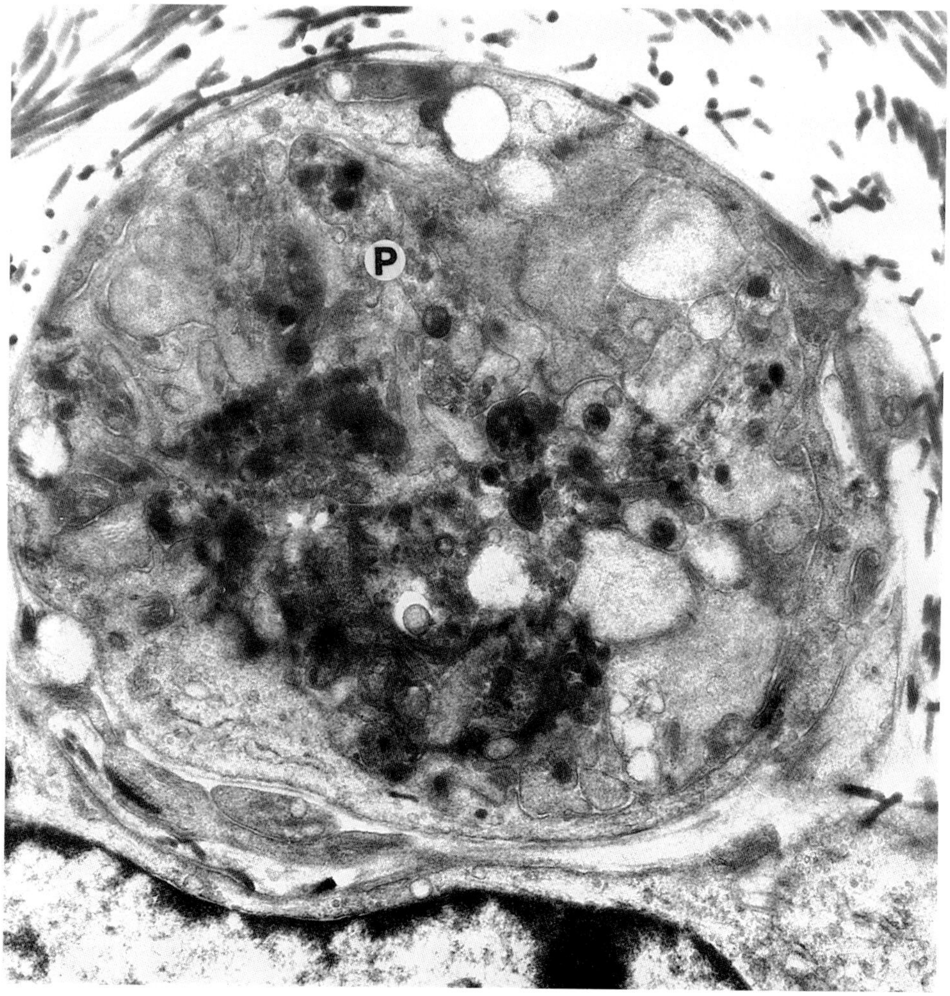

Fig. 3—Electron micrograph of a dermal blood vessel taken 30 min after administration of 100 ng Paf-acether illustrating intravascular congestion with platelet aggregates (P). × 13250

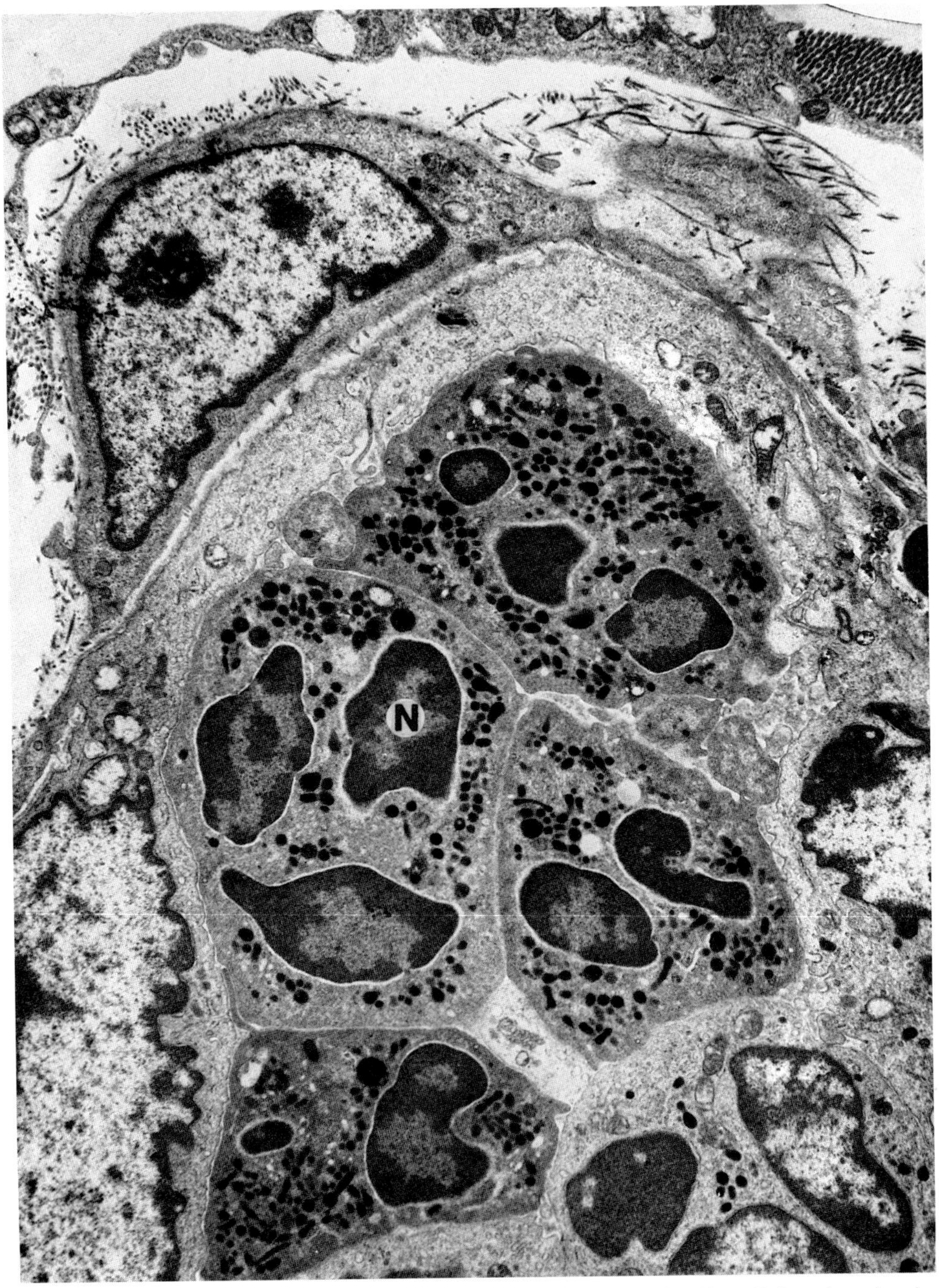

Fig. 4—Electron micrograph of skin 30 min after administration of 100 ng Paf-acether showing intravascular congestion of dermal blood vessels with neutrophils (N). ×8500

carbon labelling of vessel walls, an observation consistent with vascular leakage at these sites (Fig. 2); in addition, occasional extravasated red blood cells were seen. At 30 min, aggregates of platelets were apparent in many of the vessels (Fig. 3) and intravascular accumulation of neutrophils was frequently encountered (Fig. 4). Skin sites excised 2–8 h after intradermal injection of Paf-acether revealed a perivascular infiltrate in which neutrophils were predominant (Fig. 5). Sites of Paf-acether injection had an erythematous appearance which appeared within 30 min and persisted for at least 24 h. Skin sites excised at this time revealed substantial numbers of neutrophils, accompanied by comparable numbers of large mononuclear cells (Fig. 6). Histological examination of control sites injected with PBS–BSA or lyso-Paf did not show these inflammatory changes.

Effects of intravenous administration

Lungs removed 1 min after intravenous injection of Paf-acether exhibited intravascular accumulation both of platelets and neutrophils (Fig. 7). Substantial aggregates of platelets and neutrophils were evident throughout the pulmonary vasculature including larger arterial vessels, as well as small arterioles and capillaries (Fig. 8). Neutrophils were only evident in close proximity to platelet aggregates or as inclusions within such aggregates.

Intravenous injection of lyso-Paf (100 ng/kg) had no significant effect on circulating ^{111}In-labelled guinea-pig platelets (Fig. 9). In contrast, the same dose of Paf-acether produced a pronounced accumulation of radiolabelled platelets within the thoracic region (Fig. 9). Peak platelet accumulation occurred at approximately 1 min after the

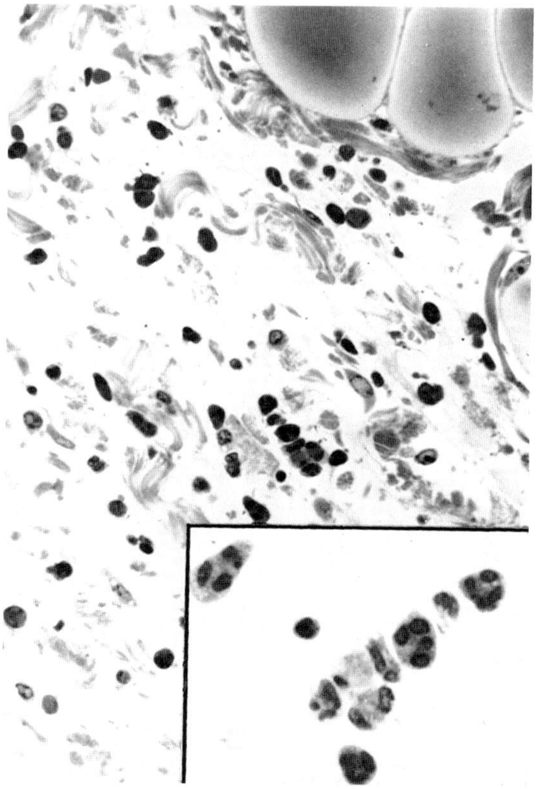

Fig. 5—Toluidine blue stained section of guinea-pig skin 8 h after intradermal administration of 100 ng Paf-acether displaying a mixed cellular infiltrate comprising predominantly neutrophils (×385). The multilobed nuclei of these cells are more closely seen at higher power (Inset, ×950)

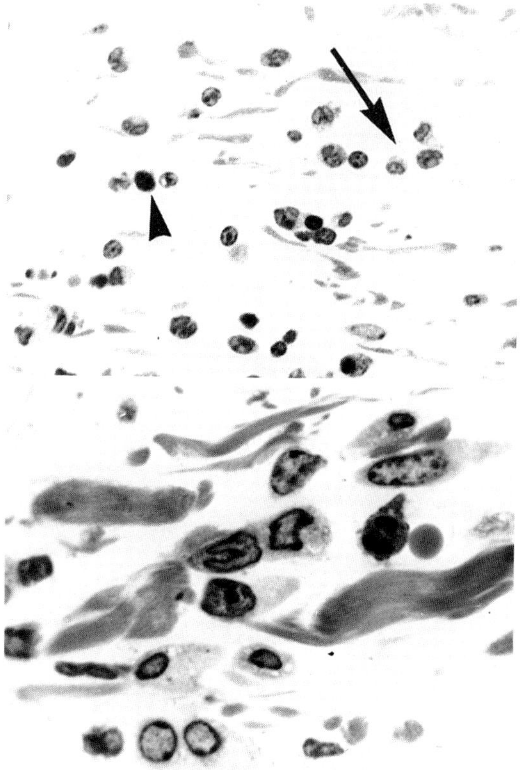

Fig. 6—Toluidine blue stained section of guinea-pig 24 h after intradermal administration of 100 ng Paf-acether showing a mixed cellular infiltrate comprising mononuclear cells (arrow) and occasional neutrophils (arrow head). ×370 (top) and ×950 (lower)

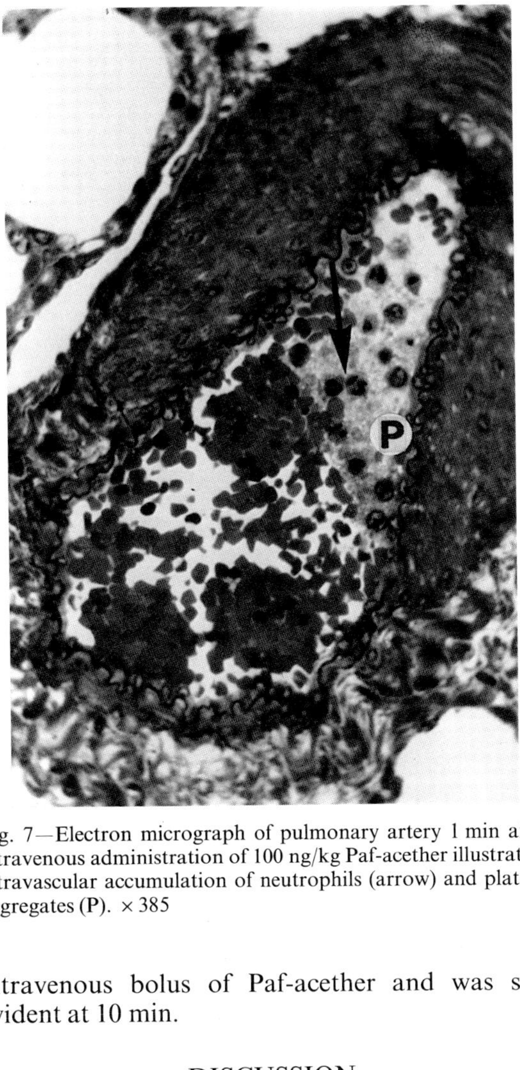

Fig. 7—Electron micrograph of pulmonary artery 1 min after intravenous administration of 100 ng/kg Paf-acether illustrating intravascular accumulation of neutrophils (arrow) and platelet aggregates (P). ×385

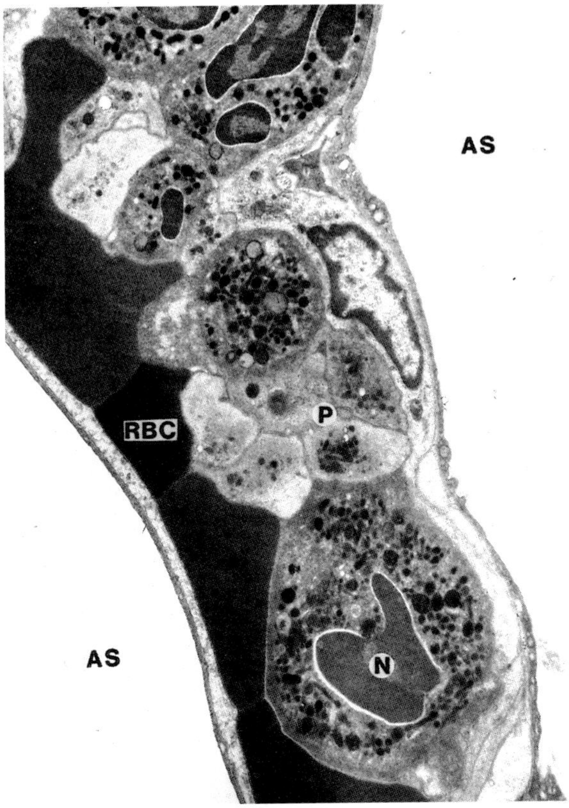

Fig. 8—Electron micrograph of a pulmonary capillary 1 min after intravenous administration of 100 ng/kg Paf-acether showing intravascular congestion with neutrophils (N), platelets (P) and red blood cells (RBC). Alveolar space (AS). ×9000

intravenous bolus of Paf-acether and was still evident at 10 min.

DISCUSSION

We have demonstrated that Paf-acether causes acute pathological changes both in the skin and the lung, in addition to persisting changes in the skin. Accumulation of platelets and neutrophils within the pulmonary vasculature, within 1 min of intravenous administration of Paf-acether, reflects the rapid thrombocytopaenia which follows Paf-acether injection[4] and accords with the direct observation of ^{111}Indium oxine labelled platelet accumulation within the thoracic region of anaesthetized animals following injection of Paf-acether (Fig. 9).[19]

Paf-acether has a range of biological properties appropriate to a mediator of asthma, and release of Paf-acether during allergic reactions[20] could

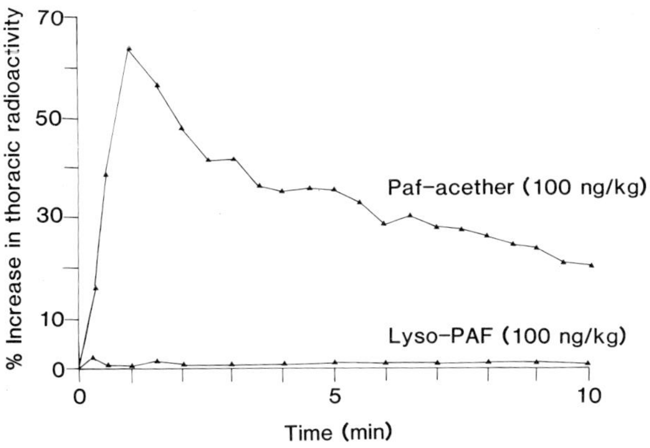

Fig. 9—The time course of accumulation of ^{111}Indium labelled platelets following intravenous injection of Paf-acether (100 ng/kg) or lyso-Paf (100 ng/kg). Responses obtained in a single representative animal have been expressed as percentage increases in ^{111}In counts above the stable basal values prior to injection

determine the platelet activation and associated bronchospasm recently observed in allergic asthmatics.[21,22] Bronchospasm may accompany activation of both platelets[4] and neutrophils[23] and since intravenous administration of Paf-acether produces neutrophil accumulation in association with platelet aggregates, the possibility arises that an interaction between these two blood elements could determine changes in lung function in response to Paf-acether.

Intradermal administration of Paf-acether promoted increased cutaneous vessel permeability demonstrated by the leakage of colloidal carbon between endothelial cells. This histological observation is consistent with the plasma protein extravasation revealed by isotopic or dye leakage studies[8,10] and the acute wheal reaction which follows intradermal administration in the forearm of man.[24] Histological evidence of platelet and neutrophil accumulation at sites of intradermal injection of Paf-acether is consistent with the retention of radioisotopically labelled blood elements in guinea-pigs.[11] Extravascular accumulation of neutrophils has been noted 2–4 h after intradermal injection of Paf-acether in rabbits.[9] The appearance of mononuclear cells in 24 hour lesions, as well as neutrophils, contrasts with rabbit skin, where no inflammatory cell infiltrate was evident at this time.[8,9] Whilst this may reflect a species difference, it should be noted that mononuclear cell accumulation is observed in human skin at 24 h.[24] Alternatively, this may result from a difference in Paf-acether preparations, since variations in chain length have been observed in Paf-acether preparations isolated from different sources.[25] The mixed cell population evident 24 h after intradermal Paf-acether was reminiscent of an Arthus response and, as it has been reported that Paf-acether release is related to immune complex deposition in the kidney,[26] it is possible that Paf-acether may contribute to Arthus type reactions in the skin. The ability of Paf-acether to effect late onset, sustained accumulation of mononuclear cells in animal and human skin suggests that this phospholipid should be considered as a potential mechanism for cellular accumulation in inflammatory dermatoses. Although we did not study inflammatory changes in the lung beyond 1 h after administration of Paf-acether, it has recently been reported that instillation of Paf-acether into the lungs of rabbits will induce inflammatory changes similar to those found in this study in guinea-pig skin.[27]

Paf-acether has been widely investigated as a potential mediator of platelet aggregation. However, being released from a range of inflammatory cell types other than platelets, and since it has acute inflammatory actions which include platelet-independent increased vascular permeability,[10] Paf-acether also has a potential role as a mediator of acute inflammation. Production of both acute and late onset responses to Paf-acether in the guinea-pig suggests that this substance should, in addition, be considered as a mediator of more persistent manifestations of inflammation and its release may contribute to the interaction between acute and late-onset allergic responses.

ACKNOWLEDGEMENTS

Financial support from Schering Chemicals (C.P.P.) and the Arthritis and Rheumatism Council (W.P.) is gratefully acknowledged.

REFERENCES

1. Benveniste J, Henson PM, Cochrane CG. Leucocyte dependent histamine release from rabbit platelets: the role of IgE, basophils and a platelet activating factor. *J Exp Med* 1972; **136:** 1356.
2. Benveniste J, Tence M, Varenne P, Bidault J, Boullet C, Polonsky J. Semi-synthèse et structure proposée du facteur activant les plaquettes (PAF): Paf-acether, un alkyl ether analogue de la lysophosphatidylcholine. *C R Acad Sci* 1979; **289:** 1037.
3. Demopoulos CA, Pinckard RN, Hanahan DJ. Platelet activating factor: evidence for 1-*O*-alkyl-2-acetyl-*sn*-glyceryl-3-phosphorylcholine as the active component (a new class of lipid chemical mediators). *J Biol Chem* 1979; **254:** 9355.
4. Vargaftig BB, Cignard M, Benveniste J, Lefort J, Wal F. Background and present status of research on platelet-activating factor (Paf-acether). *Ann NY Acad Sci* 1981; **370:** 119.
5. Godfroid JJ, Heymans F, Michel E, Redeuilh C, Steiner E, Benveniste J. Platelet activating factor (Paf-acether): total synthesis of 1-*O*-octadecyl-2-*O*-acetyl-*sn*-glycero-3-phosphorylcholine. *FEBS Letters* 1980; **116:** 161.
6. Page CP, Paul W, Dewar A, Wood LE, Basran GS, Morley J. Paf-acether: a putative mediator of asthma and inflammation. *Ag Act* 1983; **13:** (Suppl): 177.
7. Basran GS, Page CP, Paul W, Morley J. Cromoglycate (DSCG) inhibits responses to platelet-activating factor (Paf-acether) in man: an alternative mode of action for DSCG in asthma? *Eur J Pharmacol* 1983; **86:** 143.
8. Humphrey DM, McManus LM, Satouchi K, Hanahan DJ, Pinckard RN. Vasocative properties of acetyl glyceryl ether phosphorylcholine and analogues. *Lab Invest* 1982; **46:** 422.

9. Humphrey DM, Hanahan DJ, Pinckard RN. Induction of leukocytic infiltrates in rabbit skin by acetyl glyceryl ether phosphorylcholine. *Lab Invest* 1982; **47:** 227.
10. Morley J, Page CP, Paul W. Inflammatory actions of platelet activating factor (Paf-acether) in guinea-pig skin. *Br J Pharmac* 1983; **80:** 503.
11. Paul W, Page CP. Cutaneous responses to synthetic platelet activating factor (Paf-acether) in the guinea-pig. *Ag Act* 1983; **13:** 455.
12. Pinckard RN, Kniker WT, Lee L, Hanahan DJ, McManus LM. Vasoactive effects of 1-*O*-alkyl-2-acetyl-*sn*-glyceryl-3-phosphorylcholine (AcGEPC) in human skin. *J Allergy Clin Immunol* 1980; **65:** 196.
13. Pirotzky E, Page CP, Roubin R, Pfister A, Paul W, Bonnet J, Benveniste J. Paf-acether induced plasma exudation is independent of platelets and neutrophils in rat skin. *Microcirculation* 1984; **1:** 107.
14. Wedmore CV, Williams TJ. Platelet-activating factor (PAF), a secretory product of polymorphonuclear leucocytes, increases vascular permeability in rabbit skin. *Br J Pharmacol* 1981; **74:** 916.
15. Heffner JE, Shoemaker SA, Canham EM, Patel M, McMurty IF, Morris HG, Repine JE. Acetyl glyceryl ether phosphorylcholine-stimulated human platelets cause pulmonary hypertension and edema in isolated rabbit lungs. *J Clin Invest* 1983; **71:** 351.
16. Voelkel NF, Worthen S, Reeves JT, Henson PM, Murphy RC. Non-immunological production of leukotrienes induced by platelet-activating factor. *Science* 1982; **218:** 286.
17. Page CP, Paul W, Morley J. An *in vivo* model for studying platelet aggregation and disaggregation. *Thrombos Haemostas* 1982; **47:** 210.
18. Page CP, Paul W, Morley J. Platelets and bronchospasm. *Int Archs Allergy Appl Immun.* 1984; **74:** 347.
19. Page CP, Paul W, Morley J. *In vivo* aggregation of guinea-pig platelets in response to synthetic platelet activating factor (Paf-acether). *Ag Act* 1983; **13:** 506.
20. Arnoux B, Simoes-Caeioro MH, Landes A, Mathieu M, Duroux P, Benveniste J. Alveolar macrophages from asthmatics release Paf-acether and lyso-Paf-acether when stimulated with specific antigen. *Amer Rev Resp Dis* 1982; **125** (Suppl): 70 (Abstract).
21. Cella G, Girolami A. Platelet activation in antigen-induced bronchoconstriction. *N Engl J Med* 1981; **305:** 892.
22. Knauer KA, Lichtenstein LM, Franklin Adminson Jr N, Fish JE. Platelet activation during antigen-induced airway reactions in asthmatic subjects. *N Engl J Med* 1981; **304:** 1404.
23. Craddock PR, Fehr J, Brigham KL, Kronenberg R, Jacob HS. Complement and leukocyte-mediated pulmonary dysfunction in hemodialysis. *N Engl J Med* 1977; **296:** 769.
24. Archer CB, Page CP, Paul W, Morley J, MacDonald DM. Early and late inflammatory effects of Paf-acether in the skin of experimental animals and man. *J Invest Dermatol* 1983; **80:** 346.
25. Pinckard RN, McManus LM, Demopoulos C, Halonen M, Clark PO, Shaw JO, Kniker WT, Hanahan DJ. Molecular pathobiology of acetyl glyceryl ether phosphorylcholine: evidence for the structural and functional identity with platelet activating factor. *J Reticuloendothel Soc* 1980; **28:** 95.
26. Camussi G, Tetta C, Deregibus MC, Bussolino F, Segoloni G, Vercellone A. Platelet activating factor (PAF) in experimentally induced serum sickness: role of basophil derived PAF in immune complex deposition. *J Immunol* 1982; **128:** 86.
27. Camussi G, Pawlowski I, Tetta C, Roffinello C, Alberton M, Brentjens J, Andres G. Acute lung inflammation induced in the rabbit by local instillation of 1-*O*-octadecyl-2-acetyl-*sn*-glyceryl-3-phosphorylcholine or of native platelet activating factor. *Am J Pathol* 1983; **112:** 78.

JOURNAL OF PATHOLOGY, VOL. **144**: 35–44 (1984)

IMMUNOHISTOCHEMICAL LOCALIZATION OF MACROMOLECULES OF THE BASEMENT MEMBRANE AND THE PERITUMORAL STROMA IN HUMAN LARYNGEAL CARCINOMAS

Y. CAM*

Laboratoire de Biochimie, Era 959 du C.N.R.S., Faculté de Médecine de Reims, France

T. CAULET

Laboratoire Central d'Anatomie Pathologique, Centre Hospitalo-Universitaire Reims, France

G. BELLON AND G. POULIN

Laboratoire de Biochimie, ERA 959 du C.N.R.S., Faculté de Médecine de Reims, France

M. LEGROS

Service d'Oto-Rhino-Laryngologie, C.H.U. Reims, France

AND

M. PYTLINSKA

Laboratoire Central d'Anatomie Pathologique, Centre Hospitalo-Universitaire Reims, France

Received 6 January 1984
Accepted 17 April 1984

SUMMARY

Forty laryngeal carcinomas were studied by immunofluorescence with specific antisera against components of the basement membrane (type IV collagen and laminin) as well as antisera against connective tissue antigens (type V collagen and fibronectin). The basement membrane surrounding well-differentiated squamous cell carcinomas showed an appearance similar to that seen beneath normal epithelium. In contrast, marked alterations of the basement membrane were constantly observed around infiltrating and poorly-differentiated carcinomas. The staining of connective tissue components in most cases was as intense in carcinomas as in normal laryngeal mucosa. The use of antibodies to basement membrane components may help to elucidate the mechanism of invasion of connective tissues by malignant cells.

KEY WORDS—Type IV collagen, laminin, type V collagen, fibronectin, laryngeal carcinomas, basement membrane.

INTRODUCTION

Normal epithelium and vascular endothelium are surrounded by a basement membrane[1] at the boundary between the cells and the connective tissue. Intraepithelial carcinomas do not migrate through the basement membrane, in contrast to invasive carcinomas which are characterized by infiltration through the basement membranes into the underlying connective tissue. In these tumours alterations occur in the basement membrane which may eventually disappear. Once neoplastic cells have migrated into the connective tissue they may disseminate more widely. However, most of the

*Head of research I.N.S.E.R.M., France.
Addressee for correspondence: Dr Y. Cam, Laboratoire de Biochimie, Faculté de Médecine, 51 rue Cognacq Jay, 51 095 Reims Cedex, France.

0022–3417/84/090035–10$01.00

tumour cells remain localized, proliferating and developing a peritumoural stroma.[2] The basement membrane can be demonstrated by light microscopy using immunohistochemical methods with specific antibodies to its main components: laminin, type IV collagen and proteoglycans.[3-5] Other components of the extracellular matrix such as fibronectin and type V collagen can be demonstrated in the same way and show a close association with the basement membrane.[6-8] The distribution of the molecular components of the basement membrane has already been studied in several types of neoplasm.[9-12] Fibronectin and type V collagen have also been localized in different types of tumour.[13-17]

In the present work we report the distribution of type IV and type V collagens, laminin and fibronectin in laryngeal carcinomas obtained from surgical laryngectomy specimens. Sections were examined from normal epithelium adjacent to the tumours and from invasive and non-invasive areas of the carcinomas. Tissues from the intermediate areas between normal mucosa and carcinoma were also examined. By studying the distribution of four different molecules, type IV collagen and laminin usually exclusively found within the basement membrane and type V collagen and fibronectin preferentially located within the intercellular matrix, we tried to relate modification in the appearance of these structures with the invasiveness of the overlying carcinoma.

MATERIALS AND METHODS

Histological diagnoses

Forty surgical specimens of laryngectomies were examined. The histological diagnoses were as follows. Twenty-three differentiated squamous cell carcinomas without lymph node metastases. Eight differentiated squamous cell carcinomas with lymph node metastases. Eight differentiated squamous cell carcinomas with lymph node metastases. Four undifferentiated squamous cell carcinomas without lymph node metastases. Five undifferentiated squamous cell carcinomas with lymph node metastases.

Preparation of specific antisera

Pure collagens were used for this purpose. Native type IV collagen was prepared from a pepsin digest of the chorionic amniotic membranes of human placenta according to a method previously described.[18] Placental type IV collagen gave molecular weight components of 140K, 120K and 75K, when run in polyacrylamide gel electrophoresis after reduction in 5 per cent sodium dodecylsulphate.[18]

Type IV collagen was purified from the same human placental membranes as described.[19] This material showed two specific bands named α-1 (V) and α-2 (V) when run on 5 per cent SDS polyacrylamide gel as described.[20]

Type I and type III collagens isolated from pepsin digest of calf skin and human placental membranes and characterized by established procedures[21,22] were used for purifying antibodies to type IV and type V collagens and determining their characteristics.

Antisera against type IV and type V collagens were obtained by injection of the respective purified antigens to New Zealand rabbits.[23]

Antibodies to type IV and type V collagens were purified by immunosorption on CnBr-activated Sepharose 4B columns using types I, III, IV and V collagens as ligands.[23]

Anti-type IV and anti-type V collagen antibodies were identified by performing enzyme-linked immunoassays (ELISA) as described.[24]

No cross reactivity of anti-type IV collagen antibodies was noted with either of the following molecules: type I, type III and type V human collagens, human fibronectin and laminin. Similarly, no cross reactivity of anti-type V collagen antibodies was found with either of the following antigens: types I, III and IV collagens, fibronectin and laminin.

Anti-fibronectin antibodies were obtained commercially from Cappel Laboratories as the IgG fraction of anti-fibronectin serum. Purified anti-laminin antibodies were obtained from Bethesda Research Laboratories.

Fluorescent staining and electron microscopy

Samples were obtained immediately following laryngectomy from uninvolved mucosa and from superficial and deep parts of the carcinoma avoiding areas of necrosis. When possible, samples were taken from the junctional area between normal epithelium and carcinoma. Adjacent tissues were removed for routine histology. The tissues for immunohistochemical study were frozen in liquid nitrogen. Other samples were fixed in glutaraldehyde–osmium-tetroxide and embedded in epon for electron microscopy. Some samples were fixed in mixed solutions containing ruthenium red or tannic acid or alcian blue.[25] The immunohistochemical study was performed as follows.

Six μm sections were cut on a cryostat at -25°C, placed on glass slides and briefly air dried. The slides were then fixed in absolute ethanol for 10 min at 4°C. Specific antisera were applied to sections of tissues for 30 min at room temperature. The sera were diluted in phosphate buffered saline, pH7·4 in a dilution of 1/40 for anti-type IV collagen and anti-laminin, a dilution of 1/20 for anti-type V collagen and anti-fibronectin. A control section was layered with non-immune rabbit serum diluted 1/40. After incubation the sections were washed three times in buffered saline and then layered with a fluorescein isothiocyanate conjugated goat anti-rabbit immunoglobulin (Institut Pasteur, Paris), diluted 1/10. After 30 min incubation the slides were again washed three times in phosphate buffered saline. The sections were then mounted in glycerol-phosphate buffered saline mixture (10 per cent glycerol). In some cases additional slides were digested in pepsin for 10 min before incubation with the antisera. The sections were examined in a Reichert Univar microscope equipped with a fluorescence vertical illuminator. Photographs were taken on Ektachrome 400 ASA film with an automatic camera.

RESULTS

Normal mucosa

There was no staining of the cells of the epidermis by any of the antisera. Antibodies to type IV collagen gave a continuous strong linear staining at the level of the basement membrane close to the basal cell layer of the epithelium (Fig. 1). It was not possible to distinguish whether the staining was localized to the lamina densa or was present on other layers of the basement membrane. A similar staining pattern was obtained with anti-laminin serum (Fig. 2). Staining with antisera against type V collagen and fibronectin showed an uneven and discontinuous pattern that appeared to be composed of interwoven, short fibrillary structures. The

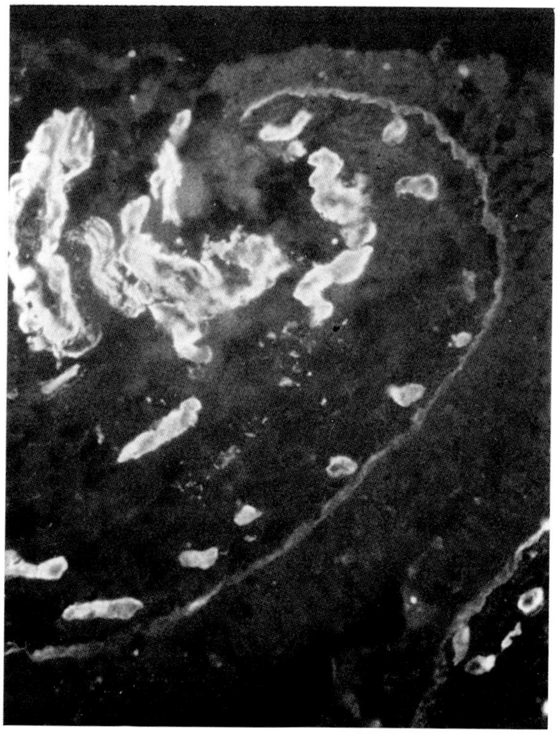

Fig. 1—Normal laryngeal mucosa. Immunofluorescence staining of type IV collagen; epithelial and vascular basement membranes are clearly visible as linear deposits. ×96

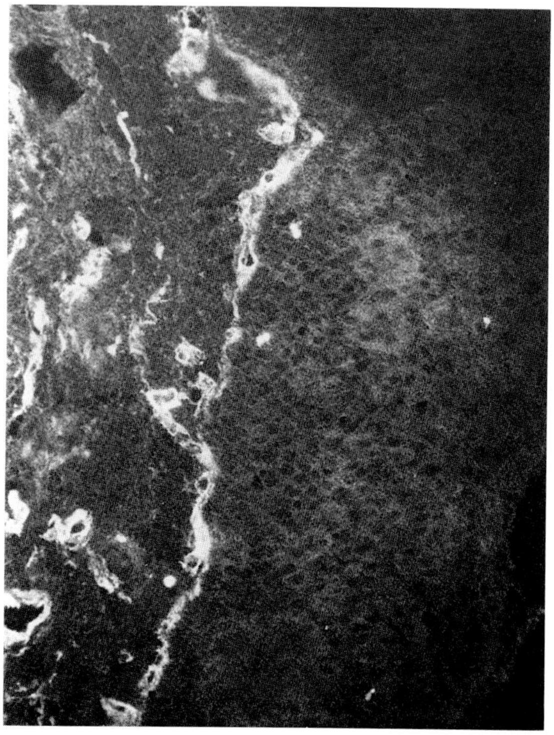

Fig. 2—Normal laryngeal mucosa. Immunofluorescence staining of laminin; epithelial and vascular basement membranes are clearly visible. ×200

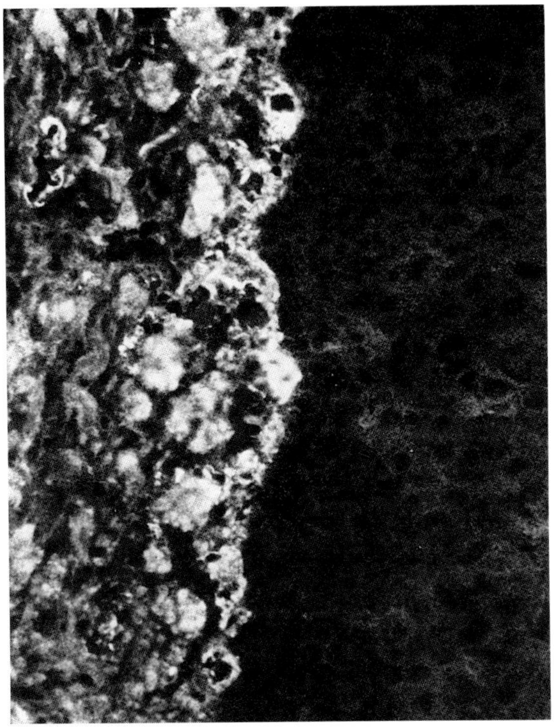

Fig. 3—Normal laryngeal mucosa. Immunofluorescence staining of type V collagen. Irregular, uneven and discontinuous fibrillar deposits are visible close to the basement membrane zone of the epithelium and the vessels. Fibrillar structures stained in the underlying connective tissue. ×200

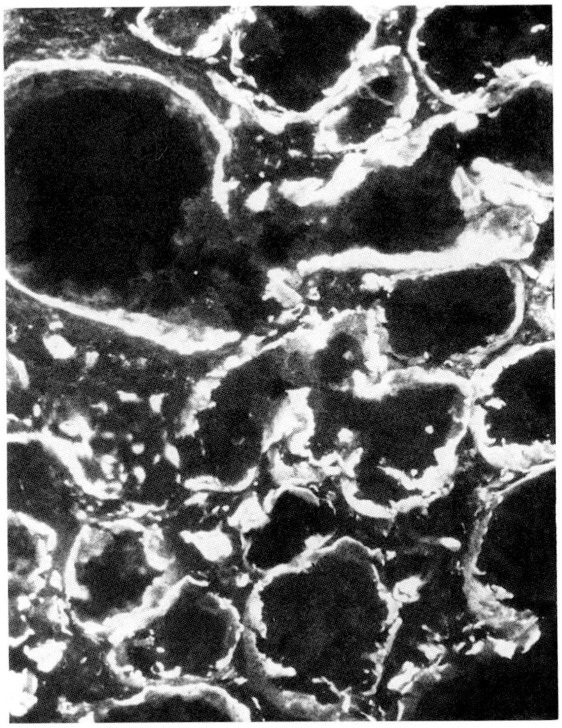

Fig. 4—Normal laryngeal mucosa. Immunofluorescence staining of type IV collagen. Sero-mucous gland basement membranes are heavily stained. ×200

basement membrane zone appeared thick and irregular. The staining appeared to be continuous with the underlying fibrillary connective tissue (Fig. 3).

The capillaries, arterioles and venules showed a different staining pattern. The results can be summarized as follows. Anti-type IV collagen and anti-laminin stained exclusively the sub-endothelial basement membrane which sometimes appeared single, sometimes double or multi-layered corresponding to the patterns seen by electron microscopy. Type V collagen showed a condensed irregular pattern in the walls of vessels. Arterioles were labelled in their whole thickness. Anti-fibronectin gave a fibrillar and often dense staining but did not always underline the basement membrane of capillaries. In larger vessels, fibronectin was seen in the media and in the perivascular tissues.

The basement membranes of sero-mucinous glands and striated muscle cells was stained strongly by anti-type IV collagen and anti-laminin (Fig. 4). Anti-fibronectin and anti-type V collagen reacted with the surrounding chorion incorporating the basement membrane to a variable extent (Fig. 5). Anti-fibronectin and anti-type V collagen strongly stained the connective tissue in a fibrillary pattern. There was no staining by anti-laminin and anti-type IV collagen within the connective tissue.

Laryngeal carcinomas

The appearances obtained with well-differentiated squamous cell carcinomas differed substantially from those seen with undifferentiated and very infiltrative carcinomas. Well-differentiated squamous cell carcinomas often showed moderate degrees of invasion in the deeper parts of the tumour. Antibodies against laminin and type IV collagen showed a similar linear staining of the basement membrane bordering the trabeculae of carcinoma. This staining was interrupted in some places giving small gaps (Fig. 6). Staining of sequential sections showed that the position of the gaps demonstrated by anti-laminin antibodies

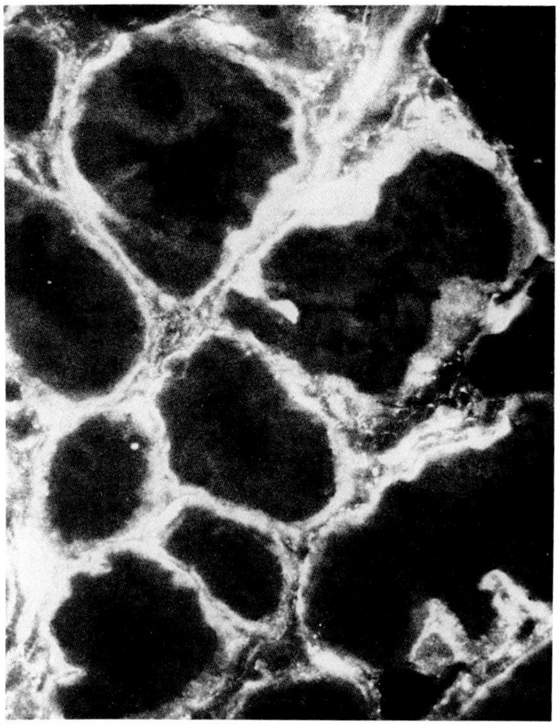

Fig. 5—Normal laryngeal mucosa. Immunofluorescence staining of fibronectin; heavy but irregular deposits are visible in seromucosal gland basement membrane zones; a faint staining is noticed at the periphery of epithelial cells. × 320

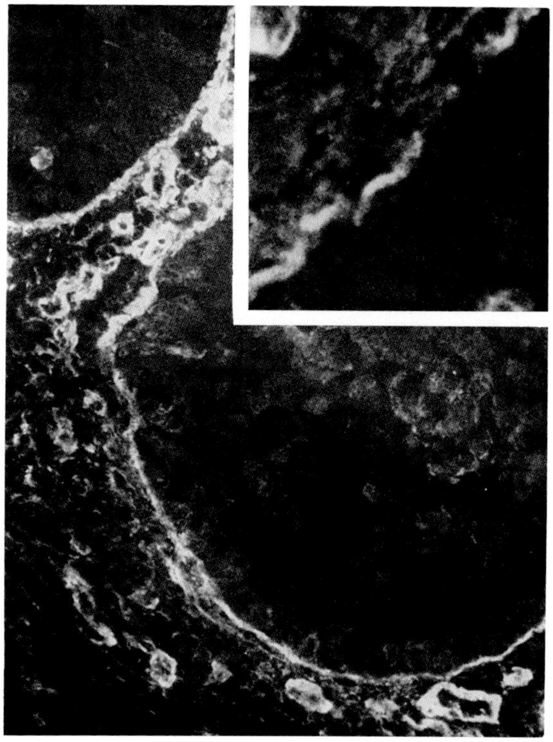

Fig. 6—Invasive and well-differentiated carcinomatous lobules. Immunofluorescence staining of type IV collagen. Linear and regular deposits, with small gaps (insert), surround the tumoral lobule. Basement membranes of the vessels are also stained. × 250, insert × 400

was the same as those demonstrated by anti-type IV collagen antibodies (Fig. 7). Tumour cells were not stained by either of these antibodies. Adjacent vessels and surrounding structures showed the same staining pattern as was seen in normal tissues.

Anti-fibronectin and anti-type V collagen antibodies strongly stained the tumour stroma (Fig. 8). The staining pattern was diffuse and fibrillary and sometimes showed a discontinuous condensation along the basement membrane (Fig. 9). The basement membrane was never well-defined by these antisera. The tumour cells were unstained.

In undifferentiated carcinomas, carcinomas with marked infiltration and areas within differentiated carcinomas in which there was infiltration antibodies against type IV collagen and laminin gave a weaker and more irregular staining of the basement membrane (Fig. 10). Sometimes they showed a linear staining but more often they disappeared almost entirely at the periphery of the tumour trabeculae (Fig. 11). The poorly-differentiated tumour lobules exhibited the weakest and most irregular staining of the basement membrane (Fig. 12).

Anti-type V collagen and anti-fibronectin sera usually showed a strong reaction pattern in the stroma of the tumour (Fig. 13) but there was no condensation of staining at the periphery of the tumour. The labelling was as intense in the tumour stroma as in the normal connective tissue for both antigens (Fig. 14). There was no staining of tumour cells by any of these antisera.

Intermediate areas

Areas of intra-epithelial spread were found adjacent to a number of the tumours. The distribution of the basement membrane components bordering on these intra-epithelial carcinomas was similar to that seen in normal mucosa. In particular, the basement membrane appeared intact without gaps.

Electron microscopy

In well-differentiated carcinomas the basement membrane appeared as a delicate dense line usually

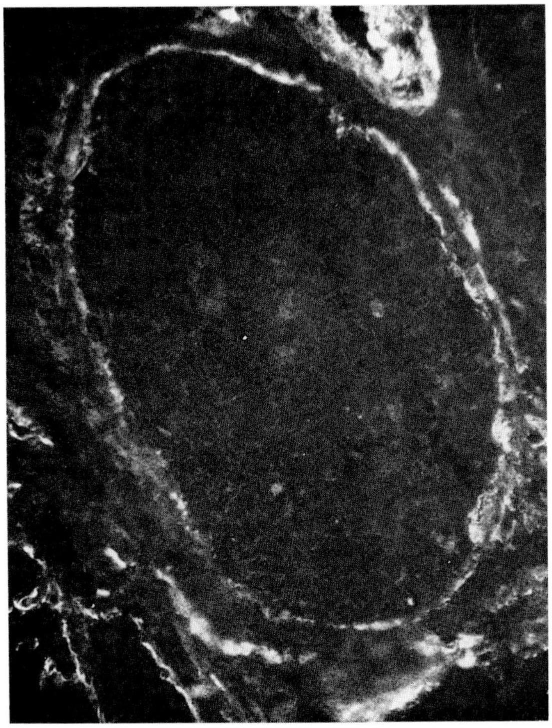

Fig. 7—Invasive and well-differentiated carcinomatous lobules. Immunofluorescence staining of laminin. Linear and regular deposits with small gaps surround the tumoral lobules. × 200

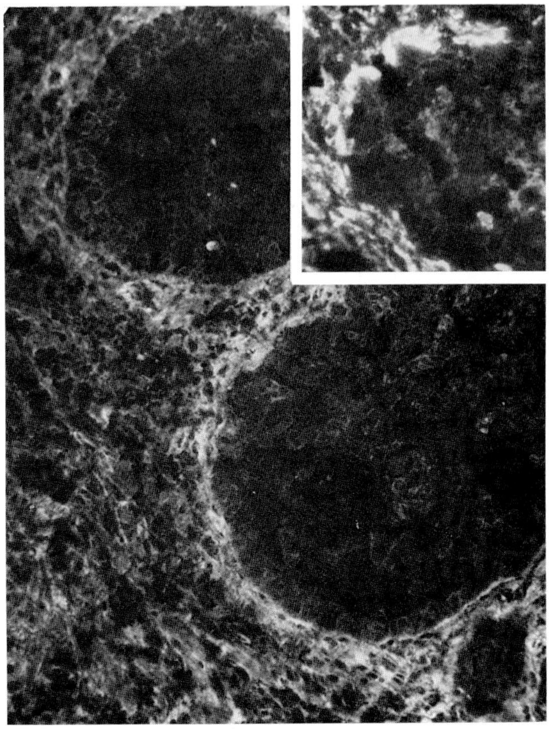

Fig. 8—Invasive and well-differentiated carcinomatous lobules. Immunofluorescence staining of type V collagen shows fibrillar deposits within the stroma and dense but discontinuous (insert) localization around the tumoral lobules. × 120, insert × 200

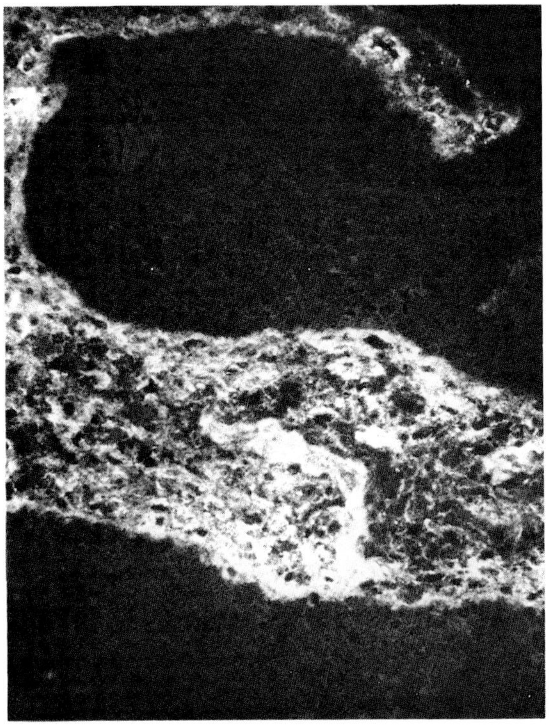

Fig. 9—Invasive and well-differentiated carcinomatous lobules. Immunofluorescence staining of fibronectin shows a distribution of this molecule similar to type V collagen around the tumoral lobules. × 128

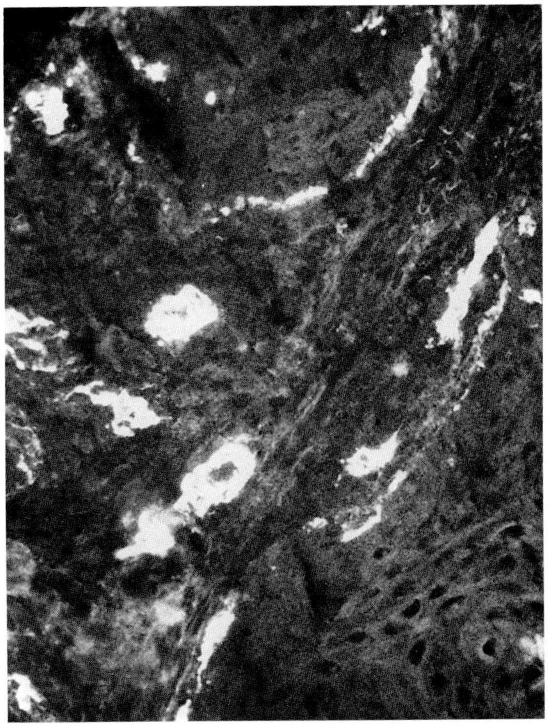

Fig. 10—Undifferentiated and infiltrating carcinoma. Immunofluorescence staining of type IV collagen shows large disruptions in the basement membranes of highly infiltrating areas. × 200

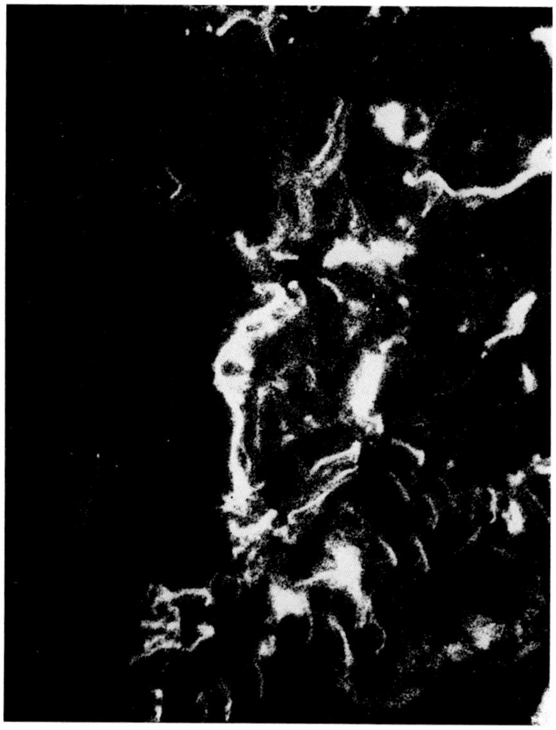

Fig. 11—Undifferentiated and infiltrating carcinoma. Immunofluorescence staining of laminin shows disrupted basement membranes. ×200

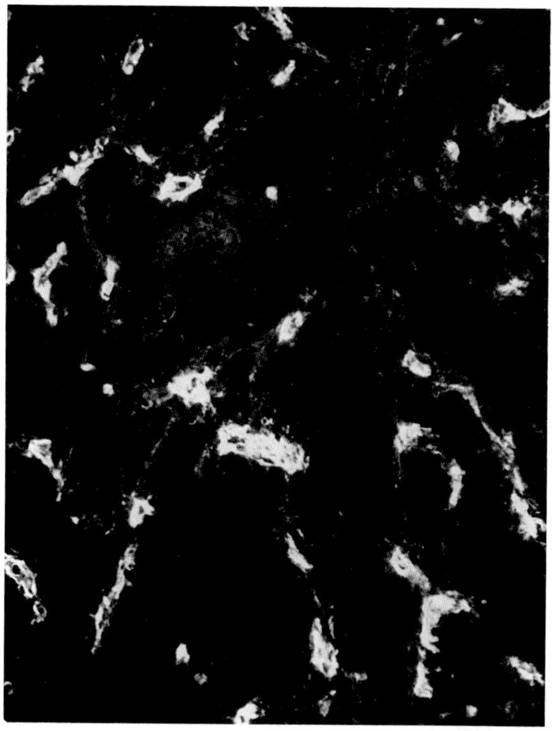

Fig. 12—Undifferentiated and very infiltrating carcinomatous area. Immunofluorescence staining of type IV collagen. No more basement membrane is clearly visible except around the vessels. ×96

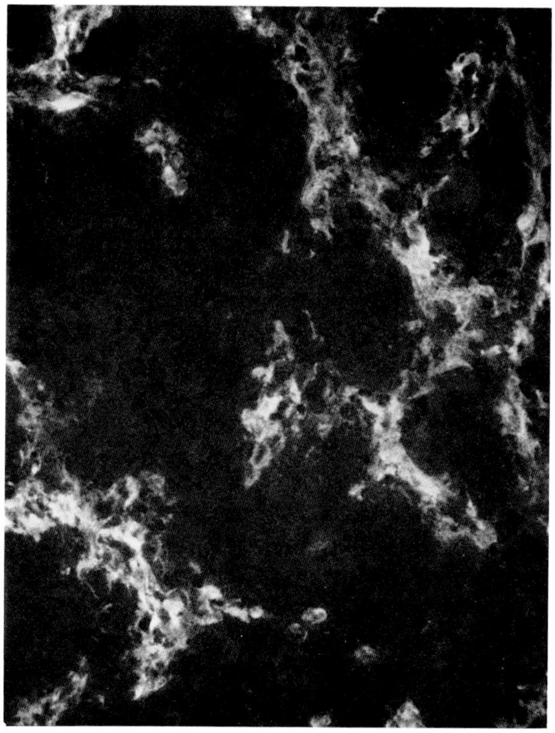

Fig. 13—Undifferentiated and very infiltrating carcinomatous area. Immunofluorescence staining of type V collagen. Fibrillar deposits are visible within the connective tissue; a dense positivity is seen around the vessels. ×200

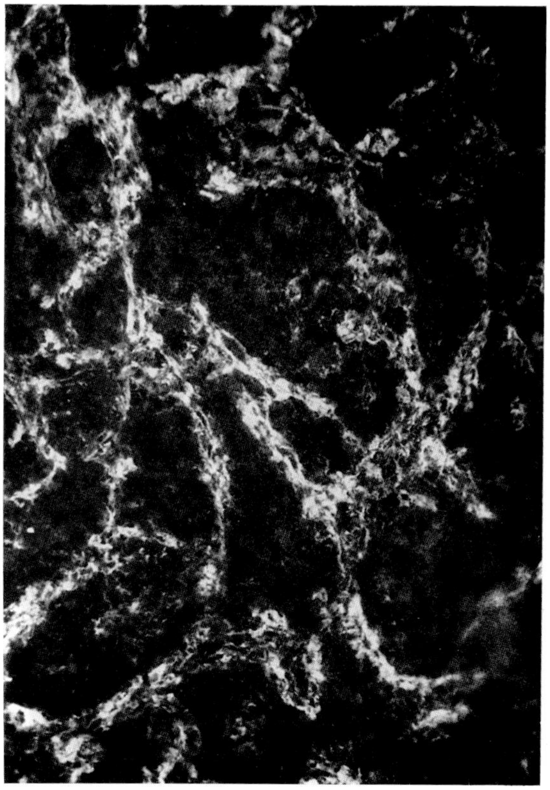

Fig. 14—Undifferentiated and very infiltrating carcinomatous area. Immunofluorescence staining of fibronectin. Fibronectin has a distribution similar to type V collagen. ×96

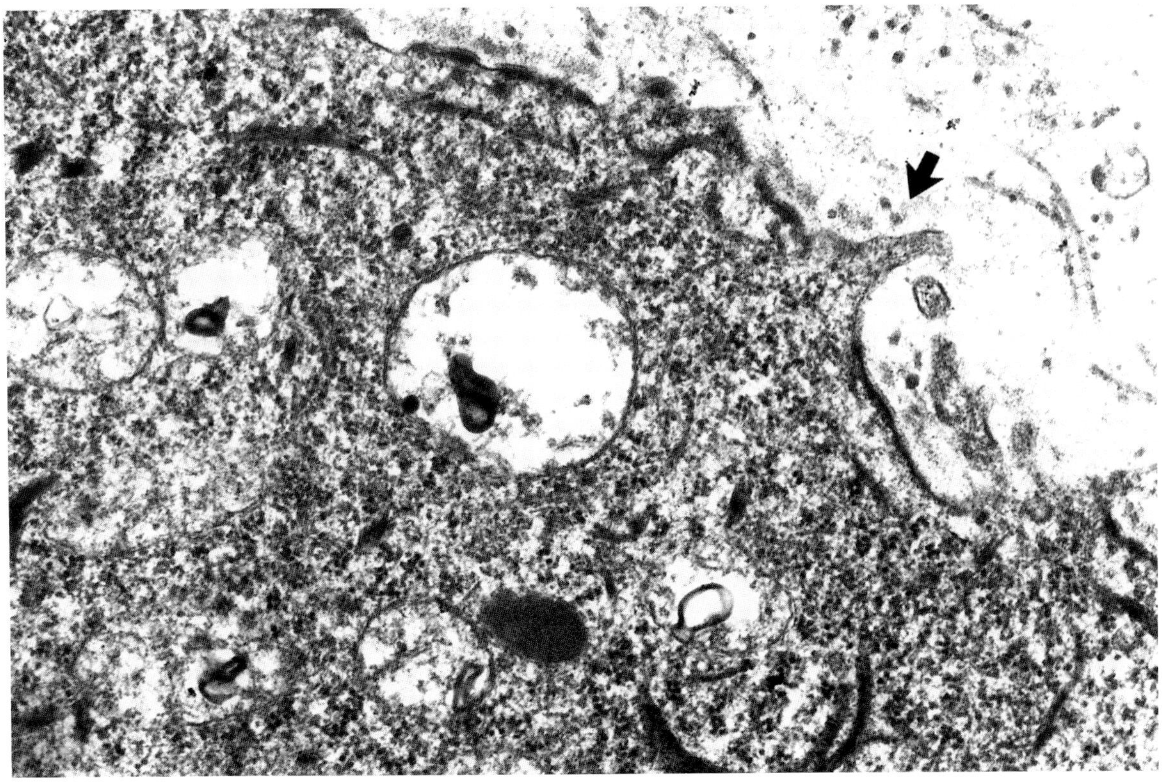

Fig. 15—Electron micrograph of an invasive well-differentiated epidermoid carcinoma lobule showing a loss of basement membrane at advancing front of infiltration (arrow). Adjacent areas have intact basement membrane structures. × 25 500

thin and continuous. It ran along the sinuosities of the cytoplasmic membrane of the tumour cells at the periphery of the lobules. However, in some places there were gaps through which small and irregular spikes of cell membrane protruded (Fig. 15). Basement membrane structures were totally absent around the tumour cell groups in the most invasive areas.

DISCUSSION

Our studies show that normal sub-epithelial and sub-endothelial basement membranes are always stained by antibodies to type IV collagen and laminin. These results are in keeping with previous studies performed on other tissues.[26–29] No study of the basement membrane antigens in laryngeal tumours has previously been reported. In this study we demonstrated a linear staining around lobules of well-differentiated squamous cell carcinomas of the larynx. Similar results have been described in tumours of the skin.[12] However, we found small gaps in the basement membrane at the periphery of carcinomatous lobules. These gaps may be related to the limited invasiveness of these well-differentiated tumours.

We observed a more or less complete loss of type IV collagen and laminin at the periphery of undifferentiated tumour lobules. The absence or decreased staining of the components of basement membranes around carcinoma lobules has been described in carcinomas of the colon and of the cervix.[11,30] Our observations are consistent with the general claim that type IV collagen and laminin disappear at the periphery of infiltrating undifferentiated tumours. We found integrity of the basement membrane in superficial areas of laryngeal carcinomas in the adjacent mucosa where the carcinomas appeared to be intra-epithelial and in some areas of epithelial dysplasia. Siegal *et al.*[9] reported in their study of human breast lesions a normal staining pattern of the basement membranes in benign and intraductal malignant epithelial tumours. The same authors[10] demonstrated alterations of the basement membrane in microinvasive lesions and a loss of these components in invasive carcinomas compared with *in situ* carcinomas. It would appear from our observations that the loss of the basement membrane is not *sine qua non* evidence of the ability of the tumour to invade the adjacent tissues since an intact basement membrane without gaps bordered some lobules of invasive well-differentiated carcinoma, while other lobules showed discontinuous staining of the basement membrane. These results corroborate previous reports concerning type IV collagen and laminin.[31–37]

Antibodies to type V collagen and fibronectin showed maximal positivity within the connective tissue between interstitial collagen bundles. In well-differentiated carcinomas these antisera stained densely but discontinuously the vicinity of the basement membrane surrounding the carcinomatous lobules. Both antigens were absent at the advancing edge of infiltrating tumours. Similar results have been observed in other solid human tumours.[11,14–16]

Our ultrastructural findings relate to our observations made by immunofluorescence staining. A basement membrane was noted at the periphery of well-differentiated carcinomas. It was discontinuous in some places where membranes of tumour cells had lost their hemidesmosomes and projected towards the surrounding connective tissue.

Tumour cells have been found to elaborate degradative enzymes of basement membranes in tissue culture.[10,38–40] *In vivo* carcinoma cells are able to migrate through basement membranes into the adjacent connective tissue and to multiply at this site establishing new carcinomatous lobules. Our observations on laryngeal carcinomas suggest that new basement membranes might appear for a while at the periphery of the new carcinomatous lobules before a later stage of local infiltration. Basement membrane loss may be related to the migratory and infiltrative properties of tumour cells. This study does not solve the problem as to whether the basement membrane loss is a primary event or secondary to tumour cell invasion of the adjacent tissues.

ACKNOWLEDGEMENTS

We are grateful to Dr R. W. Glanville of the Max Planck Institut für Biochemie (München, F.R.G.) for helpful discussion concerning the purification of collagens. We are also very thankful to Dr Y. Courtois (I.N.S.E.R.M., France) for the generous gift of laminin. We are grateful to Mrs C. Leroux, Mrs Carquin (Laboratoire d'Immunologie, C.H.U. de Reims), Mrs Menu-Guillemin and the staff of the Centre de Transfusion Sanguine de Reims for excellent technical assistance. We are also very grateful to Mr G. Boudet, Mrs N. Lefevre, C. Jeannel, B. Clement, M. Vauchelin for their excellent technical work.

REFERENCES

1. Kleinman HK, Robert JK, Martin GR. Role of collagenous matrix in the adhesion and growth of cells. *J Cell Biol* 1981; **88:** 473.
2. Graf M, Baici A, Sträuli P. Histochemical localization of cathepsin B at the invasion front of the rabbit V2 carcinoma. *Lab Invest* 1981; **45:** 587.
3. Kefalides NA, Alper R, Clarck C. Biochemistry and metabolism of basement membranes. *Int Rev Cytol* 1979; **61:** 167.
4. Timpl R, Martin GR, Bruckner P, Wick G, Wiedeman H. Nature of the collagenous protein in a tumour basement membrane. *Eur J Biochem* 1978; **84:** 43.
5. Foidart JM, Bere EW, Yaar M, *et al.* Distribution and immunoelectronmicroscopic localization of laminin, a non collagenous basement membrane glycoprotein. *Lab Invest* 1980; **42:** 336.
6. Ruoshlati E, Engvall E, Hayman EG. Fibronectin: current concepts of its structure and functions. *Collagen Rel Res* 1981; **1:** 95.
7. Martinez-Hernandez A, Amenta PS. The basement membrane in pathology. *Lab Invest* 1983; **48:** 6.
8. Warburton MJ, Mohaghan P, Ferns SA, Hughes CM, Rudland P. Distribution and synthesis of type V collagen in the rat mammary gland. *J Histochem Cytochem* 1983; **31:** 1265.
9. Siegal GP, Barsky SH, Terranova VP, Liotta LA. Stages of neoplastic transformation of human breast tissue as monitored by dissolution of basement membrane components. An immunoperoxidase study. *Invas Metastasis* 1981; **1:** 54.
10. Barsky S, Siegal GP, Jannota F, Liotta L. Loss of basement membrane components by invasive tumours but not by their benign counterparts. *Lab Invest* 1983; **49:** 140.
11. Burtin P, Chavanel G, Foidart JM, Martin E. Antigens of basement membrane and the peritumoral stroma in human colonic adenocarcinomas. Immunofluorescence study. *Int J Cancer* 1982; **30:** 13.
12. Stanley JR, Beckwith JB, Fuller RP, Katz SI. A specific antigenic defect of the basement membrane is found in basal cell carcinoma but not in other epidermal tumors. *Cancer* 1982; **50:** 1486.

13. Vaheri A, Ruoshlati E, Westermark B, Ponten J. A common cell type—specific surface antigen in cultured human glial cells and fibroblasts. Loss in malignant cells. *J Exp Med* 1976; **143:** 64.
14. Birembaut P, Gaillard D, Adnet JJ, *et al.* La fibronectine. Etude immunomorphologique de sa distribution en pathologie. *Ann Pathol* 1981; **1:** 140.
15. Labat-Robert J, Birembaut P, Robert L, Adnet JJ. Modification of fibronectin distribution pattern in solid human tumors. *Diagn Histopath* 1981; 4: 299.
16. Barsky S, Grotendorst GR, Liotta L. Increased content of type V collagen in desmoplasia of human breast cancer. *Am J Pathol* 1982; **108:** 276.
17. d'Ardenne AJ, Burns J, Sykes BC, Bennett HK. Fibronectin and type III collagen in epithelial neoplasms of gastrointestinal tract and salivary gland. *J Clin Pathol* 1983; **36:** 756.
18. Glanville RW, Rauter A, Fietzek P. Isolation and characterization of a native placental membrane collagen and its component α-chains. *Eur J Biochem* 1979; **95:** 383.
19. Bentz H, Bächinger HP, Glanville RW, Kühn K. Physical evidence for the assembly of A and B chains of human placental collagen in a single triple helix. *Eur J Biochem* 1978; **92:** 563.
20. Madri JA, Foellmer HG, Furthmayr H. Type V Collagens of the human placenta: trimer α-chain composition, ultrastructural morphology and peptide analysis. *Collagen Rel Res* 1982; **2:** 19.
21. Fujii T, Kühn K. Isolation and characterization of pepsin-treated type III collagen from calf skin. *Hoppe Seyler's J Physiol Chem* 1975; **356:** 1793.
22. Laurain G, Delvincourt T, Szymanowicz A. Isolation of a macromolecular collagenous fraction and AB_2 collagen from calf skin. *FEBS Lett* 1980; **120:** 44.
23. Wick G, Glanville RW, Timpl R. Characterization of antibodies to basement membrane (type IV) collagen in immunohistochemical studies. *Immunobiol* 1979; **156:** 372.
24. Rennard SI, Berg R, Martin GR, Foidart JM, Gehron-Robey R. Enzyme-linked immunoassay (ELISA) for connective tissue components. *Anal Biochem* 1980; **104:** 205.
25. Merker JH, Barrach HJ. The morphology of basement membrane formation. *Eur J Cell Biol* 1981; **26:** 111.
26. Laurie GW, Leblond CP, Cournil P, Martin GR. Immunohistochemical evidence for the intra-cellular formation of basement membrane collagen in developing tissues. *J Histochem Cytochem* 1980; **28:** 1267.
27. Roll FJ, Madri JA, Albert J, Furthmayr J. Co-distribution of collagen types IV and AB_2 in basement membranes and mesangium of the kidney. An immuno-ferritin study of ultrathin frozen sections. *J Cell Biol* 1980; **85:** 597.
28. Konomi H, Hori H, Sano J, *et al.* Immunohistochemical localization of type I, II, III and IV collagens in the lung. *Acta Pathol Japn* 1981; **31:** 601.
29. Sano J, Sato S, Ishizaki M, *et al.* Types I, III and IV (basement membrane) collagens in the bovine liver parenchyma: electron microscopic localization by peroxidase labelled antibody method. *Biomed Res* 1981; **2:** 546.
30. Birembaut P, Caron Y, Van Cauwenberg D, Foidart JM. Distribution of laminin, a basement membrane glycoprotein in epithelial proliferations. *Collagen Rel Res* 1983; **3:** 25.
31. Stenman S, Vaheri A. Distribution of a major connective tissue protein, fibronectin, in normal human tissues. *J Exp Med* 1978; **147:** 1054.
32. Kurkinen M, Vaheri A, Roberts P, Stenman S. Sequential appearance of fibronectin and collagen in experimental granulation tissue. *Lab Invest* 1980; **43:** 47.
33. Gay S, Martinez-Hernandez A, Rhodes RK, Miller EJ. The collagenous exocytoskeleton of smooth muscle cells. *Collagen Rel Res* 1981; **1:** 377.
34. Silver MH, Foidart JM, Pratt RM. Distribution of fibronectin and collagen during mouse limb and palate development. *Differentiation* 1981; **18:** 141.
35. Martinez-Hernandez A, Gay S, Miller E. Ultrastructural localization of type V collagen in rat kidney. *J Cell Biol* 1982; **92:** 343.
36. d'Ardenne AJ, Burns J, Sykes BC, Kirkpatrick, P. Comparative distribution of fibronectin and type III collagen in normal human tissues. *J Pathol* 1983; **141:** 55.
37. Cam Y, Bellow G, Poulin G, Caron Y, Birembaut P. Distribution of type IV collagen in benign and malignant epithelial proliferations. An indirect immunofluorescence study on the breasts, the lungs and the skin. *Invas Metastasis*, in press.
38. Liotta L, Kleinerman J, Catanzaro P, Rynbrandt D. Degradation of basement membrane by murine tumor cells. *J Natl Cancer Inst* 1977; **58:** 1427.
39. Liotta LA, Abe S, Robey GP, Martin GR. Preferential digestion of basement membrane collagen by an enzyme derived from a metastatic murine tumor. *Proc Natl Acad Sci USA* 1979; **76:** 2268.
40. O'Grady RL, Upfold LI, Stephens RW. Rat mammary carcinoma cells secrete active collagenase and activate latent enzyme in the stroma via plasminogen activator. *Int J Cancer* 1981; **50**: 509.

JOURNAL OF PATHOLOGY, VOL. **144**: 45–55 (1984)

FERRITIN DEPOSITION IN THE GLOMERULAR DEPOSITS OF FOCAL GLOMERULAR SCLEROSIS IN THE RAT

CELINE MELCION

Institut National de la Sante et de la Recherche Medicale, Hôspital Tenon, Paris, France

AND

JENNIFER SMITH AND VICTORIA CATTELL

Department of Experimental Pathology, St. Mary's Hospital Medical School, London, U.K.

Received 30 September 1983
Accepted 27 April 1984

SUMMARY

The glomerular lesions of focal sclerosis clinically associated with a steroid-resistant nephrotic syndrome, are of unknown origin. IgM and C3 deposits and electron dense material found in areas of sclerosis are not convincing evidence of an immune pathogenesis. These deposits have been studied in a rat model of focal sclerosis induced by uninephrectomy and repeated aminonucleoside administration. Sclerotic lesions closely resembling human disease developed in the remaining kidney. There was a severe progressive proteinuria. Seventy-eight days after initial aminonucleoside injection 65 per cent of glomeruli were sclerotic with IgM, IgG, C3 and fibrinogen deposits, and electron dense deposits by electron microscopy. To study macromolecule deposition in this model of focal sclerosis, ferritin uptake 4 and 24 h after intravenous ferritin given at 77 days was compared in focal sclerosis rats with control rats without sclerosis (uninephrectomy plus saline-only injections). In focal sclerosis rats sclerotic areas contained massive accumulations of ferritin. In unaffected segments of sclerotic glomeruli, and normal glomeruli of focal sclerosis rats, ferritin concentration was no different from controls. Abnormal ferritin trapping in areas of sclerosis suggests that the presence of IgM and C3 may be due to a similar mechanism, and is not indicative of an immune pathogenesis for focal sclerosis.

KEY WORDS—Aminonucleoside, mesangium, ferritin, glomerulonephritis, focal glomerular sclerosis.

INTRODUCTION

The glomerular lesions of focal glomerular sclerosis (FGS), clinically associated with a steroid-resistant nephrotic syndrome, are of unknown pathogenesis.[1] Although by immunofluorescence IgM and C3 are detectable in the sclerotic glomerular segments, and electron dense deposits are found in the same areas by electron microscopy, there is no convincing evidence that the lesions or the deposits are due to an immune reaction.

Sclerotic lesions, similar in appearance to human FGS have been studied in experimental animals using models of spontaneous sclerosis in aging rats,[2,3] sclerosis produced by removal of renal tissue[4] and chronic aminonucleoside (AMNS) administration.[5] In some of these models, there are 'deposits' similar to those of human FGS[2,3] which have been assumed to be of immunological origin. In one model described in the rat, where uninephrectomy was performed during a course of AMNS[6], increased glomerular uptake and persistence of intravenously administered human aggregated IgG was demonstrated.[7]

In the experiments reported here, the glomerular localization of intravenous ferritin in the above AMNS-nephrectomy model of FGS has been studied by electron microscopy. The aims were to study further the ultrastructure of glomerular sclerosis and the macromolecular uptake in FGS, to investigate the mechanisms involved in the formation of glomerular deposits.

0022–3417/84/090045–11$01.10

METHOD

Animals

Sprague-Dawley rats weighing 100 g at the start of the experiment were used.

Chemicals

Aminonucleoside of puromycin (Sigma) was dissolved in phosphate buffered saline to a concentration of 130 mg/ml before injection.

Ferritin—native horse Ferritin (Type I, Sigma Chemical Company Ltd., London)—concentration 100 mg/ml, was dialysed before injection as previously described.[8]

Surgical procedures

Intravenous injections were given by dorsal penile vein under ether anaesthesia. Renal biopsies and nephrectomies were performed as previously described.[9]

Processing of tissues

Tissues for light microscopy were fixed in alcoholic Dubosq's Brazil (modified Bouin's solution), processed by standard histological methods, and sections stained with haematoxylin and eosin, periodic acid–Schiff reagent, and Perls' potassium ferrocyanide method for iron (Perls' Prussian blue reaction). Tissues for immunofluorescence were snap-frozen in liquid nitrogen, cut and examined with the following rabbit anti-rat fluorescein-labelled antisera: anti-IgG, anti-IgM, anti-C3 and anti-fibrinogen. Tissues for electron microscopy were fixed, processed, cut and examined as previously described.[9]

Urinary proteins—These were determined by the sulphosalicylic acid precipitation method. Twenty-four-hour urine samples were collected at the start of the experiment, before nephrectomy, and on three subsequent occasions before the animals were killed.

Experimental protocol

There were three experimental groups: (I) aminonucleoside-nephrectomy (AMNS-N) group (15 rats), (II) aminonucleoside-nephrectomy-ferritin (AMNS-N-Fer) group (4 rats) and (III) control-nephrectomy-ferritin (control-N-Fer) group (2 rats).

The experimental protocol for the induction of glomerular sclerosis was a modification of the model previously described by Glass *et al.* in 1977.[6] Briefly, group I and group II rats were given an initial intraperitoneal injection of aminonucleoside 13 mg/100 g body weight, uninephrectomized 22 days later, and sacrificed at 78 days after three further injections of aminonucleoside 4 mg/100 g body weight on days 27, 32 and 39. Group III rats received saline injections only and were nephrectomized as in the other two groups.

Rats for ferritin experiments (groups II and III) received a single dose of intravenous ferritin 100 mg/100 g body weight on day 77. Renal biopsies were performed on the same day, 4 h after ferritin, and kidneys removed at time of death on day 78, 24 h after ferritin.

Glomerular sclerosis was recognized by light microscopy whilst glomerular ferritin deposition was assessed as heavy, light or absent from Perls'-stained sections.

RESULTS

Survival

Twenty out of 21 rats survived. The one animal which did not survive was in group I (AMNS-N). In groups I and II there were gross ascites and interstitial oedema at the time of death. Group III rats appeared normal.

Urinary protein

In AMNS-N rats the mean urinary protein rose from 5 mg/24 h at the start of the experiment to 65 mg/24 h (standard error 5·6) after nephrectomy, and finally to 670 mg/24 h (standard error 82). In control rats the mean urinary protein rose to 15 mg/24 h (standard error 3) after nephrectomy.

Renal pathology

At time of death on day 78, the single kidneys in AMNS-group and AMNS-N-Fer rats were enlarged. The cortical width was reduced, and the surfaces finely granular. Kidneys of control-N-Fer rats were enlarged but otherwise normal.

Morphology—

Aminonucleoside-nephrectomy group (group I)

Light microscopy—In this group the mean incidence of glomeruli with sclerotic lesions was 65 per cent (range 57–65 per cent). Sclerotic glomeruli were no more frequent in the juxtamedullary zone. Sclerosis was either global or segmental with appearances as previously described.[6] The remaining glomeruli appeared normal or had only a slight increase in the number of mesangial cells. There were alternating areas of small atrophic tubules, hyperplastic tubules and normal tubules, many containing homogenous eosinophilic casts, and surrounding interstitial fibrosis with some mononuclear cell infiltrates. There were no significant vascular lesions. By immunofluorescence large deposits of IgG, IgM, C3 and fibrinogen were seen in sclerotic areas whilst non-sclerosed glomeruli were negative.

Electron microscopy—Figure 1 shows the essential features of the fully developed lesion of hyalinosis and sclerosis. The overlying capsule was thickened and in Bowman's space (between capillary loops and the capsule) there were collagen fibres and wavy strands of electron dense material resembling the basket-weave of basement membranes in Alport's syndrome. Visceral epithelial cells were either absent, leaving bare areas of basement membrane, or showed extensive degenerative changes. The basement membranes were thinned and stretched over large granular subendothelial deposits. The lumina were reduced or obliterated. In patent lumina the plasma appeared denser than normal. Residual endothelium was swollen, with loss of fenestrations. The mesangial cells were reduced in number and the mesangial matrix increased with occasional collagen fibres and electron dense deposits. In non-sclerotic glomeruli and non-sclerosed segments of affected glomeruli there was partial epithelial foot process obliteration and epithelial cells contained some dense droplets. There was also a slight segmental increase in mesangial cells and mesangial matrix.

Ferritin localization—All animals in groups II and III were biopsied at 4 h and killed at 24 h after intravenous ferritin. The numbers of sclerotic glomeruli in these groups and the deposition of ferritin at 4 and 24 h after intravenous injection is summarized (Table I).

Aminonucleoside-nephrectomy-ferritin group (group II)

Light microscopy—Appearances were as described in group I. In 4 h biopsies between 13 and

Table I—Incidence of glomerular sclerosis and glomerular distribution of intravenous ferritin in control and aminonucleoside-treated rats

Group	Rat	Sclerosis %	Glomerular ferritin distribution (%) Heavy*	Light†	Absent
Aminonucleoside-nephrectomy-ferritin rats (group II)					
4 h after ferritin	1	91 (21)	89	11	0
(biopsy)	2	78 (18)	70	20	10
	3	61 (33)	39	46	15
	4	46 (13‡)	18	9	73
24 h after ferritin	1	81	74	10	16
(nephrectomy)	2	82	87	13	0
	3	92	66	19	15
	4	80	5	95	0
Control-nephrectomy-ferritin rats (group III)					
4 h after ferritin	1	4 (25)	11	61	28
(biopsy)	2	0 (28)	0	12	88
24 h after ferritin	1	3	1	73	26
(nephrectomy)	2	5	0	77	23

* Heavy—large segmental deposits.
† Light—scattered mesangial granules.
‡ Rat with minor segmental lesions.
Numbers in parentheses indicate number of glomeruli available in biopsy.

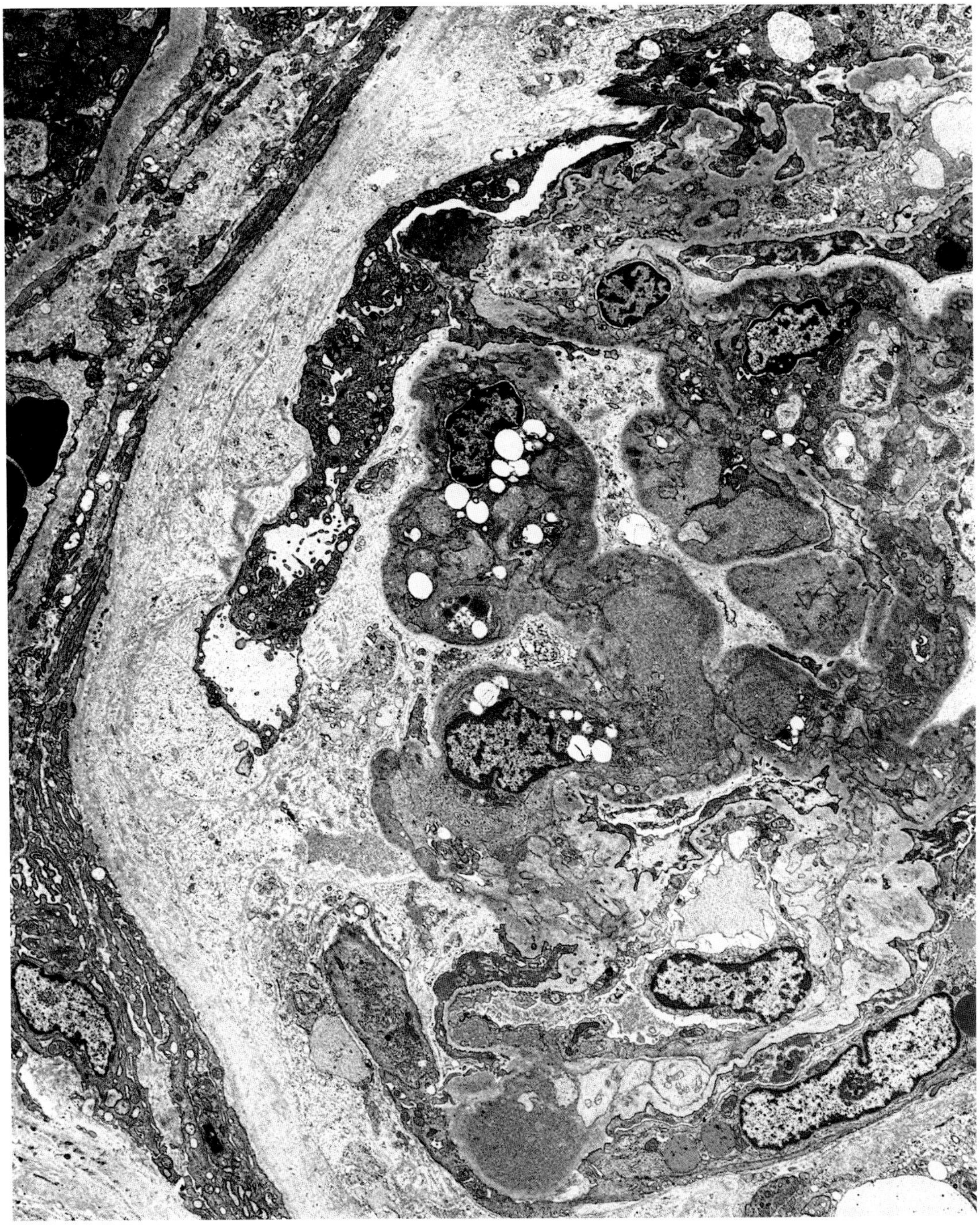

Fig. 1—Low power electron micrograph of segmental glomerular sclerosis at 78 days, in group I (AMNS-N) rat. There is loss of epithelial cells, a large capsular adhesion, and multiple electron dense subendothelial deposits. ×2960

33 glomeruli were available per biopsy. Nephrectomy specimens at 24 h showed a mean incidence of 83·8 per cent sclerosis. Greatly increased amounts of ferritin, easily identifiable in haematoxylin and eosin stained sections as brown material were seen in areas of glomerular sclerosis at 4 and 24 h. Perls' stain showed enormous subendothelial masses of ferritin (Fig. 2a) compared with control animals (Fig. 2b). The mean number of glomeruli with heavy deposits was 58 per cent at 24 h. In unaffected areas of sclerotic glomerili, and in normal glomeruli, there was either a light scattering of ferritin positive granules in the mesangium, up to five heavily laden cells per glomerulus (monocytes), or no ferritin. At 24 h some lacis areas contained ferritin. Ferritin was seen in proximal tubular cells, some peritubular capillary endothelia and interstitial cells.

Electron microscopy—Figure 3(a) shows an area of segmental sclerosis in the glomerulus of an animal *4 h* after receiving intravenous ferritin. The large subendothelial electron dense deposits contained very large numbers of ferritin particles (Fig. 3b). The lamina densa did not have ferritin particles, although ferritin was identified in many of the remaining visceral epithelial cells and in the urinary space. Ferritin was present in vacuoles of cells in the mesangium and in massive amounts within the mesangial matrix (Fig. 3c). The amounts of ferritin in sclerotic mesangial regions were much more than in normal mesangial regions, which appeared no different from the mesangium of control-N-Fer (group III) rats (Fig. 4). Capillary lumina contained ferritin particles in greater concentration in sclerotic glomeruli than unaffected glomeruli or glomeruli of control-N-Fer group rats. In some lumina monocytes were seen as previously described after intravenous ferritin adminstration.[8] There were also strands of intraluminal fibrin, an increased number of circulating platelets, and some polymorphs. From 4 to 24 h the amounts of ferritin in subendothelial dense deposits increased. Mesangial cells and mesangial matrix in sclerotic glomeruli also contained more ferritin than at 4 h (Fig. 5, 6). Some ferritin particles were still present in the lumina of sclerotic glomeruli. In non-sclerotic glomeruli the amount of ferritin in mesangial cells and matrix was less and was comparable to that in

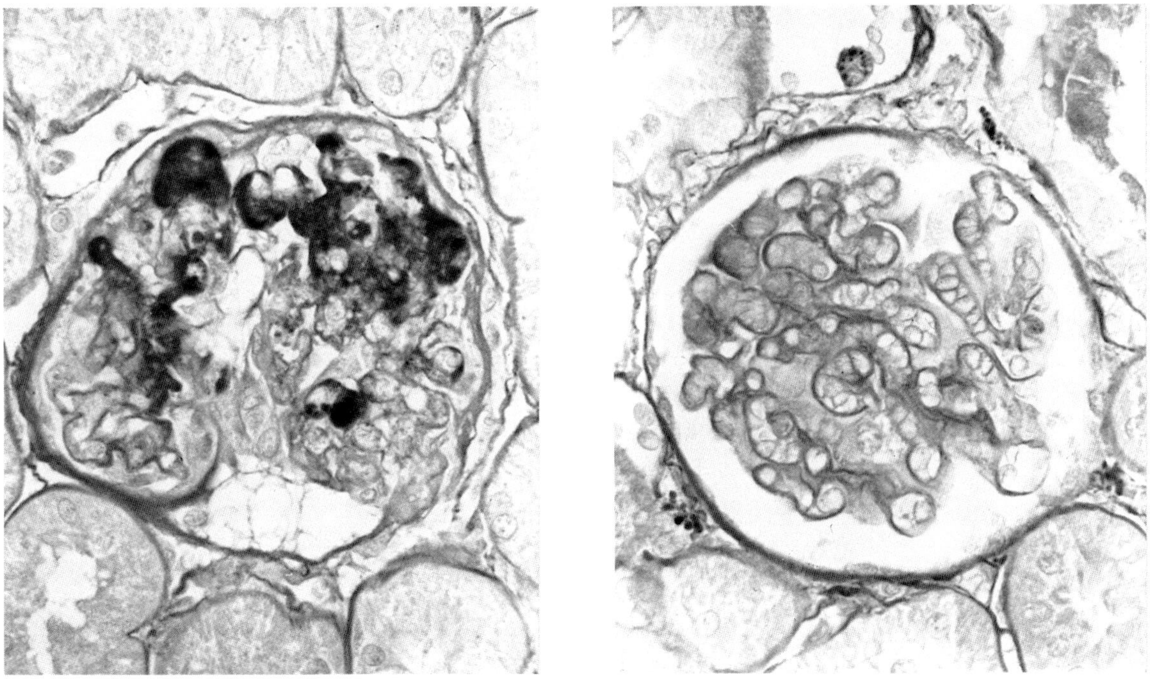

(a) (b)

Fig. 2—Glomeruli 24 h after intravenous ferritin (Perls' stain). (a) Group II (AMNS-N-Fer) rat with massive ferritin accumulation in sclerotic areas. (b) Group III (control-N-Fer) rat with no detectable ferritin in glomerulus, but three ferritin-carrying cells in the interstitium and one in a small blood vessel

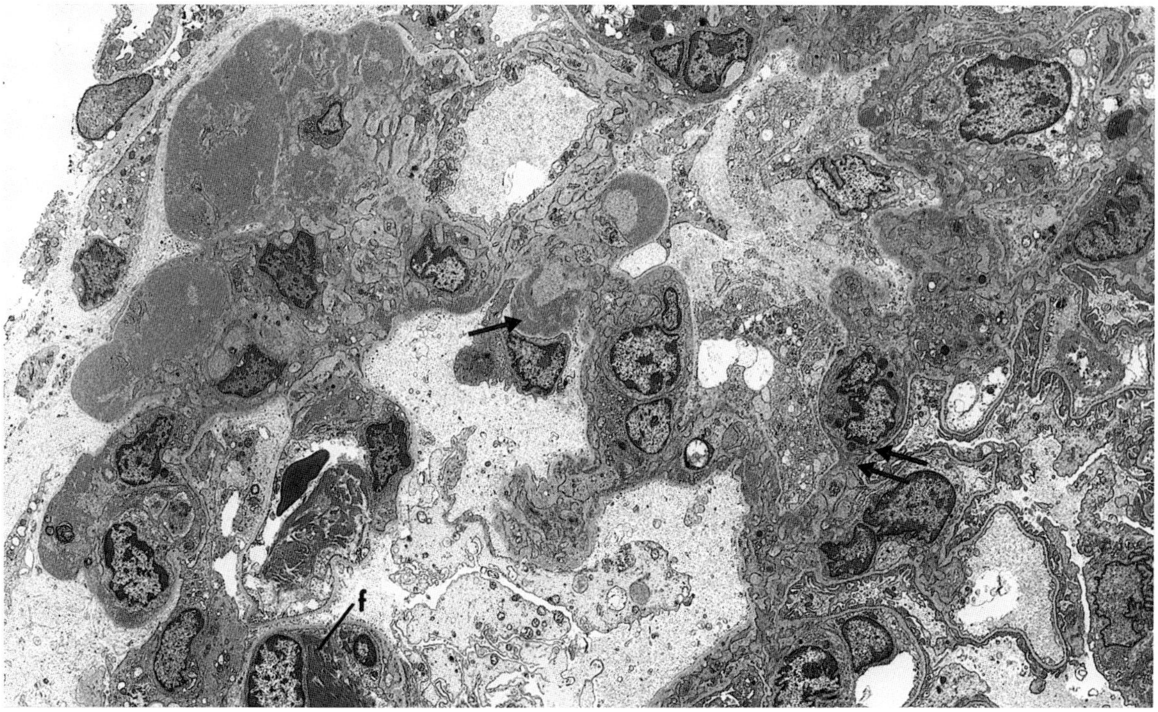

Fig. 3a—Segmental glomerular sclerosis in group II (AMNS-N-Fer) rat 4 h after intravenous ferritin. Ferritin is present in subendothelial deposits, (single arrow). There are intraluminal fibrin deposits (f)

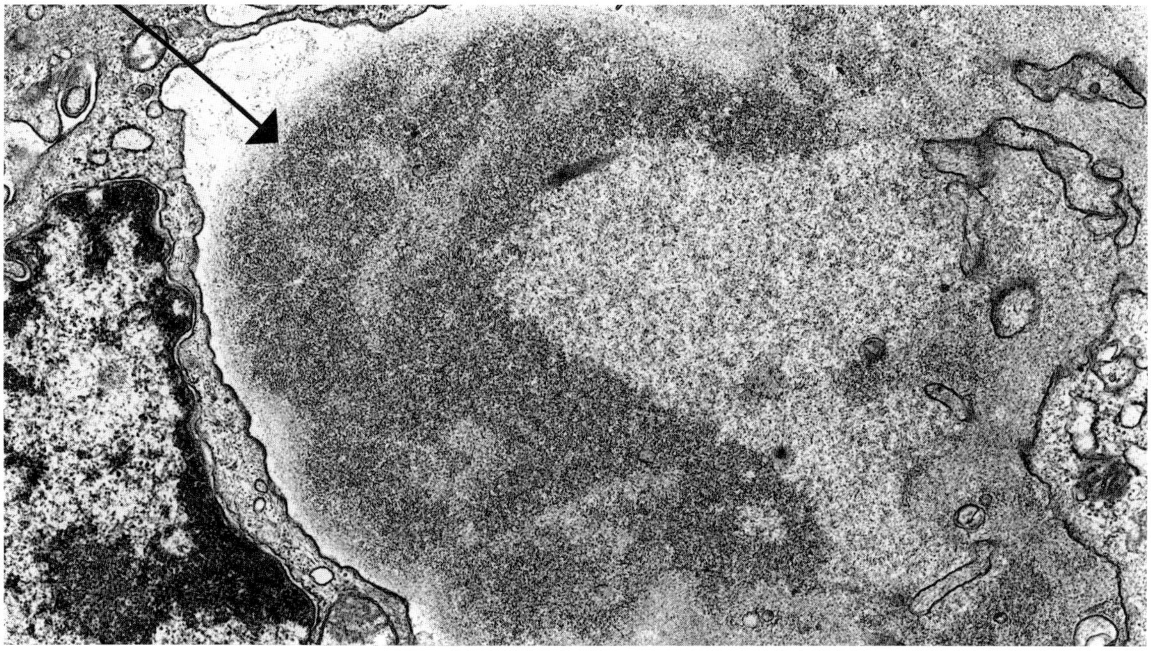

Fig. 3b—Segmental glomerular sclerosis in group II (AMNS-N-Fer) rat 4 h after intravenous ferritin. Ferritin is present in subendothelial deposits (single arrow) × 20 900

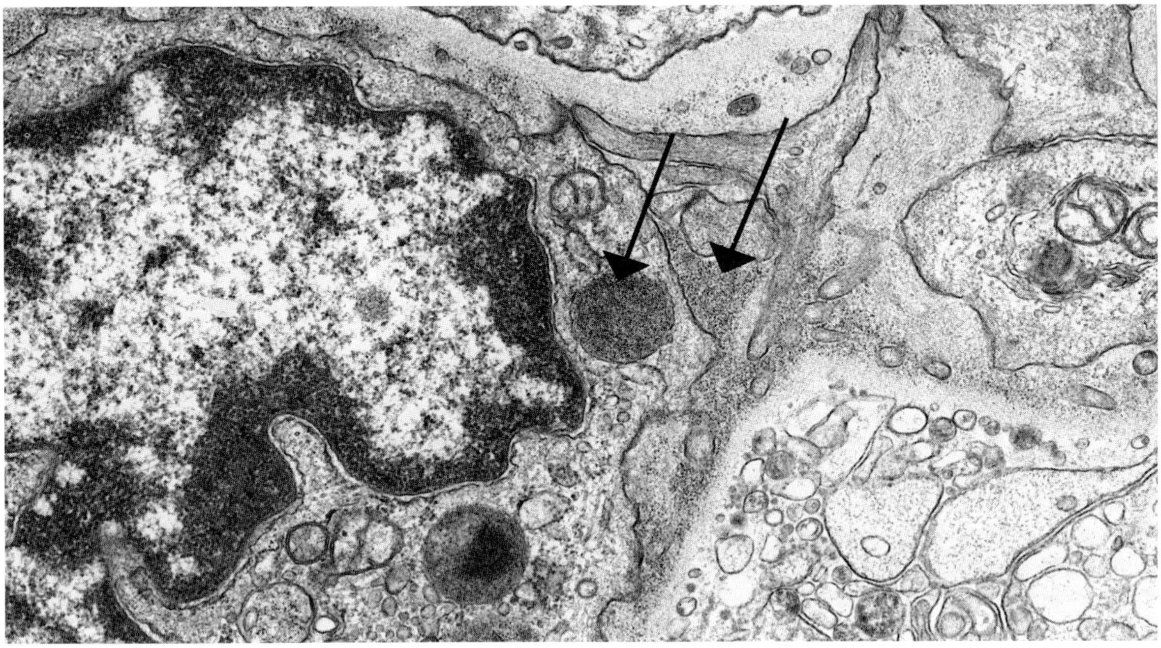

Fig. 3c—Segmental glomerular sclerosis in group II (AMNS-N-Fer) rat 4 h after intravenous ferritin. Ferritin is present in subendothelial deposits and in adjacent mesangium (double arrows) × 22 800

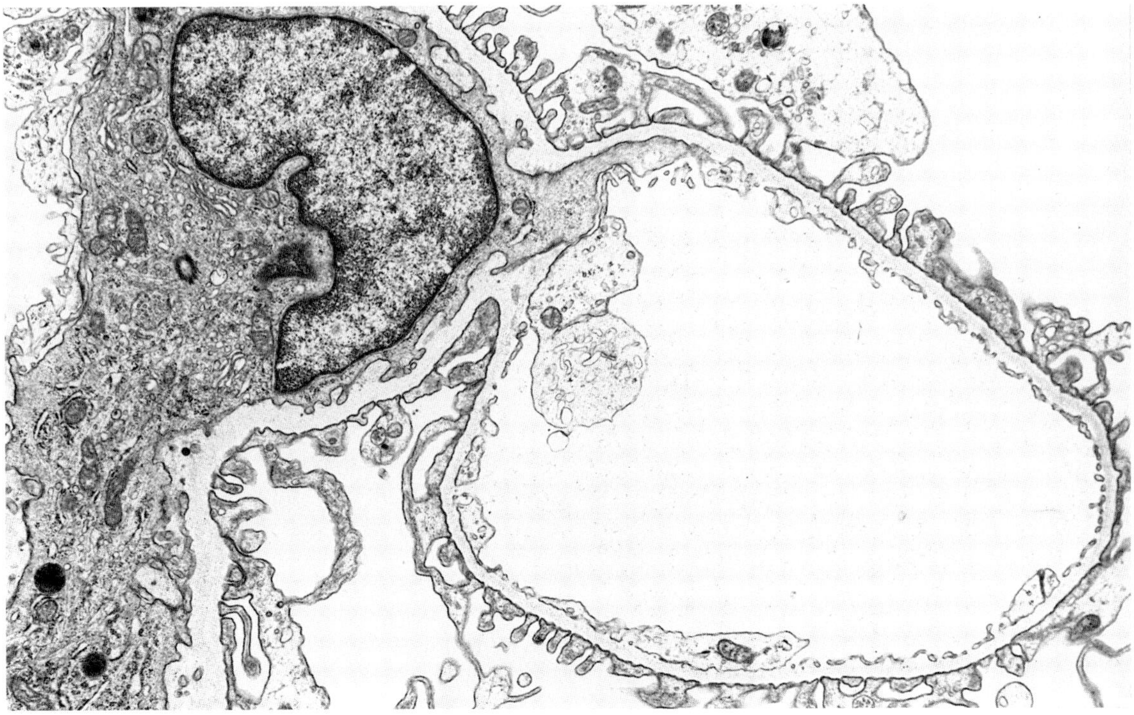

Fig. 4—Electron micrograph of mesangium and capillaries in group II (AMNS-N-Fer) rat 4 h after intravenous ferritin. In this area without sclerosis ferritin particles are scanty. Note the normal capillary walls and discrete epithelial cell foot processes. The appearances are similar to control-N-Fer rats (see Fig. 7). × 10 070

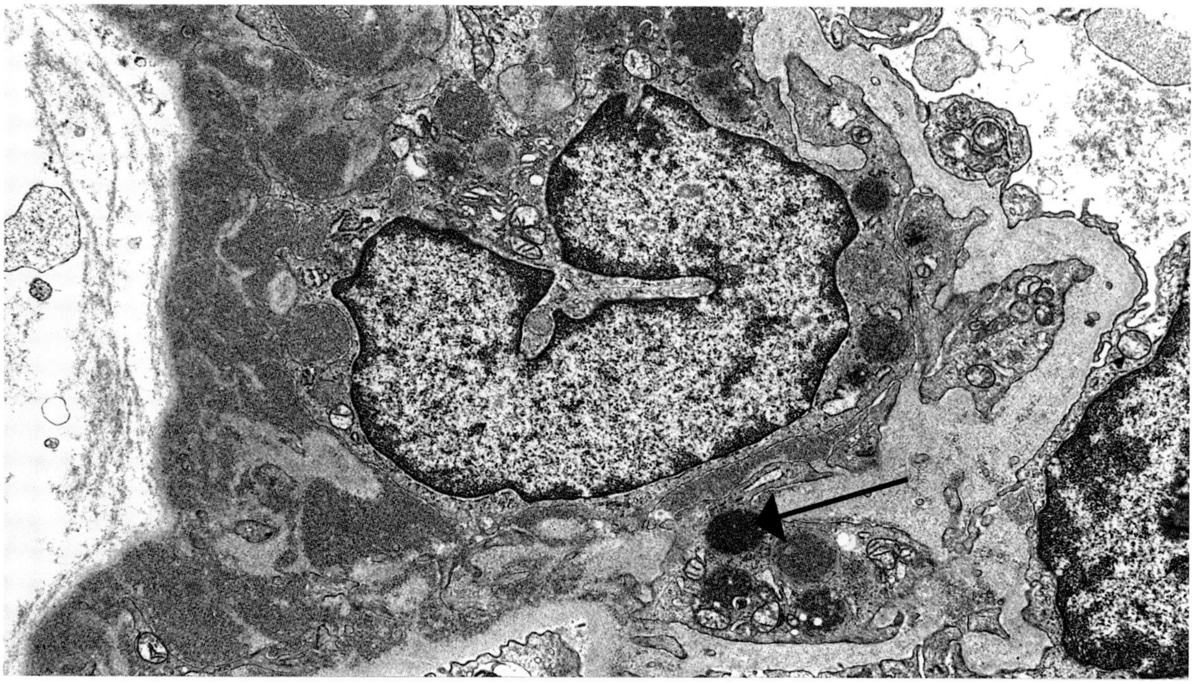

Fig. 5—Electron micrograph of mesangium of a group II (AMNS-N-Fer) rat 24 h after intravenous ferritin. Large dense masses of ferritin persist in cells, matrix and vacuoles (arrow). × 8900

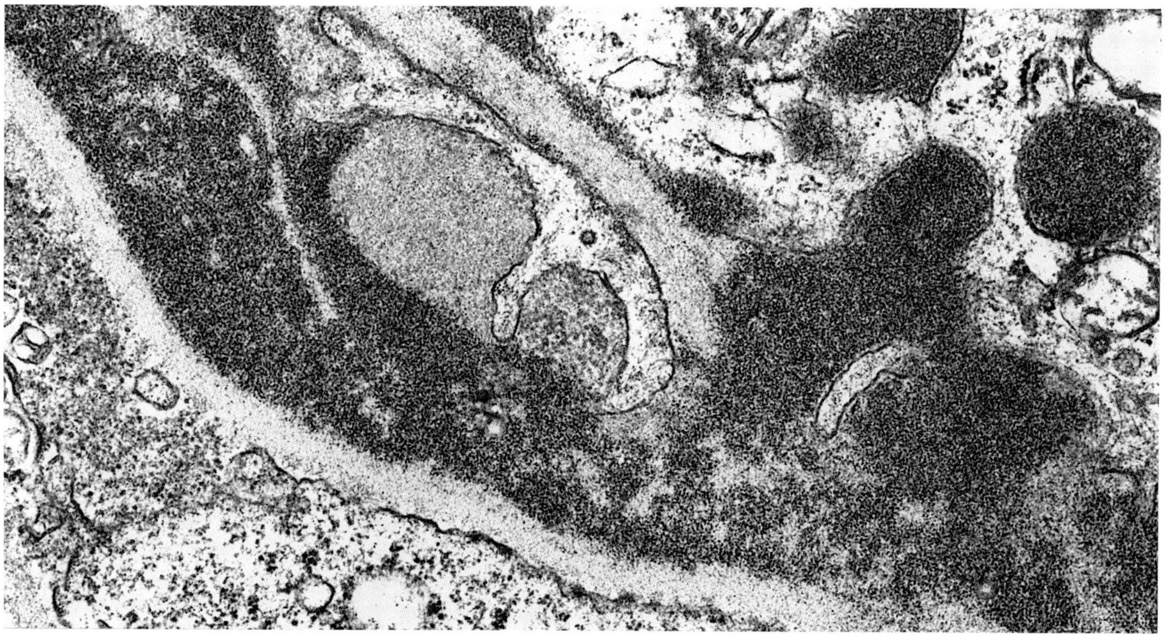

Fig. 6—Higher power electron micrograph of part of a mesangial cell and adjacent matrix from a group II (AMNS-N-Fer) rat 24 h after intravenous ferritin. Masses of ferritin particles in matrix and cell vacuoles. × 30400

control-N-Fer (group III) rats.

Control-nephrectomy-ferritin group (group III)

Light microscopy—The majority of glomeruli were normal. Up to 5 per cent glomerular sclerosis was seen, by counting large numbers of glomeruli, in the 24 h nephrectomy specimens (Table I). In contrast to group II animals, ferritin was not readily detectable in haematoxylin and eosin-stained sections. With Perls' stain up to 77 per cent (mean at 24 h—75 per cent) of glomeruli showed light mesangial staining but ferritin was undetectable in the remainder, except in one animal with heavy staining of 11 per cent of glomeruli (see Fig. 2b). Ferritin was seen in proximal tubular cells, some peritubular capillaries and some interstitial cells. No vascular lesions were seen. By immunofluorescence there were trace amounts of mesangial IgG and fibrinogen, but no IgM or C3.

Electron microscopy—At 4 h some free ferritin particles, monocytes and occasional neutrophils, were present in capillary lumina. No fibrin or platelets were seen. There was no ferritin in lamina densa or visceral epithelial cells. Ferritin was rarely seen in the subendothelium. Ferritin was present in some areas of the mesangial matrix, and in smaller amounts in mesangial cells (Fig. 7). At 24 h ferritin was rarely seen in lumina or subendothelium. As in group II rats the number of monocytes had increased from 4 h. Ferritin appeared degraded in phagosomes as in group II rats. Ferritin was present in increased amounts in cells of the mesangium compared with 4 h, but was less than in group II rats at either 4 or 24 h. There was very little ferritin left in the mesangial matrix.

DISCUSSION

In the rat, as previously described,[6] chronic aminonucleoside administration with uninephrectomy causes chronic proteinuria and lesions closely resembling human focal glomerular sclerosis. As in the human lesions there is IgM and C3 deposition in sclerotic areas. Velosa *et al.*[7] have previously shown by immunofluorescence increased glomerular deposits of intravenously administered aggregated human IgG in this model. Our results, using ferritin, extend this observation to an ultrastructural level, using a different macromolecule and show further that the exact site of abnormal

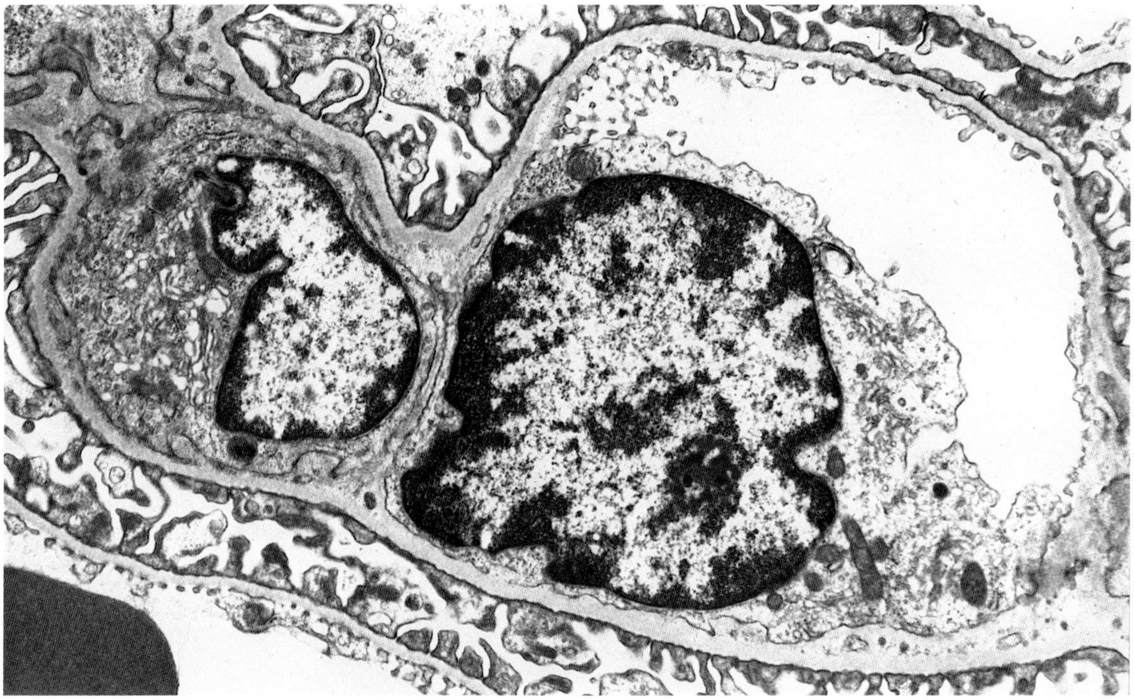

Fig. 7—Electron micrograph of mesangium and capillary in group III (control-N-Fer) rat 4 h after intravenous ferritin. Ferritin particles are scanty compared with Fig. 3c. × 10070

deposition is confined to the sclerotic segments of damaged glomeruli. Excessive ferritin was not seen in normal glomeruli or normal areas of sclerotic glomeruli in these FGS rats; in these sites it was no different from control uninephrectomized rats.

Uptake at 4 h after intravenous ferritin in scarred areas was enormously increased, suggesting abnormal haemodynamics and permeability in these areas. At 24 h after intravenous ferritin (when ferritin in controls had almost disappeared from the mesangial matrix) there were persisting masses of ferritin in sclerotic loops, which probably represent delayed removal. The similar distribution of immunoglobulins and C3 is also likely to occur due to similar mechanisms, as is the more global trapping seen in end-stage kidneys.[10]

There are several other observations from this ultrastructural study. The first is that many of the visceral epithelial cells were normal in non-sclerotic areas (Fig. 4). Previously it has been noted that polyanion loss is confined to sclerotic segments,[7] a supporting observation. Acute epithelial cell injury is a well recognized effect of acute AMNS administration,[11–13] and these findings suggest a capacity of epithelial cells to recover. Epithelial cell damage has been reported in other models of FGS occurring spontaneously[3] or following removal of functioning renal mass[4] whilst the role of chronic proteinuria remains controversial. It may be that irreversible segmental epithelial cell damage is one of the factors leading to sclerosis.

A mild increase in mesangial cells was seen in non-sclerotic areas in FGS rats, a change now recognized by morphometry and electron microscopy in some cases of human minimal change glomerular disease and in FGS.[14,15] In these areas no Ig or C3 deposition, or ultrastructural deposits were found, and there was no increased ferritin uptake. The stimulus to mesangial cell increase is, therefore, not apparent. It is possible that there is a more generalized but transient increase in macromolecule deposition following each AMNS injection, as has been well-documented after acute AMNS administration, [16–20] which is sufficient to cause persisting mesangial proliferation.

Increased plasma density was noted in abnormal loops. It is possible that this appearance indicates local haemoconcentration. This would support haemodynamic changes as contributory factors in the development of sclerosis.[21]

Finally, fibrin deposition was found in FGS rats but not in control animals. Fibrin-related-antigen has been noted previously by immunofluorescence in this model[7] and abnormal coagulation and platelet consumption[12] have been reported in human FGS.[22,23] Local endothelial trauma causing segmental thrombosis may play a role in the development of segmental scarring.

In conclusion, this study confirms that the model of AMNS plus nephrectomy closely resembles human FGS. Although the role of deposits of macromolecules in the evolution of sclerosis was not studied, this ultrastructure tracer experiment shows that once sclerosis has developed macromolecules which had no part in the formation of the initial lesions, can be trapped in areas of sclerosis.

REFERENCES

1. Cameron JS. The problem of focal segmental glomerulosclerosis. In: Kincaid-Smith, P, D'Aprice AJF, Atkins RC, eds. Progress in Glomerulonephritis. New York: Wiley Medical Publication, 1979: 209–229.
2. Couser WG, Stilmant MM. Mesangial lesions and focal glomerular sclerosis in the aging rat. *Lab Invest* 1975; **33:** 491–501.
3. Elema JD, Arends A. Focal and segmental glomerular hyalinosis and sclerosis in the rat. *Lab Invest* 1975; **33:** 554–561.
4. Shimamura T, Morrison AB. A progressive glomerulosclerosis occurring in partial five-sixths nephrectomized rats. *Am J Path* 1975; **79:** 95–101.
5. Saito T, Furuyama T, Kyogoku Y, Yamakage K, Arakawa M, Yoshinaga K. Focal glomerular sclerosis in aminonucleoside nephropathy. *J Exp Med* 1981; **133:** 349–360.
6. Glasser RJ, Velosa JA, Michael AF. Experimental model of focal sclerosis. Relationship to protein excretion in aminonucleoside nephrosis. *Lab Invest* 1977; **36:** 519–525.
7. Velosa JA, Glasser RJ, Nevins TE, Michael AF. Experimental model of focal sclerosis. II. Correlation with immunopathological changes, macromolecular kinetics and polyanion loss. *Lab Invest* 1977; **36:** 527–534.
8. Cattell V, Gaskin de Urdaneta A, Arlidge S, Collar JE, Roberts A, Smith J. Uptake and clearance of ferritin by the glomerular mesangium. 1. Phagocytosis by mesangial cells and blood monocytes. *Lab Invest* 1982; **47:** 296–303.
9. Bradfield JWB, Cattell V, Smith J. The mesangial cell in glomerulonephritis. II. Mesangial proliferation caused by Habu snake venom in the rat. *Lab Invest* 1977; **36:** 487–492.
10. Velosa JA, Miller K, Michael AF. Immunopathology

of the end-stage kidney. *Am J Path* 1976; **84:** 149–160.

11. Bretton R, Rouchon M, Bariety J. Podocytes in aminonucleoside glomerulonephritis investigated ultrastructurally with concanavalin A. *J Histochem Cytochem* 1979; **27:** 1588–1595.
12. Caulfield JP, Reid JJ, Farquhar MG. Alterations of the glomerular epithelium in acute aminonucleoside nephrosis. Evidence for formation of occluding functions and epithelial cell detachment. *Lab Invest* 1976; **34:** 43–59.
13. Nevins TE, Basgen J, Gaston T. Quantitative indices of aminonucleoside-induced nephrotic syndrome. *Kidney Internat* 1983; **23:** 188 (Abstr).
14. Schoeneman MJ, Bennett B, Greifer I. The natural history of focal segmental glomerulosclerosis with and without mesangial hypercellularity in children. *Clin Nephrol* 1978; **9:** 45–54.
15. Waldherr K, Gubler MC, Levy M, Broyer M, Habib R. The significance of pure diffuse mesangial proliferation in idiopathic nephrotic syndrome. *Clin Nephrol* 1978; **10:** 171–179.
16. Couser WG, Jermanovich NB, Belok S, Stilmant MM. Effect of aminonucleoside nephrosis on immune complex localization in autologous immune complex nephropathy in rats. *J Clin Invest* 1978; **61:** 561–572.
17. Farquhar MG, Palade GE. Glomerular permeability. II. Ferritin transfer across the glomerular capillary wall in nephrotic rats. *J Exp Med* 1961; **114:** 699–715.
18. Grond J, Elema JD. Glomerular mesangium. Analysis of the increased activity observed in experimental acute aminonucleoside nephrosis in the rat. *Lab Invest* 1981; **45:** 400–409.
19. Hoyer JR, Mauer SM, Michael AF. Unilateral renal disease in the rat. I. Clinical, morphologic and glomerular mesangial functional features of the experimental model produced by renal perfusion with aminonucleoside. *J Lab Clin Med* 1975; **85:** 756–768.
20. Seiler MW, Hoyer JR, Kreuger TE. Altered localization of protamine–heparin complexes in aminonucleoside nephrosis. *Lab Invest* 1980; **43:** 9–17.
21. Brenner BM, Meyer TW, Hostetter TH. Dietary protein intake and the progressive nature of kidney disease: the role of hemodynamically mediated glomeruler injury in the pathogenesis of progressive glomeruler sclerosis in aging, renal ablation, and intrinsic renal disease. *N Engl J Med* 1982; **307:** 652–659.
22. Futrakul P, Poshyachinda M, Mitrakul C. Focal sclerosing glomerulonephritis: a kinetic evaluation of hemostasis and the effect of anticoagulant therapy: a controlled study. *Clin Nephrol* 1978; **10:** 180–186.
23. George CRP, Slichter SJ, Quadracci LJ, Striker GE, Harker LA. A kinetic evaluation of hemostatis in renal disease. *N Engl J Med* 1974; **291:** 1111–1115.

JOURNAL OF PATHOLOGY, VOL. **144**: 57–68 (1984)

SHORT COMMUNICATION

PIGMENTED VILLONODULAR SYNOVITIS ASSOCIATED WITH PSORIATIC POLYARTHROPATHY: AN ELECTRON MICROSCOPIC AND IMMUNOCYTOCHEMICAL STUDY

JENNET M. ARCHER-HARVEY

Department of Pathology, University of Western Australia, Nedlands, Australia

D. W. HENDERSON

Flinders Medical Centre, South Australia, Australia

J. M. PAPADIMITRIOU

Department of Pathology, University of Western Australia, Nedlands, Australia

AND

M. A. M. ROZENBILDS

Flinders Medical Centre, South Australia, Australia

Received 6 February 1984
Accepted 27 March 1984

SUMMARY

A case of pigmented villonodular synovitis in a patient with psoriatic polyarthropathy was studied by means of light microscopy, electron microscopy and immunocytochemical techniques. The lesion consisted of mononuclear phagocytes with features intermediate between type A and type B cells, two types of multinucleate giant cells, an abnormal vasculature, extravasated fibrin and erythrocytes. An unexpected feature was the presence of a mononuclear cell whose cytoplasm contained intermediate filaments and reacted strongly to antisera to cytokeratins. Such a cell type has not previously been described in this condition and its significance is unclear. The findings support the theory that the pathogenesis of PVNS involves leakage of blood through abnormal vessels resulting in the local accumulation and proliferation of mononuclear phagocytes, connective tissue cells and unidentified cytokeratin positive mononuclear cells. The aetiology of the vascular damage, however, remains unknown.

KEY WORDS—Pigmented villonodular synovitis, psoriatic arthritis.

INTRODUCTION

Pigmented villondular synovitis (PVNS), a curious condition of unknown aetiology, is characterized by a diffuse villous and nodular proliferation of synovial cells and subsynovial tissue. A massive accumulation of haemosiderin and lipid in subintimal cells and multinucleated giant cell formation are striking features which have been well described in both light microscopic, [1–3] and ultrastructural studies.[4–8]

This paper describes the electron microscopic and immunocytochemical features of a case of pigmented villondular synovitis, occurring in a patient with psoriatic polyarthropathy, an association not previously reported.

CASE REPORT

A 32-year-old woman with a 2 year history of psoriatic arthropathy was admitted with dispropor-

Addressee for correspondence and reprints: J. M. Archer-Harvey, Hospital and University Pathology Services, Queen Elizabeth II Medical Centre, Nedlands, Western Australia 6009.

0022–3417/84/090057–12$01.20

tionately severe arthritis of the right knee for 3 months. Psoriasis of the scalp, ears, limbs and trunk antedated by eleven years her polyarthropathy, which involved principally the metacarpophalangeal and interphalangeal joints of the hands, and the left elbow joint.

For 4 months prior to admission she had noted malaise, lethargy, anorexia, febrile episodes and marked weight loss, and her right knee had become severely swollen and painful 2 days previously. There was clinical evidence of synovial thickening and joint effusion, with marked restriction of movement, and she was moderately anaemic (haemoglobin 9·6 g/100 ml). Serological investigations revealed no evidence of either rheumatoid or antinuclear factor, but HLAB27 antigen was demonstrated on her leukocytes.

At surgical exploration of the right knee, the synovium was extensively replaced by nodular masses of yellow-brown tissue. A diagnosis of PVNS was established on frozen section and synovectomy performed.

Her systemic symptoms improved postoperatively, but relapsed after three months, and were again associated with swelling, and severe restriction of movement of the right knee. The lateral femoral condyle was eroded, and at re-exploration there was extension of the PVNS into the musculature of the lateral aspect of the thigh. Further synovectomy, with enucleation of the proliferative synovitis from the bone erosion and thigh muscles, was performed. A synovial biopsy from the opposite knee, which contained a small effusion, revealed a chronic villous synovitis consistent with the clinical diagnosis of psoriatic arthropathy.

Six months later, because of recrudescence of the PVNS, she underwent total excision of the right knee joint, with arthrodesis and post operative radiotherapy. There has been no subsequent recurrence of the disease, but 4 years later, she remains severely disabled because of the psoriatic polyarthropathy.

MATERIALS AND METHODS

The synovectomy specimens were fixed in 10 per cent buffered formalin. Routine histological specimens were stained with haematoxylin and eosin. For immunocytochemical studies an immunoperoxidase (PAP) method was used employing antisera to muramidase, α-1-antitrypsin and cytokeratins (DAKO-immunoglobulins Copenhagen, Denmark).

Tissue fixed in 2·5 per cent glutaraldehyde in cacodylate buffer (pH 7·4), was processed for electron microscopy. It was post-fixed in 1 per cent osmium tetroxide, dehydrated in graded ethanol and embedded in Araldite. Ultrathin sections were obtained from selected and representative blocks, mounted on uncoated 200 mesh copper grids, stained with uranyl acetate and lead citrate, and examined in a Philips 201 transmission electron microscope at an accelerating voltage of 60kV.

RESULTS

Gross features

The first synovectomy specimen consisted of an irregular variegated mass of tissue 140 × 90 × 50 mm with numerous brown nodules of 10–20 mm in diameter throughout the entire specimen. In some areas the nodules were more yellow in colour and there were intervening areas of pale connective tissue.

Light microscopic features

The joint surface was covered by a layer of synovial lining cells and fibrin, overlying tissue with a nodular appearance. The nodules were cellular and composed of mononuclear cells, some with vacuolated cytoplasm, admixed with multinucleated giant cells of two types (Fig. 1). Type I possessed elongated, somewhat hyperchromatic nuclei, and densely eosinophilic cytoplasm (Fig. 2) and type II possessed larger, more vesicular nuclei with paler, less well-defined cytoplasm (Fig. 3). Type II cells were somewhat more common than type I cells, the ratio being approximately 3:2 overall, although clusters of similar type tended to be grouped together. Erythrophagocytosis was apparent, and in some regions extravasated fibrin was detectable in the intercellular spaces. There were variable, but often copious, amounts of haemosiderin pigment, particularly at the periphery of the nodules and within the intervening bands of collagenous fibrous tissue. Lipid-laden cells were sometimes seen. Active fibroblastic proliferation was apparent within the fibrous bands, together with scattered lymphoplasmacytic cells.

The appearance was considered typical of PVNS and was seen in all three surgical specimens. Extension of the disease into bone and striated muscle was confirmed in the latter surgical specimens.

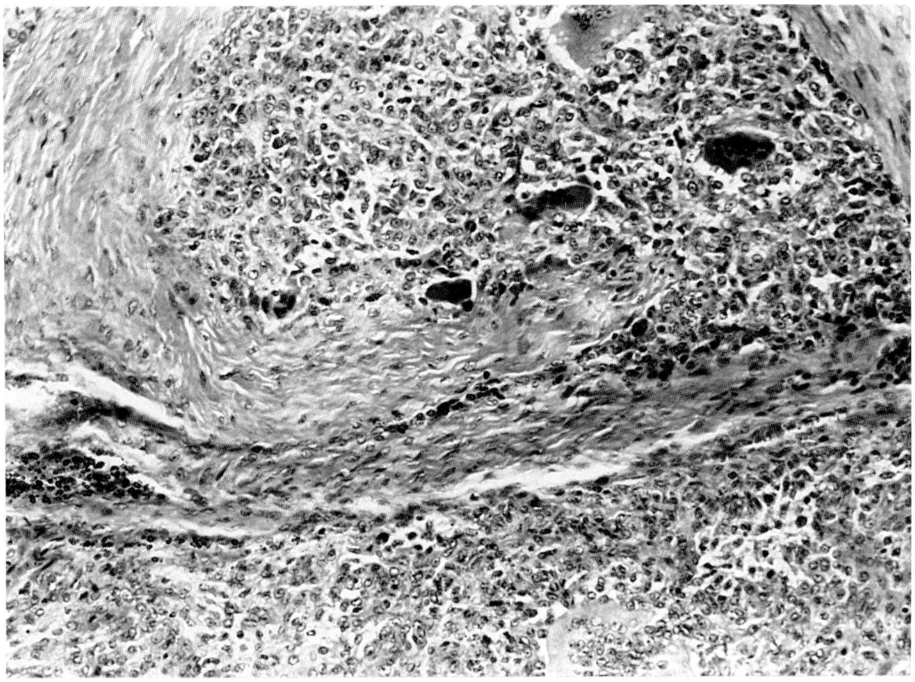

Fig. 1—Photomicrograph showing a nodular proliferation of mononuclear cells, some containing haemosiderin granules, multinucleate giant cells, and bands of fibrous tissue. Haematoxylin and eosin, × 160

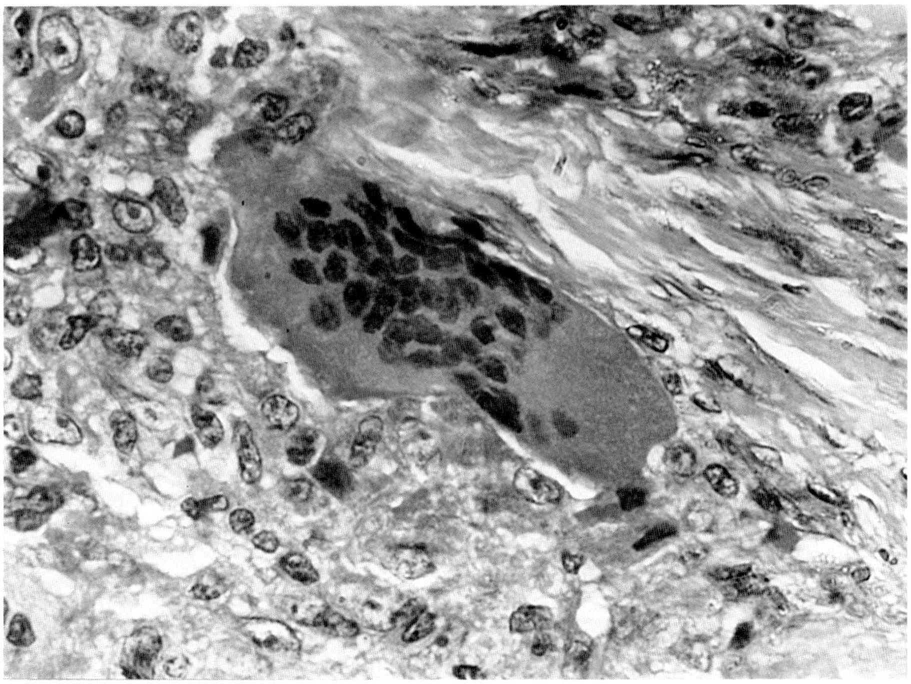

Fig. 2—Type I multinucleate giant cell and surrounding mononuclear cells. Note the hyperchromatic nuclei and densely staining cytoplasm. HE, × 640

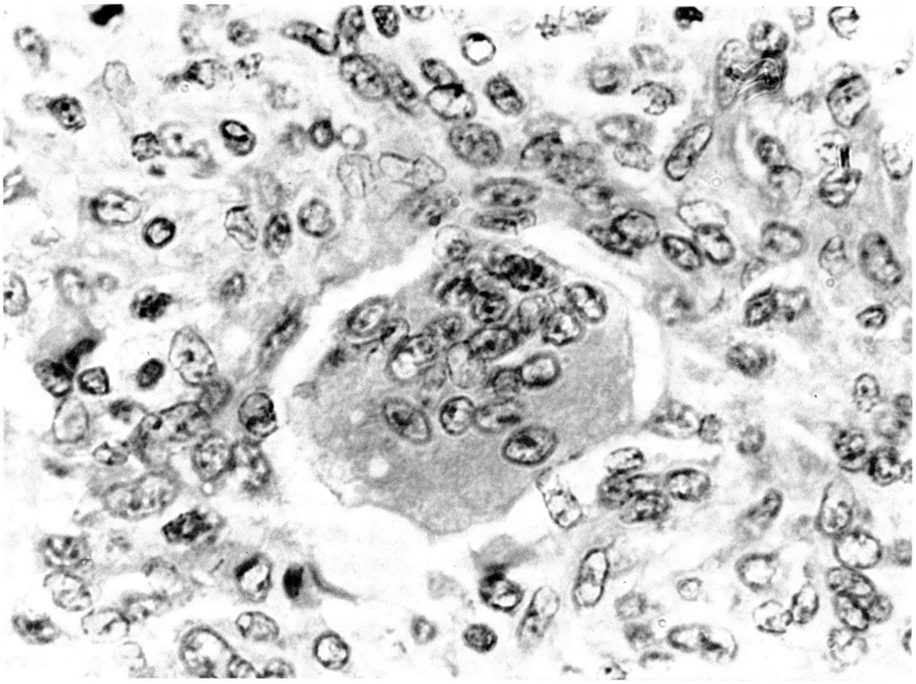

Fig. 3—Type II multinucleate giant cell. Note the large vesicular nuclei. HE, × 640

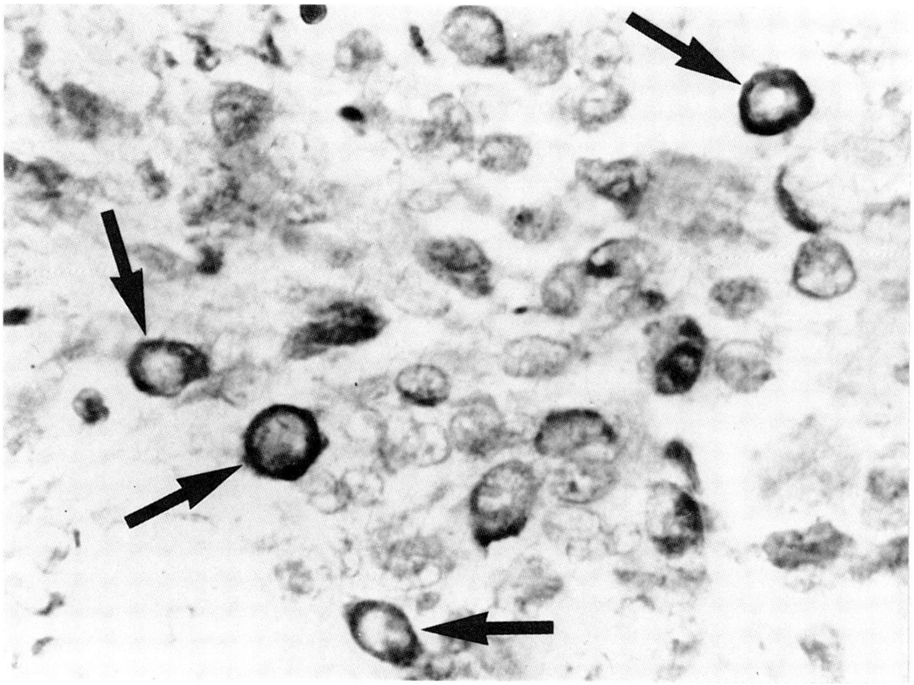

Fig. 4—Immunoperoxidase staining for cytokeratins shows a distinct perinuclear rim of reaction product (arrows) in approximately 1 in 20 of all mononuclear cells. Haematoxylin, × 640

Immunocytochemical studies

Muramidase and α-1-antitrypsin—The great majority of subsynovial macrophages contained abundant cytoplasmic granules which stained positively. Of the multinucleate giant cells, those of type I mostly showed faint peripheral cytoplasmic staining of diffuse distribution rather than granular deposits, and cells of type II showed no reaction product at all.

Cytokeratins—Many cells (approximately 1 in 20 of all mononuclear cells) showed a distinct perinuclear rim of reaction product (Fig. 4). Such cells were scattered throughout the lesion and possessed pale oval nuclei 8–11 μm in size, a prominent nucleolus, a moderate amount of cytoplasm, and exhibited no evidence of phagocytosis.

Electron microscopic features

Both intimal and subtimal tissue (Figs 5, 6) was composed mainly of a population of mononuclear cells with features intermediate between typical type A and type B cells as designated by Barland *et al.*[10] Thus, most cells contained moderate amounts of rough endoplasmic reticulum in addition to prominent Golgi complexes and many smooth-walled phagosomes (Figs 5–7). Within the phagosomes, ingested erythrocytes in various stages of degradation were detected (Figs 6–8). Siderosomes were frequently found (Fig. 7) and, in addition, free iron containing particles were present in the cytoplasm. Cell junctions were not present between these mononuclear cells. From the cell surface, many cytoplasmic processes intertwined in a complex fashion and projected into the fibrin masses (Figs 5–9). These extensions also contained many lysosomal granules and siderosomes.

Less frequently, polygonal mononuclear cells with features different from those described above were found. These were characterized by bundles of intermediate filaments in the perinuclear region of their cytoplasm (Fig. 10). In addition, they possessed moderate numbers of mitochondria, short strands of ergastoplasm, and many ribosomal rosettes. The Golgi complex was poorly developed and only a few lysosomes could be found. Phagosomes were not detected. The nuclei were mildly irregular and contained much chromatin, moderately prominent nucleoli and electron-lucent nuclear bodies. A patchy external lamina was present in some areas (Fig. 11), attached to the cell membrane with hemidesmosomes, but no convincing junctional specializations had formed.

The multinucleated cells were of two types, corresponding to the two types observed by light microscopy. Type I cells had crenated nuclei, large nucleoli, many mitochondria, abundant endoplasmic reticulum and an irregular cell surface. Type II cells had a regular smooth nuclear outline and contained fewer mitochondria and less endoplasmic reticulum than the type I. Neither type displayed evidence of phagocytosis.

Many small capillary buds were found, with slit-like lumina, containing clumps of electron-dense material, probably fibrin (Fig. 12). Fibrin was also found within caveolar invaginations of the endothelial cells, many of which were swollen. In some areas multilayering of the basal lamina of vessels was present. Within the interstitium fibrin was present in some areas as well as normal collagen and long-spaced collagen (Fig. 6).

DISCUSSION

This paper describes a clinically aggressive example of PVNS of the knee, the joint most frequently affected by this condition.[3] The disease occurred in a young woman with psoriatic polyarthropathy, an association not, to our knowledge, previously reported and on whose leukocytes HLA B27 antigen was demonstrated. Many studies have noted an increased frequency of HLA B27 in association with arthritic conditions particularly sacroiliitis.[10] Psoriatic arthropathy with or without sacroiliitis, has also been associated with a greater than expected frequency of B27.[11–15]

Bhawan *et al.*[8] have stressed the importance of microcirculatory changes in the pathogenesis of PVNS and have suggested an immune response, having as its target, endothelial cells of the local microcirculation, and possibly initiated by trauma. Our studies confirm the presence of abnormal vasculature with swollen endothelial cells and multilayering of the basal lamina. The suggestion is made that proliferation of abnormal vessels occurs, and the injured endothelium allows extravasation of fibrin and red blood cells, with subsequent erythrophagocytosis and degradation to haemosiderin in siderosomes, accounting for the pigmentation characteristically found in this condition.

The ultrastructural appearance of our case indicates proliferation of a population of mononuclear

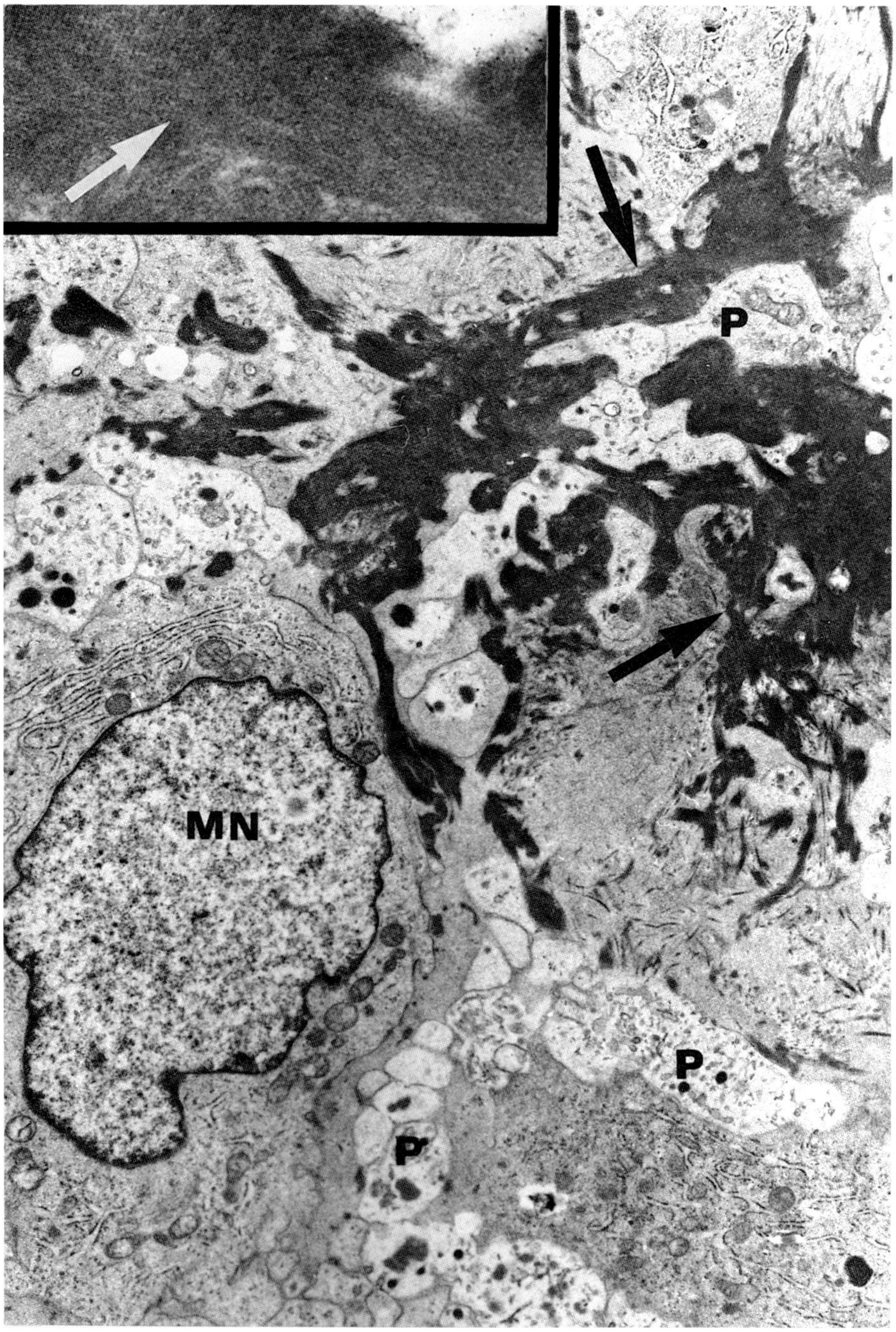

Fig. 5—Transmission electron micrograph of fibrin mass (arrows) surrounded by cytoplasmic projections (P). A mononuclear cell (MN) with long strands of endoplasmic reticulum is adjacent. (×7000). Inset: higher power view of fibrin stands showing 18 nm periodicity (white arrow) ×45000

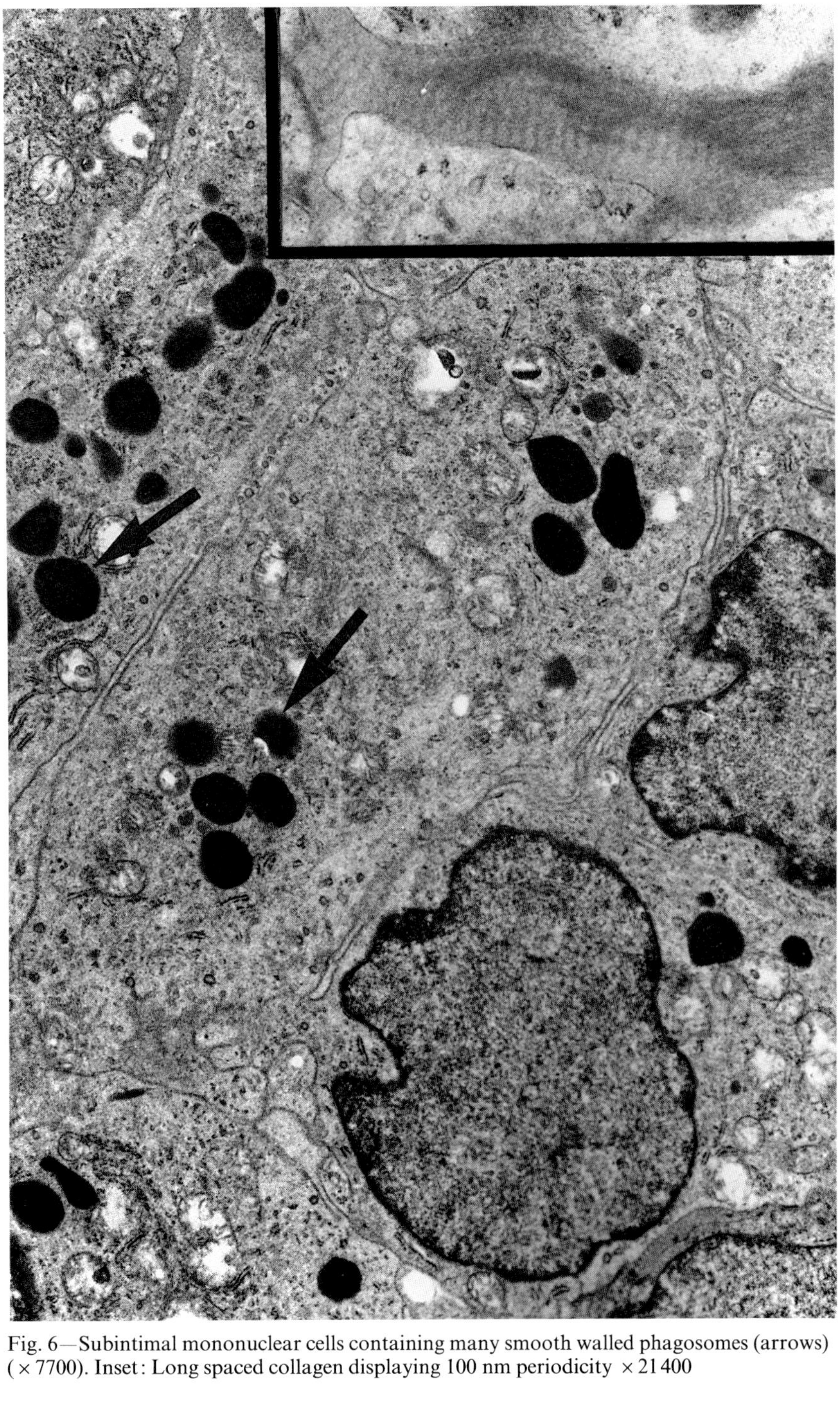

Fig. 6—Subintimal mononuclear cells containing many smooth walled phagosomes (arrows) (× 7700). Inset: Long spaced collagen displaying 100 nm periodicity × 21400

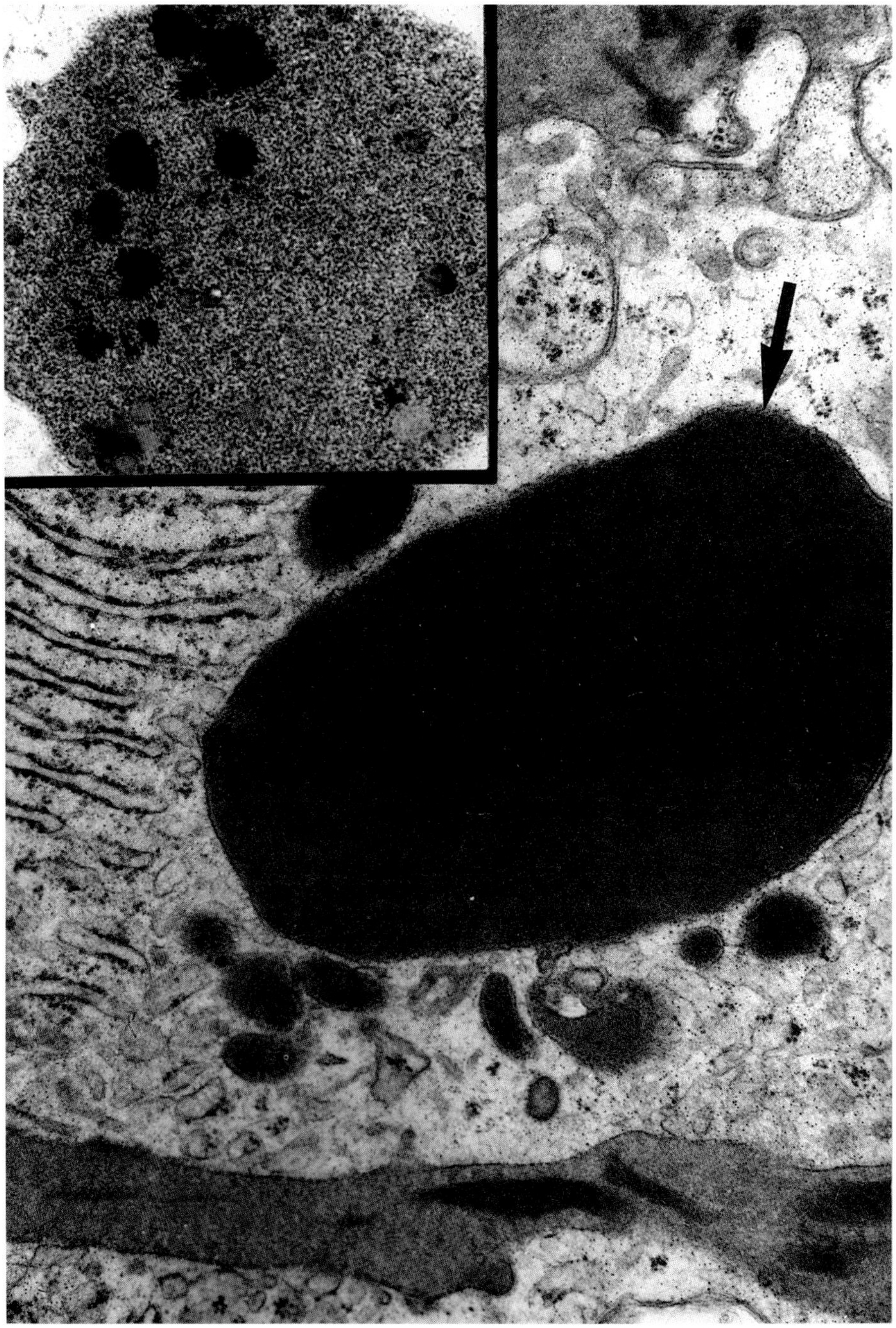

Fig. 7—Part of a mononuclear cell containing several phagosomes, some of which contain ingested erythrocytes (arrow) and abundant endoplasmic reticulum, ×32000. Inset: Siderosome. Note its granular substructure. ×38800

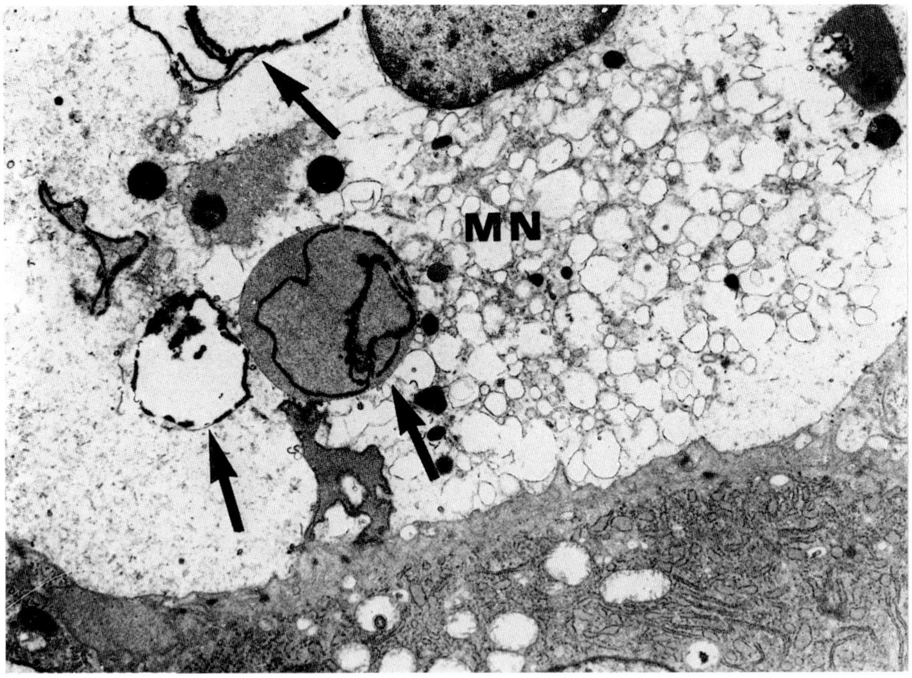

Fig. 8—Mononuclear cell (MN) with phagosomes containing erythrocytes in varying stages of degradation (arrows). × 5200

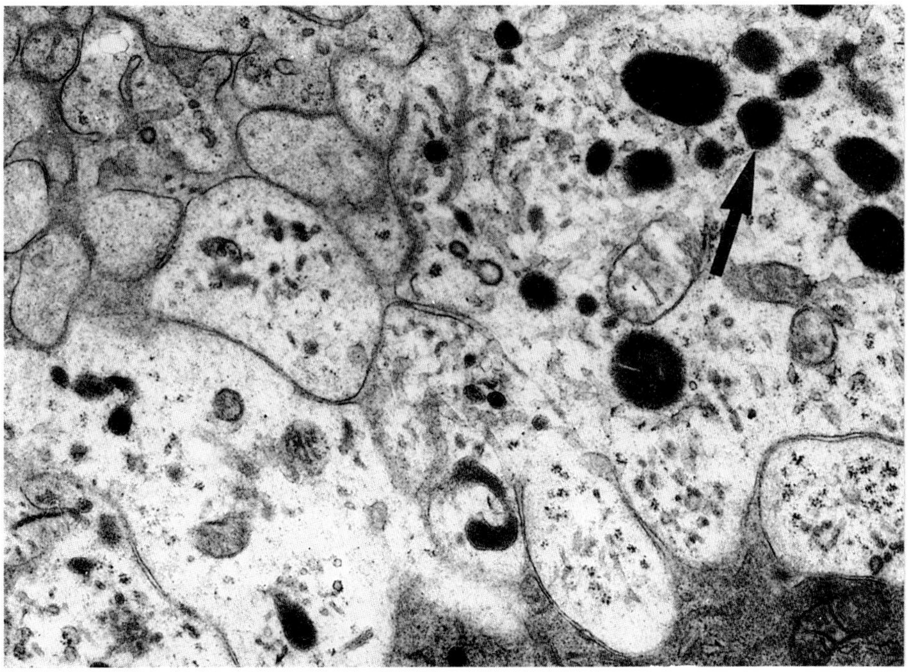

Fig. 9—Interdigitating cytoplasmic processes of mononuclear cells, some of which contain phagosomes (arrow). × 13600

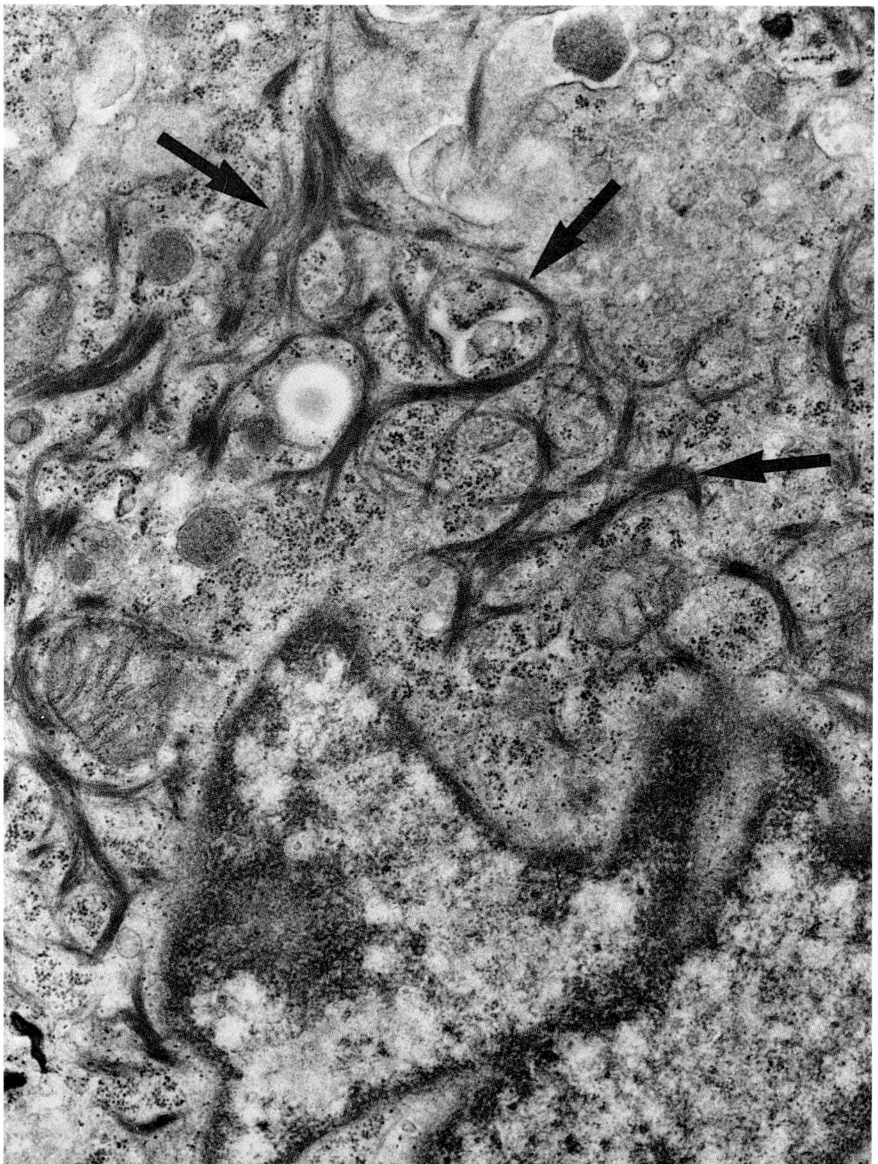

Fig. 10—Distinctive mononuclear cell containing bundles of intermediate filaments (arrows) in a perinuclear distribution. × 24000

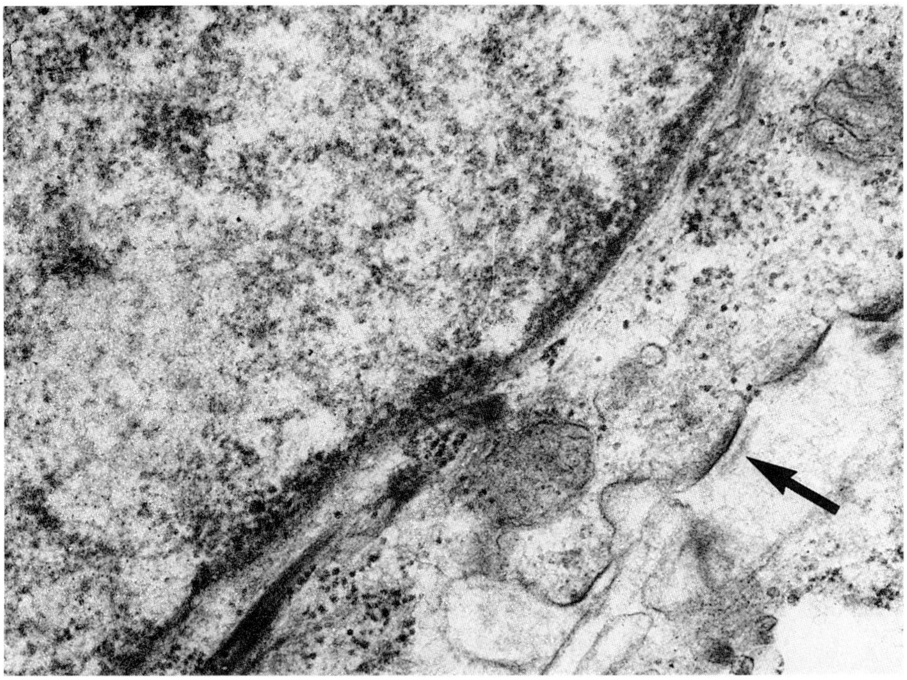

Fig. 11—Periphery of distinctive mononuclear cell showing a patchy external lamina (arrow) and hemidesmosome formation. × 42000

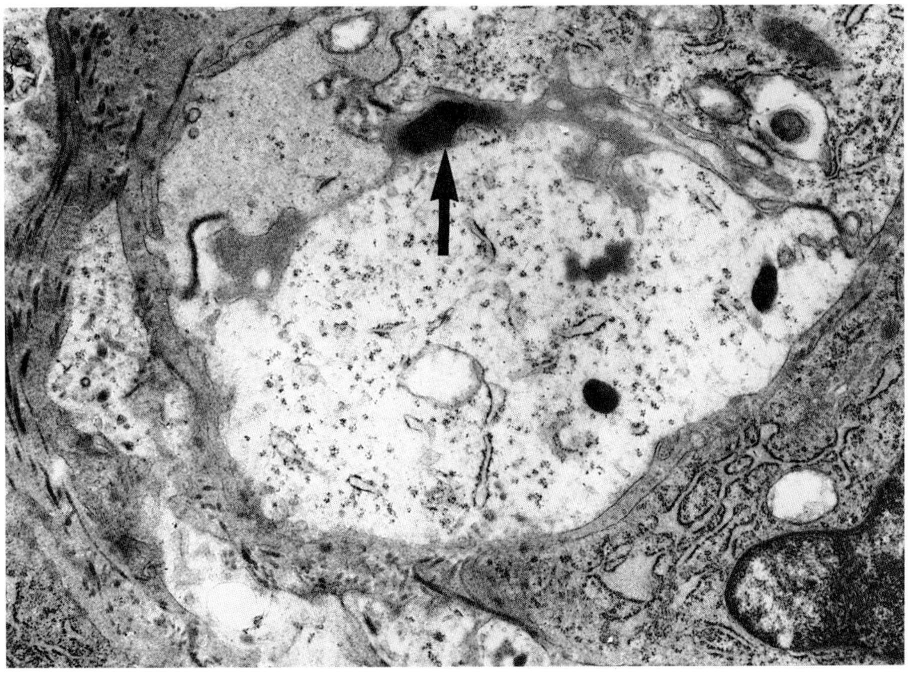

Fig. 12—Small capillary with swollen endothelial cells enclosing a narrow lumen containing electron-dense material (arrow). × 8200

cells with features intermediate between typical type A (macrophage-like) and type B (fibroblast-like) synovial cells. They virtually all exhibited evidence of phagocytosis but had, in addition, a moderate amount of rough endoplasmic reticulum. There was no clear distinction into type A and type B synovial cells. A striking feature of these cells, corresponding to Ghadially's subsynovial macrophages, was the presence of a complex labyrinth of cell processes which intertwined, and projected into fibrin masses. The presence of lysosomal granules and siderosomes in these processes suggests that they are actively involved in erythrophagocytosis, and perhaps chemotactically attracted by fibrin.

In addition, approximately 1 in every 20 of mononuclear cells showed different structural and cytochemical features from those described above. They characteristically contained intermediate filaments forming bundles around the nucleus, and a patchy external lamina. These cells most likely correspond with those showing positive staining reaction for cytokeratins. Such a cell type has not previously been described in normal human synovium and its nature and origin is open to speculation.

Multinucleated giant cells, another common component of PVNS, were frequently seen in our material. They showed, as previously described, little evidence of phagocytic activity and were of two distinct types. The significance of the two types is uncertain; it would not appear that one represents a more degenerate stage of the other as both are abundant in cytoplasmic organelles and there is no structural evidence of nuclear abnormality. Type I showed some muramidase activity but this was absent in type II cells. This may possibly reflect secretory activity by the type II cells. Evidence for secretion by murine multinucleate giant cells has been presented elsewhere.[16] Such syncytia also failed to phagocytose particulate material in their immediate environment.

ACKNOWLEDGEMENT

The authors wish to thank Professor D. Dahlin who examined the histological sections and confirmed the diagnosis.

REFERENCES

1. Jaffe HL, Lichtenstein L, Sutro CJ. Pigmented villonodular synovitis, bursitis and tenosynovitis. *Arch Path* 1941; **31**: 731.
2. Docken WP. Pigmented villonodular synovitis: a review with illustrative case reports. *Seminars in Arthritis and Rheumatism* 1979; **9**: 1.
3. Schajowicz F. Tumors and Tumor-like Lesions of Bones and Joints. New York: Springer-Verlag, 1981: 526.
4. Hirohata K. Light microscopic and electron microscopic studies of individual cells in pigmented villonodular synovitis and bursitis (Jaffe). *Kobe J Med Sci* 1968; **14**: 251.
5. Wyllie JC. The stromal cell reaction of pigmented villonodular synovitis: an electron microscopic study. *Arthritis and Rheumatism* 1969; **12**: 205.
6. Alguacil-Garcia A, Unni KK, Goellner JR. Giant cell tumor of tendon sheath and pigmented villonodular synovitis. *Amer J Clin Pathologists* 1978; **69**: 6.
7. Ghadially FN, Lalonde J-MA, Dick CE. Ultrastructure of pigmented vollonodular synovitis *J Path* 1979; **127**: 19.
8. Bhawan J, Joris I, Cohen N, Majno G. Microcirculatory changes in post-traumatic pigmented villonodular synovitis. *Arch Pathol Lab Med* 1980; **104**: 328.
9. Barland P, Novikoff AB, Hamerman D. Electron microscopy of the human synovial membrane. *J Cell Biol* 1962; **14**: 207.
10. Dawkins RL, Christiansen FT, Kay PH, Garlepp M, McCluskey J, Hollingsworth PN, Zilko PJ. Disease associations with complotypes, supratypes and haplotypes. *Immunological Rev* 1983; **70**: 5.
11. Brewerton DA, Nicholls A, Caffrey M, Walters D, James DCO. HL-A27 and arthropathies associated with ulcerative colitis and psoriasis. *Lancet* 1974; **i**: 956.
12. McCluskey OE, Lordon RE, Arnett FC Jr. HL-A27 in Reiter's syndrome and psoriatic arthritis: a genetic factor in disease susceptibility and expression. *J Rheumatol* 1974; **1**: 263.
13. Lambert JR, Wright V, Rajah SM, Moll JMH. Histocompatibility antigens in psoriatic arthritis. *Ann Rheum Dis* 1976; **36**: 526.
14. Eastmond CJ, Woodrow JC. The HLA system and the arthropathies associated with psoriasis. *Ann Rheum Dis* 1977; **36**: 112.
15. Kammer GM, Soter NA, Gibson DJ, Schur PH. Psoriatic arthritis: a clinical immunologic and HLA study of 100 patients. *Seminars in Arthritis and Rheumatism* 1979; **9**: 75.
16. Papadimitriou JM, Walters MN-I. Macrophage polykarya. *Int Rev Toxicol* 1979; **6**: 211.

JOURNAL OF PATHOLOGY, VOL. **144**: 69 (1984)

BOOK REVIEW

The Biology of Immunologic Disease. FRANK J. DIXON and DAVID W. FISHER (Eds.). Sinauer Associates Inc., Sunderland, Massachusetts, and Blackwell Scientific Publications, Oxford, 1983. No. of pages: 399. Price: £22.50. ISBN: 0 87893 1481.

This is an attractive, sturdily-bound collection of 35 articles in the style of *Scientific American* which were published originally in *Hospital Practice*. The chapters, updated in the spring of 1983, are (with two exceptions) by eminent immunologists working in the States. They deal with those recent advances in immunology which have made significant contributions to our further understanding of disease processes.

The first 14 chapters are concerned primarily with basic science. There are articles on the genetic control of the immune response and antibody structure, IgE, the identification and function of T cell subsets (although there is little coverage in the book of human T cell markers and no recent references), NK cells, macrophages, MHC restriction, tolerance and lymphocyte circulation. Then follow articles on complement, C reactive protein and the PMN as a secretory cell. Here a chapter on the interleukins would have been appropriate, in view of their diversity, biological significance and prospective clinical importance.

The third part of the book is devoted to disease-specific mechanisms and good coverage is given to HLA associations, the immunopathology of renal and neurologic disease, SLE and 'anti-receptor' diseases (Graves' disease and myasthenia gravis). The final and most stimulating section concerns the role of hybridoma technology, computers (vaccine design), cellular engineering (immune reconstitution), immunopharmocology and drug targetting.

Suggestions for further reading are provided at the end of the book, rather than at the conclusion of each chapter. The numerous colour diagrams are extremely well-produced and provide excellent teaching material. Although the typeface varies somewhat between and within chapters, this is a minor imperfection in an otherwise high quality product. The latter feature, together with the prominence of its contributors, should ensure the book has a place in most pathology and all immunology departmental libraries.

A. E. THOMSON
Department of Pathology
University of Aberdeen

ANNOUNCEMENT

THE SPECTOR SCHOLARSHIP FUND

1. It is proposed to create a fund with a capital of approximately £40,000, the interest from which is to be set aside to further the scientific and pathological interests of the members of the Society.
2. The scholarships will be known as 'Spector Scholarships'.
3. The sum of £40,000 is to be placed with Government Securities, such as 10% Treasury Stock 1992, thereby yielding a high rate of interest.
4. Of the interest, which will be of the order of £4,000 annually and derived from the capital of the Fund, half is to be re-invested, while the other half is used on an annual basis. This option should ensure that the Fund capital and subsequent interest keeps pace with the rate of inflation if it is of the order of 5%.
5. The purpose of the Spector Scholarships is to enable Society members to travel to another university, institute, hospital or academic establishment to learn methodology and techniques with which they would return to their own department. Attendance at meetings with no laboratory or practical component is not envisaged as part of the scheme.
6. The Scholarships would be available to any member of the Society, irrespective of age, to cover travel, abroad or at home, and a stay of up to 6 working days. Each Scholarship will carry a maximum value of £500. Travel and subsistence rates for this purpose will be those designated for the appropriate medical and scientific grades by a current MRC Code of Practice.
7. Applications can be received at any time by the General Secretary of the Society. Ajudication, which will occur on a 3 monthly basis, will be by the General Secretary and the Meetings Secretaries, who collectively, will have the power to recommend award or otherwise.
8. After being awarded, the Scholarship should be taken up within 1 year. A short report on the scholar's activities should be sent to the General Secretary for the Committee's attention within 6 months of completing the Scholarship.
9. The existence of the Scholarships will be advertised in the Society's journals and in papers of the Society from time to time.

PUBLISHING AGREEMENT

1. It is our custom to request authors to vest the worldwide copyright of their papers in John Wiley & Sons Limited for the full term of copyright and we would be grateful if you would confirm your acceptance of these terms by signing and returning the agreement below. We will not withhold permission for any reasonable request from you to publish any part of this paper in connection with any other work by you, provided the usual acknowledgements are given regarding copyright notice and reference to the original publication.
2. If it is appropriate, the author's employer may sign this agreement, and in any event the employer may reserve the right to use the paper internally or for promotional purposes only, by so indicating on this agreement. It is understood that proprietary rights other than copyright (including patent rights) are reserved.
3. If the author is a U.S. Government employee and this work was done in that capacity the assignment applies only to the extent allowable by U.S. law. If at least one co-author is *not* a government employee, said author should sign the agreement.
4. If the author is an employee of the British Government then HMSO will grant a non-exclusive licence to publish this paper in the Journal in any form or media provided British crown copyright and user rights (including patent rights) are reserved.
5. The author warrants that the manuscript is the author's original work, and has not been published before. (If excerpts from copyrighted works are included, the author will obtain written permission from the copyright owners and show credit to the sources in the manuscript.) The author also warrants that the article contains no libellous or unlawful statements, and does not infringe on the rights of others.
6. If the work was prepared jointly the author agrees to inform co-authors of the terms of the agreement, and to sign on their behalf.

With the qualifications listed above I assign to John Wiley & Sons Limited, the copyright of my paper entitled ______________________________

____

for publication in ______________________________

______________________________ Signed

______________________________ Date

If the paper is rejected this assignment is null and void.

JOURNAL OF PATHOLOGY, VOL. **143**: 73–79 (1984)

AMIODARONE LUNG TOXICITY: A HUMAN AND EXPERIMENTAL STUDY

F. R. COSTA-JUSSÀ

Department of Neuropathology, Institute of Neurology, Queen Square, London, U.K.

B. CORRIN

Department of Thoracic Pathology, Cardiothoracic Institute, Brompton Hospital, London, U.K.

AND

J. M. JACOBS

Department of Neuropathology, Institute of Neurology, Queen Square, London, U.K.

Received 16 February 1984
Accepted 13 March 1984

SUMMARY

This paper describes the pathology of pulmonary histiocytosis developing in a patient treated with amiodarone, and reports comparable changes in the lungs of rats and mice to which this drug had been administered. Ultrastructural studies indicate that the experimental lung changes are similar to those produced by iprindole and chlorphentermine. The patient also displayed focal necroses and an eosinophilic bronchiolitis; these may represent further effects of amiodarone on the lung.

KEY WORDS—Amiodarone lung toxicity, pulmonary histocytosis, lipid pneumonia.

INTRODUCTION

Amiodarone is widely used in the control of cardiac dysrhythmia and although generally quite safe there have recently appeared several reports of adverse reactions. The lungs may be affected and pulmonary toxicity has recently been reviewed by Rakita *et al.*[1] The pulmonary reaction is generally described as showing interstitial pneumonitis and fibrosis but in one patient, prominent foam cells were reported.[2] Another patient with such lipid pneumonia has recently been seen at the Brompton Hospital and the clinical details of this patient are recorded elsewhere.[3] The present paper describes the lung pathology of this patient and the development of similar changes in the lungs of rats and mice dosed with amiodarone.

0022–3417/84/100073–07$01.00

CASE REPORT

The clinical details of this patient have been described by Clarke *et al.*[3] Briefly, he is a 29-year-old man suffering from sinuatrial disease with paroxysmal atrial fibrillation and flutter, and treated with amiodarone (800 mg/day) for 10 months. Because of increasing breathlessness and radiographic lung opacities he underwent fibroptic transbronchial biopsy and later, open lung biopsy at which a wedge of lung 3 cm in length was resected from the left lower lobe. Both biopsies showed filling of the alveoli by foamy macrophages (Fig. 1) or occasionally, knots of granulation tissue, the appearances of an organizing endogenous lipid pneumonia. The open lung biopsy also showed interstitial oedema and low grade lymphocytic infiltration of the

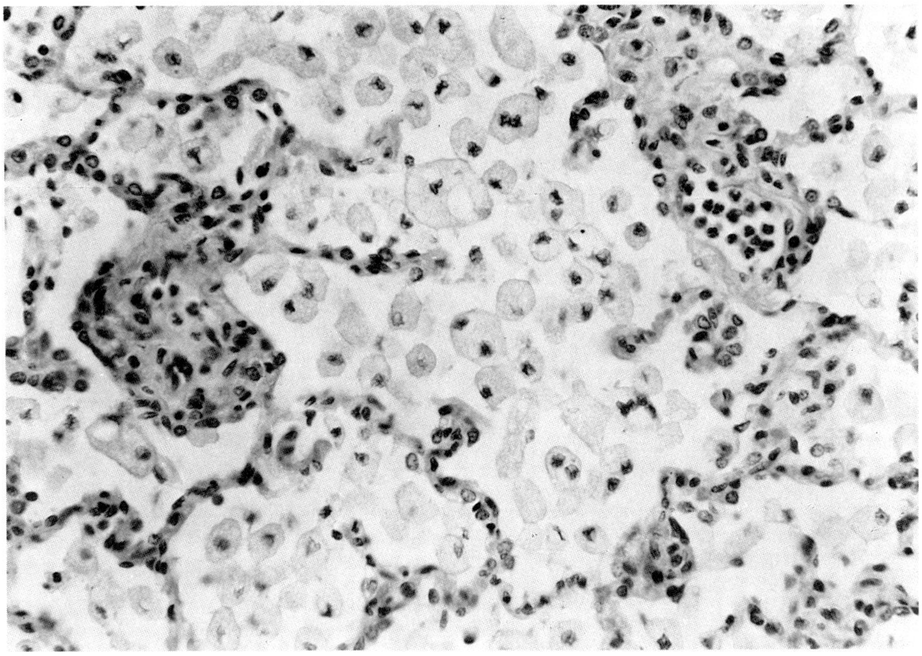

Fig. 1—Lung biopsy showing numerous foamy macrophages filling the alveoli. Haematoxylin and eosin, ×244

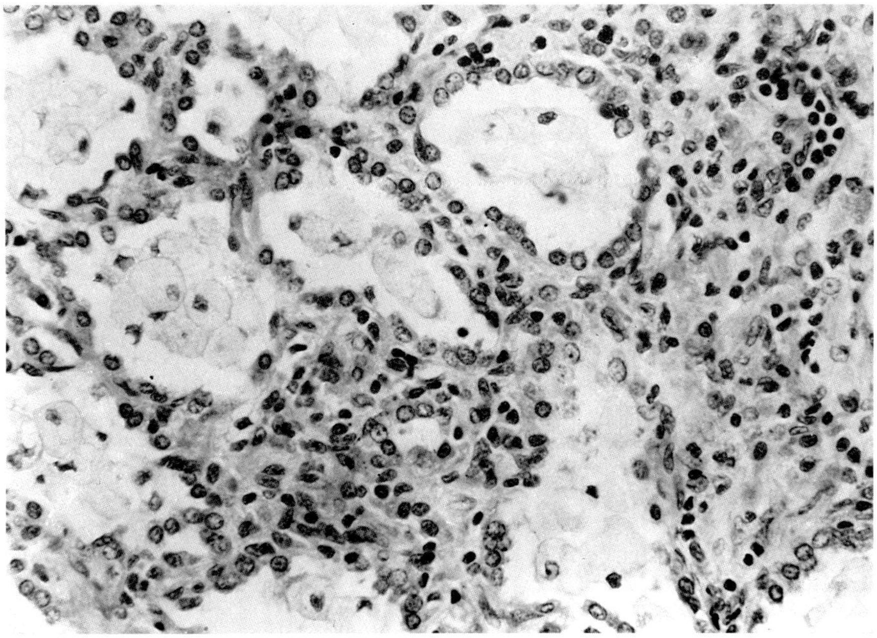

Fig. 2—Lung biopsy showing an interstitial infiltrate of lymphocytes and intra-alveolar foam cells. Haematoxylin and eosin, ×324

alveolar walls (Fig. 2) with only a little patchy interstitial fibrosis. Several bronchioles were filled by a mixed neutrophil and eosinophil exudate. Eosinophils also infiltrated the walls of the bronchioles and the peribronchiolar tissues, but were not seen away from the airways. Also evident in the open lung biopsy were occasional foci of necrosis.

EXPERIMENTAL STUDY

These experiments were undertaken to study amiodarone neuropathy, but in this paper attention is confined to incidental changes observed in the lungs. The neurological changes will be reported separately.

Materials and methods

Fifteen mice (male, Balb/c, aged about 6 weeks) were dosed with 200 mg/kg·day amiodarone suspended in 5 per cent methylcellulose for up to 3 months; seven control animals of the same strain were dosed with methylcellulose alone. Twelve young adult (Sprague Dawley) rats were given 400 mg/kg·day for up to 1 month (one animal survived for 2 months). All animals were dosed orally using an oesophageal cannula and were weighed daily.

At the end of each experiment the animals were perfused through the aorta under deep pentobarbitone (Sagatal) anaesthesia with modified Karnovsky fixative containing 3 per cent glutaraldehyde and 1 per cent paraformaldehyde in 0·07 M sodium cacodylate buffer (pH 7·3–7·4). A peristaltic pump was used to perfuse the rats whilst mice were perfused using a 20 ml syringe. Many types of tissues were examined, but only findings in the lungs are reported in this paper. The lungs were examined after dosing for more than 2 months in mice and after 3 weeks to 2 months of dosing in rats. They were removed after perfusion and immersed for a further 12–24 h in fixative. Blocks were processed into araldite and 1 μm sections were stained with toluidine blue. Ultra-thin sections were treated with uranyl acetate and lead citrate and examined in a Jeol electron microscope 100CX at 80 kV.

Some rats were perfused with formol-calcium for paraffin histology; 5 μm sections of lungs were stained with haematoxylin and eosin.

RESULTS

Body weights

Figures 3 and 4 and Tables I and II show mean weights and standard deviations of mice and rats, respectively, together with their controls. In mice, weight differences between treated and controls were significant by the third and fourth week of dosing. Failure of young treated rats to gain weight becomes marked by the end of the first week of dosing.

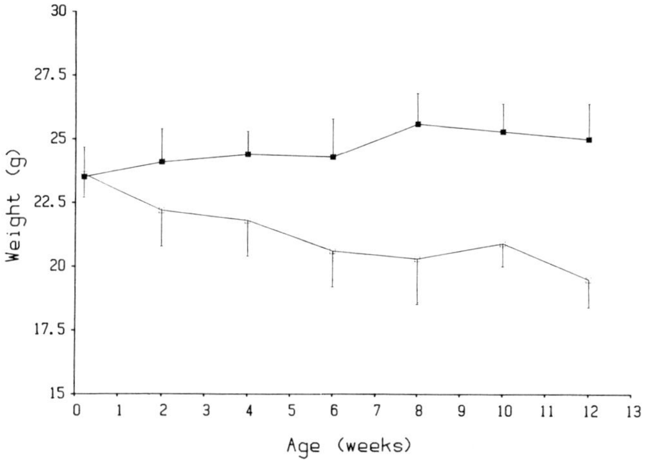

Fig. 3—Graph showing mean weights (g) and standard deviations of control mice (solid squares) and amiodarone-treated mice (open squares)

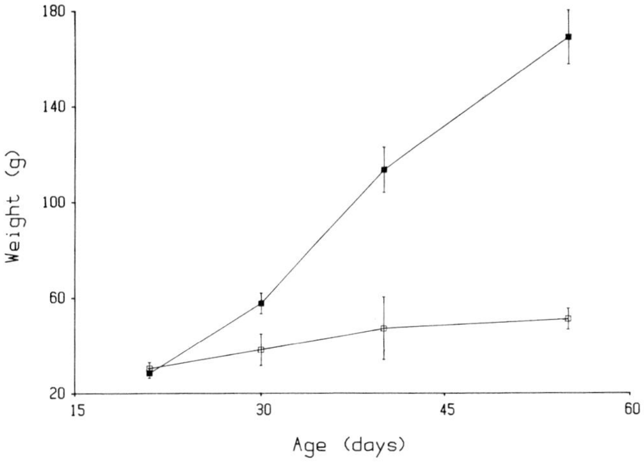

Fig. 4—Graph showing mean weights (g) and standard deviations of control rats (solid squares) and amiodarone-treated rats (open squares)

Table I—Means and standard deviations ( ) in weight (g) in control and amiodarone-dosed rats (400 mg/kg·day), 21 days old at the beginning of the experiment

Age	Control	Treated	Significance
21	28·5 (2·06) ($n=4$)	30·5 (2·5) ($n=12$)	$0·5>p>0·1$
30	57·7 (4·3) ($n=4$)	38·3 (6·6) ($n=11$)	$0·001>p$
40	113·5 (9·44) ($n=4$)	47·2 (13·1) ($n=9$)	$0·001>p$
55	169 (11·3) ($n=3$)	51·3 (4·4) ($n=3$)	$0·001>p$

Mortality

The mice survived 3 months of dosing with 200 mg/kg·day, except for some which became very sick and were killed as described above after being dosed for 10 and 11 weeks.

After dosing with 400 mg/kg·day, about 25 per cent of the young rats died over a period of 3–4 weeks. All animals appeared sick, with less motor activity, ruffled fur and marked weakness.

Light and electron microscopy

Mice—Examination of plastic sections showed a moderate increase in the numbers of alveolar macrophages. These were seen to contain dense inclusions, and electron microscopy showed that these were electron dense structures having a whorled and lamellated appearance. Small numbers of inclusions were found in endothelial cells and in type I pneumocytes. In type II pneumocytes it was difficult to distinguish drug-induced lamellated bodies from the lamellated structures which these cells normally contain.

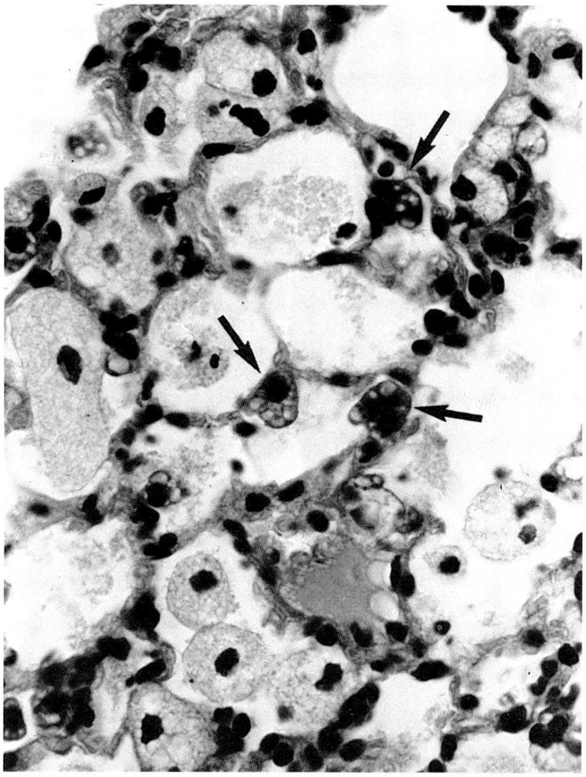

Fig. 5—Paraffin section of lung from a 42-day-old rat dosed with amiodarone (400 mg/kg·day) for 3 weeks. Several foamy macrophages are seen within the alveoli and a number of type II pneumocytes with vacuolated cytoplasm are shown (arrows). Haematoxylin and eosin, ×459

Rats—A massive proliferation of large alveolar macrophages was seen by the third week of dosing. In paraffin sections these had a foamy appearance (Fig. 5). Plastic sections (1 μm) from rats dosed for up to 2 months showed that macrophages were full of round, dense inclusions. Similar inclusions were

Table II—Means and standard deviations ( ) in weight (g) in control and amiodarone treated mice (200 mg/kg·day)

	Initial weight	2 weeks	4 weeks	6 weeks	8 weeks	10 weeks	12 weeks
Controls	23·5 (1·17) ($n=7$)	24·1 (1·3) ($n=7$)	24·4 (0·9) ($n=7$)	24·3 (1·5) ($n=6$)	25·6 (1·2) ($n=3$)	25·3 (1·1) ($n=3$)	25·0 (1·4) ($n=3$)
Treated	23·6 (0·9) ($n=15$)	22·2 (1·4) ($n=15$)	21·8 (1·4) ($n=14$)	20·6 (1·4) ($n=13$)	20·3 (1·8) ($n=13$)	20·9 (0·9) ($n=13$)	19·5 (1·1) ($n=4$)
Significance	$p>0·5$	$0·02>p>0·01$	$0·001>p$	$0·001>p$	$0·001>p$	$0·001>p$	$0·01>p>0·001$

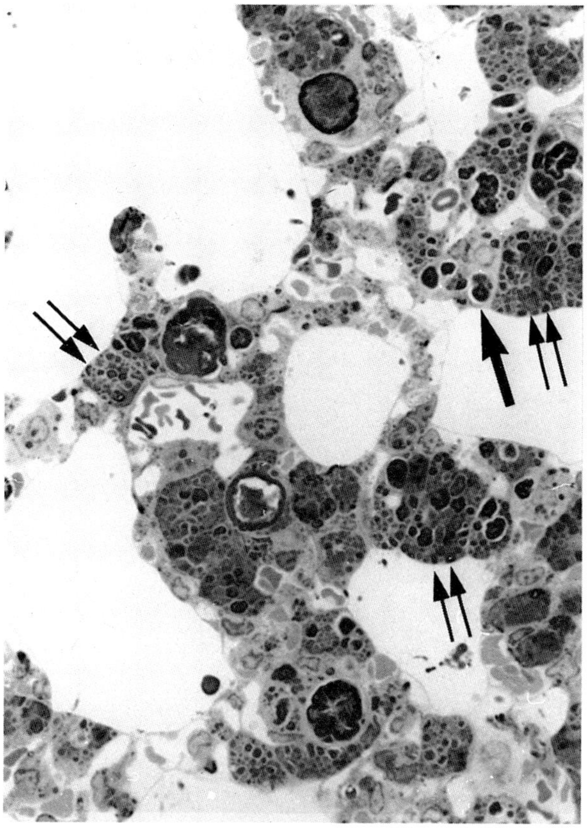

Fig. 6—Araldite section (1 μm) of lung from a rat dosed for 2 months with 400 mg/kg·day showing many inclusions, some of large size (3–14 μm), in macrophages (double arrows) and in other cell types including abnormally large inclusions in type II pneumocytes (arrow). Toluidine blue, ×485

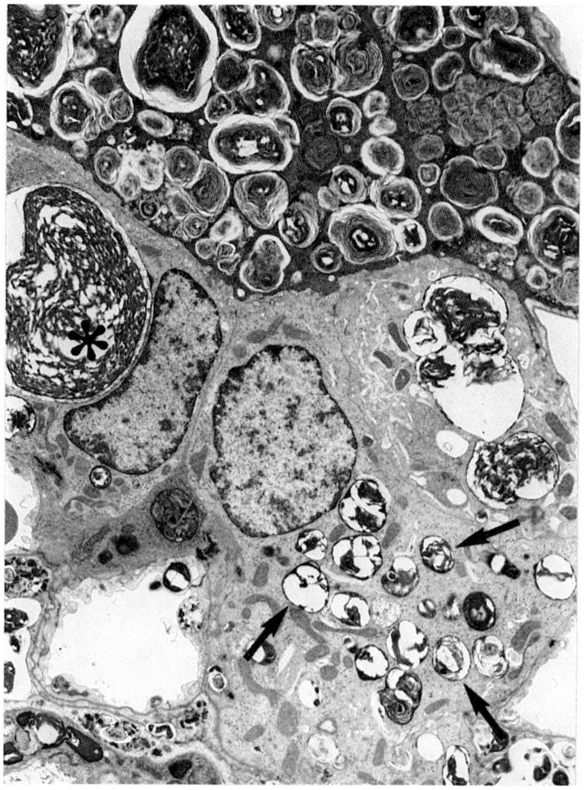

Fig. 7—Electron micrograph of lung from a rat dosed with 400 mg/kg·day for 2 months. An alveolar macrophage is packed with lamellated bodies. Type II pneumocytes with a characteristic polygonal shape are seen. These cells normally contain lamellated structures associated with surfactant (arrows), but also seen are large lamellated, drug-induced inclusions (asterisk). Inclusions are also present in capillary endothelial cells. ×3600

seen in cells within the alveolar wall (Fig. 6). Electron microscopy showed macrophages packed with lamellated inclusions, proliferation of type II pneumocytes, some containing large lamellated inclusions, and similar bodies in capillary endothelial cells and type I pneumocytes (Fig. 7). Similar inclusions in other tissues, e.g. muscle, were found to stain positively with Baker's haematein for phospholipids and electron histochemistry showed that the inclusions were associated with acid phosphatase activity.

DISCUSSION

We have reported our clinical and experimental findings together as they have one feature in common: an endogenous lipid pneumonia marked by the accumulation of foamy lipid-laden macrophages in the alveoli. This was the principal change in both patient and animals. Such histiocytosis is a well-recognized effect of certain other drugs, at least in the experimental animal. Examples include the tricyclic antidepressant drug iprindole[4–6] and the anorectic drug chlorphentermine.[7–9] Bochhardt *et al.*[10] examined a number of tissues in rats dosed with amiodarone. They found lipidosis-like alterations in lymph nodes, adrenal glands, retinal pigment epithelium and lung.

Marchlinski *et al.*[2] suggested that amiodarone toxicity in the lung in human pathology was related to the amphiphilic nature of the drug. Drugs of this type induce the formation and accumulation of lamellated bodies containing mainly phospholipids in a wide range of cell types, although there appears to be no increase in phospholipid synthesis.[11] The lamellated bodies appear to form within lysosomes and the morphogenesis of their formation has been studied in cultured neurons by Brosnan *et al.*,[12] and in cultured macrophages by Drenckhahn *et al.*[13] Further support for the lysosomal origin of these bodies comes from the demonstration within them of acid phosphatase activity.[12,14] Amphiphilic drugs have been found to cause a deficit of the lysosomal enzymes phospholipase A and phospholipase C[15] and sphingomyelinase.[16,17] The basic pathogenesis of the cytological changes in lung seems to be related to the effects of the drug upon lipid degradation by lysosomes, principally affecting the normal turnover of surfactant in macrophages. This causes the appearance of lamellated bodies in these cells and to a lesser extent in alveolar epithelial and capillary endothelial cells. Consequent upon this, alveolar macrophages increase in number and there is evidence of proliferation of type II pneumocytes.

Lamellar inclusions seen in capillary endothelial cells in the lung have also been observed in blood vessels within biopsied human sural nerves from cases of amiodarone neuropathy.[18] Similar effects upon lung capillary endothelial cells could explain the interstitial oedema seen in experimental studies with another amphiphilic drug, iprindole.[6]

Most other reports of amiodarone pulmonary toxicity describe interstitial fibrosis rather than histiocytosis and it has been suggested that the fibrosis may represent an end-stage of the histiocytosis.[19] We are sceptical of this because of our previous experimental long-term studies with iprindole in which the histiocytosis progressed to alveolar lipoproteinosis rather than widespread interstitial fibrosis.[6] Focal fibrosis in association with cholesterol pneumonitis is another long term complication of pulmonary histiocytosis but this is distinguished by the presence of cholesterol crystal clefts and attendant foreign body giant cells.[20] The diffuse alveolar damage reported in a fatal case of amiodarone pneumonitis by Darmanata *et al.*[21] is a more likely precursor of interstitial fibrosis than histiocytosis and it is conceivable that in our patient the lymphocytic infiltration (a chronic interstitial pneumonia) may represent a low grade inflammatory precursor of interstitial fibrosis. Interstitial pulmonary fibrosis is of course a well-recognized cytotoxic effect of many drugs and it is possible that histiocytosis and interstitial fibrosis represent two separate effects of amiodarone toxicity in the lung but why it should cause one rather than the other is unclear.

Note must be taken of two further features evident in our patient's lung biopsy, namely the focal necrosis and the eosinophilic bronchiolitis. No infective organisms were identified and the histological appearances suggest hypersensitivity responses; it is possible that these too are attributable to the amiodarone.

ACKNOWLEDGEMENTS

We are grateful to Dr Honey for providing the clinical information. Dr Jacobs and Dr Costa-Jussà would like to express their thanks to Professor W. Jacobson for his interest and useful discussions, and to the Brain Research Trust and Labaz for financial support. Labaz kindly supplied the amiodarone. Dr Costa-Jussà was in receipt of a scholarship from the Caixa d'Estalvis de Barcelona.

REFERENCES

1. Rakita L, Sobol SM, Mostow N, Vrobel T. Amiodarone pulmonary toxicity. *Amer Heart J* 1983; **106:** 906–916.
2. Marchlinski FE, Gansler TS, Waxman HL, Josephson ME. Amiodarone pulmonary toxicity. *Ann Intern Med* 1982; **97:** 839–845.
3. Clarke, B, Ward DE, Honey M. Pneumonitis with pleural and pericardial effusions and proximal motor neuropathy during amiodarone therapy. 1984; submitted for publication.
4. Vijeyaratnam GS, Corrin B. Pulmonary histiocytosis simulating desquamative interstitial pneumonia in rats receiving oral iprindole. *J Path* 1973; **108:** 105–113.
5. Vijeyaratnam GS, Corrin, B. Pulmonary alveolar proteinosis developing from desquamative interstitial pneumonia in long-term toxicity studies of iprindole in the rat. *Virchows Arch A Path Anat*, 1973; **358:** 1–10.
6. Vijeyaratnam GS, Corrin B. Fine structural alterations in the lungs of iprindole-treated rats. *J Path* 1974; **114:** 233–239.
7. Heath D, Smith, P, Hasleton PS. Effects of chlorphentermine on the rat lung. *Thorax* 1973; **28:** 551–558.
8. Lullmann-Rauch R, Reil GH, Rossen E, Seiler KU. The ultrastructure of rat lung changes induced by an anorectic drug (chlorphentermine). *Virchows Arch B Zellpath* 1972; **11:** 167–181.
9. Smith P, Heath D, Hasleton PS. Electron microscopy of chlorphentermine lung. *Thorax* 1973; **28:** 559–566.
10. Bockhardt H, Drenckhahn D, Lullmann-Rauch R. Generalisierte Lipidose bei der Ratte nach Behand-

lung mit Amiodaron und Zimelidin. *Verh Anat Ges* 1978; **72:** 417–418.
11. Hildebrand J, Thys O, Gerin Y. Alterations of rat liver lysosomes and smooth endoplasmic reticulum induced by the diazofluorathen derivative AC-3579. II Effects of the drug on phospholipid metabolism. *Lab Invest* 1973; **28:** 83–86.
12. Brosnan FC, Bunge MB, Murray MR. The response of lysosomes in cultured neurons to chlorpromazine. *J Neuropath Exp Neurol* 1970; **29:** 337–353.
13. Drenckhahn D, Kleine L, Lullmann-Rauch R. Lysosomal alterations in cultured macrophages exposed to anorexigenic and psychotropic drugs. *Lab Invest* 1976; **35:** 116–123.
14. MacDonald RD, Engel AG. Experimental chloroquine myopathy. *J Neuropath Exp Neurol* 1970; **29:** 479–499.
15. Matsuzawa Y, Hostetler KY. Inhibition of lysosomal phospholipase A and phospholipase C by chloroquine and 4,4′-*bis* (diethyl-aminoethoxy) diethyldiphenylethane. *J Biol Chem* 1980; **255:** 5190–5194.
16. Albouz S, Boutry J-M, Dubois G, Bourdon R, Hauw JJ, Baumann N. Lipid and lysosomal enzymes in human fibroblasts cultured with perhexiline maleate. *Naunyn-Schiedeberg's Arch Pharmacol* 1981; **317**: 173–177.
17. Sakuragawa N, Sakuragawa M, Kuwabara T, Pentchev PG, Barranger JA, Brady RO. Niemann–Pick disease experimental model: sphingomyelinase reduction-induced by AY-9944. *Science* 1977; **196:** 317–319.
18. Jacobs JM, Costa-Jussà FR. Human and experimental amiodarone neuropathy. *Neuropath Appl Neurobiol* 1983; **9:** 332 (Abstract).
19. Sobol SM. Amiodarone pulmonary toxicity (in discussion). *Amer Heart J* 1983; **106:** 915.
20. Corrin B, King E. Experimental endogenous lipid pneumonia and silicosis. *J Path* 1969; **97:** 325–330.
21. Darmanata JI, van Zandwijk N, van Royen EA, Mooi WJ, Plomp TA, Jansen HM, Durrer D. Amiodarone pneumonitis: three further cases with a review of published reports. *Thorax* 1984; **39:** 57–64.

JOURNAL OF PATHOLOGY, VOL. **144:** 81–87 (1984)

IMPROVED CHIMAERIC MOUSE MODEL CONFIRMS THAT RESIDENT PERITONEAL MACROPHAGES ARE DERIVED SOLELY FROM BONE MARROW PRECURSORS

A. R. MURCH, MIRANDA D. GROUNDS AND J. M. PAPADIMITRIOU

Department of Pathology, University of Western Australia, Queen Elizabeth II Medical Centre, Nedlands 6009, Western Australia, Australia

Received 6 February 1984
Accepted 29 March 1984

SUMMARY

The origin of resident peritoneal macrophages was studied in radiation mouse chimaeras with and without reconstitution of the peritoneum with viable isogeneic peritoneal cells. The selection of host and donor strains were such that the isoenzymes of glucose-6-phosphate isomerase could be used to distinguish host from donor bone marrow derived cells. It was found that the resident peritoneal macrophages were completely replaced by bone marrow donor derived cells within 5–6 weeks. There was little difference between the results from mice which had been additionally reconstituted with peritoneal cells and those which were not.

KEY WORDS—Peritoneal macrophages, radiation mouse chimaeras.

INTRODUCTION

While there is general agreement that exudate peritoneal macrophages are derived directly from circulating monocytes,[1,2] the origin of resident peritoneal macrophages is still in question. Two theories have been proposed: one suggests that resident peritoneal macrophages form a separate, self-replicating population (see Daems[2] for a review), while the other proposes that resident macrophages, like exudate macrophages, originate in the bone marrow, and are continuously replenished from that source (see van Furth[1] for a review).

The use of radiation chimaeras to study the origin of peritoneal macrophages[3–6] has provided strong support for the theory of bone marrow origin. In these experiments the bone marrow of irradiated hosts was replaced with donor marrow from a different strain. In the peritoneum of such chimaeras donor macrophages steadily replaced resident host macrophages over a period of about 6 weeks, until finally only donor macrophages could be identified in the resident population. The weakness of these experiments is that any potential population of dividing host cells in the peritoneum will have been destroyed by irradiation. In addition, cell markers used to distinguish host from donor macrophages in these studies were not entirely satisfactory: Virolainen[5] used the cytogenetic marker, T_6, which can only differentiate between dividing cells and thus is selective; Balner,[3] and Goodman[4] distinguished cells from two strains of mice using the cytotoxic activity of specific antisera where non-specific death of some cells can be a complicating factor, and Haller *et al.*[6] used differences in genetically determined susceptibility to murine influenza virus.

In the present experiments the criticisms of the radiation chimaera model are overcome by replacing irradiated host peritoneal cells with healthy isogeneic peritoneal cells and a different cell marker is employed. The mouse strains used were each homozygous for one of the two isoenzyme

0022–3417/84/100081–07$01.00

forms of glucose-6-phosphate isomerase (GPI; E.C. 5.2.1.9) which enables cells of the two strains to be identified by distinct isoenzyme mobilities on starch gel electrophoresis. GPI isoenzymes are effective markers for the nuclei which code for them and have been widely used as cells markers.[7,8] By injecting donor bone marrow cells from animals homozygous for one GPI isoenzyme into host animals homozygous for the other form, it was possible to determine whether resident peritoneal macrophages are an independent self-perpetuating cell population or are replaced by circulating bone marrow derived cells.

METHODS

The mouse strains C3H (homozygous for the electrophoretically fast GPI isoenzyme) and AKR (homozygous for the slow isoenzyme) were maintained as inbred colonies: these strains are compatible (H-2k) at the H-2 locus.[9] All experimental animals were 10–12-week-old males.

Whole body irradiation (800 rads, Siemens deep x-ray; 200 kV; 1 mm Cu half value layer; 0·5 Cu filter; 83·2 rad/min) was given to unanaesthetized mice in a lidded Perspex box. Experimental animals were divided into two groups designated A and B: group A had only bone marrow reconstitution, whereas group B had bone marrow and peritoneal cell reconstitution. AKR bone marrow cells (and in mice of group B also C3H peritoneal cells) were injected within four hours of irradiation. Marrow cells were obtained from mice by syringing thoroughly cleaned femurs with phosphate buffered saline, pH 7·1 (PBS). Cells were washed once with PBS, passed through Miracloth (Calbiochem) to remove clumps, and approximately 5×10^6 cells in 0·2 ml PBS injected into tail veins of irradiated C3H mice.

Peritoneal cells, rich in resident macrophages (typically 60 per cent macrophages and 35 per cent lymphoid cells[10]) were obtained by washing peritoneal cavities of C3H mice with 2 ml PBS. Cells were concentrated by centrifugation, and injected in 0·5 ml PBS into the peritoneal cavity of C3H mice (group B). Cells from two donor mice were used for each host (approximately $2–4 \times 10^6$ cells). Poor survival of many mice beyond 20 days was attributed to mild 'graft versus graft' disease, resulting from C3H lymphocytes in the injected peritoneal washings interfering with reconstitution by AKR marrow cells. To circumvent this problem, another group of 10 mice (designated B* in Table II) were injected with a purified population of peritoneal macrophages. Peritoneal washings were settled in a Petri dish for 2 h, adherent macrophages washed by pipetting PBS vigorously over the surface of the dish to remove loosely attached lymphocytes, then macrophages scraped off with a rubber policeman, washed and concentrated by centrifugation for injection as above. Dye exclusion tests using trypan blue showed that approximately 40 per cent of the macrophages obtained this way were viable. Each animal received approximately 2×10^5 viable macrophages.

At varying times after irradiation, mice were killed by cervical dislocation. To obtain bone marrow cells, one femur was thoroughly cleaned of adherent tissue, cut longitudinally, and the marrow scraped out directly on to a small piece of Whatman No. 1 filter paper (approximately 1×5 mm). Peritoneal cells were lavaged with 2 ml PBS and in many instances peritoneal cells from paired mice were pooled. Cells were pelleted, resuspended in culture medium consisting of MEM (Flow Laboratories, Sydney) +10 per cent fetal calf serum (Flow Laboratories, Sydney), and allowed to settle in 35 mm Petri dishes at 37°C for either 4 h or overnight. The supernatant was pipetted vigorously over the surface to remove loosely attached cells, spun, and this cell pellet collected on to a piece of filter paper. Peritoneal macrophages adhering to the Petri dish[11] were rinsed twice with PBS, scraped off with a rubber policeman, spun and the pellet collected on to a piece of filter paper. Samples were stored in sealed containers at −20°C.

Pieces of filter paper were inserted directly into an 11 per cent starch gel, and electrophoretic separation and visualization of GPI isoenzyme bands was performed as described by Grounds *et al.*[12] The relative proportions of fast and slow isoenzyme bands were visually graded and band size indicated on a scale from (+) to + + + + +; where no isoenzyme band was detected, this was indicated by −.

A control experiment was set up to determine whether injected macrophages remained in the peritoneum or were rapidly dispersed or destroyed. Three C3H mice were irradiated as in the other experiments, and approximately 2×10^5 settled AKR macrophages were injected into the peritoneum. At 6 days (before the mice began to die of radiation effects) the peritoneal cells were collected, and macrophages separated for electrophoresis as before.

RESULTS

Isoenzyme patterns of mice were examined from 3 to 61 days after irradiation. The results of 37 mice from five experiments are shown in Tables I and II: 24 mice (group A) were reconstituted with AKR bone marrow (Table I), and 13 mice (group B) with AKR bone marrow and C3H peritoneal cells (Table II).

Bone marrow

GPI isoenzyme patterns of irradiated C3H bone marrow reconstituted with AKR cells were similar in all mice (Tables I and II). AKR isoenzyme was not detected at day 3, but was present by day 5 (Fig. 1, A_3). The proportion of AKR isoenzyme increased rapidly and was usually equal to, or greater than that of host C3H isoenzyme by day 7 (Fig. 1, A_5). From day 7 the small amount of host isoenzyme present in bone marrow samples (Fig. 1, B_8) was attributed to persisting host red blood cells which, unlike white blood cells, are known to survive for several months after irradiation.[13]

Non-adherent peritoneal cells

Non-adherent cells from the peritoneum of mice are largely lymphocytes (85 per cent) with occasional polymorphs, mast cells and degenerate mesothelial cells.[10] In group A, where peritoneal cells were not replaced after irradiation, bone marrow derived AKR isoenzyme was not detected in samples of non-adherent cells examined at 3 or 5 days, and only a trace amount was visible in one of two samples examined at day 7. However, by day 15, AKR isoenzyme predominated. The small proportion of host isoenzyme present in samples after this time was probably due to contaminating red blood cells since these were always seen in peritoneal washings. Host C3H isoenzyme had almost disappeared by day 49.

In group B, where mice were reconstituted with C3H peritoneal cells, isoenzyme patterns similar to

Table I—(Group A) Isoenzyme results of irradiated C3H mice reconstituted with AKR bone marrow

Mouse	Days after irradiation	GPI isoenzyme patterns: Bone marrow		Non-adherent peritoneal cells		Peritoneal macrophages	
		C3H	AKR	C3H	AKR	C3H	AKR
$*A_1$	3	+++	−				
A_1	3	+++	−	+	−	−	−
$*A_2$	5	++	+				
A_2	5	++	+	+++	−	+	−
$*A_3$	5	++	+				
A_3	5	+++	+	+++	−	−	−
A_4	7	+	++	+	−	+	(+)
$*A_5$	7	++	++				
A_5	7	+++	+++	++	(+)	++	−
A_6	9	+	++	++	+	(+)	−
$*A_7$	10	++	++				
A_7	10	+	+++	++	+	++	+
A_8	12	+	+++	+	+	+	+
A_9	15	+	+++	(+)	++	(+)	+
A_{10}	21	+	+++	(+)	+	+	++
$*A_{11}$	24	+	+++				
A_{11}	24	+	+++	+	+++	+	+++
A_{12}	31	++	+++++	−	+	+	+++
A_{13}	35	+	++++	+	+++	−	+++
A_{14}	38	++	+++++	−	+	−	+++
$*A_{15}$	49	++	+++				
A_{15}	49	+	++	(+)	+++	−	−
$*A_{16}$	61	+	++				
A_{16}	61	−	++	−	++	−	(+)

*In these samples peritoneal cells from two mice were pooled to increase isoenzyme detection in macrophages and non-adherent cells. Bone marrow samples from the individual mice were run separately.

Table II—(Group B) Isoenzyme results or irradiated C3H mice reconstituted with AKR bone marrow and with C3H peritoneal cells

Mouse	Days after irradiation	GPI isoenzyme patterns: Bone marrow C3H	Bone marrow AKR	Non-adherent peritoneal cells C3H	Non-adherent peritoneal cells AKR	Peritoneal macrophages C3H	Peritoneal macrophages AKR
B_1	7	++	+++	+	(+)	++	+
B_2	9	++	+++	++	++	(+)	−
B_3	12	++	++++	+	+	+++	+++
B_4	15	+	++++	++	++	++	++
B_5	20	++	++++	++	++	+	+
B_6*	21	++	++++	+	++	+	++
B_7	34	+	+++	++	++	++	++
B_8	35	(+)	+++++	++	+++	+	+++
B_9	40	++	++++	++	+++	−	+++
B_{10}*	42	++	+++++	(+)	++	+	+++
B_{11}	47	++	+++++	+	+++	−	+++
B_{12}*	49	+	+++++	+	++	−	+
B_{13}*	56	+	+++++	(+)	+++	−	++

* Series B with purified peritoneal macrophages.

group A were found up to day 12. From day 15 the proportion of C3H isoenzyme was higher than in group A (Fig. 1, day 35 cf. B_8 with A_{13}) and this was attributed directly to implanted C3H cells, particularly lymphocytes. The poor survival of mice in this series beyond day 20 was probably also due to these viable C3H lymphocytes resulting in mild 'graft versus graft' reaction. In group B* where mice were reconstituted with purified peritoneal macrophages containing few or no lymphocytes, there were few deaths, and samples of non-adherent cells contained a smaller proportion of C3H isoenzyme (Table II, cf. B_6 with B_5) and were similar to group A (cf. Tables II and I, B_6 and A_{10}).

Peritoneal macrophages

More than 90 per cent of peritoneal cells adhering to a Petri dish are macrophages.[11] Bone marrow derived AKR macrophages were not detected in the peritoneum before day 7 and even at this time were not found in one of three samples. In some early samples of peritoneal macrophages little or no GPI activity was detected, which was the result of excessive lysing of macrophages and consequent loss of enzyme during collection. This was corrected by more gentle cell collection. In group A, the proportion of AKR isoenzyme was greater than C3H isoenzyme from day 15. A small amount of C3H isoenzyme was detected up to day 31, but by day 35 only AKR isoenzyme was present (Fig. 1, A_{13} cf. B_8), indicating that irradiated C3H macrophages do not survive beyond this time.

In group B, where peritoneal macrophages were replenished with viable C3H cells, the proportion of C3H macrophages was high, as expected. In contrast to group A, similar amounts of C3H and AKR isoenzyme were present from days 12 to 34, although, there were only traces of C3H isoenzyme in samples collected after this time. The time of disappearance varied slightly between animals: though not detected in samples taken at day 40, 47, or 49, C3H isoenzyme was present in one sample at day 42 (Table II).

In control C3H mice injected with purified AKR peritoneal macrophages but without AKR marrow reconstitution, peritoneal macrophages collected 6 days after transplantation showed equal proportions of AKR and C3H GPI isoenzyme indicating that donor macrophages remained in the peritoneum for at least this period.

DISCUSSION

The results show that in both groups of mice (A and B) there is steady replacement of C3H peritoneal macrophages by bone marrow derived AKR cells from about day 7 (when marrow transplants begin to take) until day 35 (Group A) or after day 42 (Group B) when only AKR cells were detec-

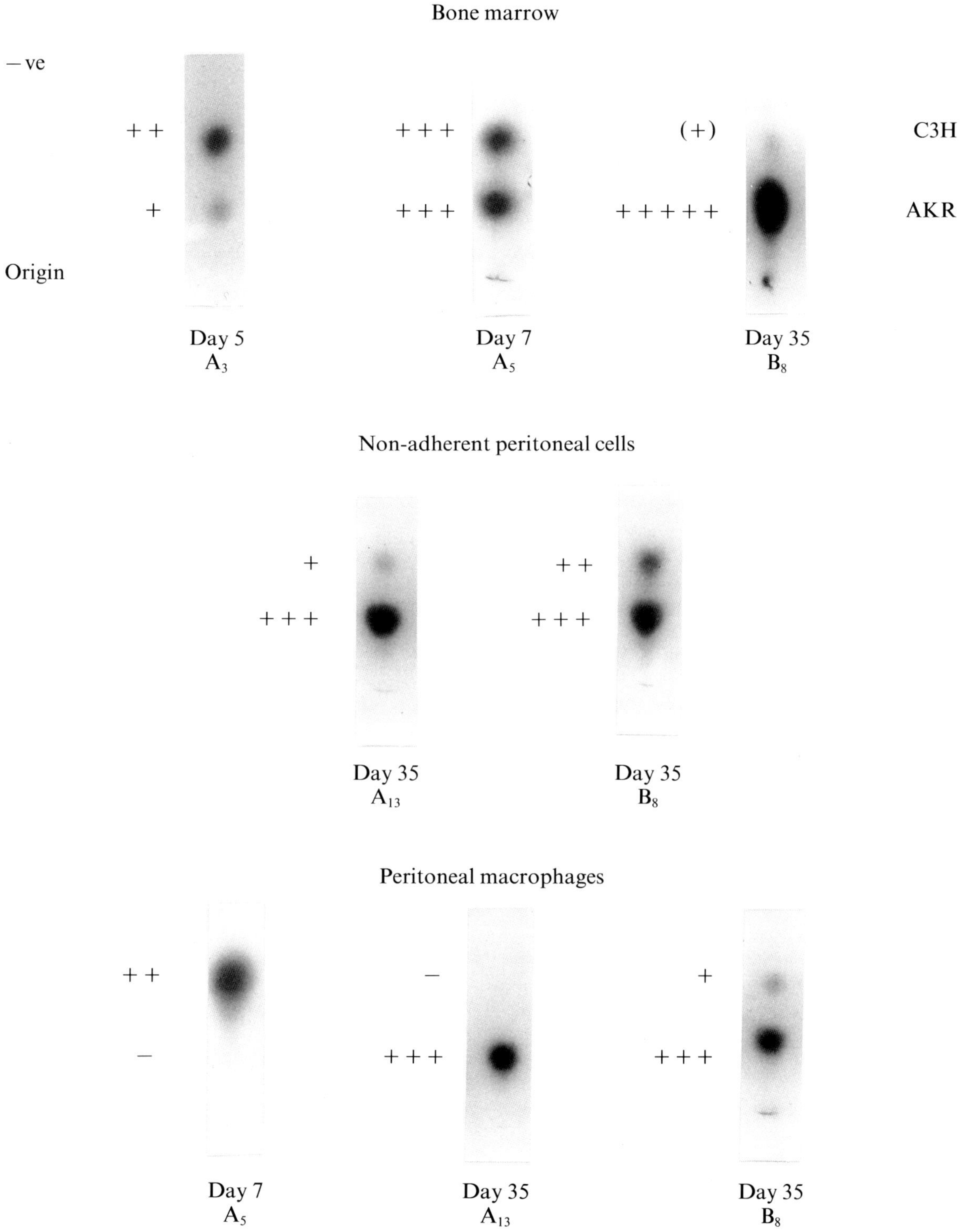

Fig. 1—Starch gel electrophoresis patterns of GPI isoenzymes. (See Tables I and II and text for details)

ted. The disappearance of C3H peritoneal macrophages in Group B, where healthy peritoneal cells were injected into the peritoneum following irradiation, shows that dividing cells of the peritoneum do not significantly contribute to this population of resident macrophages. This is an important finding since previous work using radiation chimaeras (see Introduction) can be criticized on the basis that the capacity of possible host macrophage precursors in the peritoneum to divide would have been destroyed by irradiation. One possible objection to the present experiments is that an inadequate number of cells may have been used to repopulate the irradiated peritoneum. The total number of cells in the murine peritoneum in the normal steady state is not known, nor is the proportion of progenitor cells (if any), but the $2–4 \times 10^6$ cells injected in the present experiments closely approximates the number of cells which can be obtained by thorough washing of the peritoneum.[2] Even if the number of precursor cells reinjected is significantly lower than the number present in the normal steady state, they would still be expected to contribute to the repopulation of the peritoneum. Moreover, the electrophoretic technique used is sensitive enough to detect even a very small contribution. That the transplanted peritoneal macrophages remain viable in the peritoneum for at least 6 days is demonstrated by the significant amounts of AKR isoenzyme detected in irradiated C3H mice injected with AKR peritoneal macrophages but without AKR bone marrow transplants. The disappearance of C3H peritoneal macrophages by day 35 in group A compared to about day 42 in group B suggests that irradiation shortens the life of resident macrophages.

Our results lend no support to the idea that macrophages resident in the peritoneal cavity are a predominantly self-replenishing population (review, Daems[2]). It should be noted that the use of radiation chimaeras does leave open the possibility that resident macrophages might derive from stem cells lying within tissues of the peritoneum, such as the omentum milky spots: any contribution of such dividing cells would be prevented by irradiation and would not be overcome by reconstitution with healthy peritoneal washings. Available evidence suggests that milky spot cells which give rise to resident peritoneal macrophages, are in turn derived from blood-borne monocytes from the marrow, however, the possibility of a milky spot macrophage stem cell has not been excluded.[14,15]

In conclusion, these results confirm those of Balner[3] and show that in the mouse, resident peritoneal macrophages are of bone marrow origin, and that they turn over completely within a period of 5–6 weeks.

ACKNOWLEDGEMENT

This work was supported by grants from the National Health and Medical Research Council of Australia.

REFERENCES

1. van Furth R, Diesselhoff-den Dulk Martina MC, Raeburn, JA, van Zwet TL, Crofton R, Blusse van Oude Alblas A. Characteristics, origin and kinetics of human and murine mononuclear phagocytes. In: van Furth R, ed. Mononuclear phagocytes: Functional Aspects. The Hague 1980: 279.
2. Daems WT. Peritoneal macrophages. In: Carr I, Daems WT, eds. The Reticuloendothelial System: A Comprehensive Treatise. Vol. 1. New York 1980: 57.
3. Balner H. Identification of peritoneal macrophages in mouse radiation chimeras. *Transplantation* 1963; **1:** 217.
4. Goodman JW. On the origin of peritoneal fluid cells. *Blood* 1964; **23:** 18.
5. Virolainen M. Hematopoietic origin of macrophages as studied by chromosome markers in mice. *J Exp Med* 1968; **127:** 943.
6. Haller O, Arnheiter H, Lindenmann J. Natural genetically determined resistance towards influenza virus in hemopoietic mouse chimeras: role of mononuclear phagocytes. *J Exp Med* 1979; **150:** 117.
7. Chapman VM, Whitten WK, Ruddle FH. Expression of paternal glucose phosphate isomerase (GPI-1) in pre-implantation stages of mouse embryo. *Devel Biol* 1971; **26:** 153.
8. Murch AR, Grounds Miranda D, Marshall CA, Papadimitriou JM. Direct evidence that inflammatory multinucleate giant cells form by fusion. *J Path* 1981; **137:** 177.
9. Staats Joan. Standard nomenclature for inbred strains of mice: sixth listing. *Cancer Res* 1976; **36:** 4333.
10. Carr I. The Macrophage. London: 1973: 6.
11. Mosier DE. Separation of murine macrophages by adherence to solid substrates. In: Adams DO, Edelson PJ, Koren H, eds. Methods for Studying Mononuclear Phagocytes. New York 1981: 179.
12. Grounds Miranda D, Partridge TA, Sloper JC. The contribution of exogenous cells to regenerating skeletal muscle: an isoenzyme study of muscle allografts in mice. *J Path* 1980; **132:** 325.
13. Grounds Miranda D. Skeletal muscle precursors do not arise from bone marrow cells. *Cell Tissue Res* 1983; **234:** 713.

14. Beelen RJH, Fluitsma DM, Hoefsmit ECM. The cellular composition of omentum milky spots and the ultrastructure of milky spot macrophages and reticulum cells. *J Reticuloendothel Soc* 1980a; **28:** 585.

15. Beelen RJH, Fluitsma DM, Hoefsmit ECM. Peroxidatic activity of mononuclear phagocytes developing in omentum milky spots. *J Reticuloendothel Soc* 1980b; **28:** 601.

JOURNAL OF PATHOLOGY, VOL. **144**: 89–100 (1984)

THE CUMULATIVE SCANNING ELECTRON MICROSCOPIC CHANGES IN BABY MOUSE LUNGS FOLLOWING PRENATAL AND POSTNATAL EXPOSURES TO NICOTINE

NAI-SAN WANG, MOY-FONG CHEN AND DEAN E. SCHRAUFNAGEL

McGill University, Department of Pathology, Lyman Duff Medical Sciences Building, 3775 University Street, Montreal, P.Q. H3A 2B4, Canada

AND

YU-TUNG YAO

Department of Pathology, National Taiwan University School of Medicine, Taipei, Taiwan

Received 22 March 1984
Accepted 2 April 1984

SUMMARY

Half of the offspring from nicotine exposed and control mother mice were cross-fostered at birth to form four groups of those exposed to nicotine only during the gestational period (NC), only during the lactational period (CN), throughout both periods (NN), or exposed to none (CC). Nodular mucosal bulges (neuroepithelial bodies, NEB) were found in all groups; their number decreased with the increase in the age in the control group (CC). The bulges were large and irregular in all nicotine exposed groups, especially in the NN group. Although they also decreased in number with age, NEB were significantly retained and abnormal in the NN group compared with the NC and CC groups on day 30 ($p < 0{\cdot}01$). In addition, the bronchioles were tortuous in the nicotine exposed groups probably due to the expansion of mucosal depressions, pits, and fenestrations. In mice, maternal exposures to a small dosage of nicotine throughout both gestational and lactating periods appear to induce more baby lung changes than when the exposure to nicotine is limited to either period alone. More importantly, nicotine induced baby lung changes observed on day 5 appear to regress by day 30, if the exposure to nicotine is discontinued at birth.

KEY WORDS—Nicotine toxicity, mouse lungs, lung development.

INTRODUCTION

The rate of office visits and hospital admissions of children from smoking mothers is significantly higher than that of children from non-smoking mothers, mainly due to the increase in the incidence of bronchitis and pneumonia during the first year of life.[1–3] Acute and prolonged impairments of lung functions of the former have also been reported.[4] Most studies, however, cannot differentiate the effect of smoking during pregnancy and the effect of the infant's or child's passive exposure to cigarette smoke after birth.[5]

Among the many compounds present in the cigarette smoke, nicotine, carbon monoxide and the polycyclic aromatic hydrocarbons are most likely to affect the fetus and placenta;[6] nicotine probably crosses the placenta most readily although all three accumulate in the fetus and placenta.[7–9] The structural alterations induced by these agents, the morphological aspects of the functional impairments, are largely unknown. We have previously shown that maternal oral intake of nicotine in mice

Supported in part by the Medical Research Council of Canada and The Quebec Thoracic Society.

Addressee for correspondence and reprints: Dr Nai-San Wang, Associate Professor of Pathology, Department of Pathology, McGill University, Lyman Duff Medical Sciences Building, 3775 University Street, Montreal, P.Q. H3A 2B4, Canada.

0022–3417/84/100089–12$01.20

throughout the gestational and lactating periods do not alter the number of alveoli in the fetal and baby mice. The bronchi and bronchioles of the offspring, however, show some tortuosity with an increase in the number of mucosal nodular bulges (neuroepithelial bodies, NEB) at the branching site, and pits and depressions in the small bronchioles.[10] In this study we compared the pulmonary changes of mouse babies following maternal oral intake of low dose nicotine during gestational, lactating or both periods.

MATERIAL AND METHODS

Sixteen female Charles River white mice were fed with lab chow. Eight received tap water *ad lib* and another eight received tap water with 1 mg/l nicotine, prepared daily, all through the experimental period. The amount drunk was recorded daily.

Following observation for 2 weeks on the above-mentioned regime, the female mice were mated with untreated male mice. Baby mice were cross-fostered within 24 h of their birth between four mothers in the non-nicotine and four mothers in the nicotine fed groups. Thus, four litters of baby mice formed each of the following groups.

(A) Baby mice who remained with their own non-nicotine mother (control, CC).

(B) Baby mice from a nicotine mother fostered by a non-nicotine mother (NC).

(C) Baby mice from a non-nicotine mother fostered by a nicotine mother (CN).

(D) Baby mice who remained with their own nicotine mother (NN).

Eight control mother mice formed group E (MC) and eight nicotine mother mice formed group F (MN).

All animals were weighed three times weekly. Baby mice were killed on days 5, 15, and 30 by pentobarbital injections. Mother mice were also sacrificed on day 30 postpartum. The lungs were fixed by intratracheal inflation of 3 per cent glutaraldehyde in 0·1 M sodium cacodylate buffer at pH 7·4, or 4 per cent formaldehyde in phosphate buffered saline at 10 cm (day 5), or 20 cm (days 15 and 30) H_2O pressure for 18–24 h. The lung volume was obtained after inflation fixation, by the method of Scherle.[11] The lungs were sliced coronally at 1 to 2 mm thickness.

For light microscopy (LM) all right lung slices from each animal were processed routinely and embedded in paraffin. Sections (7 μm thick) were stained with haematoxylin and eosin. For scanning electron microscopy 2–3 slices of the left lower lobe (LLL) from each animal were dehydrated with graded acetone and dried with CO_2 using the critical point method.[12] The dried tissues were coated with a 20 nm layer in gold and examined with a scanning electron microscope (SEM). For transmission electron microscopy (TEM) glutaraldehyde-fixed tissues (LLL) and 4–6 blocks of lungs already examined with the SEM from all groups at each age were processed as before.[13]

The maturation of the baby lung was assessed by counting the number of alveolar intercepts on a straight line, marked on the eye piece of a light microscope, placed from a terminal bronchiole perpendicular to the nearest lobular septum or pleura, modified from the method of Emery and Mithal.[10,14] At least four well-delineated terminal bronchioles were evaluated in each lung slice (a total of 12 or more per case) at × 100 magnification.

With the SEM, the bronchial surface was surveyed; the number of mucosal nodular bulges was recorded using the number of bronchi branching sites as the denominator. The surface depressions and fenestrations were assessed and the number of macrophages in each well-delineated terminal bronchiole was recorded. Data obtained from different groups were compared using the Student *t*-test.

The morphology of Clara, ciliated and other cells, both on the mucosal surface as well as in the interstitium, especially those in the bulges and the bronchioloalveolar junction, were evaluated with a TEM.

RESULTS

The total number of baby mice was 171, ranging between 42 and 44 offspring from four mother mice in each group. No baby mice were lost during the cross-fostering or thereafter. The mother mice drank 10–15 ml of water per day. No difference in the amount drunk was noted between groups or before or after delivery in the same group.

Lung volumes and body weights

The lung volumes and body weights are shown in Table I. The body weights are similar between groups at the same age, including the mother mice, except in the group D (NN) on day 30. The lung volume was slightly small in group B (NC) on day

Table I—The lung volume and body weight afer 5, 15 and 30 days

Group	5 days V	5 days BW	5 days V/BW	15 days V	15 days BW	15 days V/BW	30 days V	30 days BW	30 days V/BW
(A) C-C	0·26±0·07	3·29±0·58(14)	7·95	0·49±0·08	9·78±0·74(14)	5·02	1·21±0·06	25·17± 3.20(14)†	4·81
(B) N-C	0·21±0·05	3·24±0·37(13)	6·48	0·46±0·04	9·48±0·71(15)	4·83	1·24±0·05	25·12± 2·51(16)	4.94
(C) C-N	0·24±0·03	3·14±0·53(13)	7·63	0·47±0·04	9·81±0·83(14)	4·78	1·23±0·05	24·57± 2·16(15)	4·99
(D) N-N	0·26±0·04	3·23±0·26(12)	7·92	0·49±0·04	9·58±0·87(15)	5·12	1·22±0·05	22·83± 2·12(16)†	5·36
(E) MC*							1·37±0·05	36·85± 1·45(8)	3·72
(F) MN*							1·43±0·05	37·29± 2·56(8)	3·83

Average and standard deviation.
Number of baby mice in parentheses.
V_l, Lung volume in mm³.
BW, Body weight in grams.
* Mother mice killed on day 30 postpartum.
† $p<0{\cdot}05$.
For C-C, N-C, C-N, and N-N, MC, and MN, please see Material and Methods.

5 but became comparable with other groups on days 15 and 30. No difference in lung volumes was noted between the two groups of mother mice.

Alveolar intercepts and light microscopy

The number of alveolar intercepts almost doubled between days 5 and 15, and increased approximately 1·25 times between days 15 and 30 in all baby groups (Table II). The number of intercepts of baby mice on day 30 was comparable with that of mother mice.

No overt bronchiolitis or emphysematous changes were found in any baby lungs. The bronchial and bronchiolar walls were more undulant in the nicotine-exposed groups; they were mostly straight in the control groups.

SEM findings

In the control groups (CC), the surface of large bronchi showed a high ratio of ciliated to non-ciliated cells. Focal mucosal dome-shaped elevations 20–30 μm in diameter were present mainly at the bronchial or bronchiolar bifurcations and occasionally also between bifurcations (neuroepithelial bodies, NEB) (Figs 1a, b). The surface of the NEB was non-ciliated with loosely scattered microvilli. Cells with a smaller surface area on NEB usually showed crowded microvilli.[15] NEB were most frequent on day 5; the number decreased by day 15 and they were rare at day 30 (Table III).

Table II—The number of alveolar intercepts after 5, 15 and 30 days

Group	5 days	15 days	30 days
(A) C-C	4·75±2·06	7·59±1·66	9·16±2·17
(B) N-C	4·02±0·97	8·17±1·06	10·20±2·10
(C) C-N	4.06±0·99	7·91±1·27	10·42±2·04
(D) N-N	4·13±0·57	7·88±0·78	9.23±1·99
(E) M-C			10·61±2.50
(F) M-N			10·22±2·15

Average and standard deviation.
Please see Material and Methods for the groups.

The small bronchioles in the control groups (CC) resembled branching straight tubules with smooth walls. The ciliated cells were reticular around the protruded cellular processes of Clara cells reaching the bronchioloalveolar junction. The transition from the bronchiolar to alveolar epithelium was abrupt, forming a straight or slightly curved line (Fig. 2a). One, occasionally more, macrophages were found in approximately half of terminal bronchioles of all ages in the control group (Table III).

In all nicotine groups (B, C, D) slight tortuosity of bronchial walls and focal loss of ciliated cells were found; some of the non-ciliated areas were slightly elevated from the bronchial surface. Focal surface unevenness, transverse ridges, and dilatation were more common in the small bronchioles, especially in group D (NN) on days 15 and 30 (Fig. 2b). Although the number of NEB also decreased with the increase in age, as in the control group A (CC) (Table III), there were significant differences in their numbers between group D (NN) and group A on days 5 and 30, and also between groups D and B (NC) on day 30 ($p<0{\cdot}01$). NEB were frequently found in pairs near the inlet of a bronchus. They appeared to be slightly altered in groups B (NC), and C (CN), but were most bizarre in shape, larger than 50 μm in size with ciliated cells,

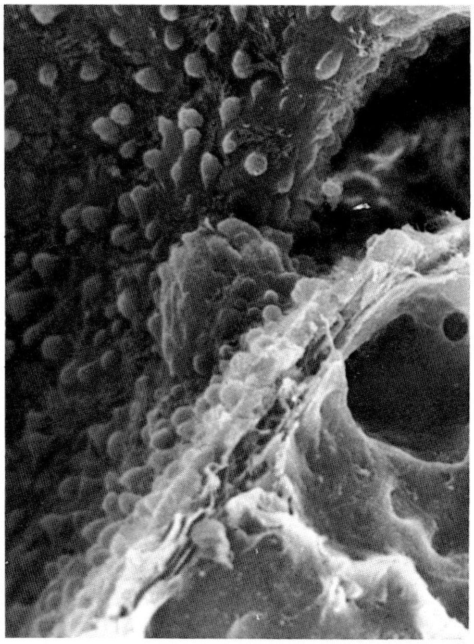

(a)

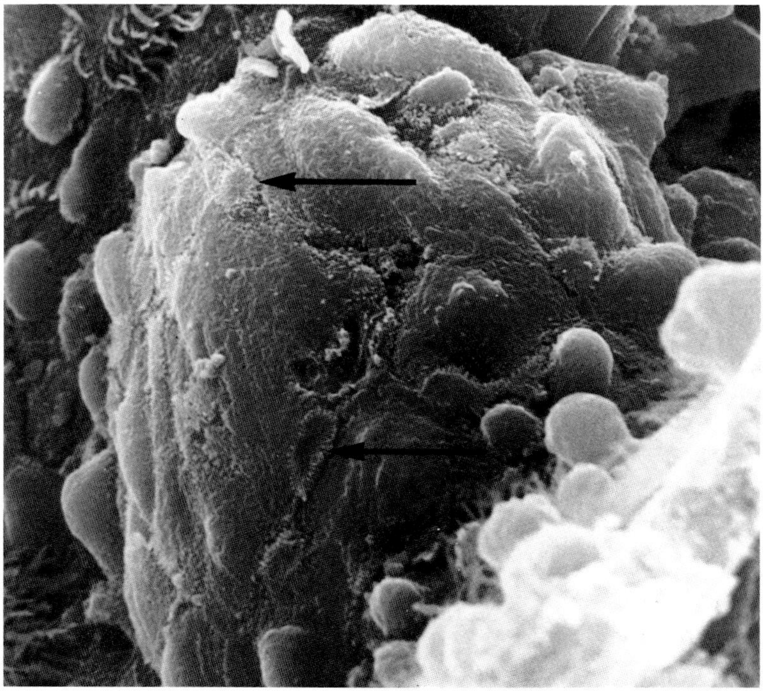

(b)

Fig. 1—A dome-shaped bulge (neuroepithelial body, NEB) at the bronchial bifurcation of a control mouse. Microvilli are sparse but appear to concentrate more on the neuroendocrine cell with smaller cellular surface area (arrows). SEM group A (CC) day 5 (a) × 630; (b) × 3416

Table III—The changes in the bronchus and bronchiole and 5, 15 and 30 days

	Macrophages*			Bulge†		
Group	5 days	15 days	30 days	5 days	15 days	30 days
(A) C-C	0·44±0·16	0·66±0·37	0·40±0·17‡	1·28±0·32‡	0·86±0·55	0·17±0·17§
(B) N-C	0·61±0·32	0·68±0·25	0·92±0·33‡	1·58±0·27	0·96±0·79	0·18±0·21§
(C) C-N	0·38±0·20	0·54±0·11	0·71±0·34‡	1·13±0·25	0·84±0·19	0·34±0·28
(D) N-N	0·35±0·33	0·75±0·48	1·16±0·34‡	1·83±0·92‡	1·00±0·32	0·51±0·37§

Average and standard deviation.
*The number of macrophages per terminal bronchiole.
†Per bronchial bifurcation.
‡$p<0.01$ between groups B, C, or D and group A.
§$p<0.01$ between groups D and A or B.

in group D (NN) (Figs 3, 4). Pits and depressions were common in association with the bizarre bulge. Rare, small bulges were found in only two out of eight nicotine fed mother mice.

Depressions, pits, and fenestrations of the terminal bronchiole appeared small in the control group (Fig. 2a). The depressions and fenestrations in the nicotine groups varied in size and shape; some appeared to be in the process of fusing with each other (Fig. 2b). The surface of some large depressions showed capillaries and resembled the surface of alveoli. Macrophages were generally rare although their numbers were significantly increased in all nicotine exposed groups on day 30 (Table III). They were frequently found adjacent to depressions of fenestrations. In the nicotine exposed groups, islands of Clara and ciliated cells were away from the proximal bronchiole resulting in an irregular bronchioloalveolar junction. Pits, depressions and fenestrations were rare in the terminal bronchioles of all adult mouse lungs.

TEM findings

Neuroepithelial bodies were confirmed on all bulges originally localized by a SEM and then reprocessed and studied by a TEM (Figs 5a, b). Because of the double processing, some fine structural details, especially cell membranes, were less than ideal. Isolated neuroendocrine (NE) cells were, however, found in random TEM specimens. The NEB in the control mice were formed by a combination of non-ciliated Clara cells and NE cells with cytoplasmic 'neurosecretory granules' and fibrils (Figs 5a, 6a). Nerve-like structures were occasionally seen. The bizarre shaped NEB in nicotine-treated baby mice were sometimes pedunculated (Fig. 5b) and had more cells than normal NEB, including ciliated cells and poorly-differentiated cells with ovoid or notched nuclei and scanty organelles (Fig. 6b). Isolated epithelial cell necrosis and detachment, and neutrophils or lymphocytes were occasionally present in the bronchial and bronchiolar mucosa.

The interstitium beneath the bulge usually showed closely abutted smooth muscle bundles in cross-section, fibroblast-like cells, nerve bundles, and small vessels. The muscle bundles appeared hyperplastic in the nicotine-treated groups. Neutrophils, mast cells and lymphocytes were rare but probably slightly increased in number in the nicotine-treated groups.

The depressions, pits, and larger fenestrations seen by SEM were found to be either focal flattening or thinning of the bronchial lining cells or various sized bronchioloalveolar communications by TEM. Capillaries were identified in the depressions seen by SEM. Complete denudation of the lining cells exposing the interstitium to the air was not seen. The occasional macrophages, seen by SEM, were confirmed with the TEM. They were usually adjacent to fenestrae or mucosal bulges.

DISCUSSION

We found an increased number of large and bizarre shaped nodular mucosal bulges (NEB) in the bronchi and bronchioles of baby mice, in our previous study, following maternal oral intake of a relatively large dose of nicotine.[10] These findings were confirmed in this study despite the relatively low dose of nicotine, and despite the fact that the maternal weights, litter sizes, and birth weights of the offspring were unaffected. A significant increase in the number of NEB and bizarre changes in these were, however, found only in group D (NN) at day 30; by then the baby mice were exposed to nicotine all

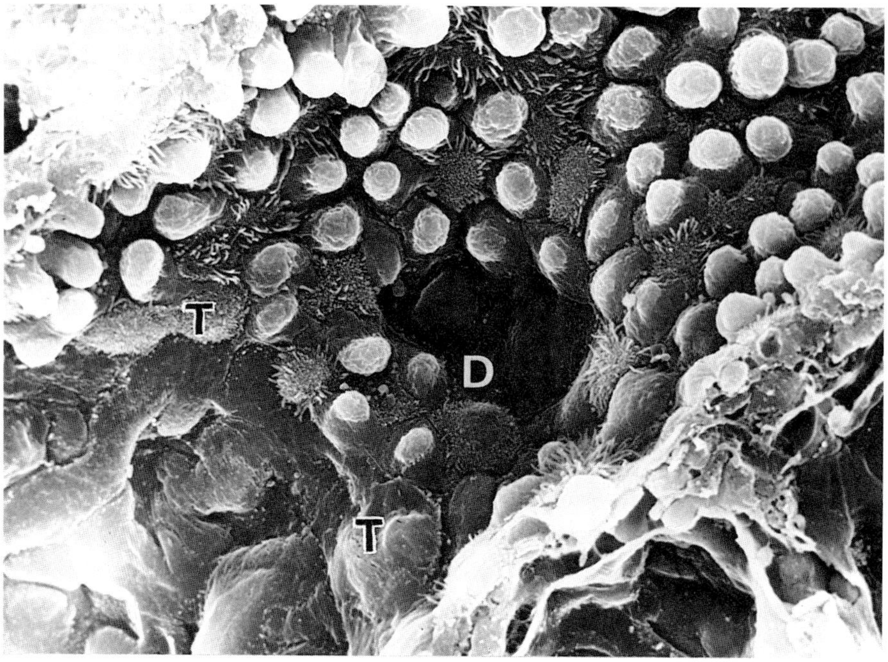

(a)

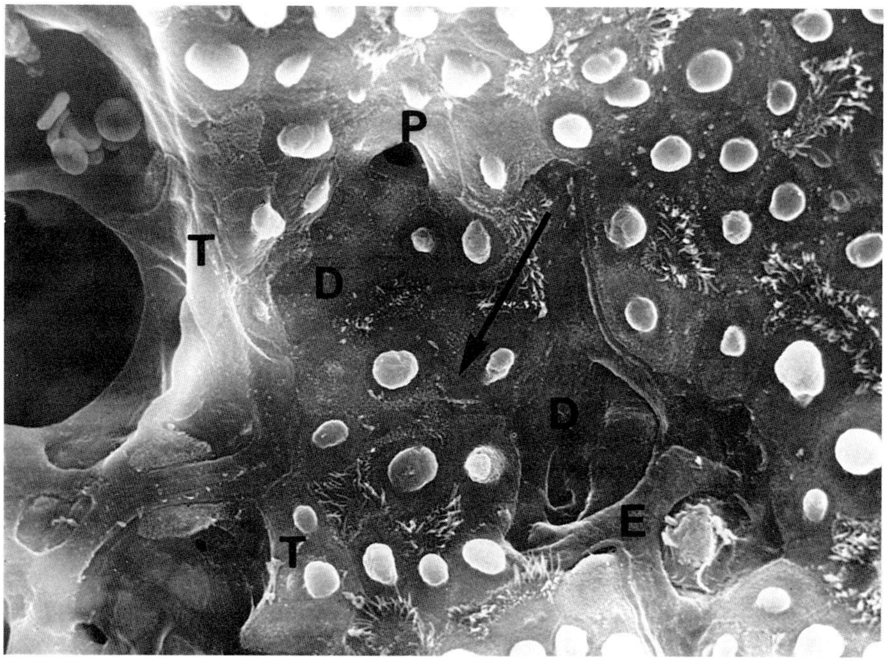

(b)

Fig. 2—Depressions (D) are usually small and found near the smooth bronchioloalveolar junction (T) in the control mouse (a). They are variable in size and shape in the nicotine mouse showing branching band-like capillaries (E) or sunken and uneven surface devoid of microvilli (b). The depressions are almost fused with each other (arrow) and the bronchioloalveolar junction is irregular. One edge of the depression is also fenestrated (P). SEM (a) group A (CC) day 30 × 1330; (b) group D (NN) day 30 × 1330

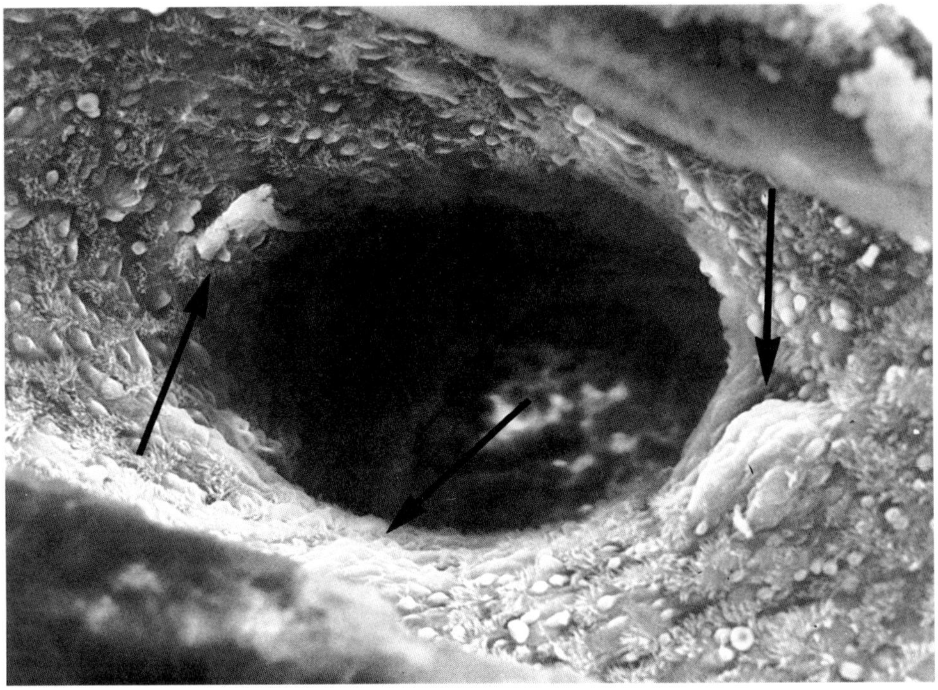

Fig. 3—Nodular mucosal bulges (NEB) are frequently present in pairs or more (arrows) near the inlet of the bronchus showing different degrees of nodular elevations and deformities. A bulge with adjacent fenestration is also present. SEM Group D (NN) day 15 × 810

through the prenatal and lactating periods. The changes were less severe in group C (CN) and were comparable to the control group in group B (NC) at day 30, indicating that mild fetal bronchial changes induced by nicotine may recover if further exposure to nicotine, after birth, is avoided.

The nicotine concentration of 1 mg/l in the drinking water was probably beyond the taste detection limit of mice and the amount of water drunk was not different between our control and nicotine groups. The amount of nicotine taken by each mother mouse was in the range of 0·3–0·5 mg/kg·day, or roughly equivalent to smoking 1–1·5 packs of average cigarettes daily in humans. Nicotine reaches the fetus by crossing the placenta and the baby through maternal milk.[16]

Dome-shaped bulges at the branching site of the bronchus have been identified as neuroepithelial bodies (NEB) in fetuses, newborns and young babies of a few species of mammals as well as humans.[15,17–20] They are formed by conglomerates of neuroendocrine (NE) and non-ciliated Clara-like cells with probable nerve fibres.[15,20] Although not proven in all species, the NE cells may contain serotonin, bombesin or calcitonin, and NEB are suspected to regulate regional ventilation as well as perfusion.[18,20] The proofs of these speculations are, however, not yet conclusive. NEB are relatively uncommon in the lung of adults although scattered NE cells are common.[21] The reason for this presumably physiologic regression of NEB from the bronchial surface or dispersion of NE cells is unknown.

The NEB have been reported to be sensitive to nicotine, hypoxia and also a variety of pharmacologic agents in rabbits.[20] The large and bizarre bulges that we had found in the nicotine-exposed baby mice were most likely deformed NEB, because of their location and ultrastructure. Normal NEB may be quite varied in size and shape ranging from 15 × 20 to 30 × 50 μm in mice.[22] We, however, have not seen any reports of normal mouse lungs which have bizarre, branching NEB, well over 50 μm in size, with ciliated and basaloid cells as seen in the nicotine exposed group (D).

The atypical transformation of NEB is likely to be due to the direct humoral or indirect neural effects of nicotine or its metabolic products, since nicotine stimulates all cholinergic nerve endings[23] and may also accumulate along the bronchi.[24] These assumptions remain to be clarified. However,

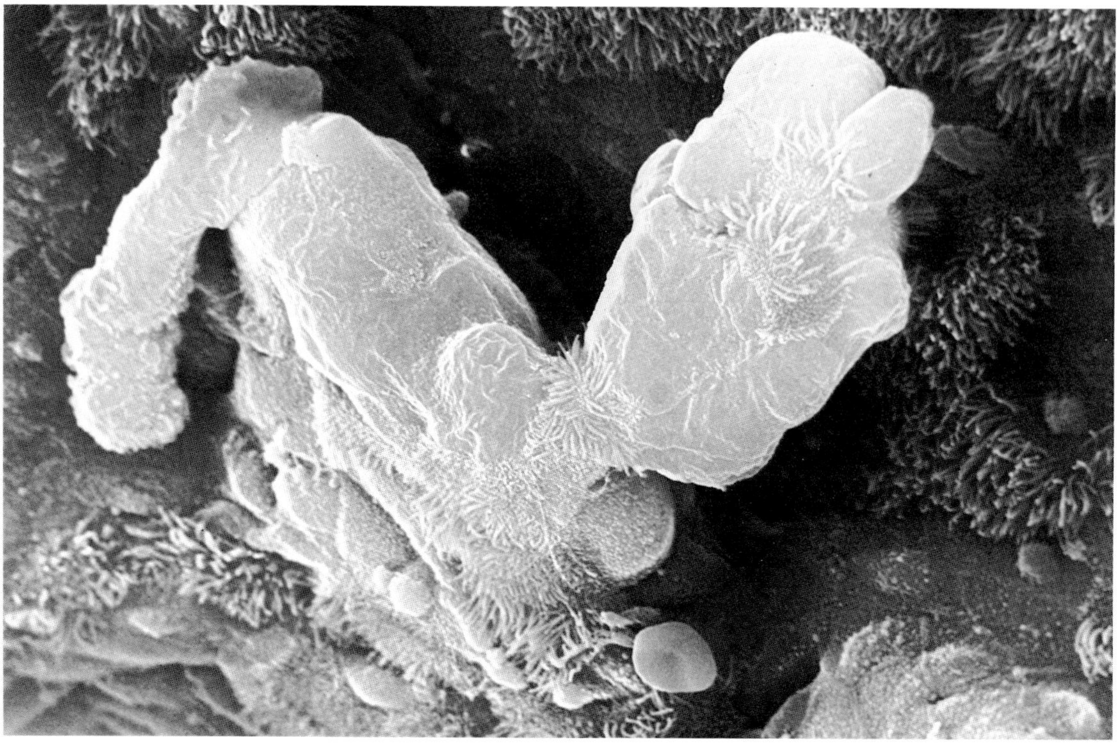

Fig. 4—Large, bizarre shaped bulges (NEB) tend to be pedunculated or branching and have smooth surfaced cells alternating with ciliated cells. Macrophages, red blood cells, foreign particles or pits may be found adjacent to the bulge. SEM group D (NN) day 30 × 3200

nicotine may also weaken the normal cleansing and defence mechanisms of the airway and render the animals more susceptible to infection. Since ozone or other irritants may induce focal mucosal hyperplasia with aggregates of Clara and NE cells,[21,25] reactive changes from infection or other extrinsic factors should also be considered. This seems unlikely in our animals since apart from a few macrophages, no overt bronchitis or bronchiolitis was seen by light microscopy.

If NEB indeed regulate the regional ventilation and perfusion and were deranged by nicotine, abnormal discharges of NEB may cause irregular contraction and relaxation of smooth muscle cells in the airway and vessels. The changes of the bronchial and bronchiolar surface, therefore, may be related to the degree of the derangement of the smooth muscle contraction.

The doubling of the radial linear count in all groups between days 5 and 15 suggests an apparent eight-fold (2^3) increase in the alveolar number. The $1{\cdot}25^3$-fold increase between days 15 and 30 indicates a further doubling of the number of alveoli suggesting that alveolar multiplication does not cease around day 15 in mice. Despite some difficulties that may be encountered in the intra- and inter-observer variability, the method of Emery and Mithal[14] is a relatively simple and a reasonably satisfactory way to assess lung development.[26] Our estimation of alveolar numbers showed no apparent difference between all groups.

The development and multiplication of alveoli are primarily through subdivision of the primary saccule by secondary crests in early babyhood.[27] Although surface depression and fenestration of the small bronchiole have also been suggested as an alternative means of alveolar mutliplication,[28] how much the alveolarization of the bronchiole actually contributes to the formation of new alveoli is uncertain. Macrophages are frequently associated with depressions and fenestrations in our mice and in young human lungs.[28] This and the similarities between the surface changes found in large bronchi (Figs 3, 4) and in small bronchioles, and also in adult human lungs[29] suggest that at least some of them are pathological alterations.

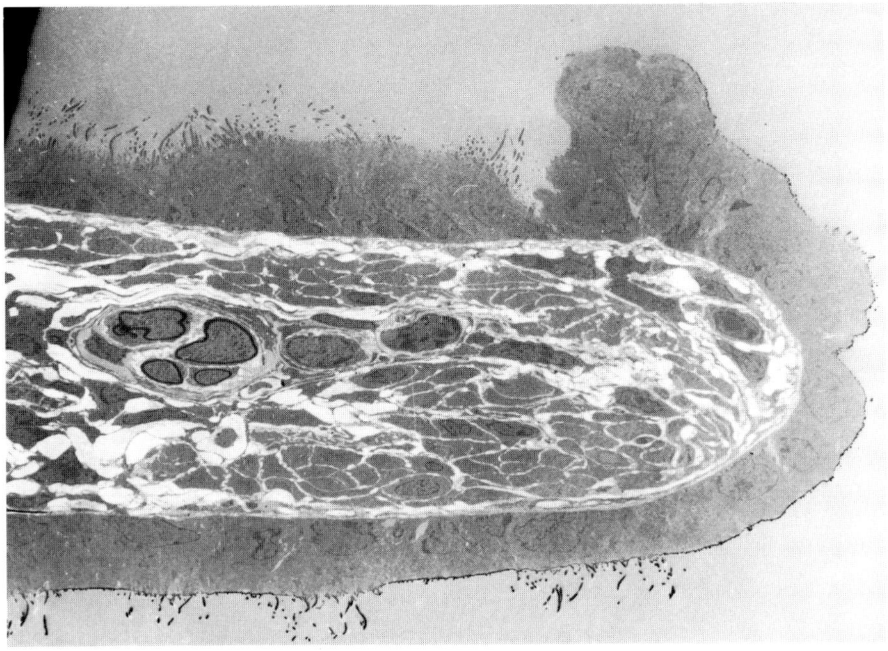

(a)

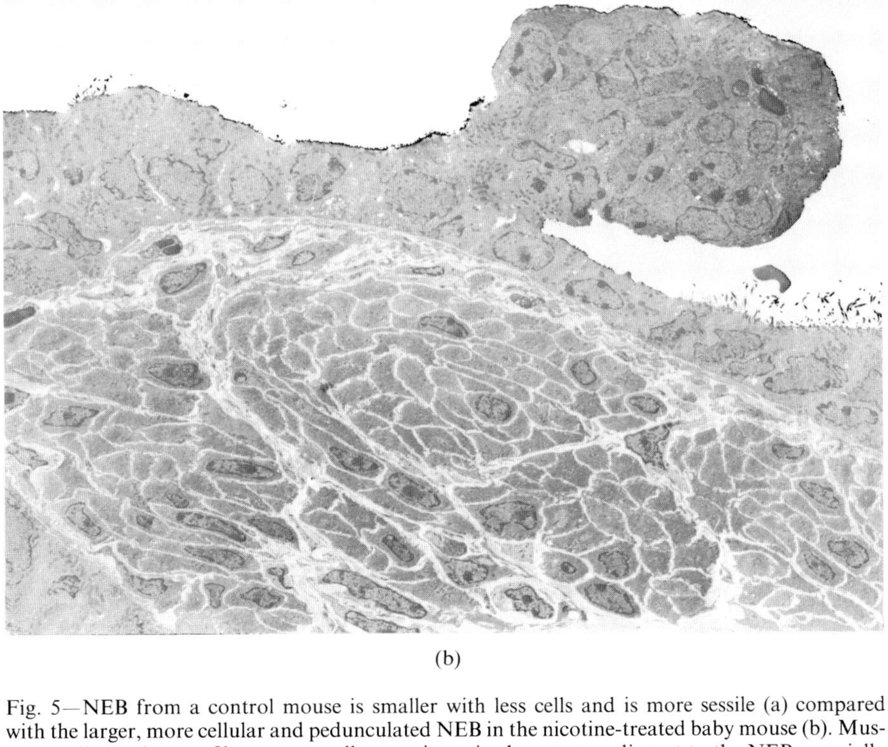

(b)

Fig. 5—NEB from a control mouse is smaller with less cells and is more sessile (a) compared with the larger, more cellular and pedunculated NEB in the nicotine-treated baby mouse (b). Muscle bundles and nerve fibres are usually prominent in the stroma adjacent to the NEB especially in the nicotine mouse. TEM of tissue originally processed for SEM (a) group A (CC) day 30 × 1440; (b) group D (NN) day 30 × 1406

In the nicotine groups the irregularities of the bronchioloalveolar junction, especially the severence of segments of bronchiolar epithelium away from their progenitor bronchiole, are probably caused by the extension and fusion of depressions and fenestrations. Whatever the mechanism, the disrupted continuity of ciliary flow may affect the cleansing of the terminal airway and perpetuate the local disease.

Bulges were small and rarely seen in both groups of mother mice. They were also rarely encountered in adult human lungs.[29] Although the mechanisms are not completely clear, NEB in the fetal and baby mouse lungs, appear to be especially sensitive to nicotine, as other developing organs are to many drugs and other noxious agents which may not cause maternal ailments but cross the placenta to affect the fetus.[30] As well as differences in sensitivity the nicotine effect in the baby mouse lung could be dose-dependent and cumulative as in the

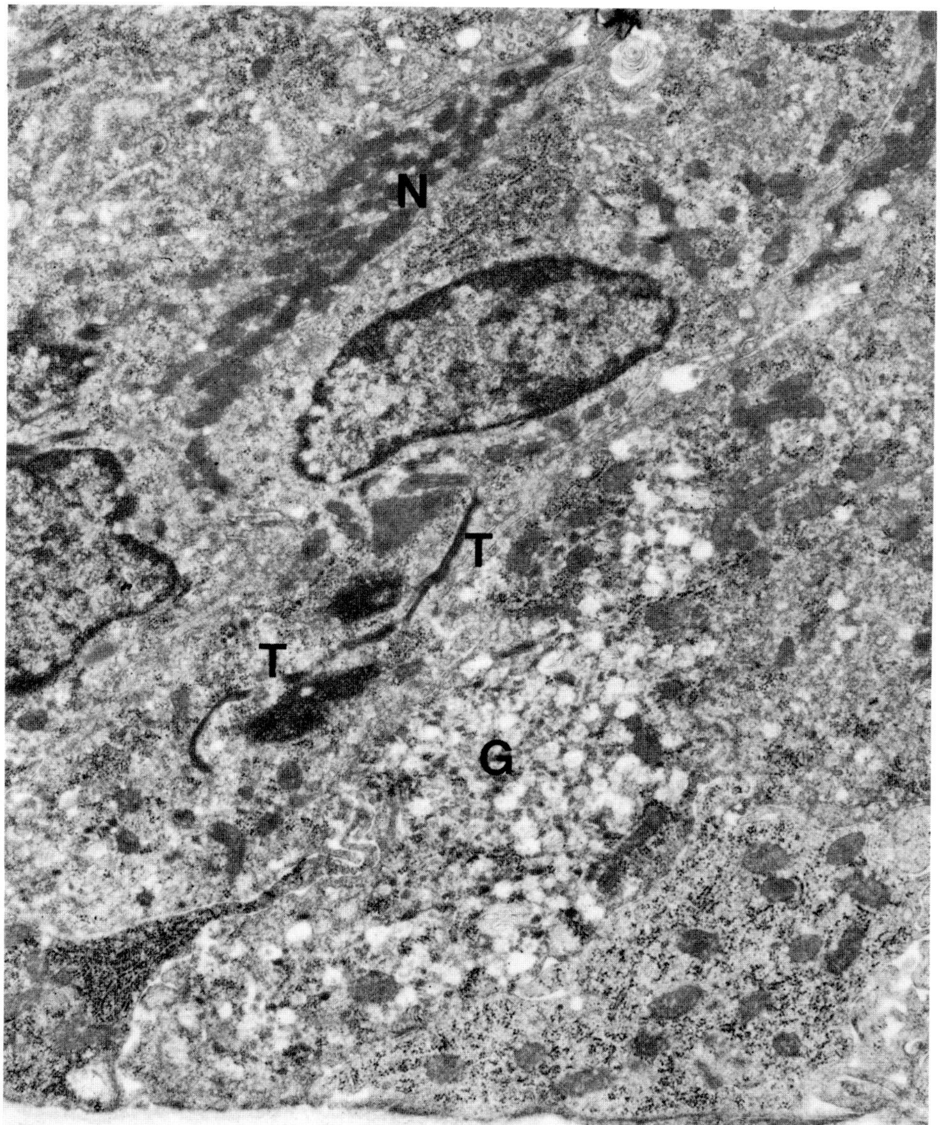

Fig. 6—(a) Normal NEB have many tonofilaments (T) and neurosecretory granule (G) containing cells. Nerve-like structures (N) are also seen. TEM of tissue originally processed for SEM. Group A (CC) day 15 × 11 900

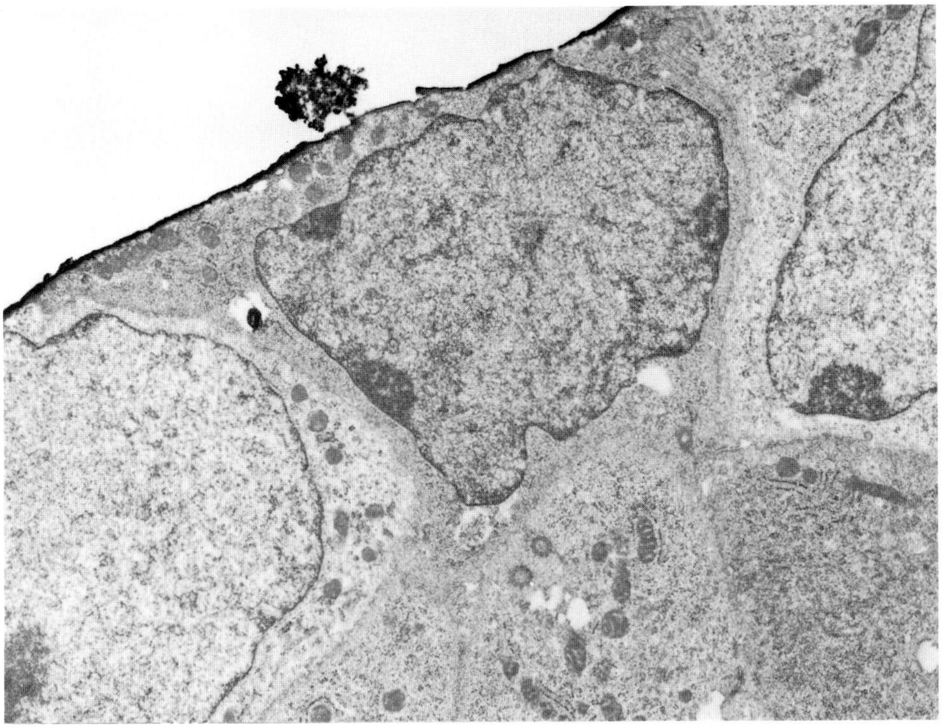

Fig. 6—(b) Abnormal NEB which have areas of large nucleated cells with few cytoplasmic organelles. The dark line on the surface of the cells is the gold coating of the SEM specimens. TEM of tissue originally processed for SEM. Group C (CN) day 30 × 12716

adult lung. The functional and long-term effects of these airway changes in the baby mice are unclear.

ACKNOWLEDGEMENTS

We wish to thank Monique Charbonneau for her technical assistance and Grace Pawelec for typing the manuscript.

REFERENCES

1. Colley JRT. Respiratory symptoms in childhood and parental smoking and phlegm production. *Brit Med J* 1924; **2:** 201–204.
2. Harlap S, Davies AM. Infant admissions to hospital and maternal smoking. *Lancet* 1974; **i:** 527–532.
3. Rantakallio P. Relationship of maternal smoking to morbidity and mortality of the child up to the age of five. *Acta Paediatr Scand* 1978; **67:** 621–631.
4. Yarnell JWG, St Leger AS. Respiratory illness, maternal smoking habit and lung function in children. *Brit J Dis Chest* 1979; **73:** 230–236.
5. Abel EL. Smoking during pregnancy: a review of effects on growth and development of offspring. *Human Biol* 1980; **52:** 593–625.
6. The health consequences of smoking for women: a report of the Surgeon General. *U.S. Department and Human Services* 1978; 229.
7. Longo LD. The biological effects of carbon monoxide on the pregnant woman, fetus, and newborn infant. *Am J Obstet Gynecol* 1977; **129:** 69–103.
8. Suzuki K, Horiguchi T, Comas-Urrutia AC, Mueller-Heubach E, Morishima HO, Adamsons K. Placental transfer and distribution of nicotine in the pregnant rhesus monkey. *Am J Obstet Gynecol* 1974; **119:** 253–263.
9. Welch RM, Gommi B, Alvares AP, Conney AH. Effect of enzyme induction on the metabolism of benzo (*a*)pyrene and 3-methyl-4-monomethylaminoazobenzene in the pregnant and fetal rats. *Cancer Res* 1972; **32:** 973–978.
10. Wang NS, Schraufnagel DE, Chen MF. The effect of maternal oral intake of nicotine on the growth and maturation of fetal and baby mouse lungs. *Lung* 1983; **161:** 27–38.

11. Scherle W. A simple method for volumetry of organs in quantitative stereology. *Mikroskopie* 1970; **26:** 57–60.
12. Cohen AL, Marlow DP, Garner GE. A rapid critical point method using fluorocarbons (Freons) as intermediate and transitional fluids. *J Microsc* 1968; **7:** 331–342.
13. Wang NS. The surface appearance of some lung tumors, mesothelioma and their precursor lesions. Scanning Electron Microscopy/1980/III, SEM Inc., AMF O'Hare (Chicago), II. 69–88.
14. Emery JL, Mithal A. The number of alveoli in the terminal respiratory unit of man during late intrauterine life and childhood. *Arch Dis Child* 1960; **35:** 544–547.
15. Hung KS, Chapman AL, Mestemacher MA. Scanning electron microscopy of bronchiolar neuroepithelial bodies in neonatal mouse lungs. *Anat Rec* 1979; **193:** 913–926.
16. Wilson JR. The effect of nicotine on lactation in white mice. *Am J Obstet Gynecol* 1942; **43:** 839–844.
17. Cutz E, Chan W, Sonstegard KS. Identification of neuro-epithelial bodies in rabbit fetal lungs by scanning electron microscopy: a correlative light, transmission and scanning electron microscopic study. *Anat Rec* 1978; **192:** 459–466.
18. Cutz E, Chan W, Track NS. Bombesin, calcitonin and leu-enkephalin immunoreactivity in endocrine cells of human lung. *Experimentia* 1981; **37:** 765–767.
19. Lauweryns JM, Peuskens JC. Neuroepithelial bodies (neuroreceptor or secretory organs?) in human infant bronchial and bronchiolar epithelium. *Anat Rec* 1972; **172:** 471–481.
20. Lauweryns JM, Cokelaere M, Deleersnyder M, Liebens M. Intrapulmonary neuro-epithelial bodies in newborn rabbits. Influence of hypoxia, hyperoxia, hypercapnia, nicotine, reserpine, L-DOPA and 5-HTP. *Cell Tissue Res* 1977; **182:** 425–440.
21. Kleinerman J, Marchevsky Am, Thornton J. Quantitative studies of APUD cells in airways of rats. *Am Rev Respir Dis* 1981; **124:** 458–462.
22. Hung KS. Development of neuroepithelial bodies in pre- and postnatal mouse lungs: scanning electron microscopic study. *Anat Rec* 1982; **203:** 285–291.
23. Volle RL, Koelle GB. Ganglionic stimulating and blocking agents. In: Goodman LS, Gilman A, eds. The Pharmacological Basis of Therapeutics. Toronto: The Macmillan Company 1970: 585–600.
24. Lindquist NG, Ullberg S. Autoradiography of intravenously injected ^{14}C-nicotine indicates long-term retention in the respiratory tract. *Nature* 1974; **248:** 600–601.
25. Eustis SL, Schwartz LW, Kosch PC, Dungworth DL. Chronic bronchiolitis in nonhuman primates after prolonged ozone exposure. *Am J Pathol* 1981; **105:** 121–137.
26. Cooney TP, Thurlbeck WM. The radial alveolar count method of Emery and Mithal: a reappraisal 1—postnatal lung growth. *Thorax* 1982; **37:** 572–579.
27. Amy RWM, Bowes D, Burri PH, Haines J, Thurlbeck WM. Postnatal growth of the mouse lung. *J Anat* 1977; **124:** 131–151.
28. Boyden EA. Development of the human lung. In: Quarrei I, ed. Brennemann's Practice of Pediatrics. Vol. IV, Chapter 64. Hagerstown, MD: Harper & Row, 1972: 1–12.
29. Wang NS, Ying WL. The pattern of goblet cell hyperplasia in human airways. *Hum Pathol* 1977; **8:** 301–311.
30. Naeye RL. Environmental influences on the embryo and fetus. In Hill RB, Terziam JA, eds. Environmental Pathology: An Evolving Field. New York: Alan R. Liss Inc., 1982: 111–128.

JOURNAL OF PATHOLOGY, VOL. **144**: 101–108 (1984)

THE BINDING OF PEROXIDASE-LABELLED LECTINS TO HUMAN BREAST EPITHELIUM II—THE REACTIVITY OF BREAST CARCINOMAS TO WHEAT GERM AGGLUTININ

ROSEMARY A. WALKER

Department of Pathology, Clinical Sciences Building, Leicester Royal Infirmary, P.O. Box 65, Leicester LE2 7LX, U.K.

Received 23 January 1984
Accepted 11 May 1984

SUMMARY

The binding of peroxidase-labelled *wheat germ agglutinin* (WGA) to a series of 125 human breast carcinomas has been studied. Routine fixation and processing has been shown to have no deleterious effect on reactivity. In contrast to the homogeneous binding of WGA to normal and hyperplastic human breast previously reported, the binding of WGA to breast carcinomas exhibits heterogeneity. This is of two forms: (1) in relation to cell reactivity, which is significantly correlated to tumour differentiation, with fewer cells reacting in those carcinomas showing loss of histological differentiation; (2) with regard to the interaction between WGA and specific saccharides of cellular glycan-components, binding to sialic acid appearing to be of significance to varying degrees in some carcinomas but not in others nor, as previously reported, in normal breast. The alteration in WGA–saccharide interaction is an indicator of the heterogeneity of the carbohydrate chains of glycoproteins within neoplastic cells of the same tumour and between carcinomas. The other finding of note has been that of the significant association between heterogeneity of cellular reactivity to WGA and the presence of axillary lymph node metastasis, but a lack of correlation between virtual absence of reactivity and nodal metastasis.

KEY WORDS—Breast carcinoma, lectin histochemistry, tumour heterogeneity.

INTRODUCTION

The glycosylated components of the cell membrane have been implicated in a variety of cellular reactions, such as the binding of hormones, and cell–cell and cell–substrate interactions.[1,2] Alterations in these properties could be highly significant in the development and progression of the neoplastic process. This consideration has stimulated investigation of the lipid- and protein-bound carbohydrates of malignant cells,[3–5] with differences in relation to normal cells being noted.

Lectins, because of their affinities for specific sugars, have proved to be useful tools for the investigation of the cell membranes of normal and malignant cells.[6] One such lectin is *wheat germ agglutinin* (WGA), a protein which binds to *N*-acetyl-D-glucosamine but has a higher affinity for the di- and trisaccharides of this hexosamine.[7] Recent studies have demonstrated that WGA also interacts with sialic acid.[8] WGA has been shown to agglutinate tumour cells to a greater degree than comparable normal cells[9] and to bind more readily to transformed cells.[10] These findings indicate that there could be differences in the expression of *N*-acetyl-D-glucosamine and/or sialic acid between normal and malignant cell membranes. Bramwell and Harris[11] describe the presence, in several tumour cell lines, of an abnormal membrane glycoprotein which binds less WGA than glycoproteins of the same molecular mass isolated from comparable normal cell membranes.

A previous study[12] of normal and hyperplastic human breast, utilizing tissue sections as opposed to cell lines, has shown that peroxidase-labelled WGA consistently binds to both acinar and ductal

0022–3417/84/100101–08$01.00

epithelium, and that the reactivity of such tissue is unaffected by routine fixation and processing. This approach is therefore suitable for the investigation of human breast carcinomas and has been utilized in the present study. The findings have been compared to those previously obtained for non-malignant breast, to tumour differentiation and to the presence or absence of local lymph node metastasis.

MATERIALS AND METHODS

Materials

Tissue was available from 125 breast carcinomas surgically excised from the same number of patients at Leicester Royal Infirmary between May 1981 and October 1983. Samples from each case were frozen in isopentane cooled in liquid nitrogen, with parallel slices being fixed in 4 per cent formaldehyde in 0·15M soldium chloride for 18–30 h. Tissue from the majority of specimens was also fixed in Bouin's fluid for not more than 24 h. The frozen material was stored in liquid nitrogen. The fixed tissue was dehydrated, cleared and embedded in paraffin wax.

Wheat germ agglutinin was conjugated to horse-radish peroxidase type VI, and then analysed by double affinity chromatography as previously described.[12] All reagents were obtained from Sigma Chemical Co. Ltd. unless otherwise stated.

Method

Frozen tissue from 80 of the carcinomas was examined. Sections (6–8 μm) were cut in a cryostat at −20°C and air-dried for 60 min at 40°C. Paraffin sections of all fixed material were de-waxed, rehydrated and rinsed in Tris–saline buffer (pH 7·6). Endogenous peroxidase was not blocked. All sections were incubated with WGA-peroxidase at a concentration of 5 μg/ml for 60 min at room temperature, then rinsed and washed in Tris–saline buffer. Peroxidase was localized using the diamino-benzidine (DAB)–hydrogen peroxide reaction,[13] and the nuclei counterstained with Mayer's haemalum.

Controls

These were as follows. (i) Serial sections of both frozen and fixed tissue were incubated with WGA-peroxidase absorbed with 0·1 M *N*-acetyl-D-glucosamine. (ii) Sections from formalin-fixed tissue of 60 of the carcinomas, selected at random, were treated with neuraminidase from *Vibro cholera* (Koch-light Ltd.) for 18 h at 37°C prior to incubation with WGA-peroxidase. (iii) Serial sections from formalin-fixed tissue of 10 cases were treated with 0·01 M, 0·05 M or 0·1 M *N*-acetyl neuraminic acid and *N*-acetyl-D-glucosamine after the application of WGA-peroxidase but prior to washing and localization with DAB. Sections from the same cases were tested with WGA-peroxidase absorbed with 0·05 M *N*-acetyl neuraminic acid.

Histology

Haematoxylin and eosin-stained sections of all carcinomas were examined for classification. Histological differentiation was assessed using a modification of the grading system of Bloom and Richardson.[14] Lymph nodes were available for examination in 89 cases.

RESULTS

Pattern of staining

The carcinomas could be divided into three categories; those in which all or the majority of tumour cells showed evidence of binding of WGA, designated *many*; carcinomas in which there were mixtures of positive and negative cells, either intermingled or in clusters, classified as *moderate*; and tumours in which only a small number of cells reacted, categorized as *few*. The numbers of carcinomas within each group is shown in Table I.

The cellular site of staining was either at the periphery, focally within thc cytoplasm or as a partial diffuse cytoplasmic reaction (Fig. 1). In areas of tubular differentiation the reaction was in relation to the lumina (Fig. 2) but peripheral staining could also be identified in solid groups of cells (Fig. 3). The focal staining was often perinuclear

Table I—The correlation between the proportion of cells reacting and histological differentiation

Proportion of cells	Grade I	Grade II	Grade III	Total
Many	10	40	4	54
Moderate	1	35	18	54
Few	0	8	9	17
Total	11	83	31	125

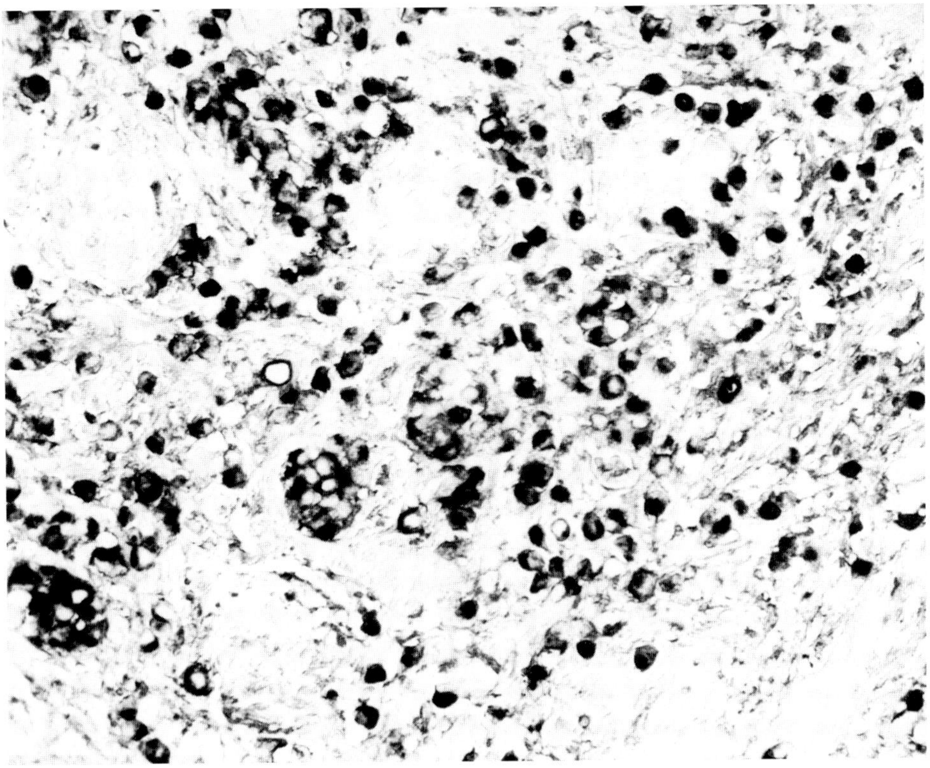

Fig. 1—Carcinoma with many cells reacting, most of which show cytoplasmic staining. ×220

and appeared to be in relation to the Golgi body (Fig. 4). Intracytoplasmic luminal staining was also a feature.

Fixation and controls

No differences were found between the frozen and fixed material in relation to the proportion and intensity of cell reactivity.

There was no evidence of staining in the sections treated with WGA-peroxidase absorbed with *N*-acetyl-D-glucosamine. A reduction in stromal staining was generally seen in sections treated with neuraminidase prior to WGA-peroxidase, but the effect on cellular staining was variable. With 28 of the 60 carcinomas tested in this way no difference was seen in the staining obtained with WGA-peroxidase. In five carcinomas there was a generalized slight reduction in intensity of staining but no effect on the proportions of cells reacting (Figs 5a, b). Fifteen tumours had a patchy reduction in staining, involving both intensity and proportion of reactive cells. A marked reduction in reactivity was seen in six cases and in the remaining six tumours there was complete loss of staining by WGA-peroxidase after neuraminidase treatment.

There was no evidence of staining in the sections treated with WGA-peroxidase absorbed with *N*-acetyl neuraminic acid. In the displacement studies using differing molar concentrations of *N*-acetyl-D-glucosamine and *N*-acetyl neuraminic acid there was no evidence of staining in any tumour after the application of 0·05 M and 0·1 M *N*-acetyl-D-glucosamine and only very weak staining of a few cells after the use of a 0·01 M solution. The findings after the use of *N*-acetyl neuraminic acid varied between tumours. After 0·1 M *N*-acetyl neuraminic acid there was a marked reduction or no staining. Treatment with 0·05 M sialic acid resulted in either a marked, patchy or little reduction in staining, whilst 0·01 M solution had either little effect or caused some reduction of the reaction. The findings correlated with those noted in the same carcinoma after the use of neuraminidase. In those tumours in which the low molar concentration of *N*-acetyl neuraminic acid caused some alteration in staining there was little effect on normal breast tissue present within the sections.

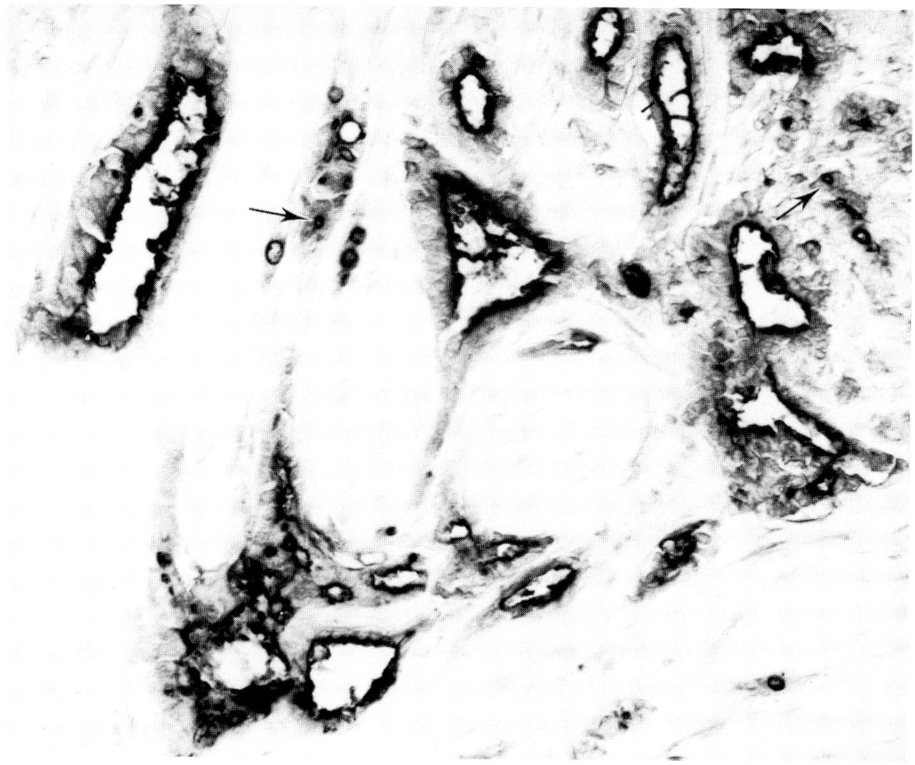

Fig. 2—Well-differentiated carcinoma in which the site of staining is predominantly the luminal periphery of the cells. Intracytoplasmic luminal staining is also present (→). ×220

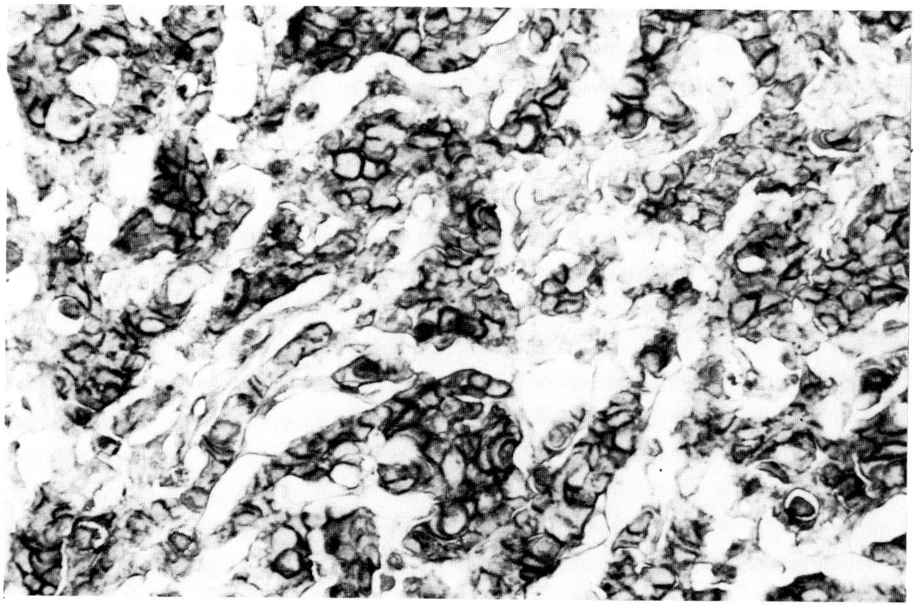

Fig. 3—The majority of the cells in this moderately differentiated carcinoma show binding of WGA-peroxidase to the cell periphery. ×220

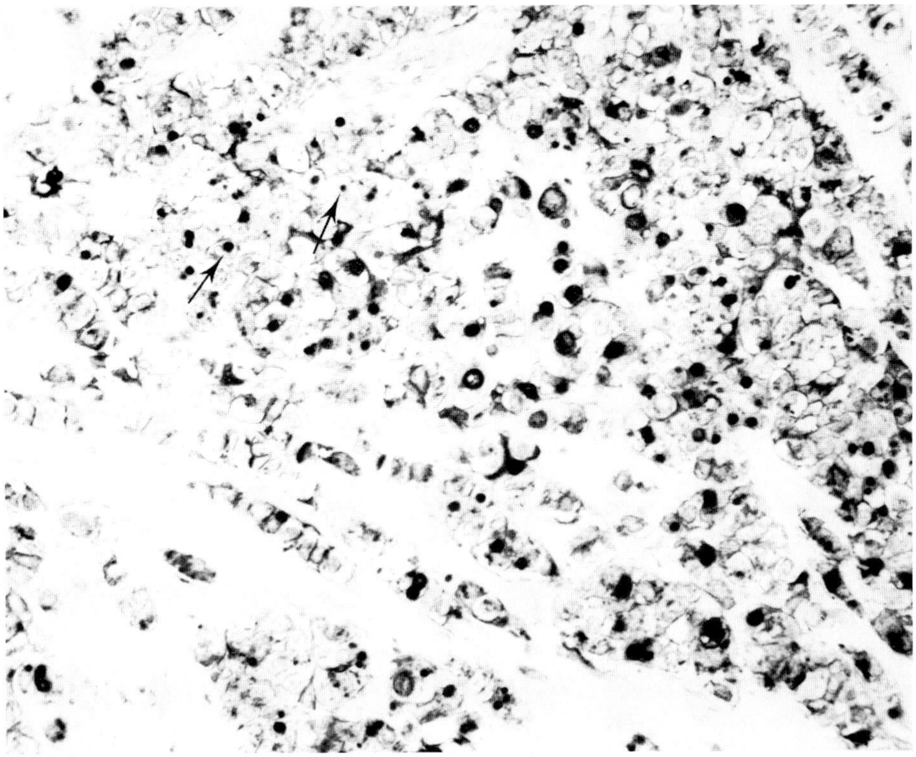

Fig. 4—A focal cytoplasmic reaction is present in many of the cells (→), although some show peripheral or a more diffuse cytoplasmic staining. ×220

Correlation with type and differentiation

The three tubular carcinomas had many cells reacting and the site of staining was at the luminal periphery of the cells. All four mucinous carcinomas had staining of the mucin. Of the ten infiltrating lobular carcinomas, five had many cells reacting, four a moderate number and one few. Staining was predominantly focal or of intracytoplasmic lumina.

The number of tumours within each histological grade is shown in Table I, as is the correlation between the proportion of cells reacting and differentiation. There is a significant relationship between the degree of reactivity of the carcinomas and histological differentiation ($p<0.001$).

There was no correlation of the effect of neuraminidase on staining with the extent of reactivity, the type of carcinoma or the degree of differentiation.

Table II—The correlation between the proportion of reactive cells and axillary lymph node status

Proportion of cells reacting	Metastasis to lymph node	Lymph node free from metastasis
Many	11	25
Moderate	25	15
Few	5	8

Correlation with axillary lymph node status

Of the 89 carcinomas in which there was definite knowledge of the node status, 41 had metastasized. The relationship between the proportions of cells reacting and the presence or absence of lymph node metastasis is shown in Table II. There is a significant correlation between decreased reactivity and the presence of lymph node metastasis ($0.02>p>0.01$).

The node status was known for 41 of the carcinomas tested with neuraminidase. The cases showing the different patterns of reactivity after sialic acid cleavage were equally divided between those tumours that were node negative and node positive.

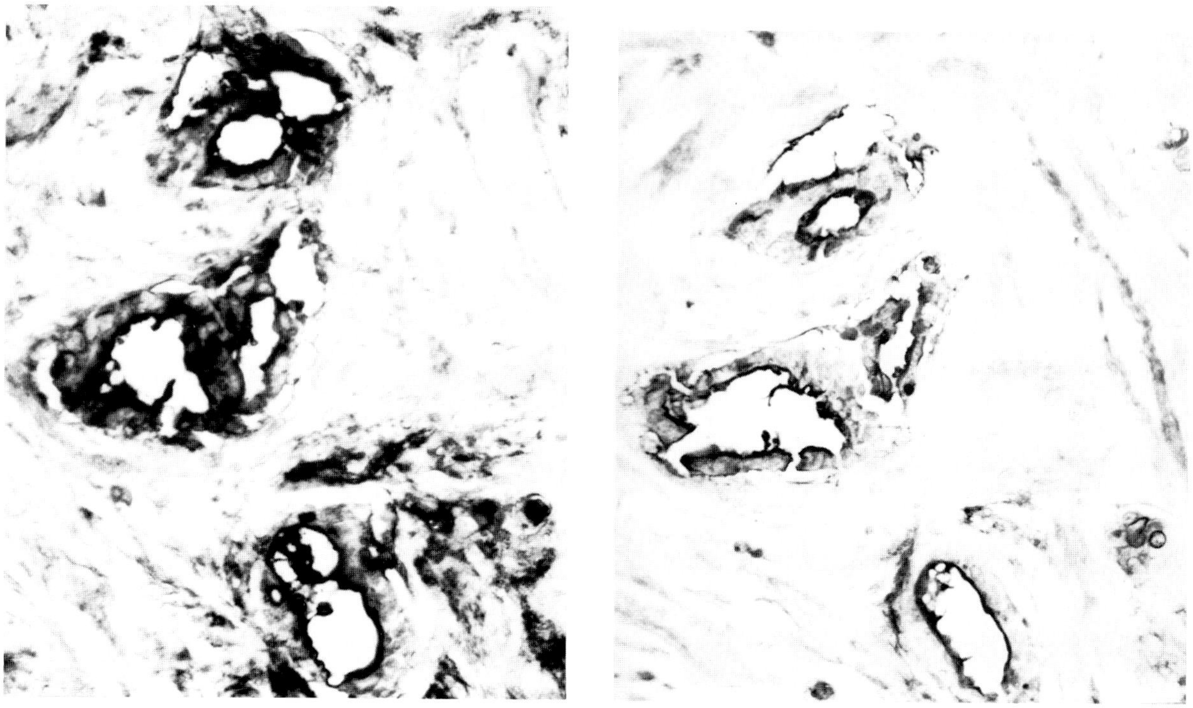

Fig. 5—(a) Carcinoma reacted with WGA-peroxidase showing prominent staining of the luminal periphery and of the cytoplasm of some cells, ×290. (b) Serial section of the same tumour which has been treated with neuraminidase prior to the application of WGA-peroxidase, showing a reduction in staining and loss of the cytoplasmic reaction. ×209

DISCUSSION

This study has shown that unlike normal and hyperplastic breast tissue[12] there is heterogeneity of binding of WGA to breast carcinomas, with the extent of reactivity paralleling the degree of histological differentiation. A difference in the cellular site of staining was also noted, with focal and partial diffuse cytoplasmic reactions occurring in carcinomas whereas this is not a feature of benign breast. A similar variation in cell staining was noted by Franklin[15] in the small number of carcinomas he examined with WGA. However, even though there is a highly significant correlation between many cells staining and good histological differentiation there are some poorly differentiated tumours in which the majority of cells react.

Earlier studies concerned with the agglutination[9] and binding[10] of normal and transformed cells by lectins recorded an increased reactivity of tumour cells with WGA, which is not supported by this study utilizing tissue sections. The findings correspond more to those of Bramwell and Harris[11] who detected an abnormal membrane glycoprotein in several tumour cell lines which bound less WGA than that of normal cells.

The binding of WGA to normal and hyperplastic breast can be inhibited by *N*-acetyl-D-glucosamine but is unaffected by neuraminidase,[12] indicating that sialic acid has little or no role in the interaction. Although the staining of all carcinomas was blocked by *N*-acetyl-D-glucosamine the effect of neuraminidase ranged from a total loss of staining to no alteration of reactivity and this bore no relation to the extent of staining, the grade of the tumour or the nodal status. The competition studies with the two sugars indicated that *N*-acetyl-D-glucosamine had a greater affinity for the lectin. Displacement procedures using differing molarities of sugars give more information about the relative binding affinities of the lectin, and are to be preferred to absorption studies in assessing specificity, but even with these it is difficult to be certain as to what WGA is interacting with in a cell-bound glycoprotein. The investigations that showed that WGA interacted with sialic acid[8] used isolated sugars and glycoproteins in agglutination inhibition and double diffusion methods, and it is obviously difficult to directly transpose the findings to tissue sections. Debray *et al.*[16] after considering the results of their inhibition studies concluded that the interactions between WGA and cell-surface glycoconjugates are very complex and have to be interpreted with care. What can be suggested from the controls undertaken in this study is that there are differences in the binding characteristics of WGA between carcinomas, and that in some it is quite different to that of normal human breast.

This study clearly shows that there are two forms of heterogeneity of binding of WGA within breast carcinomas: (1) in relation to the number of reactive cells; (2) with regard to the glycosylated components of cell constituents. Micro-heterogeneity of the glycan part of glycoproteins is well-recognized,[17] but the heterogeneity of oligosaccharides of glycoproteins from transformed and malignant cells is more marked and differs from that occurring in normal cell glycoproteins,[18–20]. This may explain the second point with regard to WGA binding.

The other finding of interest in this study has been that of the relationship between decreased WGA reactivity and axillary lymph node metastasis. However, this finding did not appear to relate to those carcinomas in which only a few cells reacted; in this group those tumours with no evidence of local lymph node metastasis were in excess. Studies on defined tumour cell lines have found alterations in metastatic behaviour to be associated with changes in cell surface glycosylation.[21,22] Increases in metastatic capacity have been associated with an increase in the total amount of cell surface sialylation and with differences in the positioning of sialic acid in glycoconjugates.[23–25] In the present study there was no correlation between the differing effects of neuraminidase on WGA binding to carcinomas and lymph node metastasis. It would seem that the alterations in glycan structure relating to sialic acid and WGA interaction do not appear to have been a factor in determining metastatic potential. Price and Tarin[26] found decreased agglutinability of metastatic mouse mammary tumour cells with WGA which was not present in the original primary tumours. Lectin agglutination and binding may not be directly related,[1] but an assessment of WGA-binding of the lymph node metastases from the primary breast carcinomas considered in this study could be rewarding.

Little information with regard to prognosis is available since the tumours assessed were surgically removed between 1981 and 1983. However, since there does appear to be a correlation between altered WGA binding and local lymph node metastasis, its relationship to prognosis is worthwhile pursuing.

ACKNOWLEDGEMENTS

I am grateful to Miss S. J. Day for excellent technical help; Mrs G. Holmes for secretarial assistance; Ms B. Jordan for help with photography and Professor F. Walker for his constructive comments in the preparation of this manuscript. Financial assistance was gratefully received from the Trent Regional Health Authority.

REFERENCES

1. Nicolson GL. Transmembrane control of the receptors on normal and malignant cells. *Biochim Biophys Acta* 1976; **458:** 1–57.
2. Hughes RC. *Membrane Glycoproteins.* London: Butterworths, 1976.
3. Hakomori S. Structures and organization of cell surface glycolipid dependency on cell growth and malignant transformation. *Biochim Biophys Acta* 1975; **419:** 55–89.
4. Critchley DR. Glycolipids as membrane receptors important in growth regulation. In: Hynes RO, ed. Surfaces of Normal and Malignant Cells. New York: John Wiley, 1979: 63–101.
5. Warren L, Buck CA, Tuszynski GP. Glycopeptide changes and malignant transformation. A possible role for carbohydrate in malignant behaviour. *Biochim Biophys Acta* 1978; **516:** 97–127.
6. Rapin AMC, Burger MM. Tumor cell surfaces: general alterations detected by agglutinins. *Adv Cancer Res* 1974; **20:** 1–74.
7. Nagata Y, Burger MM. Wheat germ agglutinin molecular characteristics and specificity for sugar binding. *J. Biol Chem* 1974; **249:** 3116–3122.
8. Bhavanandan VP, Katlic AW. The interaction of wheat germ agglutinin with sialo glycoproteins the role of sialic acid. *J Biol Chem* 1979; **254:** 4000–4008.
9. Aub JC, Sanford BH, Cote MN. Studies on reactivity of tumor and normal cells to a wheat germ agglutinin. *Proc Natl Acad Sci USA* 1965; **54:** 396–399.
10. Cronin AP, Biddle F, Sanders FK. Wheat germ agglutinin conjugated with fluorescein isothiocyanate: staining of normal and transformed Chinese hamster cells. *Cytobios* 1970; **2:** 225–231.
11. Bramwell ME, Harris H. An abnormal membrane

glycoprotein associated with malignancy in a wide range of different tumours. *Proc R Soc Lond B* 1978; **201**: 87–106.

12. Walker RA. The binding of peroxidase labelled lectins to human breast epithelium. I—Normal, hyperplastic and lactating breast. *J Pathol* 1984; **142**: 279–291.
13. Graham RC, Karnovsky MJ. The early stages of absorption of injected horseradish peroxidase in the proximal tubules of mouse kidney; ultrastructural cytochemistry by a new technique. *J Histochem Cytochem* 1966; **14**: 291–302.
14. Walker RA. The binding of fluorescent-labelled concanavalin A to human breast tissue—a marker of differentiation. *J Pathol* 1983; **140**: 255–265.
15. Franklin WA. Tissue binding of lectins in disorders of the breast. *Cancer* 1983; **51**: 295–300.
16. Debray H, Decout D. Strecker G, Spik G, Montreuil J. Specificity of twelve lectins towards oligosaccharides and glycopeptides related to *N*-glycosyl proteins. *Eur J Biochem* 1981; **117**: 41–55.
17. Sharon N. Complex Carbohydrates. Massachusetts: Addison-Wesley, 1975.
18. Ogata SI, Muramatsu T, Kobata A. New structural characteristics of the large glycopeptides from transformed cells. *Nature* 1976; **259**: 580–582.
19. Takasaki S, Ikehira H, Kobata A. Increase of asparagine-linked oligosaccharides with branched outer chains caused by cell transformation. *Biochem Biophys Res Commun* 1980; **92**: 735–742.
20. Litin BS, Grimes WJ. Heterogeneity of sialoglycoproteins purified from normal and malignant cells. *Cancer Res* 1983; **43**: 2131–2137.
21. Finne J. Tao TW, Burger MM. Carbohydrate changes in glycoproteins of a poorly metastasizing wheat germ agglutinin-resistant melanoma clone. *Cancer Res* 1980; **40**: 2580–2587.
22. Dennis J. Donaghue TP, Florian H, Kerbel RS. Apparent reversion of stable *in vitro* genetic markers detected in tumour cells from spontaneous metastases. *Nature* 1981; **292**: 242–245.
23. Skipski VP, Carter SP, Terebus-Kekish OI, Podlaski Jr FJ, Peterson RHF, Chester Stock C. Ganglioside profiles of metastases and of metastasizing and nonmetastasizing rat primary mammary carcinomas. *J Natl Acad Sci* 1981; **67**: 1251–1258.
24. Yogeeswaran G, Salk PL. Metastatic potential is positively correlated with cell surface sialylation of cultured murine tumor cell lines. *Science* 1981; **212**: 1514–1516.
25. Altevogt P, Fogel M, Cheingsong-Popov R, Dennis J, Robinson P, Schirrmacher V. Different patterns of lectin binding and cell surface sialylation detected on related high- and low-metastatic tumor lines. *Cancer Res* 1983; **43**: 5138–5144.
26. Price JE, Tarin D. Lectin agglutinability of mammary tumours with differing metastatic colonization potentials. *Differentiation* 1981; **20**: 264–269.

JOURNAL OF PATHOLOGY, VOL. **144**: 109–117 (1984)

THE BINDING OF PEROXIDASE-LABELLED LECTINS TO HUMAN BREAST EPITHELIUM III—ALTERED FUCOSE-BINDING PATTERNS OF BREAST CARCINOMAS AND THEIR SIGNIFICANCE

ROSEMARY A. WALKER

Department of Pathology, Clinical Sciences Building, Leicester Royal Infirmary, PO Box 65, Leicester LE2 7LX, U.K.

Received 23 March 1984
Accepted 13 April 1984

SUMMARY

Tissue sections from 80 human breast carcinomas have been examined for evidence of binding of the two fucose-specific lectins, *Lotus tetragonolobus* and *Ulex europeus I*, with enzymes utilized as an indicator system. Both single-staining and double-staining methods (*Lotus tetragonolobus-peroxidase* and *Ulex europeus I-alkaline phosphatase*) have been employed. In contrast to normal breast in which there is consistent reactivity of all epithelium with *Lotus tetragonologus* a variable loss of binding has been found within carcinomas. Surprisingly, this bears no relationship to tumour differentiation; nor does it correlate with local lymph node metastasis. *Ulex europeus I* has a variable reactivity with carcinomas, as it does with normal breast epithelium, and this likewise has no correlation with differentiation. However, a relationship has been found between specific patterns of binding and axillary lymph node status. The value of using two lectins with the same major sugar specificity but having different binding affinities is illustrated in this study, in which differences in behavioural characteristics have been identified between fucose-containing glycoconjugates having minor structural variations.

KEY WORDS—Breast cancer, lectins, fucose.

INTRODUCTION

Alterations in the oligosaccharide component of glycolipids and glycoproteins of malignant cells when compared to those of normal cells are well documented.[1,2] Such modifications may contribute to the changes in cell growth and cell control which are a feature of neoplasia. L-Fucose is a common component of *O*- and *N*-linked glycoproteins and glycolipids.[3] Changes in the fucosylation of glycoproteins and glycolipids or murine mammary tumours have been reported and have been related to tumourigenicity[4–6] and metastatic phenotype.[7] There have been no comparable studies of human breast tumours. Serum L-fucose levels have been estimated in patients with breast cancer but reports have varied as to the significance of the elevation.[8–10]

Lotus tetragonolobus (LTA) and *Ulex europeus I (UEA)* are lectins which bind specifically to L-fucose. However, their reactivities differ and this is related to the linkages of the sugars to which L-fucose is attached in oligosaccharide chains.[11] The binding of *UEA* can be inhibited by the monofucosyl oligosaccharide of the 'type-1' blood group chain (L-Fuc-(1→2)-β-Gal-(1→4)-βGlcNAc-) and by that of the 'type-2' blood group chain (L-Fuc-(1→2)-β-Gal-(1→3)-βGlcNAc-) whereas *LTA* binding is not inhibited by the 'type-1' chain oligosaccharide and the difucosyl 'type-2' chain is more active. The use of these two lectins can, therefore, distinguish fine differences in the glycan structure of cell-surface glycoconjugates.[12]

A previous study[13] of normal and hyperplastic human breast tissue using these lectins labelled with peroxidase has shown that *LTA* consistently binds

0022–3417/84/100109–09$01.00

to ductal and acinar epithelium whereas the reactivity of the tissue to *UEA* varies between cases. Marked alterations in the binding of *LTA* were found after fixation and processing necessitating the use of frozen tissue samples.

In this study the binding of *LTA* and *UEA* to a series of human breast carcinomas has been considered, with specific reference to alterations from the patterns obtained in normal breast, and correlation with tumour differentiation and local lymph node spread.

MATERIALS AND METHODS

Materials

Tissue was available from 80 breast carcinomas surgically excised from the same number of patients at Leicester Royal Infirmary between May 1982 and October 1983. Samples from each case were frozen in isopentane cooled in liquid nitrogen, with parallel slices fixed in 4 per cent formaldehyde in 0·15 M sodium chloride solution for 18–30 h. The frozen tissue was stored in liquid nitrogen. The fixed tissue was dehydrated, cleared and embedded in paraffin wax.

LTA and *UEA* were conjugated to horseradish peroxidase type VI as previously described.[13] *UEA* was also coupled to alkaline phosphatase type VII by the one-stage glutaraldehyde method of Voller *et al.*[14] All reagents were obtained from Sigma Chemical Co. Ltd.

Methods

Single staining—Sections (6–8 μm) were cut from the frozen tissue in a cryostat at −20°C and dried for 60 min at 4°C. Serial sections were incubated with *LTA-peroxidase* (30 μg/ml) or *UEA-peroxidase* (10 μg/ml) for 60 min at room temperature, rinsed and washed in Tris–saline buffer (pH 7·4) and the peroxidase localized by the diaminobenzidine (DAB)–hydrogen peroxide reaction. Mayer's haemalum was used as a nuclear counterstain. At least two separate blocks of tissue were examined from each case, and for several cases three samples were assessed.

Formalin-fixed paraffin-embedded tissue sections were de-waxed and rehydrated. Endogenous peroxidase was not blocked. The effect of enzyme treatment was assessed by incubating parellel sections with 0·1 per cent trypsin (Difco 1:250) solution, pH 7·8, for 30 min at 37°C, followed by thorough washing. Untreated and treated sections were then incubated with *LTA-peroxidase* or *UEA-peroxidase* in the same manner as frozen sections.

Controls were the incubation of serial sections with *LTA-peroxidase* absorbed with 0·1 M fucose, α-methyl-D-mannoside or *N*-acetyl-D-glucosamine, and *UEA-peroxidase* absorbed with 0·1 M fucose. For some carcinomas displacement of *LTA-peroxidase* from the section by the three sugars was also undertaken.

Frozen sections of 20 carcinomas were treated with alcohol or alcohol and xylene for varying periods of time ranging from 30 to 120 min, stained with *LTA-peroxidase* and the reactions compared with those seen in untreated frozen material. A similar procedure was performed for 10 cases which were subsequently reacted with *UEA-peroxidase*; three of the carcinomas were also assessed for the effect on *LTA* binding.

Double staining—Ten carcinomas were selected on the basis of the results obtained with the single staining procedure. Serial frozen sections were prepared as above and incubated with *LTA-peroxidase*, *UEA-alkaline phosphatase* and *LTA-peroxidase* plus *UEA-alkaline phosphatase*. Endogenous alkaline phosphatase was inhibited by the use of 1 mM levamisole.[15] The alkaline phosphatase was demonstrated using a simultaneous capture method;[16] this was followed by the DAB reaction. Controls were the incubation of sections with the appropriate conjugate plus 0·1 M fucose. The single and double stained sections were examined using two microscopes and a comparison bridge.

Histology—Haematoxylin and eosin stained sections of all carcinomas were assessed for classification and for differentiation using a modification of Bloom and Richardson's grading criteria.[17] The axillary lymph node status was known for 56 cases.

RESULTS

Fixation and controls

There was marked loss of binding of *LTA* in fixed, embedded tissue when compared to frozen material, and this was unaffected by the use of trypsin. All assessments of the extent of reactivity of carcinomas were, therefore, made from frozen section preparations.

The staining achieved in fixed, processed tissue with *UEA-peroxidase* was considerably less than that seen in frozen material, but in 46 of the carcinomas the use of trypsin resulted in a marked

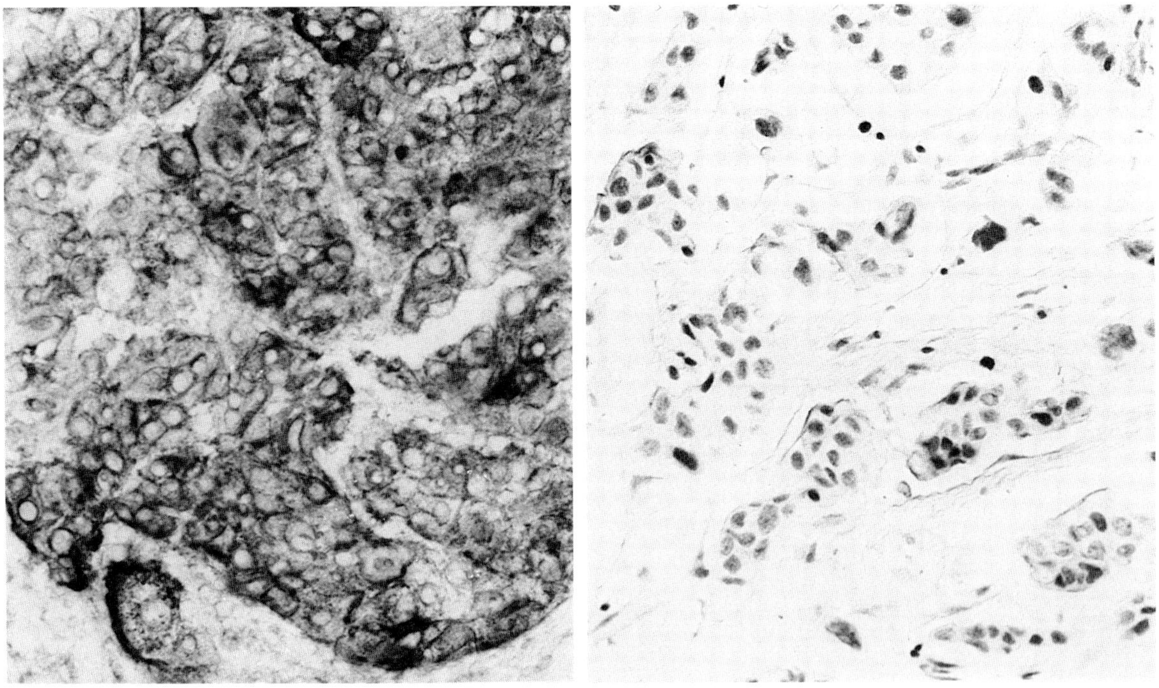

(a) (b)

Fig. 1—(a) Frozen section of a carcinoma stained with *UEA-peroxidase* showing a reaction in the majority of cells of varying intensity. × 220. (b) Trypsinized formalin-fixed paraffin-embedded section of same carcinoma also reacted with *UEA-peroxidase* but showing little evidence of staining. × 220

increase in the number of reactive cells, such that the results in the frozen and fixed tissue became similar. In 15 tumours there was a reduction in the number of positive cells in the fixed tissue, despite trypsinization, and for 19 of the 80 carcinomas there was a marked difference in reactivity in comparison to frozen material (Figs 1a, b). Because of this variation between carcinomas assessments of reactivity were taken from frozen sections; this also gave comparability with *LTA-peroxidase*.

There was inhibition of staining with *LTA-peroxidase* and *UEA-peroxidase* by 0·1 M fucose. A variable reduction in staining with *LTA-peroxidase* occurred with the use of 0·1 M *α*-methyl-D-mannoside and 0·1 M *N*-acetyl-D-glucosamine but staining was unaffected if displacement procedures were used.

Treatment of frozen sections with alcohol and alcohol plus xylene prior to the application of *LTA-peroxidase* resulted in:

No difference in staining	5 cases.
Slight reduction	3 cases.
Patchy reduction in reaction	5 cases.
Virtual absence of staining	7 cases (Figs 2a, b).

and for *UEA-peroxidase*

No difference in staining	2 cases.
Slight reduction	3 cases.
Patchy reduction in reaction	4 cases.
Marked reduction in staining	1 case (Figs 3a, b).

Three of the carcinomas were assessed for the effect on binding of both lectins; the reduction in staining with *UEA-peroxidase* was less than *LTA-peroxidase* in all three. Nine of the 10 carcinomas tested for effect on *UEA* binding showed a marked reduction in staining in fixed, processed tissue, although this was not so apparent in the treated frozen sections. In several instances normal breast tissue was also present within the samples; alcohol treatment had no effect on its reactivity with *LTA* nor *UEA*.

Pattern of staining

The carcinomas could be divided into four categories in relation to the extent of reactivity with the individual lectins: *many* in which all or the majority of cells showed evidence of binding; *moderate*, when there were mixtures of positive and negative cells,

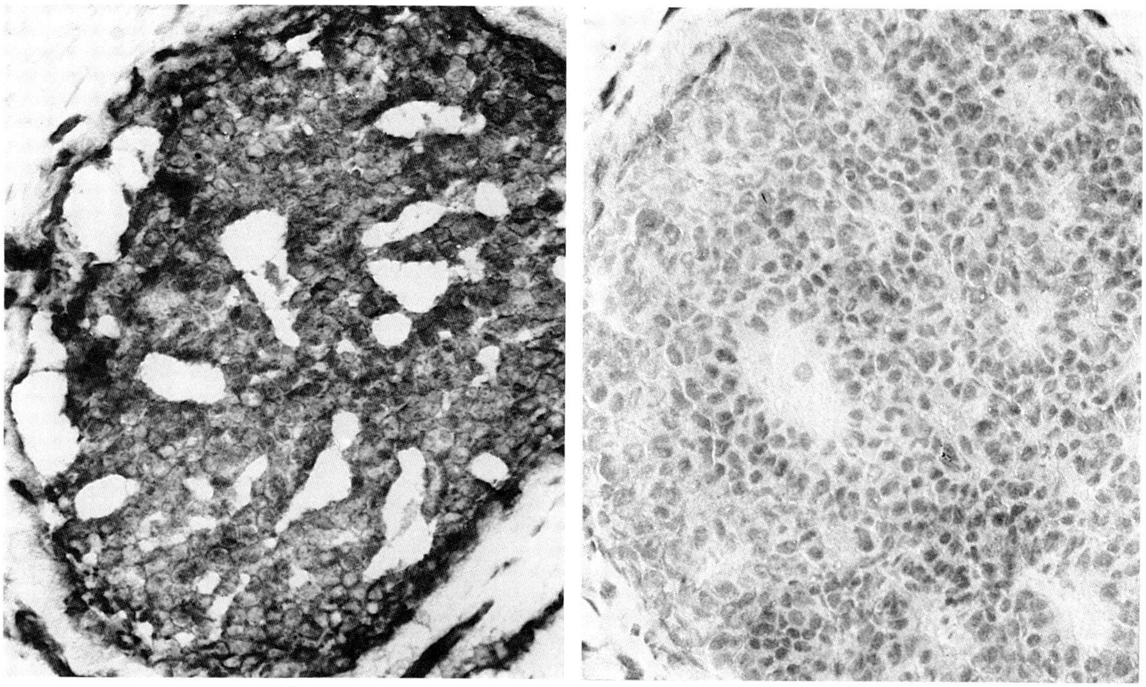

(a) (b)

Fig. 2—(a) Majority of cells showing evidence of binding of *LTA-peroxidase* in air-dried frozen section. ×220. (b) Serial frozen section which has been treated with alcohol for 60 min followed by *LTA-peroxidase*, showing complete loss of staining. ×220

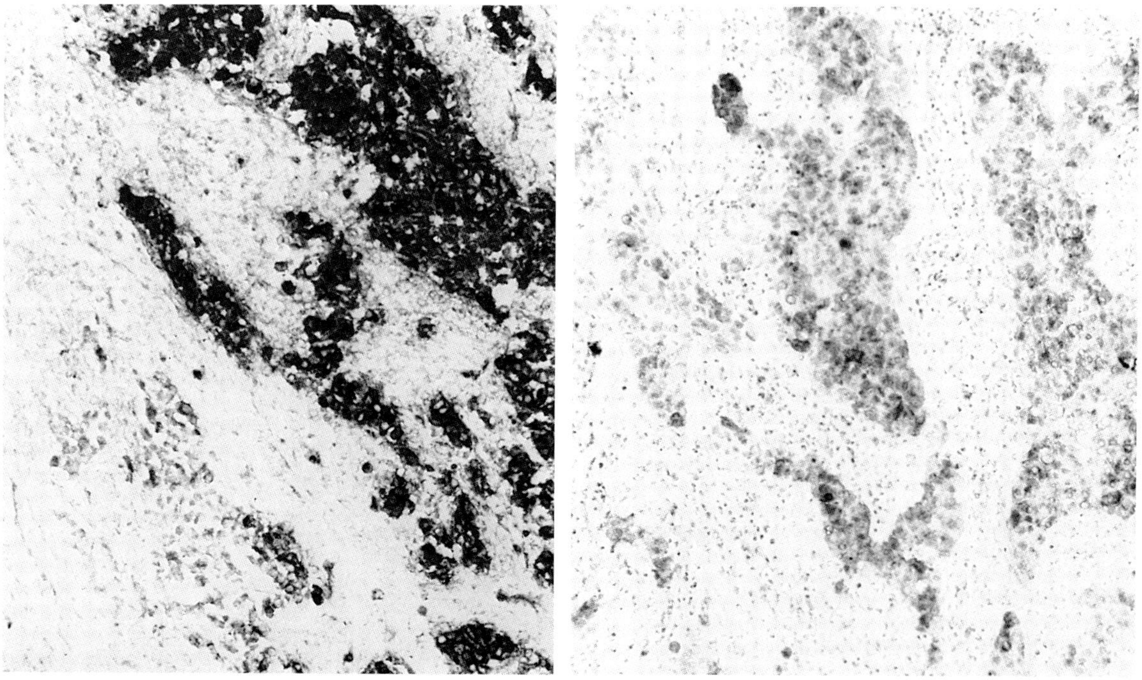

(a) (b)

Fig. 3—(a) Prominent reaction with *UEA-peroxidase* in air-dried frozen section of a carcinoma. ×87. (b) Marked reduction in reaction in serial section treated with alcohol prior to *UEA-peroxidase*. ×87

Table I—The numbers of carcinomas having a specific qualitative degree of reactivity for *LTA* and *UEA*

Proportion of cells reacting	Numbers of carcinomas (%) *LTA*	*UEA*
Many	16 (20)	30 (37·5)
Moderate	30 (37·5)	21 (26·25)
Few	22 (27·5)	21 (26·25)
Negative	12 (25)	8 (10)

Table II—The comparison of the extent of reactivity with *LTA* and *UEA* in individual carcinomas

Proportion of cells reacting *LTA*	*UEA*	Number of carcinomas (%)
Moderate/many	Moderate/many	28 (35)
Moderate/many	Few/negative	18 (22·5)
Few/negative	Moderate/many	23 (28·75)
Few/negative	Few/negative	11 (13·75)

either intermingled or in clusters; *few*, if only a small number of cells reacted; and *negative*.

There was little variation in the extent of reactivity between different blocks of frozen tissue from the same case.

The numbers of carcinomas within each group for both *LTA* and *UEA* are shown in Table I. The comparison of the binding of the two lectins with individual carcinomas is recorded in Table II. The number of tumours having a moderate number or many reactive cells is similar for both lectins (46, *LTA*; 51, *UEA*), although a marked reactivity for *UEA* was twice that for *LTA*. Over half the carcinomas (51·25 per cent) showed different patterns of binding for the two lectins; the *moderate* or *many* category with one, but the *few* or *negative* category for the other (Figs 4a, b, 5a, b).

Comparisons of individual cell reactivity to the lectins obtained from examination of single-stained serial sections were confirmed in double-stained sections. By definition, those tumours having many cells reacting with *LTA* and *UEA* had a similar cellular pattern of staining; this was also apparent in carcinomas having many cells binding one lectin and a moderate number the other. That individual cells bound both lectins was demonstrated by the double-staining method in which an orange-brown reaction product could be seen which differed from the deep red colour product of alkaline phosphatase and the brown reaction production of peroxidase.

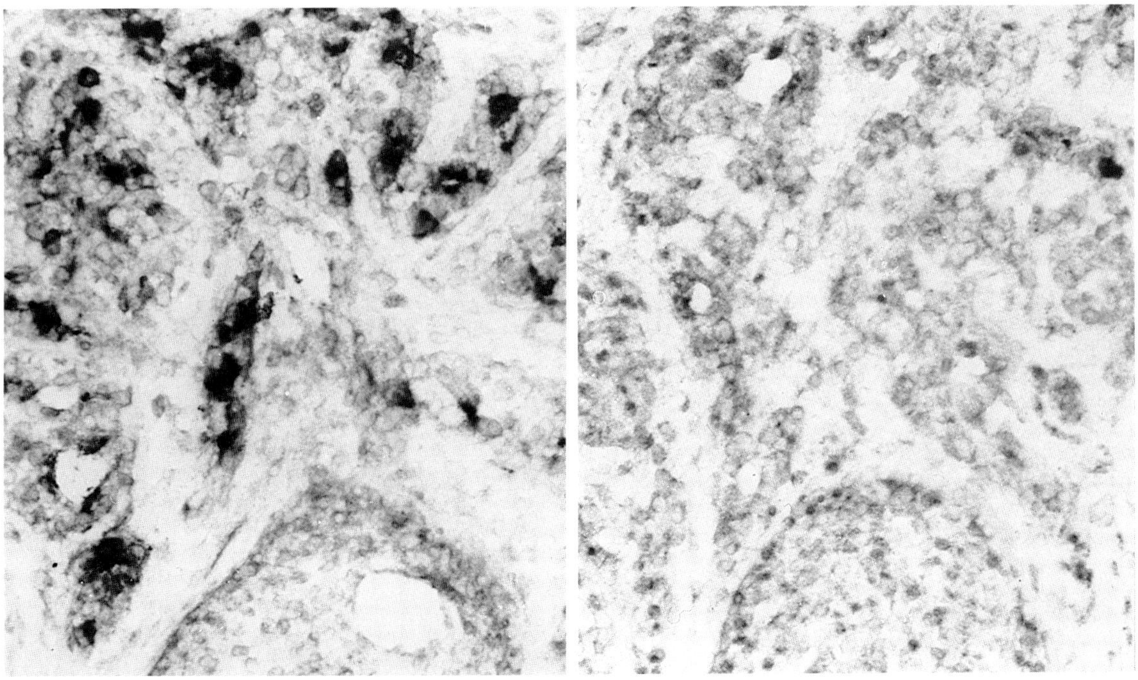

(a) (b)

Fig. 4—(a) Reaction with *UEA-peroxidase* in a frozen section of a carcinoma showing a moderate number of cells staining. × 220. (b) Serial section of the same tumour tested with *LTA-peroxidase*; there are few cells reacting. × 220

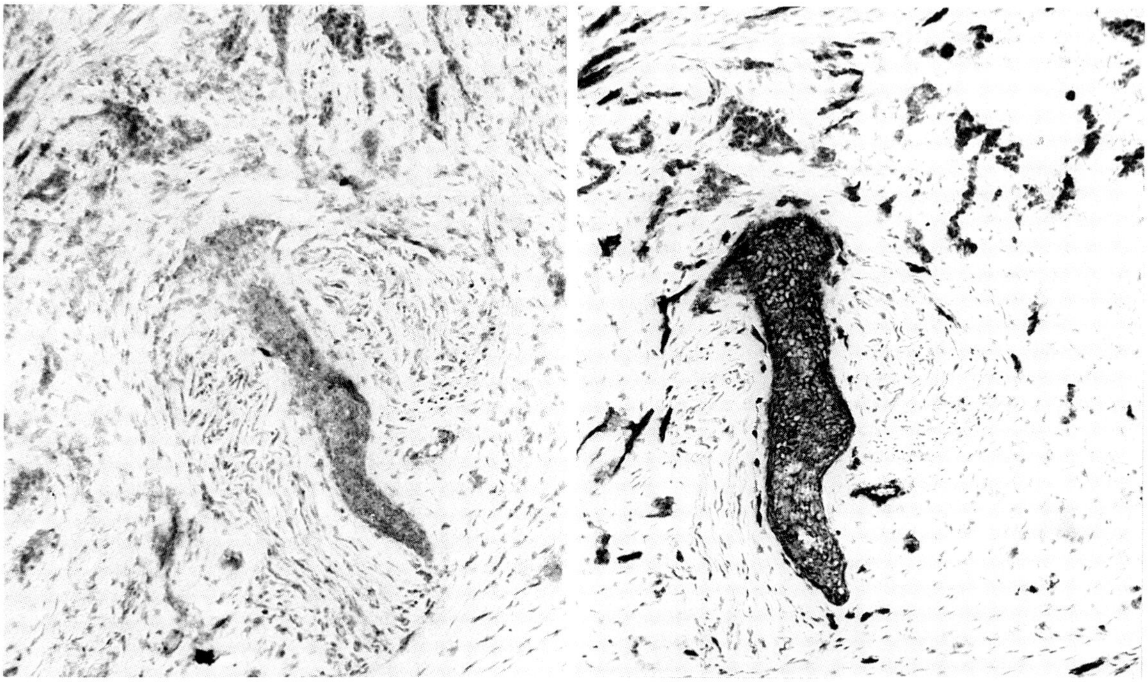

(a) (b)

Fig. 5—(a) A few cells reacting with *UEA-peroxidase* in a frozen section of a carcinoma. ×87. (b) Many cells staining with *LTA-peroxidase* in a serial frozen section of the same tumour. ×87

In those carcinomas with moderate numbers of cells binding both lectins, or moderate numbers for one and few for the other, it was apparent that the sites of lectin reactivity were often different. This was confirmed by the double-staining procedure.

Correlation with type and differentiation

There were four mucinous carcinomas, three of which showed similar staining of mucin with both lectins, the other only reacting with *UEA*. Of the six infiltrating lobular carcinomas, one showed little reactivity, four had little evidence of binding of *LTA* but a moderate number or many positive cells with *UEA* and the other showed the converse. The one tubular carcinoma had a marked reactivity with *LTA* but little evidence of binding of *UEA*. The remaining carcinomas were of the otherwise unspecified infiltrating duct type.

The correlation between the extent of reactivity with *LTA* and *UEA* within carcinomas and histological differentiation is shown in Table III. There is no significant relationship between the degree of binding of *LTA* and tumour differentiation ($0{\cdot}10 > P > 0{\cdot}05$) nor with *UEA* ($P < 0{\cdot}50$). Four of the six well-differentiated tumours had a moderate number or many cells reactive with *LTA* but were negative or had only a few cells that bound *UEA*; the other two well-differentiated tumours showed the converse. There was an even distribution of the paired staining patterns within the other two histological grades.

Table III—The correlation between the proportion of cells within a carcinoma reacting with *LTA* and *UEA* and histological differentiation

Grade	Total No.	*LTA* Neg.	*LTA* Few	*LTA* Mod.	*LTA* Many	*UEA* Neg.	*UEA* Few	*UEA* Mod.	*UEA* Many
I	6	1	1	1	3	1	3	1	1
II	47	11	13	14	9	5	9	14	19
III	27	0	8	15	4	2	9	6	10

Table IV—The extent of reactivity with *LTA* and *UEA* and the comparison between the two lectins in relation to axillary lymph node status

Axillary lymph Node metastasis	*LTA* Neg.	Few	Mod.	Many	*UEA* Neg.	Few	Mod.	Many	*LTA* Neg/Few *UEA* Neg/Few	Neg/Few Mod/Many	Mod/Many Neg/Few	Mod/Many Mod/Many
Present	6	4	13	6	3	11	1	14	5	5	10	9
Absent	3	8	9	7	1	6	9	11	1	10	7	9

Correlation with axillary lymph node status

The relationship between the extent of reactivity with *LTA* and *UEA*, plus the paired binding patterns for the two lectins, and the presence or absence of axillary lymph node metastasis is shown in Table IV. There is no significant correlation between the degree of binding of *LTA* and axillary lymph node status ($P<0\cdot05$), but there is for *UEA* ($0\cdot05>P>0\cdot02$). This is due to more cases with a moderate number of cells binding *UEA* being node-negative, and those tumours with little reactivity being node-positive. Comparison of the binding patterns of the two lectins with node status reveals that the tumours which were generally unreactive were more likely to have metastized, whereas those carcinomas unreactive with *LTA* but having moderate or marked binding of *UEA* were less likely to have spread to local lymph nodes.

DISCUSSION

This study illustrates the value of using two probes that have slight differences in their affinity for the same simple sugar, and confirms the view obtained from agglutination-inhibition studies[12] that with their use fine differences in the glycan component of cell glycoconjugates can be distinguished. The use of *LTA* alone could have suggested that in some breast carcinomas there is an absence of L-fucose-containing glycoproteins or glycolipids but this can be refuted by the demonstration of prominent reactivity with *UEA* in such tumours. Even when there is a lack of reactivity with both lectins in carcinomas it is probably better to confine statements to an absence or modification of the fucosyl oligosaccharides to which these lectins have a high affinity, rather than a total absence of L-fucose.

Modifications in the binding of *LTA* are, therefore, a feature of breast malignancy, since reactivity with this lectin is a constant feature of normal and hyperplastic breast epithelium.[13] However, the position of *UEA* is less clear since the reactivity of normal breast epithelium like that of tumours is variable.[13] Further differences between non-malignant and malignant epithelium can be extrapolated from fixation data. Although *LTA* binding can only be demonstrated in frozen sections of breast tissues the staining achieved in normal epithelium is unaffected by treatment with alcohol, whereas the reaction in 35 per cent of the carcinomas tested was shown to be markedly reduced. Similarly with *UEA* a marked difference between frozen sections and fixed processed tissue was found for 24 per cent of carcinomas, which had not previously been noted for non-malignant tissue.[13] The findings suggest that extraction of fucose-containing glycan-conjugates is occurring; these could be glycolipid in nature, absent or present in only small amounts in normal breast tissue and certain carcinomas. There have been few definitive studies which have considered whether glycolipid composition of tumours *in vivo* differs from that of the normal parent tissue,[18] and none have been related to human breast, although gastric carcinomas have been shown to accumulate less-complex precursor fucose-containing glycolipids.[19]

The comparison of serial sections clearly demonstrates the heterogeneity of binding of the two lectins within carcinomas, and this has been confirmed by the use of double-stained sections. The latter method is to be advocated for the determination of multiple or single binding sites at the cell level. The findings are evidence for the variability in glycan components between cells of the same tumour.

Although *LTA* binding occurs with all normal breast epithelium[13] no correlation could be found between the reactivity of carcinomas with *LTA* and tumour differentiation. The lack of relationship between *UEA* binding and differentiation is less surprising, in view of the unpredictable reactivity of normal epithelium.

There is no correlation between the pattern of *LTA* binding to carcinomas and local lymph node metastasis. However there is a relationship between such metastasis and *UEA* binding. Those tumours having a virtual absence of reactivity with *UEA* are more likely to have spread, whereas those carcinomas with a moderate number of cells binding *UEA* are less likely to have metastized. This indicates that the oligosaccharide chains to which *UEA* preferentially binds have a direct or indirect part in the development of the metastatic process. Deficiency of fucosylation has been related to metastatic capacity in murine tumours.[7] It is difficult to explain why heterogeneity of *UEA* binding is more significant than a consistent reaction. One problem in using lectins is that the actual glyconjugates to which they bind cannot be identified, only the specific sugar groups and these can be common to several glycoproteins or glycolipids. Differences in *UEA* binding between tumours may reflect differences in the presence or absence of several glyconjugates. Another factor which can affect lectin binding is minor variations in the composition of oligosaccharide chains, not necessarily involving the lectin-specific sugar. Such micro-heterogeneity occurs more frequently in carcinomas.[20]

The application of these lectins to tissue sections is limited by the need for fresh specimens. However, they are of value in identifying functional differences between fuco-conjugates present in breast carcinomas, namely that modifications of *LTA* binding sites are a feature of neoplasia whereas changes in *UEA* binding sites relate to metastatic capacity. Such findings indicate areas worthy of further study using other approaches.

ACKNOWLEDGEMENTS

I am grateful to Sheila M. Day for excellent technical assistance; Mrs G. Holmes for secretarial work; Ms B. Jordan for photographic help; and Professor F. Walker for helpful criticism in the preparation of this manuscript. Financial assistance was gratefully received from Trent Regional Health Authority.

REFERENCES

1. Warren L, Buck CA. The membrane glycoproteins of the malignant cell. *Clin Biochem* 1980; **13:** 191–197.
2. Hakomori S. Structures and organization of surface glycolipid dependency on cell growth and malignant transformation. *Biochim Biophys Acta* 1975; **417:** 55–89.
3. Beyer TA, Rearick JI, Paulson JC, Prieels JP, Sadler JE, Hill RL. Biosynthesis of mammalian glycoproteins, glycosylation pathyway in the synthesis of nonreducing terminal sequences. *J Biol Chem* 1979; **254:** 12531–12541.
4. Smets LA, VanBeek WP, VanNie R. Membrane glycoprotein changes in primary mammary tumors associated with autonomous growth. *Cancer Lett* 1977; **3:** 133–138.
5. Richards CS, Medina D, Butel JS, Steiner MR. Correlation of surface fucopeptide patterns with tumorigenicity of mouse mammary epithelial cells. *Cancer Res* 1981; **41:** 4967–4972.
6. Steiner MR, Richards CS, Butel JS, Medina D. Correlation of amino acid fucoside labelling patterns with tumorigenicity of mouse mammary epithelial cells. *Cancer Res* 1983; **43:** 2628–2631.
7. Dennis JW, Kerbel RS. Characterization of a deficiency in fucose metabolism in lectin-resistant variants of a murine tumor showing altered tumorigenic and metastatic capacities *in vivo*. *Cancer Res* 1981; **41:** 98–104.
8. Rosato FE, Seltzer M, Mullen J *et al.* Serum fucose in the diagnosis of breast cancer. *Cancer* 1971; **28:** 1575–1579.
9. Barlow JJ, Dillard PH. Serum protein-bound fucose in patients with gynecologic cancers. *Obstet Gynecol* 1972; **29:** 727–734.
10. Wilkinson EJ, Hause LL, Sasse EA, Pattillo RA, Milbrath JR, Lewis JD. Carcinoembryonic antigen and L-fucose in malignant and benign mammary disease. *Am J Clin Pathol* 1980; **73:** 669–675.
11. Pereira MEA, Kisailus EC, Gruezo F, Kabat EA. Immunochemical studies on the combining site of the blood group H-specific lectin 1 from *Ulex europeus* seeds. *Arch Biochem Biophys* 1978; **185:** 108–115.
12. Debray H, Decout D, Strecker G, Spik G, Montreiul J. Specificity of twelve lectins towards oligosaccharides and glycopeptides related to *N*-glycosylproteins. *Eur J Biochem* 1981; **117:** 41–55.
13. Walker RA. The binding of peroxidase-labelled lectins to human breast epithelium. I—Normal, hyperplastic and lactating breast. *J Pathol* 1984; **142:** 279–291.
14. Voller A, Bidwell DE, Bartlett A. Enzyme immunoassay in diagnostic medicine. Theory and practice. *Bull WHO* 1976; **53:** 55–65.
15. Ponder BA, Wilkinson MM. Inhibition of endogenous tissue alkaline phosphatase with the use of alkaline phosphatase conjugates in immuno-histochemistry. *J. Histochem Cytochem* 1981; **29:** 981–984.
16. Malik NJ, Daymon ME. Improved double immunoenzyme labelling using alkaline phosphatase and horseradish peroxidase. *J Clin Pathol* 1982; **35:** 1092–1094.

17. Walker RA. The binding of fluorescent-labelled concanavalin A to human breast tissue—a marker of differentiation. *J Pathol* 1983; **140:** 255–265.
18. Critchley DR. Glycolipids as membrane receptors important in growth regulation. In: Hynes RO, ed. Surfaces of Normal and Malignant Cells. Chichester: John Wiley, 1979: 63–101.
19. Hakomori S, Koscielak J, Bloch H, Jeanloz R. Immunologic relationship between blood group substances and a fucose-containing glycolipid of human adenocarcinomas. *J Immunol* 1967; **98:** 31–38.
20. Ogata SI, Muramatsu T, Kobata A. New structural characteristics of the large glycopeptides from transformed cells. *Nature* 1976; **259:** 580–582.

JOURNAL OF PATHOLOGY, VOL. **144**: 119–129 (1984)

UNEXPECTED INORGANIC ELEMENTS IN ORAL LESIONS: RESULTS OF X-RAY ENERGY SPECTROSCOPY (XES) ON PARTICULATE MATTER IN PARAFFIN SECTIONS

DAVID A. LEVISON,* PETER R. CROCKER, GARRY LEE, NEIL A. SHEPHERD AND ADRIAN P. SMITH

Department of Histopathology, St. Bartholomew's Hospital and Medical College, London EC1A 7BE, U.K.

Received 22 April 1984
Accepted 1 June 1984

SUMMARY

X-ray energy spectroscopy (XES) of all particulate matter found by light microscopy in histological sections of 222 oral lesions revealed a much wider range of elements than expected from dental amalgam. Subsequent XES of a variety of endodontic materials, impression materials and toothpastes indicated possible sources for virtually all elements identified in the histopathological lesions. The range of materials identified is tabulated; histopathological lesions and probable source substances are correlated; light microscopic pointers to the elemental nature of particulate matter in sections are indicated—titanium and bismuth have characteristic appearances; possible implications of local implantation and large scale ingestion of such substances are discussed.

KEY WORDS—XES, oral lesions, particulate matter, paraffin sections.

INTRODUCTION

The so-called amalgam tattoo[1] and apical granuloma[2] are lesions familiar to histopathologists. Until recently we tended to assume that all particulate matter seen in such lesions, especially if it appeared black in a light microscopic paraffin section, was derived from amalgam. Dental amalgam is a multiphasic material consisting predominantly of silver (Ag), mercury (Hg) and tin (Sn) as three main intermetallic compounds, the γ phase (Ag_3Sn), the γ_1 phase (Ag_2Hg_3) and the γ_2 phase (Sn_7Hg_8) with small amounts of the copper tin phases Cu_3Sn and Cu_5Sn_6.[3,4] Other elements have been found by XES in association with amalgam in tissues viz. selenium (Se), sulphur (S), chlorine (Cl), iron (Fe) and zinc (Zn).[5]

Because of the above body of knowledge on amalgam—particularly its content of and association with a wide variety of inorganic elements—one of us (P.R.C.) thought it would be a useful exercise to examine an amalgam tattoo with our recently acquired x-ray energy spectroscopy (XES) apparatus. A paraffin section of a biopsy of cheek confidently reported as an amalgam tattoo was submitted for XES analysis (case 46 in Fig. 1). To our consternation at the time the only element identifiable by XES was titanium (Ti). That finding stimulated this study.

MATERIALS AND METHODS

Haematoxylin and eosin (H and E) stained paraffin sections of all oral biopsies received from the hospital dental department in 1980, 1981 and 1982 were examined specifically for the presence of particulate matter by light microscopy with and without cross polarized light. To these were added sections from four cases seen before 1980: one of these, referred to above, was the case which stimulated this study, and the others we had on record as containing particulate matter. Material from a total of 222 patients was screened comprising 138 apical granulomas, 39 apical cysts, 4 tooth sockets, 1 tooth, 36 'other gum lesions', 6 'other jaw

* Addressee for correspondence.

0022–3417/84/100119–11$01.10

lesions' and 8 lip and cheek lesions. The 66 cases found to contain particulate matter were then examined as described previously,[6] briefly as follows. The particulate matter located by light microscopy in the H and E stained section was photographed. The coverslip was then removed, the section coated with carbon in a Nanotech CC2 carbon coater, and placed in a Jeol 35CF scanning electron microscope fitted with a backscattered electron detector, a Kevex Unispec System 7000 XES unit, and a Dapple Microplus data processor. The previously photographed area was identified in the secondary electron and backscattered electron images. The particulate matter was then analysed by XES at 25 kV for periods of 100 sec. An adjacent non-particle-containing area of the section was always examined in the same way so that the background spectrum coming through from the supporting glass (predominantly silicon (Si), magnesium (Mg) and calcium (Ca)) could then be compared with and subtracted from the spectra obtained from the particles. As we have previously identified aluminium (Al) and bromine (Br) in haematoxylin and eosin stain (unpublished), wherever Al was identified (no Br was identified in any of these cases), further sections were recut from the relevant blocks, stained with neutral red and then submitted to the analytical process outlined above. In this study Al, when present, was found in both H and E and neutral red stained sections. In one case (case 45) there was sufficient particulate material present in the block to allow infra-red spectroscopic analysis in a Perkin Elmer 577 infra-red spectrophotometer.

Samples of all endodontic materials used by the dental departments of this and King's College Hospitals (courtesy of Dr B. M. Eley) and in the surgery of a practising dental surgeon (Mr L. D. Payne, LDS, BDS London) were obtained and examined by XES. The materials in paste form were spread on a carbon stub and allowed to dry and those in powder form were sprinkled onto a drop of colloidal graphite (dag) on a carbon stub, allowed to dry then carbon-coated and examined in the scanning electron microscope as above. The materials examined in this way were: Kerr MPC Base and Catalyst, Kerr Hydrex Base and Catalyst, Kerr Cavitec Base and Accelerator, Kerr Tubli-Seal Base and Catalyst (all Kerr Manufacturing Co, Division of Sybron Corporation, Romulus, Michigan 48174, U.S.A.), three separate samples of Caulk Dycal Base and Catalyst (The LD Caulk Co., Division of Dentistry, International Inc., Milford, Delaware 19963, U.S.A.), Poly-F and Kalzinol lesion bonded zinc oxide/eugenol (both De Trey), zince cement improved powder type 1 (S. S. White Ltd, Harrow, Middlesex), Bipp (Evans Medical Ltd, Speke), Alvogen gauze, Composite A and B and Quick Set ZnO_2 (all B. M. Eley), zinc oxide (as supplied by Pharmacy), Ledermix Cement and Hardener, and Ledermix Paste (both Lederle Laboratories Division, Cyanamid of Great Britain Ltd, Gosport, Hampshire), Endomethasone root canal sealer and Devitalising Paste (both Specialities Septodent, 29 Rue des Petites Ecuris, 75010 Paris) and N_2 Root Canal Sealer (made in Switzerland by Indrag AGSA, distributed in U.K. by Courtin Ltd., Capel, Surrey). Samples of amalgam were not analysed by XES as this has previously been exhaustively performed.[4,7]

Fourteen samples of popular brands of toothpaste were obtained for analysis from local chemists. Each sample was washed three times in water to remove the sweeteners and binding substances and leave the bulk abrasive powder for analysis. A drop of each was then dried on a graphite stub and examined by XES as above. A 'disc' of each was also examined by infra-red spectroscopy as above. The toothpastes examined in this way were Macleans, Co-op Fluoride, Colgate, Gordon Moores Cosmetic, Crest (one sample bought in 1977 and one in 1984), Close-up, Cherish, Gibbs SR, Signal, Boots Fluoride, Aquafresh, Pearldrops and Euthymol.

Four samples of dental impression material were also examined by XES. These were Impregum (ESPE GMBH, Fabrik Pharmazeutischer Praparate, D-8031, Seefeld/Oberbay), Alginate (Bayer Dental, D-5090, Lauerkuscn), Polysulphide impression material (Kerr, Switzerland—U.K. distributors: Cottrell and Company, 15–17 Charlotte Street, London W1P 2AA) and Silicone (Davis, Schottlander and Davis, London EC1).

RESULTS

Biopsies

Table I summarizes the overall results of the biopsy survey. The 66 specimens listed as 'tested by XES' are all the specimens in which particulate matter was seen by light microscopy. Fifteen of these were completely negative on XES indicating that the particulate matter was composed of elements below sodium (Na) (atomic number 11) in the Periodic Table and was, therefore, of organic

Table I—Oral lesions examined for particulate matter

Specimen	Total no. screened by light microscopy	No. tested by XES	No. positive for inorganic elements*
Apical granuloma†	138	51	37
Apical cyst†	39	10	6
Tooth socket	4	1	1‡
Tooth	1	0	0
All other gum lesions	26	2	2§
All other jaw lesions	6	0	0
Lip and cheek lesions	8	2	1¶
	222	66	47+4 Fe only

*For details see Fig. 1.
†A rather artificial separation but in line with clinical impression.
‡An amalgam related lesion (case 44, Fig. 1).
§Calcified connective tissue of uncertain histogenesis (case 45, Fig. 1) and a foreign body reaction to titanium (case 46, Fig. 1).
¶A ruptured mucous retention cyst of lip related to bismuth (case 47, Fig. 1).

nature. The probable source of iron in the four iron-only cases is the breakdown of haemoglobin following haemorrhage in the region of previous dental work. We have, therefore, not included these four cases in the detailed breakdown of 47 cases in Fig. 1. All 47 cases in Fig. 1 show the presence of exogenous inorganic material; some also contain iron which may well be endogenous.

Figure 1 shows that amalgam and barium sulphate were the commonest XES findings. Amalgam was identified in various forms: in 11 cases Ag, Sn and Hg, in two Ag and Sn, in one only Sn, and one

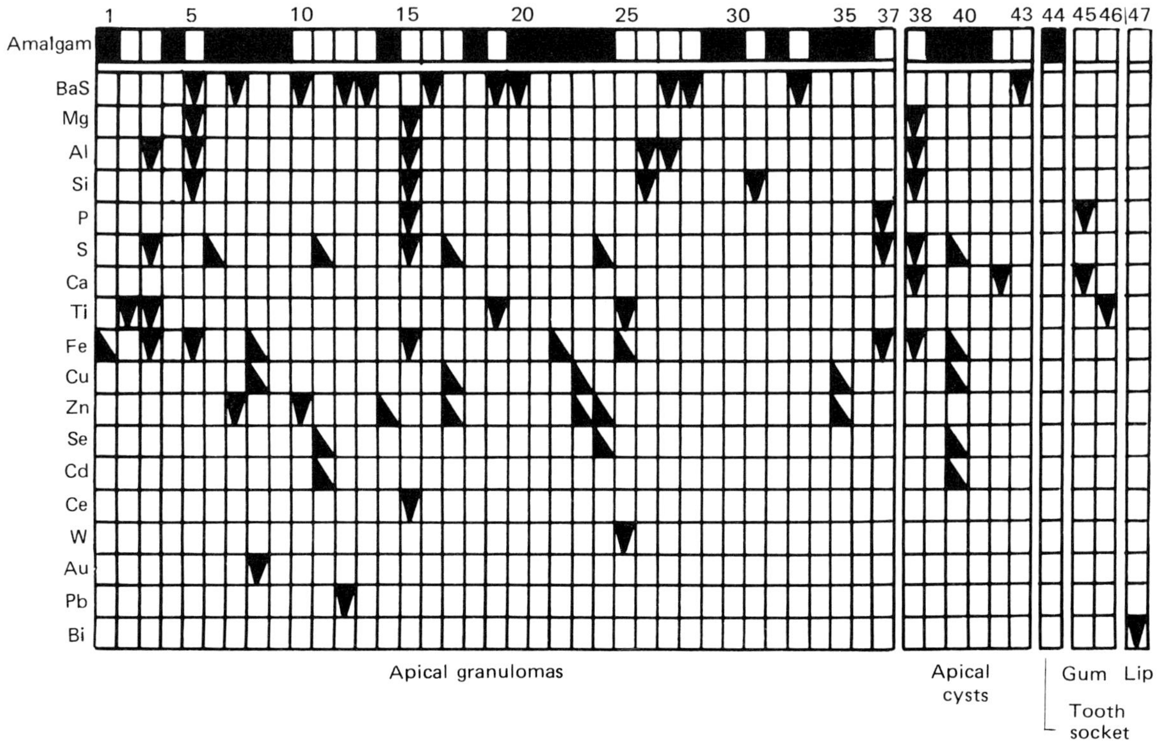

Fig. 1—Positive XES results on oral biopsies. ◣, Elements designated by this symbol are considered related to amalgam—see text. ▼, Elements designated by this symbol are considered not related to amalgam

only Hg. Other elements were found less frequently. Some of these are related to amalgam, either being present in small quantities in certain preparations viz. copper and zinc, or concentrated from endogenous sources e.g. sulphur with silver[5] and selenium with mercury and silver.[8] Other elements cannot be amalgam-related or endogenous, e.g. aluminium, titanium and bismuth (Bi). Larger amounts of Zn are probably not derived from amalgam. As Figs 2–6 show, it is possible to recognize several of these different materials in histological sections by light microscopy. Amalgam, when all three elements or whenever silver was present appeared black (Fig. 2). It was non-refractile under cross polarized light but when large clumps were present, a weak refractile glow could be seen round the edge of the clump. In the one case where mercury alone was detected by XES, it appeared brown rather than black by light microscopy and in the one case where tin was identified on its own it appeared as brown granules within macrophages. Silver, mercury and tin particles all appeared non-refractile.

Barium sulphate in histological sections is characteristically recognized by light microscopy as small (approximately 1 μm diameter) weakly doubly refractile pale yellow particles in macrophages (Fig. 3). However, in some cases (e.g. case 10 in Figs 1, 4) it was present as larger colourless brightly doubly refractile particles. Such an appearance of barium sulphate in sections has been recently described.[9]

By light microscopy zinc in sections appeared as finely divided dark brown refractile particles (Fig. 4). In the predominantly Zn-containing case illustrated in Fig. 4 there were also present larger brightly doubly refractile particles of barium sulphate. Titanium in sections had a characteristic light microscopic appearance comprising small brown/black granules, often aggregated together in clumps (Fig. 5A). The clumps appeared a delicate pink colour when viewed under cross polarized light while individual granules showed white birefringence (Fig. 5B). If there is sufficient titanium in a section, it can be recognized by naked eye examination in oblique daylight where it appears white (as opposed to similar quantities of amalgam which appear black). In fact the clinical lesion may look white as case 46 in Fig. 1 was sent by the dental surgeon as a 'white area on gum ?retained calcium hydroxide'. Bismuth had a dramatic and characteristic appearance in histological sections: under low

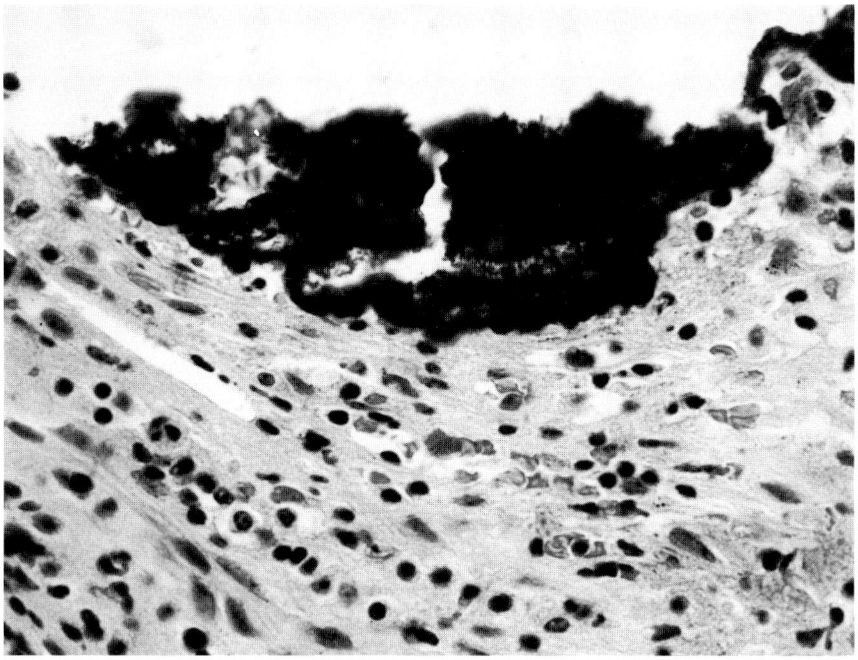

Fig. 2—Light microscopic appearance of a large clump of amalgam with associated non specific chronic inflammatory response in an apical granuloma (case 32, Fig. 1). The amalgam appears black and was non-refractile. H and E, × 630

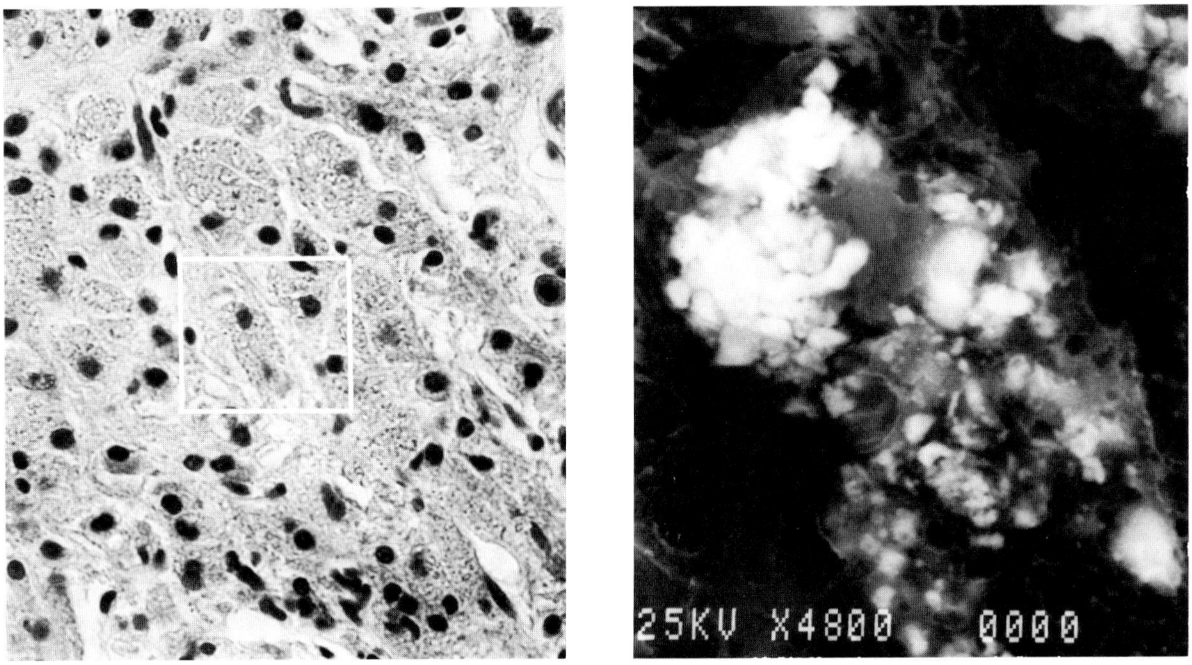

(A) (B)

Fig. 3—(A) Classic light microscopic appearances of finely granular barium sulphate in macrophages in an apical granuloma (case 33, Fig. 1) ×630. (B) The secondary electron image (SEI) of the boxed area in (A) showing BaS particles < 1 μm in diameter

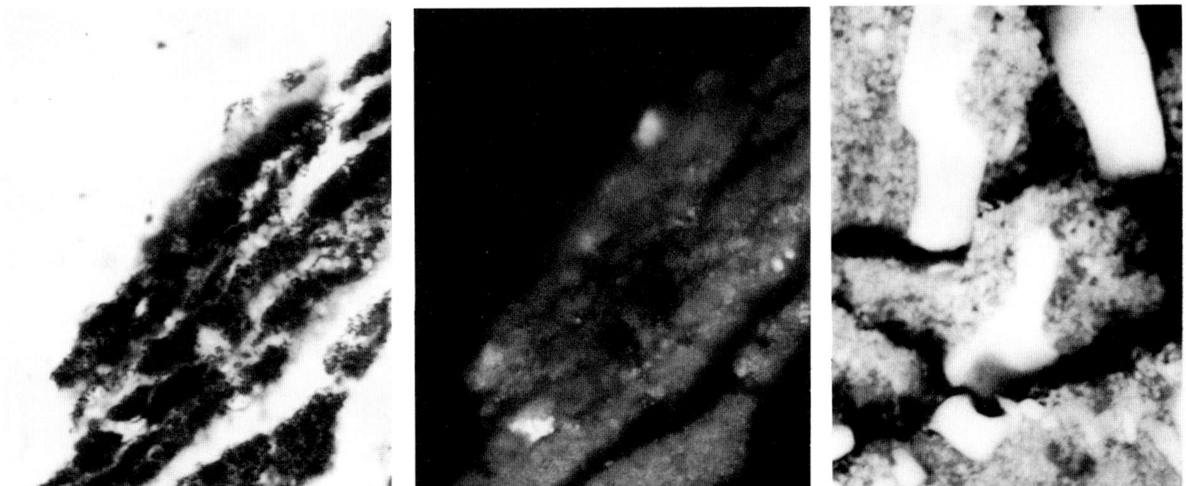

(A) (B) (C)

Fig. 4—(A) Normal light, (B) cross polarized light, and (C) the backscattered electron image (BEI) appearances of a field in case 10, Fig. 1, containing mostly Zn—the dark material in A and background granular material in C, and large particles of BaS—the bright areas in B and the large light particles in C. (A) and (B), ×630; (C), ×3600

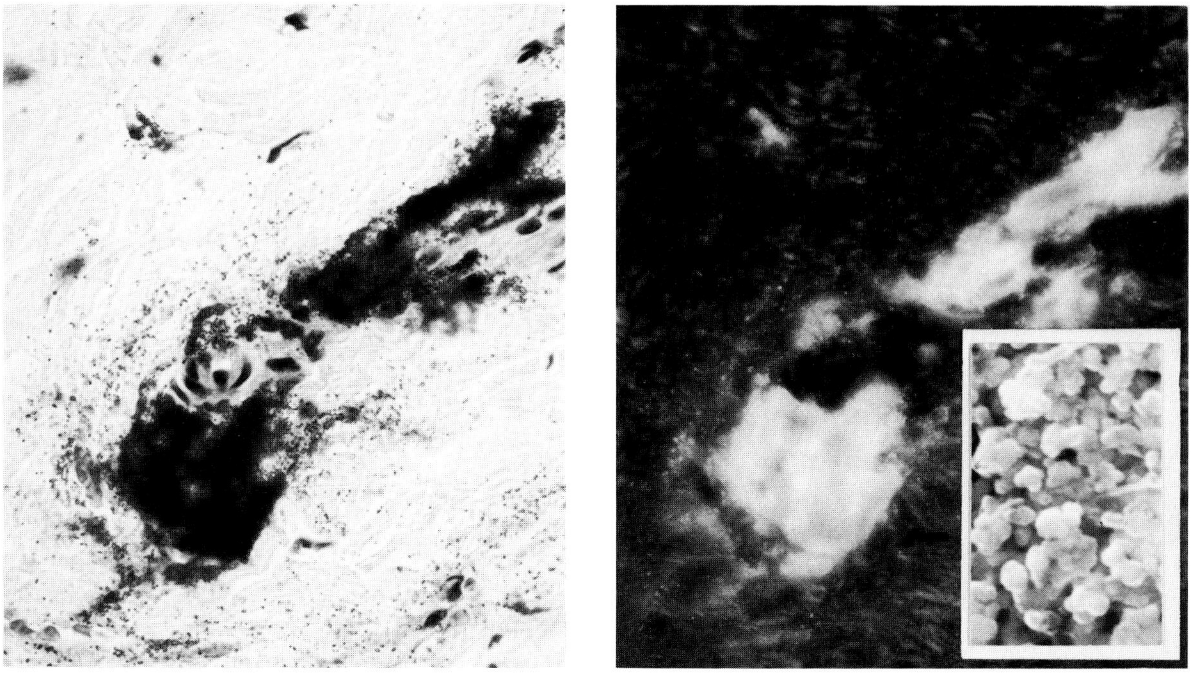

(A) (B)

Fig. 5—(A) Normal light and (B) cross polarized light appearances of titanium (Ti) in a gum lesion (case 46, Fig. 1). The clumps and particles in (A) appeared brown/black and in (B) the clumps glowed pale pink while the small particles were bright white. H and E, × 630. Inset, SEI × 10 000 of rounded granules of titanium in this section

power it presented as blackish clumps; on higher power these resolved into aggregates of yellowish brown coarsely granular particules which were brightly doubly refractile under cross polarized light (Fig. 6). None of the other elements detected and listed in Fig. 1 had characteristic light microscopic appearances.

Selected secondary electron image (SEI) and backscattered electron image (BEI) appearances of the compounds and elements described above are illustrated along with the light microscopic appearances in Figs 3–6. The BEI was particularly useful in identifying areas for XES as the intensity of the signal in the BEI is proportional to atomic weight and so varies with different underlying inorganic elements.

The inflammatory reaction associated with the different materials detected was very variable. Its intensity and quality did not appear to relate specifically to either the quantity or the nature of the foreign material present. The full range of light microscopic appearances previously described in association with amalgam was observed.[1,5,10] In one of the two cases containing only titanium (case 46—Fig. 1) some of the pigment was associated with virtually no active inflammatory response—it appeared embedded in fibrous tissue—while in other areas titanium particles appeared to be the central focus of a brisk inflammatory reaction and some were present within macrophages. The other case containing titanium alone (case 2—Fig. 1) showed very little inflammation directly related to the particles, but a brisk inflammatory response in other parts of the section. In the one case with bismuth alone (case 47—Fig. 1) there was a macrophage response related to the edges of the clumps of bismuth particles but very little other evidence of inflammation. Zinc was never seen in isolation and was associated with very variable non-specific chronic inflammatory reactions.

Case 45 in Fig. 1, with calcium (Ca) and phosphorus (P) identified on XES, is the only one in which there was sufficient material in the block for IR spectroscopy. This showed the material to be calcium carbapatite. This was a peculiar area of calcified connective tissue of uncertain pathogenesis in gum.

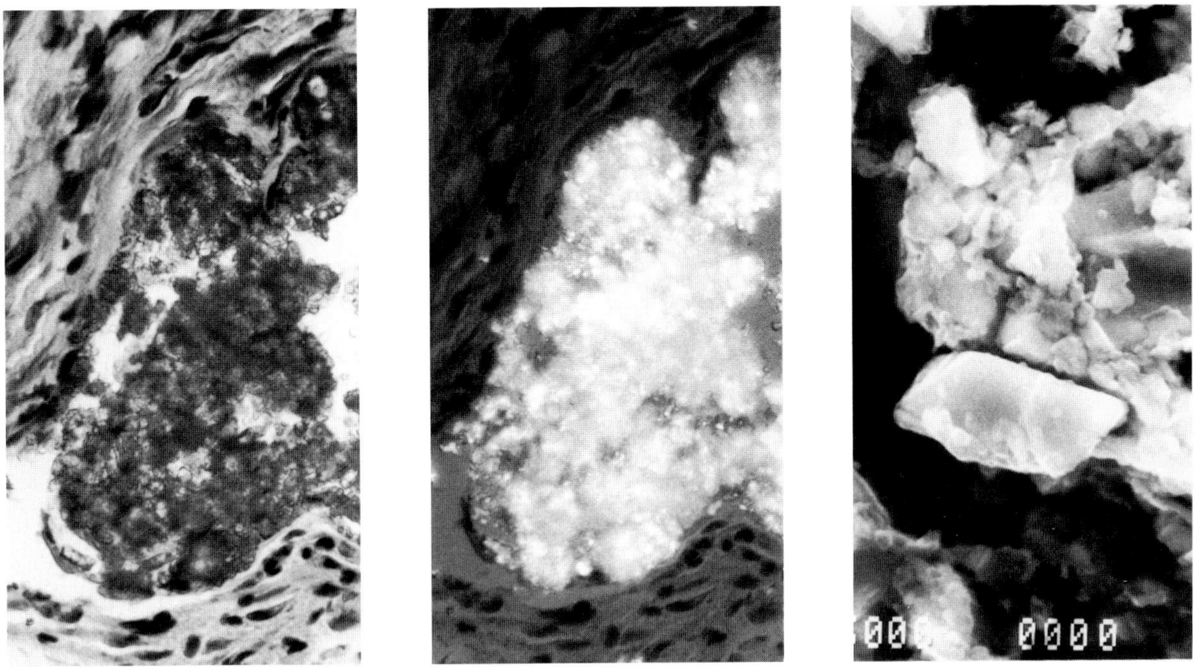

(A) (B) (C)

Fig. 6—(A) Normal light, (B) cross polarized light and (C) SEI appearances of bismuth (Bi) in a lip lesion (case 47, Fig. 1). The coarsely granular Bi-containing material appeared yellowish-brown in normal light, was strongly doubly refractile (B), and composed of irregular shaped and sized granules (C). (A) and (B), × 630; (C) × 6000

Endodontic materials

The inorganic elements identified by XES in the compounds examined are shown in Table II. IR spectroscopy was also done on most of these compounds, but the complex nature of the mixtures of substances involved did not produce readily identifiable spectra. We, therefore, decided to compare the composition of the compound as stated on its container or wrapping with our XES findings, noting 'expected' and 'detected' elements as shown in Table II. As the table shows, we found many more inorganic elements than 'expected'. The only 'expected' element which we failed to find was bismuth in N_2 root canal sealer. This may have been because bismuth made up only a tiny percentage of the mixture according to the N_2 label, though we did spend several hours searching in an attempt to eliminate this anomaly.

Backscattered electron images of Tubli-Seal Base and MPC Base are illustrated (Fig. 7A, B). The brighter particles contain the higher atomic weight elements. As in the sections and as expected, the BEI was more useful than the SEI in locating areas containing different elements which were then identified by XES.

Toothpastes

All 14 toothpaste samples were analysed by infrared spectroscopy and XES and the results are displayed in Table III. The elements we 'expected' to detect by XES were based on the IR findings and were almost exactly as expected, the only additional finding being titanium in Euthymol, Gibbs SR and Signal.

The SEIs of all toothpastes showed them to be composed of fine particles, the basis of the abrasive property of toothpaste. Figure 8 is a composite picture of the SEIs of three selected toothpaste samples showing the range of appearances of different types of particle. The BEI did help to pick out the areas containing titanium which were brighter than the background, again because titanium was the highest atomic weight element present. Titanium appeared to be present in relatively small quantities and is presumably there as a whitening agent.

Impression media

The results of XES on the four impression media examined are displayed in Table IV. The main point to note is the very large number of elements present in Alginate.

Table II—XES analysis results on endodontic materials

Sample	Stated formula	XES Expected	XES Detected
Alvogen (gauze)	—	?	Ca
Bipp	Bismuth iodoform paraffin paste	?I Bi	I-traces Bi
Cavitec	—	?	Zn
Composite A	—	?	Si
Composite B	—	?	Si
Devitalising paste	Organic	?	Mg Al Si S Fe
Dycal Base*	Radioopaque calcium hydroxide	Ca	S Ca Ti W
Dycal Base†,‡	Radioopaque calcium hydroxide	Ca	P Ca Zn W
Dycal Catalyst*	Radioopaque calcium hydroxide	Ca	S Ca Ti Zn
Dycal Catalyst†,‡	Radioopaque calcium hydroxide	Ca	S Ca Ti Zn
Endomethasone	Organic + radioopaque excipient	?	S Zn I Ba Pb
Hydrex Base	Calcium hydroxide	Ca	S Ca Ba
Kalzinol	Zinc oxide	Zn	Zn
Ledermix Cement	Organic	?	Ca Zn
Ledermix Paste	Organic	?	Si Cl Ca Zn
MPC Base	Calcium hydroxide	Ca	S Ca Ba
MPC Catalyst	Calcium hydroxide	Ca	Organic
N2	Titanium, zinc, lead, bismuth	Ti Zn Pb Bi	Ti Zn Pb
Poly F	Zinc oxide	Zn	Zn
Quick Set ZnO_2	Zinc oxide	Zn	Zn
Zinc cement	Zinc oxide	Zn	Zn
Tubli-Seal base	—	?	Zn Bi
ZNO_2	Zinc oxide	Zn	Zn

*,†,‡ Three separate samples of Dycal Base and Catalyst.

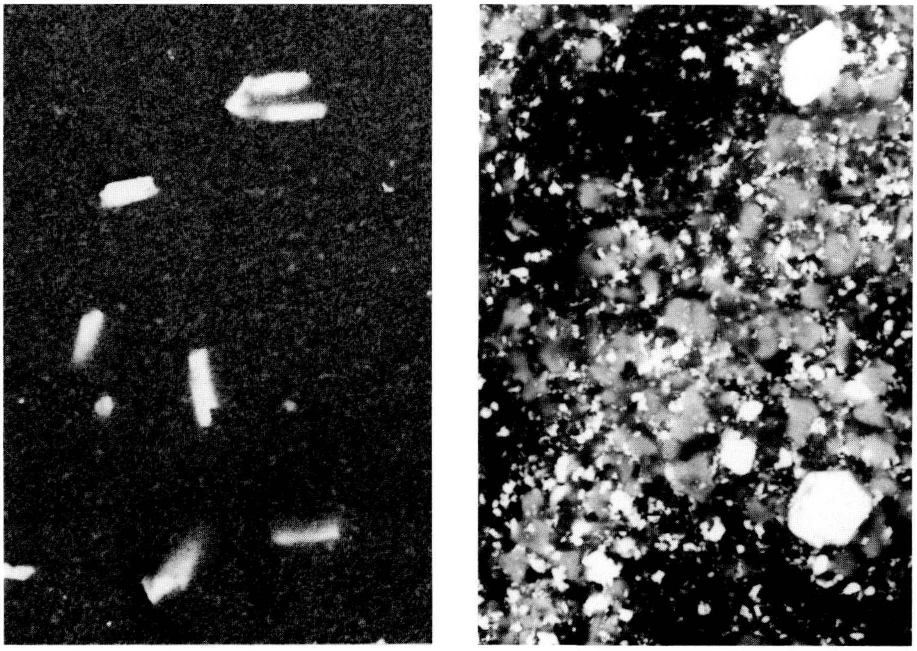

(A) (B)

Fig. 7—BEIs of (A) Tubli-Seal base and (B) MPC base. In A the fine granular particles in the background on XES are Zn and the large bright particles Bi. In (B) the dull background material is Ca and the bright particles are BaS. × 1000

Table III—Infra-red and XES analysis results on toothpastes

Brand of toothpaste	IR spectrum*	XES Expected	XES Detected
Aquafresh	Silicon dioxide, calcium carbonate	Si Ca	Si Ca
Boots Fluoride	Silicon dioxide, calcium carbonate	Si Ca	Si Ca
Boots Mildmint Fluoride	Silicon dioxide, calcium carbonate	Si Ca	Si Ca
Cherish	Silicon dioxide	Si	Si
Closeup	Silicon dioxide	Si	Si
Colgate	Calcium carbonate	Ca	Ca
Co-op Fluoride	Calcium carbonate	Ca	Ca
Crest '1977'	Calcium pyrophosphate (β)	P Ca	P Ca
Crest '1984'	Silicon dioxide	Si	Si
Euthymol	Calcium dihydrogen phosphate	P Ca	P Ca Ti
Gibbs SR	Aluminium hydroxide	Al	Al Ti
Gordon Moores Cosmetic	Calcium carbonate	Ca	Ca
Macleans	Calcium carbonate	Ca	Ca
Pearl Drops	Aluminium hydroxide, calcium phosphate	Al P Ca	Al P Ca
Signal	Aluminium hydroxide	Al	Al Ti

*IR Spectrum nearest match in *Atlas of Infrared Spectra of Inorganic Compounds*, Richard A. Nyquist and Ronald O. Kagel, New York and London: Academic Press, 1971.

DISCUSSION

Our findings show that although most inorganic particulate matter in oral lesions is derived from amalgam, much is not. Most of this appears to be derived from endodontic materials, but some possibly comes from toothpaste or even impression medium. We decided that whenever we detected only very tiny (i.e. sub light microscopic) amounts of Cu, Zn, Se, S, Cl and Fe, that these were most likely to be present as a result of the nearby presence of amalgam.[5] On that basis we designated them with a specific symbol in Fig. 1. The other element designated by that symbol and the one with the most tenuous association with amalgam is cadmium (Cd). Our reasons for allocating Cd to this group are that it is often associated with Se,[11] it was associated with Se on both occasions that it was

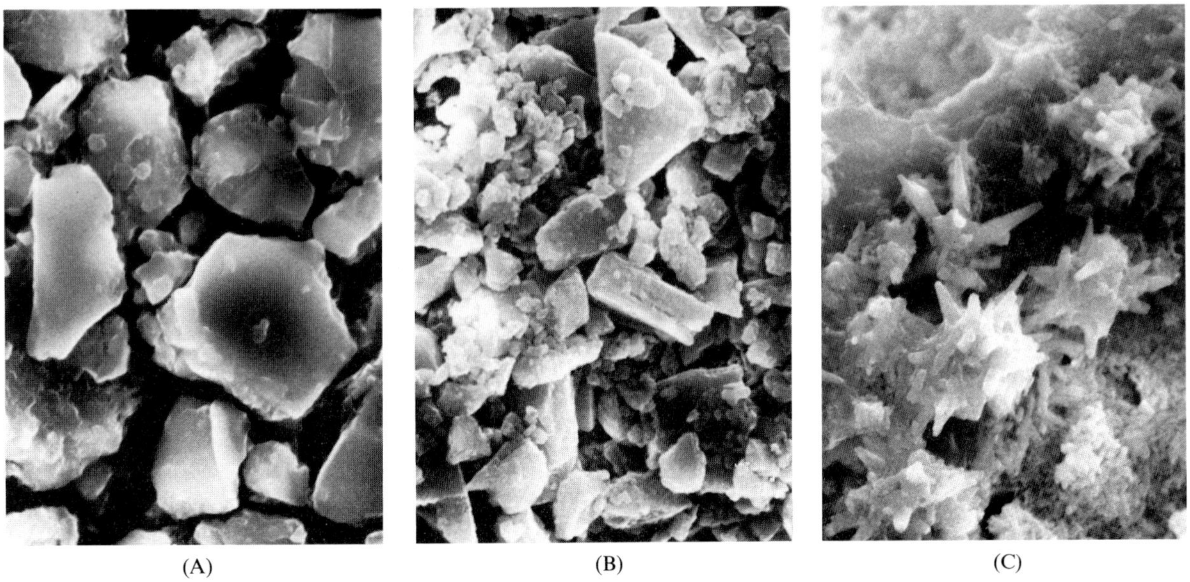

(A) (B) (C)

Fig. 8—SEIs of three toothpastes (A) Signal, (B) Crest 1977 and (C) Macleans. Infra-red spectroscopy showed (A) to be aluminium hydroxide (XES—Al), (B) to be calcium pyrophosphate β (XES—Ca, P), and (C) to be calcium carbonate (XES—Ca). × 1800

Table IV—XES results on impression materials

Impression material	XES
Alginate	Mg Al Si S K Ca Ti Fe
Impregum	Si S Cl
Polysulphide	Si S Ca (Zn Pb)*
Silicone	Mg Si S Ca

* Diffusely finely dispersed 0·5–2·0 μm particles.

seen by us, and Se is known to aggregate in relation to Hg and Ag.[8] We may be wrong to relate Cd to amalgam here but Cd is one of only three elements (see below) which does not appear in any of the endodontic, toothpaste or impression materials analysed. Larger amounts (readily detectable by light microscopy) of Zn we consider most unlikely to be derived from amalgam and much more likely to be derived from one of the endodontic materials. That is why Zn is sometimes recorded in Fig. 1 as amalgam-associated and sometimes not. Fe on five occasions and S on four occasions are recorded as not associated with amalgam. This is because they were identified on these occasions without amalgam or any other amalgam associated elements being detected and along with other elements suggesting origin in an endodontic material such as devitalizing paste or impression medium such as Alginate. Au, though not present in any of the dental materials examined by us has, of course, a variety of uses in dentistry. Cerium (Ce) is the third and only other element appearing in Fig. 1 and not present in any of Tables II, III, or IV. We do not know its source but note in our copy of the *Merck Index* that it is used in ceric fluoride as a fluorinating agent.[11]

Whether or not any of the particulate matter identified by us in these lesions, actually caused the development of the lesion is difficult to prove. However, in the only two areas where systematic study has so far been possible, there seems incontravertible evidence that such material can cause inflammatory lesions: amalgam has been thoroughly investigated experimentally and shown to produce such lesions when implanted in the tissues[5] and barium sulphate—though remarkably non-irritant in general—is widely accepted as capable of producing inflammatory lesions if it becomes impacted in the tissues of the gastrointestinal tract[12] and elsewhere.[13,14] Barium salts other than the sulphate are known to be highly toxic and it is worthy of note and comforting that we did not find barium unassociated with sulphur. It does seem reasonable to us to suggest that titanium in case 46 and as described above, was the cause of the inflammatory lesion as this was not an apical granuloma, no other likely cause was identified, and the most active area of inflammation was centred on titanium particles.

We were rather surprised to find how seldom the complete range of elements identifiable by XES was named on the product label. A notable exception to this general rule is N_2 Root Canal Sealer (Indrag AGSA, Switzerland) which lists all of the various elements we could identify by XES (see Table II), and Bi which we could not find on XES despite repeated searches. This discrepancy is most likely due to sampling in our view as Bi is only a very minor component of this product according to the label. From the point of view of sampling error, this approach of ours (viz. doing scanning electron microscopy and XES on the actual light microscopic paraffin section) is vastly superior to traditional transmission electron microscopical methods and more direct than the serial sectioning technique devised by Harrison and Davies.[15]

The material which, we are informed, is the most widely used cavity lining material and incidentally which was the only sample supplied to us by all three of our sources, viz. Caulk Dycal Base (and catalyst) contains a veritable Pandora's box of inorganic elements (Table II) and this is certainly not indicated on the label. The manufacturer presumably considers, probably correctly, that such information is not required by the dental surgeon and unlikely to be important other than in exceptional circumstances.

Both from our analytical results and from a knowledge of the way it is used we think that toothpaste seldom contributes to particulate matter in oral lesions. However, it is a possible source and of note that titanium, the stimulus for this study, is present in three brands of toothpaste as well as two endodontic samples (Tables II and III). The variety of types of the bulk abrasive powders used in toothpastes is of note and we were particularly interested to discover that several brands have silicon dioxide as a main constituent. This certainly provides another possible source of ingestion of significant quantities of silica in addition to regular ingestion of magnesium trisilicate. Should a patient who produces urinary tract stones of silicon dioxide[16] deny ingesting antacids then it might be worthwhile investigating his use of toothpaste.

We should hope that our comments on the light microscopic appearances of the different types of particulate matter in sections might help histopathologists to identify correctly more of such material. The pale yellowish weakly doubly refractile finely granular appearance of barium sulphate is well known, but it can easily be overlooked or misinterpreted if its presence is unexpected. Larger particles of barium sulphate are less widely recognized by histopathologists, are present in the double contrast agent E-Z-HD used in upper gastrointestinal radiography and have only recently been properly identified in tissue lesions.[9] Larger particle forms of barium sulphate do appear to be incorporated in some endodontic materials e.g. MPC Base (Fig. 8B), and this seems to us the likeliest source of such particles of barium sulphate in oral lesions. Titanium and bismuth have very characteristic light microscopic appearances as described and illustrated, and we have found the practice of holding a paraffin section in oblique light and observing its greyish appearance to the naked eye, to be very reliable and helpful in the preliminary identification of titanium. Zinc containing material has a less distinctive light microscopic appearance but from our description it might at least be possible to suggest its presence and distinguish it from other possible foreign material in a section.

Finally we think it worth bearing in mind that although the wide variety of particulate matter we have identified in oral lesions may be pathologically relatively unimportant in the mouth *per se*, the knowledge that such materials are being used in the mouth, are present there for very long periods in some cases, and are presumably swallowed, may be of importance elsewhere in the gastrointestinal tract.

ACKNOWLEDGEMENTS

We should like to thank the Dental Surgeons attached to St. Bartholomew's Hospital who supplied all the biopsy material examined, the North East Thames Regional Health Authority, the Wellcome Trust and the St. Bartholomew's Hospital Joint Research Board who together financed the purchase of our analytical apparatus, Dr A. J. Blackshaw who took part in early stages of this work, Mrs Dawn O'Keefe for expert photographic assistance and Miss Helen Trussler for her customary secretarial excellence.

REFERENCES

1. Weathers DR, Finc RM. Amalgam tattoo of oral mucosa. *Arch Dermatol* 1974; **110:** 727–728.
2. Lucas RB. The teeth and periodontal tissues. In: Symmers WStC, ed. Systemic Pathology, 2nd ed. Vol. 3. Edinburgh, London, New York: Churchill Livingstone, 1978: 978.
3. Ryge G, Fairhurst CW, Fischer CH. The present knowledge of the setting of dental amalgam. *Int Dent J* 1960; **11:** 181–185.
4. Mahler DB, Adey JD, Van Eysden J. Quantitative microprobe analysis of amalgam. *J Dent Res* 1975; **54:** 218–226.
5. Eley BM. Tissue reactions to implanted dental amalgam, including assessment by energy dispersive x-ray microanalysis. *J Path* 1982; **138:** 251–272.
6. Crocker PR, Toulson E, Levison DA. Particles in paraffin sections demonstrated in the backscattered electron image (BEI). *Micron* 1982; **13:** 437–446.
7. Eley BM. Soft tissue reactions to dental amalgam; an experimental and human study, including electron probe x-ray microanalysis. PhD Thesis 1980. University of London.
8. Underwood EJ. Trace Elements in Human and Animal Nutrition, 4th ed. New York, San Fransisco, London: Academic Press, 1977: 302–387, 444–445, 449–451.
9. Levison DA, Crocker PR, Smith AP, Blackshaw AJ, Bartram CI. The varied light and scanning electron microscopic appearances of barium sulphate in smears and histological sections. *J Clin Path* 1984; **37:** 481–487.
10. Harrison JD, Rowley PSA, Peters PD. Amalgam tattoos: light and electron microscopy and electron-probe microanalysis. *J Path* 1977; **121:** 83–92.
11. The Merck Index. An Encyclopaedia of Chemicals and Drugs, 8th ed. Stecher PG, ed. Rahaway, NJ: Merck and Co. Inc. 1968: 187, 223.
12. Morson BC, Dawson IMP. Gastrointestinal Pathology, 2nd ed. Oxford: Blackwood Scientific Publications, 1979: 578.
13. Kay S. Tissue reaction to barium sulphate contrast medium. *Arch Path* 1954; **57:** 279–284.
14. Mahboubi S, Gohel VK, Dalinka MK, Cho SY. Barium embolisation following upper gastrointestinal examination. *Radiology* 1974; **iii:** 301–302.
15. Harrison JD, Davies KD. A method for the identification of the particulate material in biopsies of the oral tissues. *Brit Dent J* 1982; **153:** 327–329.
16. Levison DA, Crocker PR, Banim S, Wallace M. Silica stones in the urinary bladder. *Lancet* 1982; **i:** 704–705.

JOURNAL OF PATHOLOGY, VOL. **144**: 131–147 (1984)

ANGIOFOLLICULAR LYMPH NODE HYPERPLASIA (CASTLEMAN'S DISEASE): AN IMMUNOHISTOCHEMICAL AND ENZYME-HISTOCHEMICAL STUDY OF THE HYALINE-VASCULAR FORM OF LESION

E. L. JONES*, J. CROCKER, J. GREGORY, MARY GUIBARRA AND R. C. CURRAN

Department of Pathology, Medical School, University of Birmingham, Birmingham, U.K.

Received 9 April 1984
Accepted 30 May 1984

SUMMARY

Tissues from five cases of angiofollicular lymph node hyperplasia have been studied. All had the histological structure of the hyaline-vascular type of lesion; large numbers of very compact lymphoid follicles were distributed evenly throughout a highly vascular tissue. The follicles were characterized by their small size, a vascular poorly cellular and frequently hyalinized centre, and a 'tight' concentric mantle of small lymphocytes arranged in layers producing an 'onion-skin' appearance. The interfollicular tissue was characterized by the large numbers of small vessels mainly hyalinized capillaries and a few high endothelial venules and the presence of variable numbers of lymphocytes, plasma cells, immunocytes and immunoblasts. The immunoperoxidase method demonstrated polytypic cytoplasmic immunoglobulin in the small numbers of centroblasts and plasma cells within the follicle centres and in the plasma cells and immunocytes in the interfollicular tissue. Large numbers of suppressor T cells were present in the interfollicular areas and only scattered helper T cells were seen within the lymphocyte mantles. A strong reaction for factor VIII-related antigen was seen in the endothelium of the interfollicular high endothelial venules but only a weak reaction in the vessels in the follicle centres. A concentric distribution pattern of the dendritic reticulum cells was seen with the metalophil impregnation method of Marshall and with the enzyme histochemical methods for acid α-naphthyl acetate esterase and 5′-nucleotidase. This pattern differs from the zonal distribution of these cells seen in reactive lymphoid follicles. The nature and possible pathogenesis of AFLNH are discussed and contrasted with reactive hyperplasia.

KEY WORDS—Angiofollicular lymph node hyperplasia, immunohistochemistry, enzyme-histochemistry.

INTRODUCTION

Giant lymph node hyperplasia was first described in 1956 by Castleman *et al.*[1] The morphological features of the condition have been well-documented[2,3] and two forms have been recognized, the hyaline-vascular and the plasma cell types.[4] The hyaline-vascular type is characterized by small follicles and a highly vascular interfollicular tissue. There are usually no clinical symptoms. The plasma cell type, which accounts for less than 10 per cent of the cases, is characterized by large numbers of mature plasma cells in the interfollicular tissue, and there is usually also a systemic syndrome that includes polyclonal hypergammaglobulinaemia, anaemia and fever.

The precise nature of the lesion remains unknown and the descriptive term of angiofollicular lymph node hyperplasia (AFLNH) is still appropriate. There are several reports of phenotypic analysis of the cells based on immunofluorescence[5,6] and immunoperoxidase studies[7,8] but enzyme-histochemical techniques do not seem to have been applied.

The present study is concerned with five cases of

*Addressee for correspondence: Dr E. L. Jones, Department of Pathology, Medical School, University of Birmingham, Birmingham B15 2TJ, U.K.

0022–3417/84/100131–17$01.70

Table I—Clinical features of the five patients

Case	Sex	Age (years)	Site	Size (cm)	Duration of mass (years)
1	Female	19	Cervical	3 × 3	1
2	Female	22	Cervical	5 × 5	13
3	Female	23	Cervical	4 × 3	4
4	Male	23	Cervical	4 × 4	7
5	Male	19	Cervical	3 × 2·5	1

the hyaline-vascular type and the aims were to determine the distribution of a number of plasma proteins, most notably immunoglobulin (Ig) and a number of cellular enzymes in AFLNH by immunohistochemical and enzyme-histochemical methods in an attempt to shed further light on the nature of the condition.

MATERIALS AND METHODS

Tissues were obtained over a 7-year period (1978–1984) from five patients aged 19–23 years (Table I). They were collected fresh from the operating theatre, within a few minutes of surgical removal. The lesions were situated in the neck: close to the sternomastoid in the posterior triangle in cases 2, 3, 4 and 5 and in the supraclavicular region in case 1. They ranged from 3 to 5 cm in diameter (Table I). Each lesion was an encapsulated, well-demarcated lobulated roughly spherical mass of firm consistency. Each was cut transversely through its short axis. The cut surface was creamy-white and nodular in appearance. Slices approximately 2 mm thick were cut with a degreased razor blade or disposable microtome knife and placed in a fixative solution.

Tissues from cases 2, 3 and 4 were fixed for 24–48 h at 20°C in formol–saline. Tissues from cases 1 and 5 were fixed for 2 days at 20°C in 4 per cent formaldehyde in 0·135 M phosphate buffer to which 5 per cent acetic acid had been added.

After fixation the tissues were dehydrated in ethanol (24 h), cleared in chloroform (6–9 h) and impregnated with Paraplast (12–24 h). Sections (2–4 μm thick) were cut and stained by the following methods: haematoxylin and eosin, Gordon and Sweet's method for reticulin, van Gieson's solution, and periodic acid–Schiff (PAS) sequence. Sections of the same thickness were used for immunohistochemistry but for Marshall's method[9] the sections were 8 μm thick.

Immunohistochemistry

Paraffin sections—The unlabelled antibody peroxidase–antiperoxidase (PAP) method was applied to paraffin sections to detect Ig ($\gamma,\mu,a,\delta,\kappa,\lambda$ chains), transferrin, lysozyme, al-antitrypsin, al-antichymotrypsin, factor VIII-related antigen and J chain.*

The titres of the specific polyclonal antibody used in the first stage of the PAP sequence were generally 1 in 100 for κ and λ chains; 1 in 400 for γ chain; 1 in 100 for a chain; 1 in 100 for μ chain; 1 in 40 for δ chain; 1 in 50 for J chain; 1 in 200 for transferrin; 1 in 100 for lysozyme; 1 in 100 for al-antitrypsin; 1 in 100 for al-antichymotrypsin; and 1 in 50 for factor VIII-related antigen (for details of the PAP method and of controls used, see Curran and Gregory[10]). Paraffin sections of the tissues fixed in formaldehyde–acetic acid solution (cases 1 and 5) reacted well with the PAP method but those fixed in formol–saline had to be trypsinized prior to the PAP method.[10,11]

Cryostat sections—Tissue slices 2–3 mm thick from cases 1 and 5 were quenched in isopentane cooled in liquid nitrogen and stored at −70°C. Cryostat sections 5 μm thick were air-dried at room temperature for 1 h and fixed in acetone at 4°C for 20 min.

The unlabelled PAP method was applied to cryostat sections using polyclonal antisera to detect Ig light (κ and λ) and heavy (μ and δ) chains. The titres of the specific antibody used in the first stage of the PAP procedure were 1 in 200 and 1 in 400 for μ chains: 1 in 100 for δ chains and 1 in 500 and 1 in 1000 for κ and λ chains. A two-stage indirect immunoperoxidase sequence was used with

*The antibodies for Ig ($\gamma,\mu,a,\delta,\kappa,\lambda$ chains), transferrin, lysozyme al-antitrypsin, al-antichymotrypsin and factor VIII-related antigen were obtained from Dakopatts Mercia Brocades Ltd. The antibody of J chain was obtained from Nordic Immunoglobulin Laboratories Ltd.

monoclonal antisera to detect T cells* the titres of the antibodies used in the first stage were 1 in 20 for pan T cells and 1 in 40 for suppressor T cells.

Enzyme-histochemistry

Fixation—Slices of fresh tissue 2 mm thick from cases 1, 2, 3 and 5 were placed in cold (4°C) 10 per cent formol–calcium. After 24–48 h the slices were transferred to cold (4°C) gum-sucrose and snap-frozen in liquid nitrogen. Cryostat sections (6 μm thick) were cut and reacted for the following enzymes.

α-Naphthyl acetate esterase (ANAE)
The reaction was performed with α-naphthyl acetate as a substrate and hexazotized *p*-rosaniline as the coupling agent.[12,13]

Alkaline phosphatase (AP)
The substrate was naphthol-AS-B1-phosphate (disodium salt) with simultaneous coupling to fast blue BB salt at pH 9–9·3.[14]

5′-Nucleotidase (5′-NT)
Adenosine-5′-monophosphate (sodium salt) was the substrate in the heavy metal sulphide precipitation technique.[15]

RESULTS

Histology

Each lesion consisted of many small lymphoid follicles evenly distributed throughout a highly vascular stroma. The structure was uniform, with no separate cortex and medullary zones.

The lymphoid follicles varied only slightly in size. The centre of each follicle was poorly cellular and the small lymphocytes present around the follicle were arranged in concentric layers to produce an 'onion-skin' appearance (Fig. 1). A thick-walled hyalinized arteriole entered the follicle centre usually radially (Fig. 2) and similar vessels were often numerous in the lymphocyte mantle. The vessels within the centres were obvious in H & E sections but more clearly demonstrated in the reticulin and haematoxylin–van Gieson (Fig. 2) preparations. The hyaline material in the vessels was PAS-positive.

In cases 1 and 2 occasional reactive lymphoid follicles with true germinal centres were present but the large majority of follicle centres lacked the zonal pattern of normal reactive follicles, and in them mitoses were infrequent and histiocytic reticulum cells (HRC) inconspicuous.

Much of each centre was occupied by whorls of 'endothelial' cells which appeared to be extensions of the lining cells of the hyalinized arterioles entering the centres. These stained weakly with the PAS reaction. Small numbers of centrocytes and centroblasts, and other cells of uncertain nature, were also present: their nuclei were pale, oval and vesicular and the appearances suggested that they were mainly dendritic reticulum cells (DRC) and occasional HRC (Fig. 1). A small number of the follicles was almost completely hyalinized and 'burnt-out' (Fig. 3). The metalophil method revealed scanty DRC and a few large round histiocytic cells scattered randomly throughout the centres (Fig. 4). Within the lymphocyte mantles (Fig. 4) there were fairly numerous branching dendritic and fibroblastic cells.

The interfollicular tissue had an extensive reticulin meshwork which superficially resembled that of a normal lymph node. However, the number of blood vessels was much greater than in the normal node and formed a dense arborizing network. Many of the vessels were capillaries but some had the structure of high endothelial venules (HEV) readily identified by their cuboidal endothelial cell lining, the presence of infiltrating lymphocytes, and the surrounding reticular sheath. Many of the vessels were fibrous and hyaline (Fig. 5). The hyaline material was PAS-positive. In addition the number of thick muscular-walled arteries was considerably greater than usually seen in reactive lymph nodes. In contrast to the intense vascularity was the complete absence of lymphatic sinuses, confirmed by the metalophil method.

The interfollicular stroma contained lymphocytes, large numbers of small immature plasma cells (B-immunocytes), mature plasma cells and scattered large immunoblasts. Moderate numbers of eosinophils were also present. The metalophil preparations revealed many branching dendritic and fibroblastic reticulum cells (Fig. 6) in the interfollicular stroma.

*The monoclonal T cell antibodies for pan T cells (UCHT-1) and suppressor T cells (B941) were kindly donated by Professor I. A. M. MacLennan, Department of Immunology, Medical School, Birmingham, U.K.

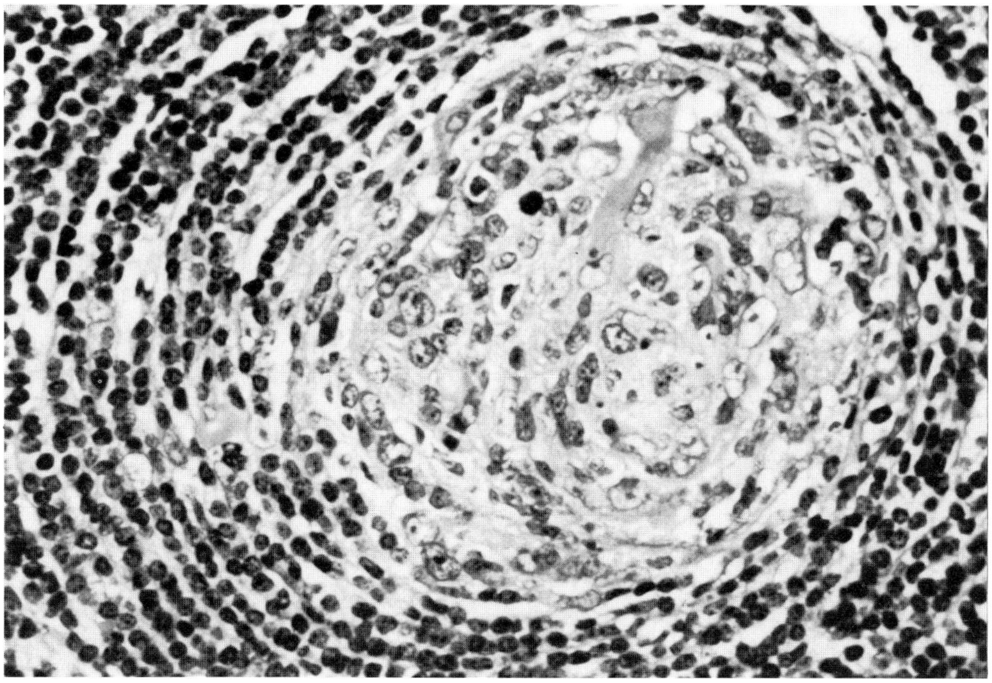

Fig. 1—Follicle composed of hyalinized vessel (top). Note tight concentric layering of lymphocytes in mantle zone ('onion-skin' appearance). ×422

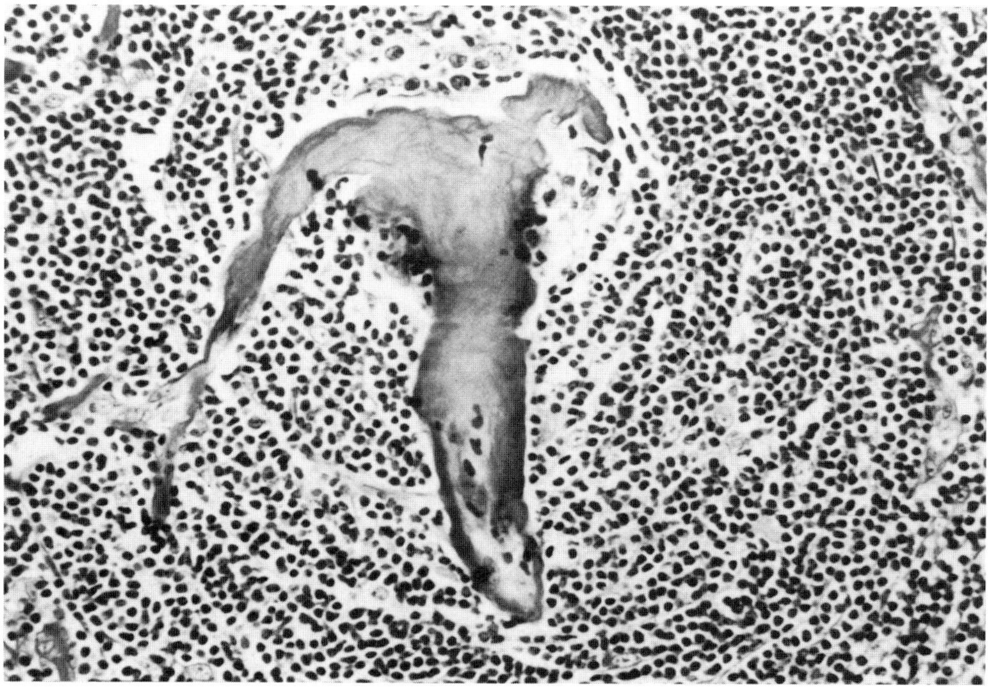

Fig. 2—Large hyalinized vessel running radially into the follicle. HVG, ×264

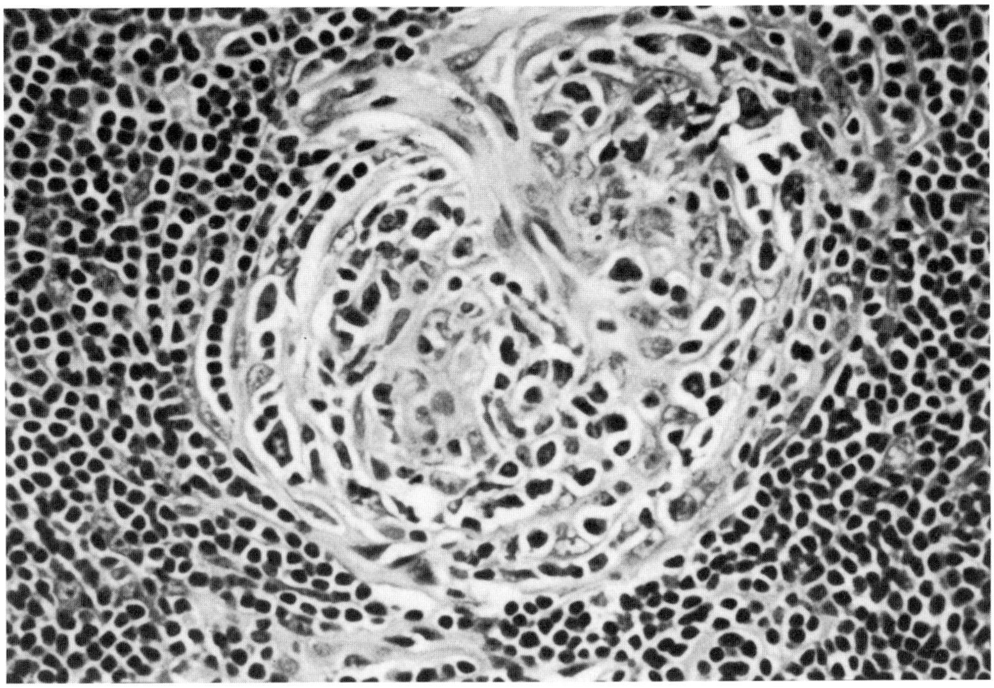

Fig. 3—A partially fibrosed follicle centre ('burnt-out' appearance). Note the reduction in numbers of cells in centre. ×422

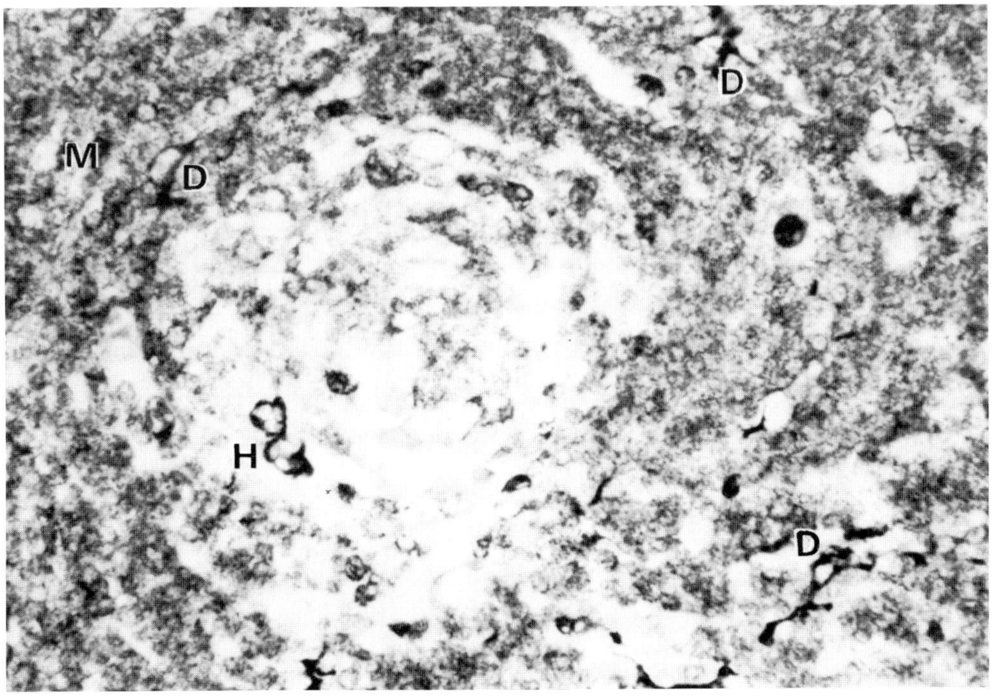

Fig. 4—Follicle containing a few rounded histiocytic reticulum cells (H). Within the mantle (M) branching dendritic reticulum cells are seen (D). Marshall's metalophil method, ×422

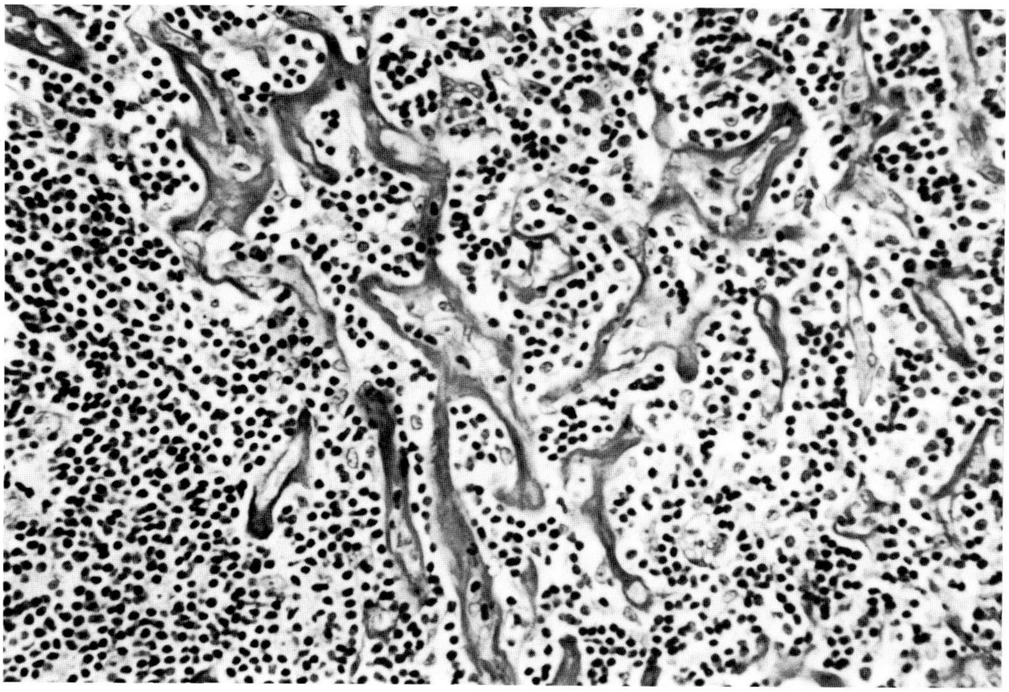

Fig. 5—Interfollicular area showing network of hyalinized arborizing capillaries. HVG, ×264

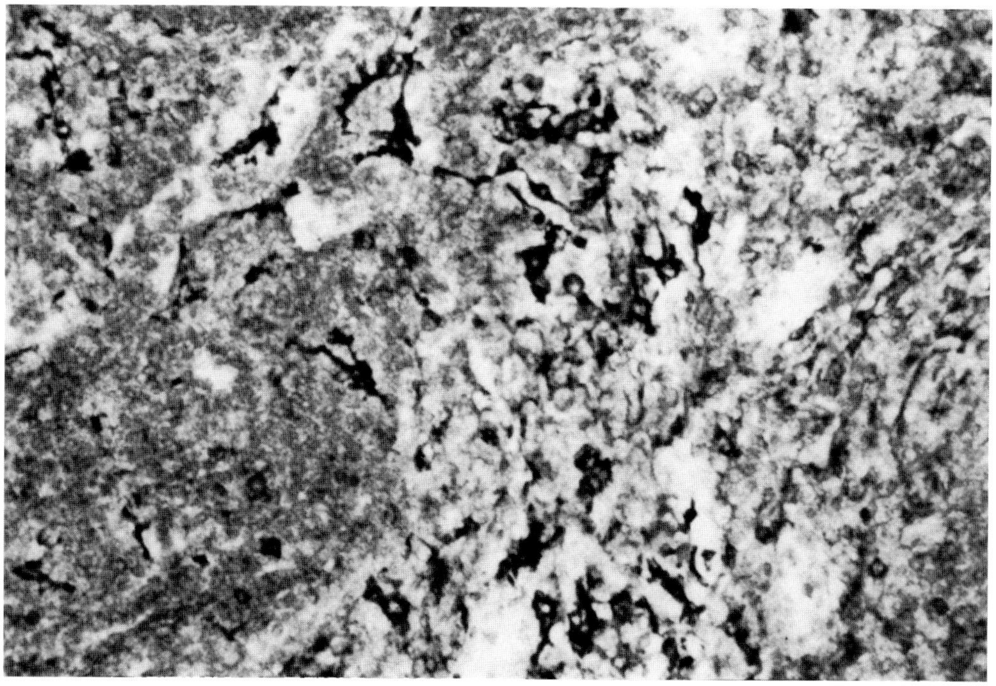

Fig. 6—Numerous branching dendritic and fibroblastic reticulum cells are lying between two follicles. Marshall's metalophil method, ×264

Immunohistochemistry

Immunoglobulin—In cryostat sections of cases 1 and 5, surface immunoglobulin (μ,δ,κ and λ chains) was present on the small lymphocytes of the follicle mantles (Fig. 7); and a faint reaction for the same sIg was also detectable in trypsinized paraffin sections of the other three cases. Within the follicle centres, small numbers of cells showed a polytypic staining pattern for cytoplasmic Ig (cIg): most were plasma cells but a few were centroblasts. The majority stained for γ chain (Fig. 8), a lesser number for α chain, and fewest for μ chain. Approximately twice as many cells reacted for κ chain as for λ chain. J chain was also detectable in small numbers of plasma cells. Most follicle centres gave a weak reaction for extracellular γ chain and for μ chain (Fig. 9). In the interfollicular areas some cells contained polytypic cIg in high concentration ($\gamma \gg \alpha\mu$; $\kappa > \lambda$ chains) (Fig. 10): most were immature B-immunocytes, with a small number of plasma cells and immunoblasts. Some of the cIg-containing immunocytes were clustered around the DRC (Fig. 10). Some of the plasma cells also reacted positively for J chain.

Lysozyme, αl-AT and αl-ACT—In the follicle centres the hyalinized arterioles were negative for lysozyme, αl-AT and αl-ACT but occasional HRC reacted weakly. The endothelium of the HEV and capillaries was also negative. In the interfollicular areas, small numbers of cells, presumably various types of histiocytes, reacted for lysozyme and αl-AT, as did the numerous eosinophils and polymorphs.

Factor VIII-related antigen—The arterioles entering the follicles in the mantle were weakly positive for factor VIII-related antigen, but a few plasma cells alongside the vessels were strongly positive (Fig. 11). In the interfollicular areas the endothelium of the HEV gave a strong granular reaction (Fig. 12), whereas the hyalinized capillaries were generally negative.

T cells—In the two cases reacted with monoclonal T cell antisera large numbers of T cells were found in the interfollicular areas (Fig. 13). The majority of these cells were of the suppressor subtype. Within the lymphocyte mantles but not the follicle centres occasional scattered helper T cells were present.

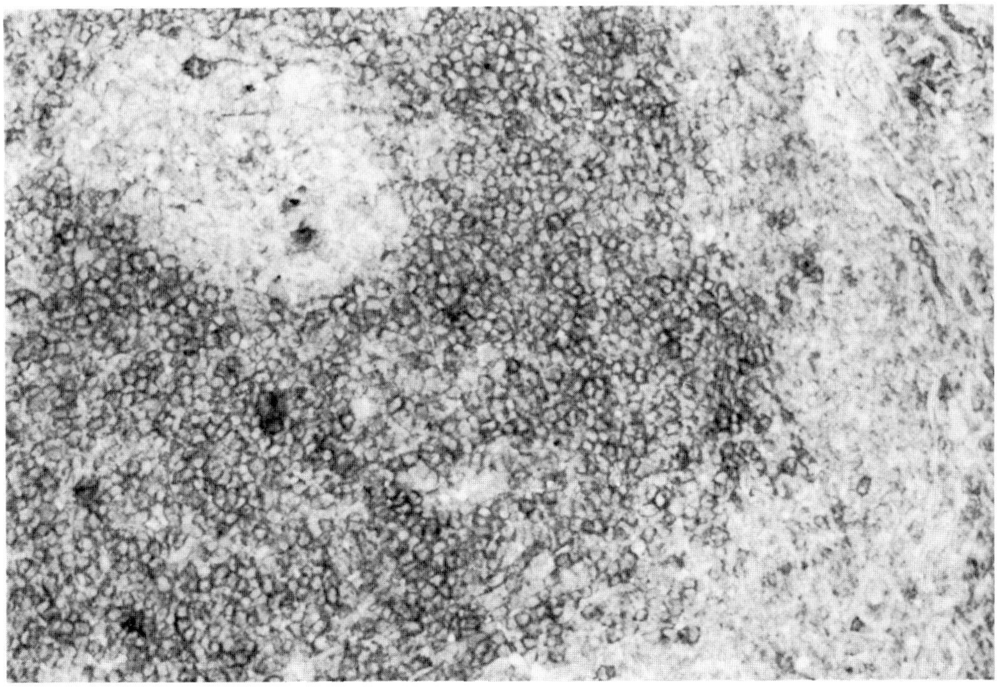

Fig. 7—Cryostat section of follicle. The lymphocytes of the mantle zone show surface Ig (κ chain). PAP method for κ chain, $\times 264$

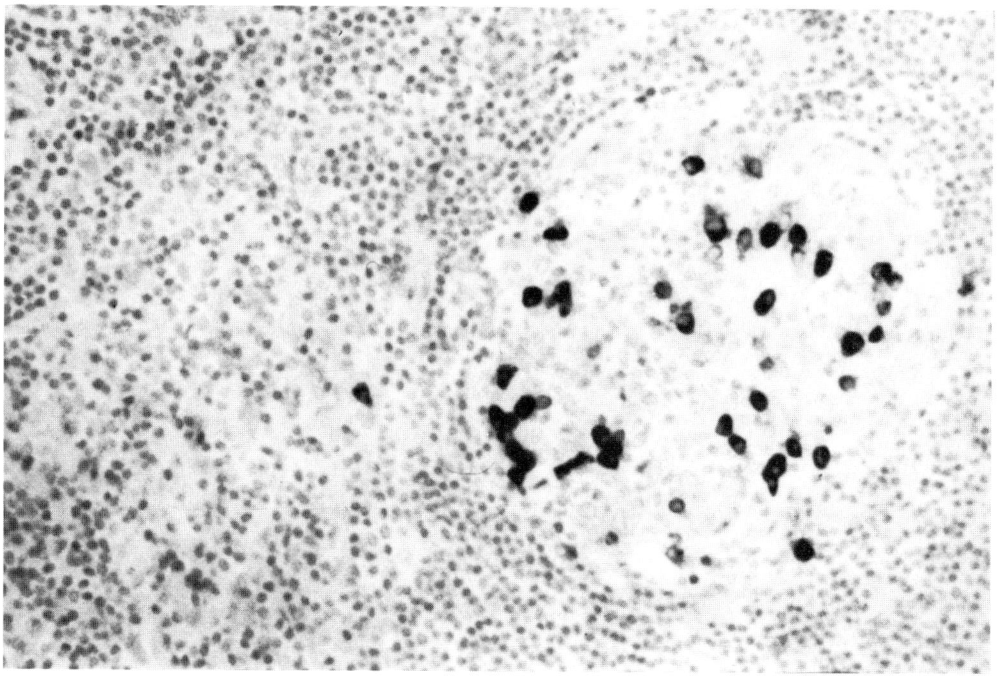

Fig. 8—Follicle centre showing plasma cells and a few centroblasts containing cytoplasmic Ig in high concentration (black). PAP method for γ chain, $\times 264$

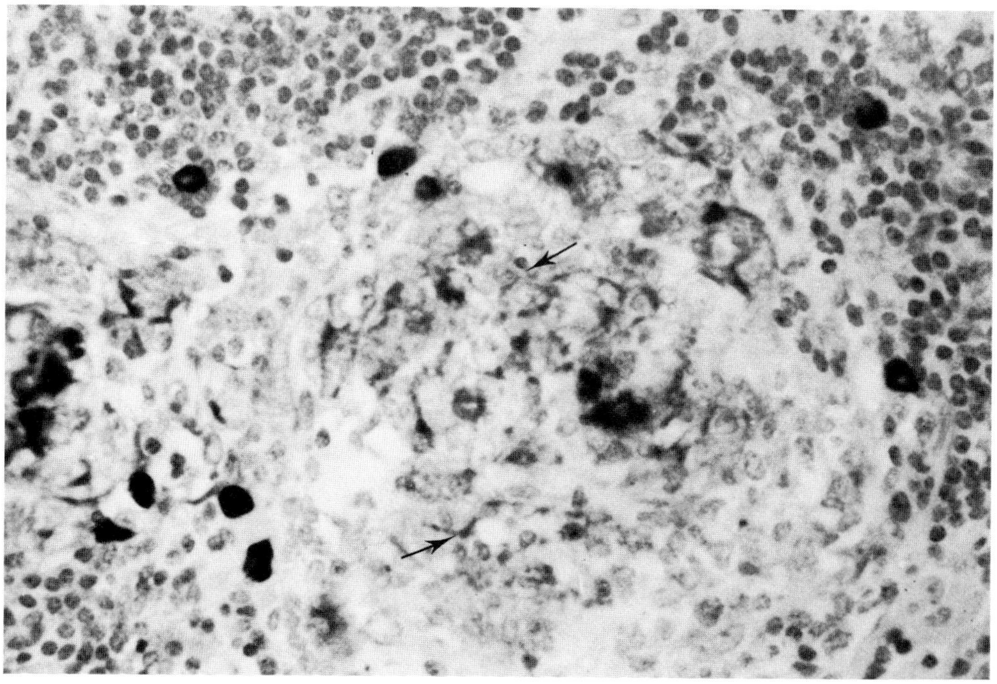

Fig. 9—Close-up of follicle, showing several plasma cells and centroblasts with cytoplasmic Ig (μ chain) within and around the centre. A faint reticular pattern is present centrally (arrows) which represents low concentrations of extracellular Ig (μ chain). PAP method for μ chain, $\times 422$

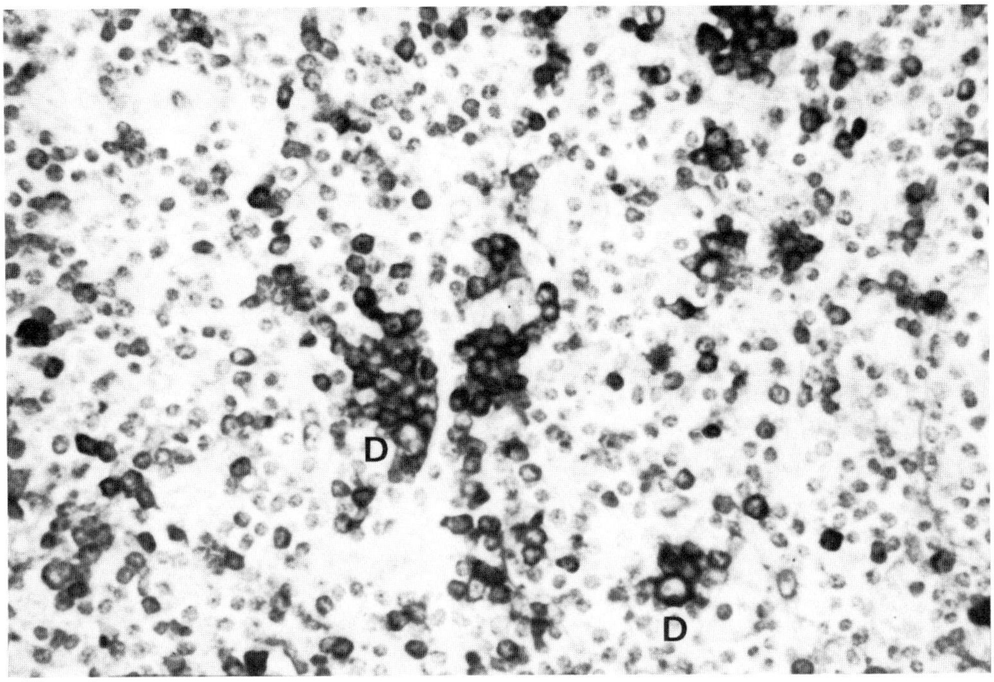

Fig. 10—Interfollicular area. Clusters of B-immunocytes reacting for Ig (κ chain) are closely associated with dendritic reticulum cells (D). Many small lymphocyte-like cells, plasma cells and immunoblasts reacting for Ig (κ chain) are present. PAP method for κ chain, $\times 422$

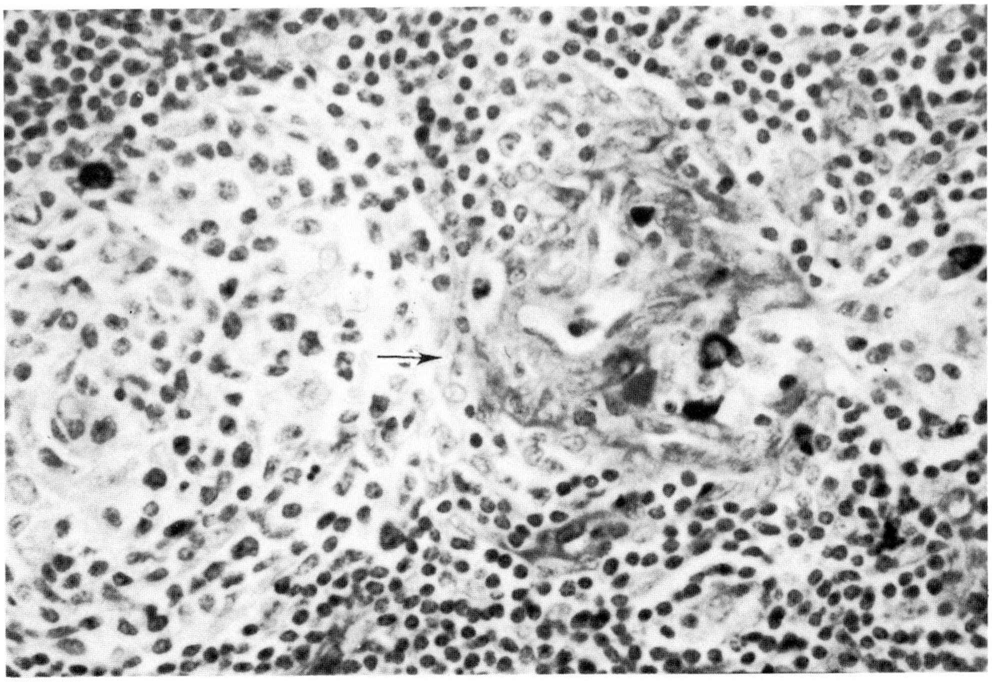

Fig. 11—Follicle with large branching arteriole (arrow) which is weakly positive for factor VIII-related antigen entering pale centre. A few strongly stained plasma cells (black) are present. PAP method for factor VIII-related antigen, $\times 422$

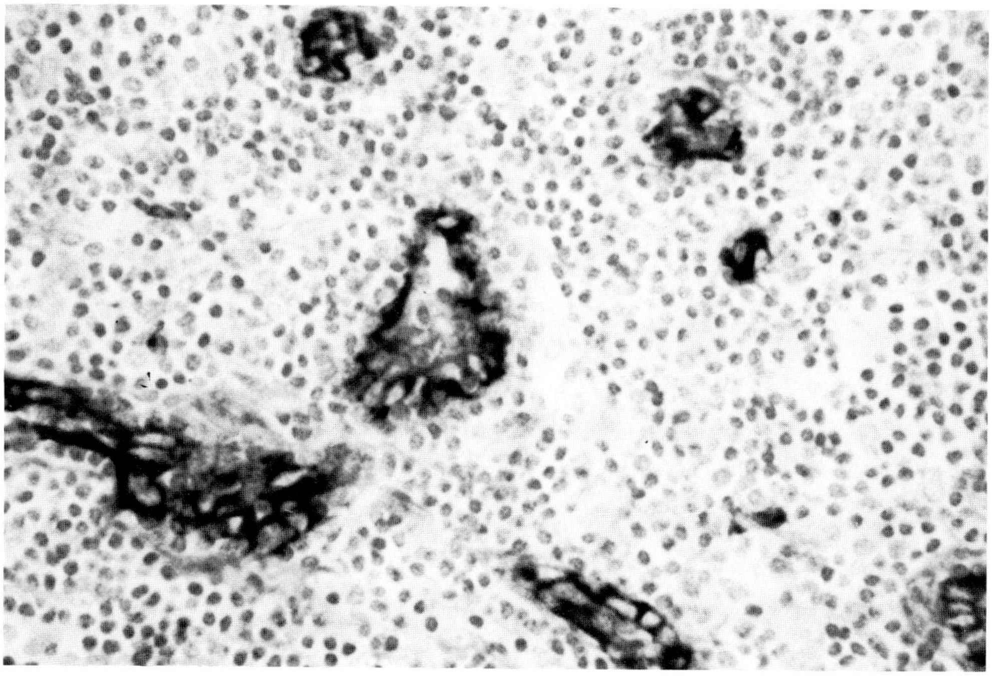

Fig. 12—Interfollicular area. Close-up of high endothelial venules reacting strongly for factor VIII-related antigens. PAP method for factor VIII-related antigen, × 422

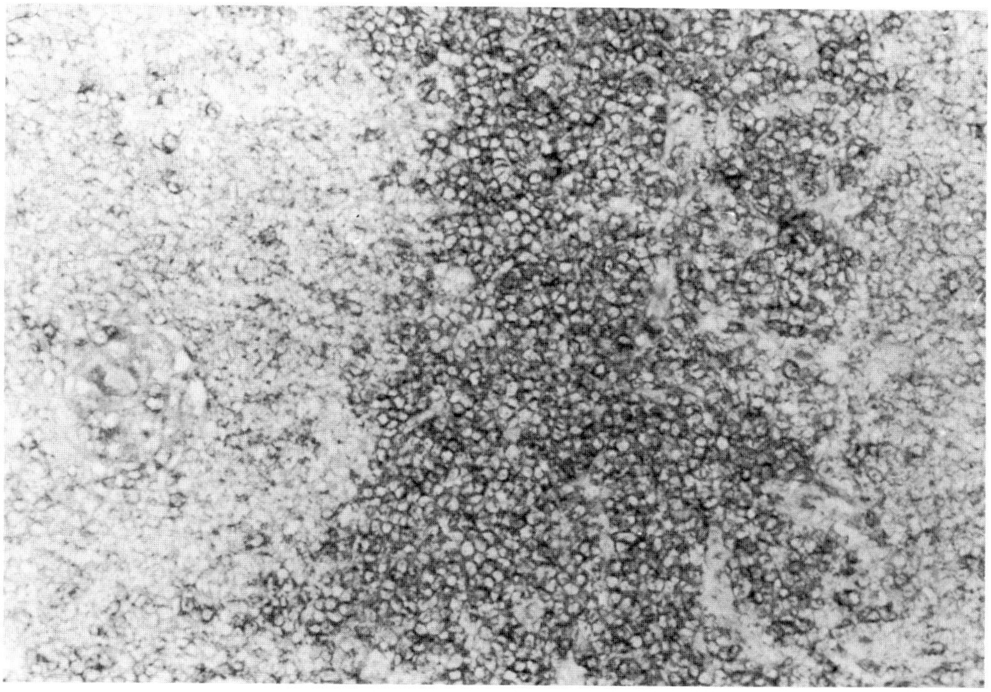

Fig. 13—Cryostat section of interfollicular area and part of two follicles. Large numbers of T cells are present between the follicles. Indirect (two-stage) IP method for Pan T cells, × 264

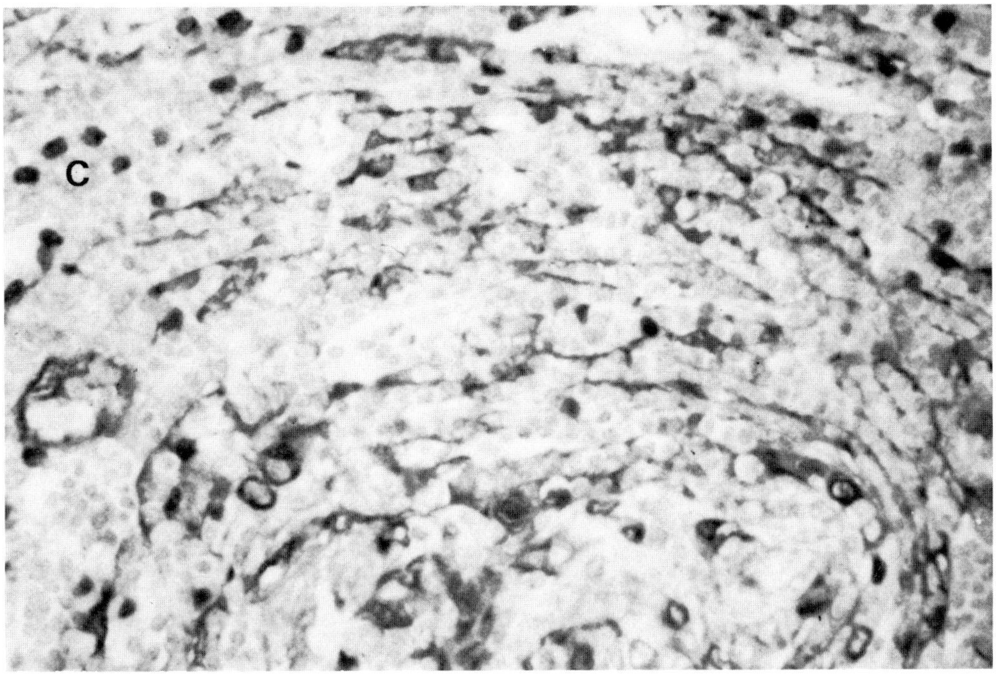

Fig. 14—Close-up of part of follicle centre and lymphocyte mantle. It shows many transferrin-containing branching and rounded reticulum cells of various types, as well as smaller numbers of transferrin positive immunocytes (C). PAP method for transferrin, ×422

Transferrin—Transferrin was detectable in low concentration in many dendritic, histiocytic and fibroblastic reticulum cells in and around the follicles, and in moderate numbers of immunocytes (Fig. 14). In the interfollicular area large numbers of immunocytes and HEV endothelium reacted in the same way (Fig. 15).

Enzyme-histochemistry

α-Naphthyl acetate esterase (ANAE)—A positive reaction was seen in the elongated cells in and around the follicles (Fig. 16), and in occasional more rounded cells within the follicle centres. In most follicles the endothelium of the entering blood vessel was weakly positive. Scattered lymphoid cells with punctate ANAE activity were seen in the follicle mantles but lymphocytes bearing one or two 'dots' of enzyme activity were much more numerous in the interfollicular areas. There were also very many branching and elongated cells showing a weakly- to moderately-positive reaction in these regions. The endothelium of the numerous small blood vessels was weakly ANAE-positive.

Alkaline phosphatase (AP)—In the follicles the cells failed to react and only the blood vessel endothelium reacted positively as did the large numbers of small branching blood vessels and the large abnormal vessels in the interfollicular areas (Fig. 17).

5′-Nucleotidase (5′-NT)—In the follicles closely-packed concentrically-arranged DRC reacted positively (Fig. 18), to produce a pattern similar to that obtained with the ANAE-method. The larger histiocytic cells were not stained. In the interfollicular areas, the 5′-NT reaction revealed scattered slender branching cells (Fig. 18).

DISCUSSION

Terminology

The names applied to AFLNH include lymph nodal hamartoma[16], angiofollicular mediastinal lymph node hyperplasia,[17] and benign lymphoid mass of probably hamartomatous nature,[18] or simply 'Castleman's disease'. This variety of names

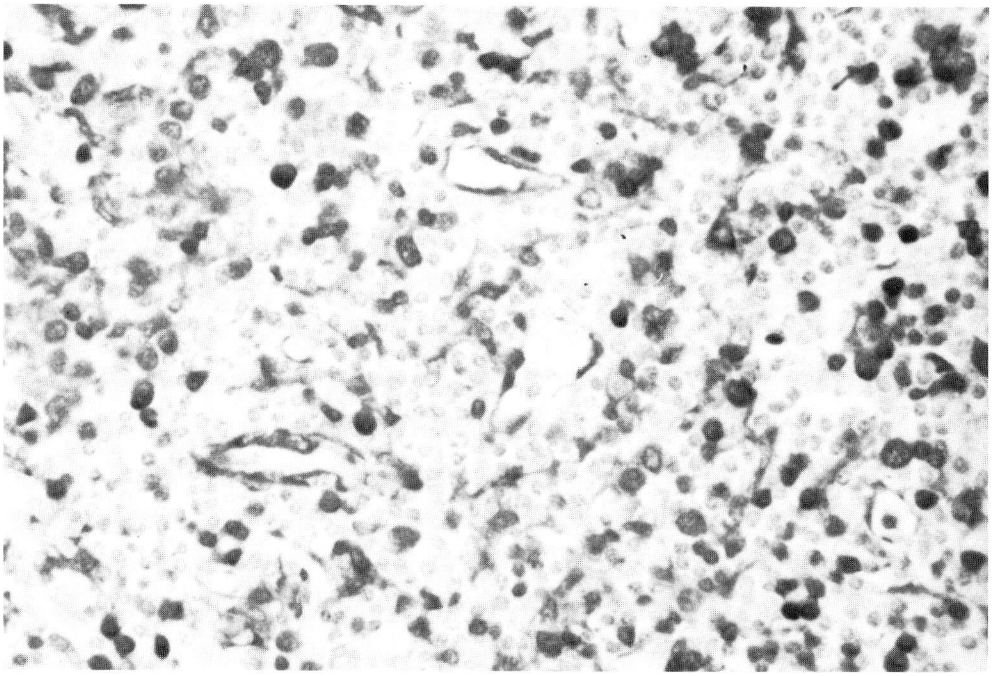

Fig. 15—Interfollicular area, with immunocytes and reticulum cells of various types giving a positive reaction for transferrin. The vascular endothelium has also reacted. PAP method for transferrin, ×422

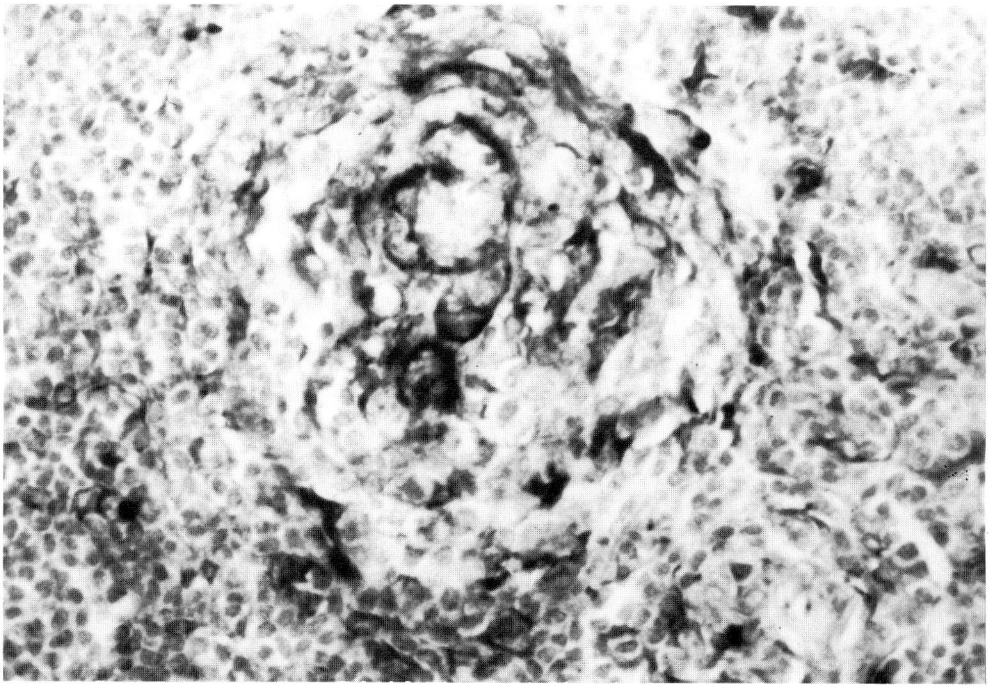

Fig. 16—Cryostat section of follicle reacted for α-naphthyl acetate esterase (ANAE). It shows circumferentially arranged ANAE-positive cells in the centre, mantle zone and interfollicular area. ANAE method, ×422

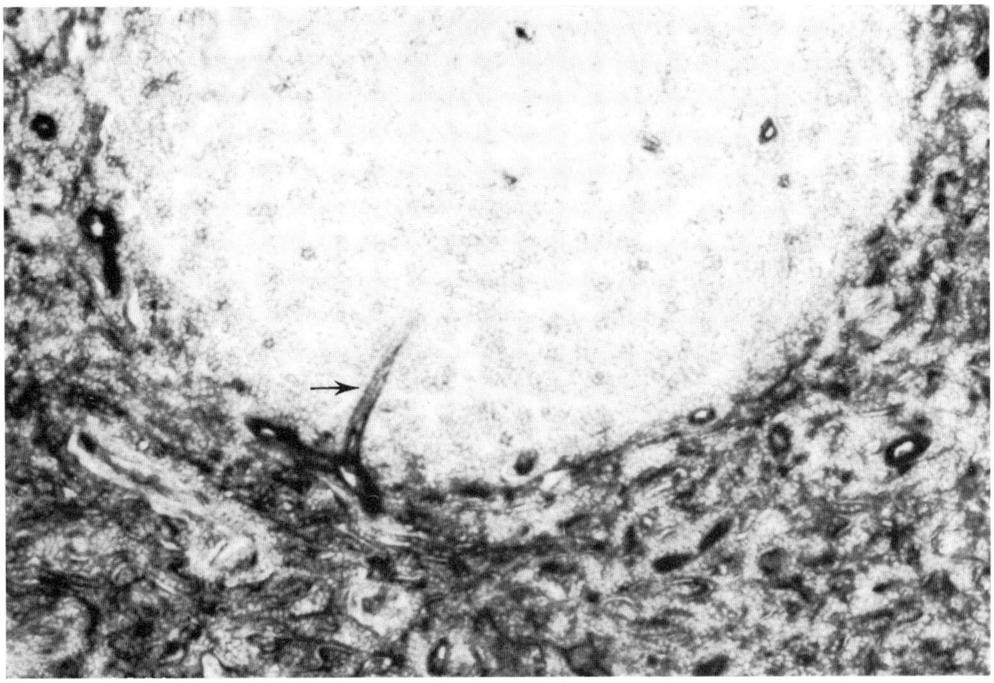

Fig. 17—Cryostat section of follicle and interfollicular area reacted for alkaline phosphatase (AP). There are numerous strongly-positive vessels around the follicles. The follicle centre is negative apart from an occasional vessel entering it (arrow). AP method, ×264

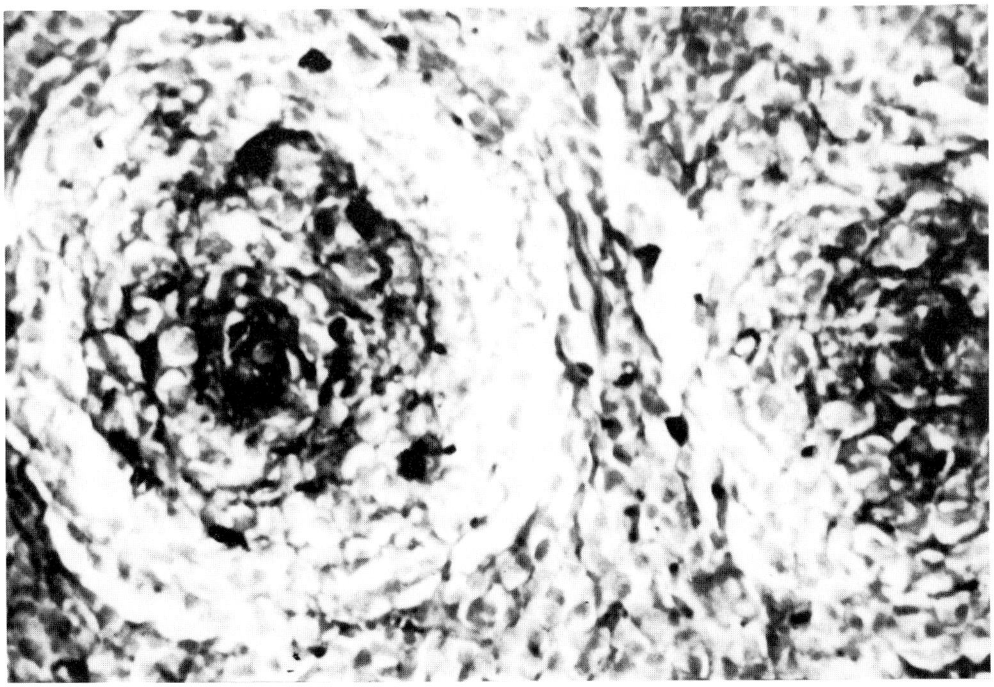

Fig. 18—Two lymphoid follicles reacted for 5′-nucleotidase (5′-NT). Closely-packed branching 5′-NT positive cells, arranged in a concentric pattern are present in the centres. Scattered positively reacting dendritic cells are also present between the follicles. 5′-NT method, ×422

confirms that the nature of AFLNH is still uncertain; and the term angiofollicular lymph node hyperplasia (AFLNH) is therefore probably as apt as any of the others.

In support of the idea that the lesion represents a lymphoid hamartoma[18–24] is the predilection of the lesion for the mediastinum. Extramediastinal and multicentric disease has however been reported[8,20] and although it usually involved lymph nodes extranodal locations have been reported.[21] The neck is the site in 14 per cent, the abdomen in 11 per cent and the axilla in 4 per cent. Our five cases presented with swellings in the neck. Typically for AFLNH, none of our patients had systemic symptoms, all were young adults (age range 19–23 years (mean 21·2 years)) and the masses had been present for some time, range 1–13 years (mean 5·2 years).

Although Castleman *et al.*[1] stated that their patients had 'asymptomatic large benign hyperplastic lymph nodes that resembled thymomas', from the presumed resemblance of the hyaline foci in the follicle centres to Hassall's corpuscles, it would seem that the AFLNH is more likely to be mistaken for either reactive follicular hyperplasia (RH) or centroblastic–centrocytic follicular lymphoma.

Reactive follicles have three distinct zones which gives the follicle polarity: a basal zone consisting predominantly of centroblasts, numerous mitoses and frequent HRC, a middle zone of centrocytes and DRC; and a corona of lymphocytes, usually eccentrically arranged around the germinal centre and sharply demarcated from it.[25–27] The follicles in our cases of AFLNH were unmistakably different: they were small, with poorly cellular centres and a corona of concentric layers of small lymphocytes producing an 'onion-skin' appearance. The follicle consisted of whorls of proliferating endothelial cells, with very few centroblasts, centrocytes and reticulum cells present. There was therefore no zonal structure and the follicles lacked polarity. The presence of a zonal structure in reactive follicles was also obvious in the pattern of distribution of DRC as revealed by the metalophil method.[25–27] We did not systematically measure the follicle sizes in our 5 cases but there is no doubt that the follicles in AFLNH are generally smaller and more uniformly round than reactive follicles which are often ovoid.[25] This conforms with the results of Anagoustou and Harrison[2] who found that the follicles in their six cases of AFLNH had a mean diameter between 355 and 480 μm, whereas the follicles in six cases of reactive hyperplasia had a mean diameter of 610 μm.

The interfollicular tissue was even more strikingly different from that in reactive lymphoid tissue, being composed to a large extent of a dense arborizing network of vessels, particularly well seen in the PAS-sequence. The vessels were predominantly hyalinized capillaries, scattered HEV and occasional thick-walled muscular arteries. The presence of variable numbers of eosinophils was also distinctive, being unusual in either RH or centroblastic–centrocytic lymphoma.

Enzyme-histochemistry

The ANAE method also helped to emphasize the differences between the follicles in AFLNH and those in reactive follicles.[12] In reactive follicles the method reveals a zonal structure whereas in AFLNH there is a concentric arrangement of fine, slender ANAE-positive cells which are probably true DRC.[28] In the interfollicular areas in AFLNH there were also many branching ANAE-positive cells with fine slender processes; these are also probably mainly DRC, although many may also be genuine branching HRC. The similarity between the staining reactions seen with ANAE and 5′-NT in AFLNH is probably significant (see below).

The ANAE reaction has been shown to serve as a 'marker' for certain types of T-lymphocytes,[12,29–32] but very few such cells were observed in the follicles of AFLNH. There were large numbers in the interfollicular areas however, a distribution pattern similar to that of reactive lymphoid tissue.[12]

ANAE also demonstrates clearly the 'littoral' and 'reticular' cells of the sinuses in reactive lymph nodes[33] and the absence of these types of cells in AFLNH was very obvious.

The alkaline phosphatase technique was equally helpful but in a different way: it revealed the network of blood vessels in the interfollicular tissue and the blood vessels entering the follicles uniquely well. In human lymph nodes HEV do not react for alkaline phosphatase whereas the capillaries and arterioles do,[34] and our results suggest therefore that the majority of the interfollicular vessels were capillaries along with a few HEV and the occasional arteriole.

5′-Nucleotidase demonstrated the same features in AFLNH as the ANAE-reaction, including a strongly-positive reaction on DRC and in similar fashion gave a staining pattern that differed markedly from reactive follicles.[28,35]

Immunohistochemistry

Comparatively few studies have been made of the immunological characteristics of the cells in AFLNH. Immunoperoxidase studies have shown a polyclonal staining pattern in the plasma cells.[7,8] Our own results are in accord with these studies. The presence of surface Ig on most of the lymphocytes in the follicle mantles confirms that these are B lymphocytes; and the distribution of cells containing Ig did not differ significantly from the pattern seen in reactive nodes:[25] the numbers of cIg-containing cells were smaller and in follicle centres the network for μ chain was less prominent than in reactive germinal centres. The immunocytes and plasma cells in the interfollicular areas gave a similar polytypic staining pattern ($\gamma \gg \alpha > \mu$; $\kappa > \lambda$) as the cells in the follicles. In contrast to the arterioles in the follicles, the HEV showed a strong positive granular reaction for factor VIII-related antigen, an antigen synthesized by endothelial cells.[36–39] The significance of this result is not known. The positive staining of a few plasma cells with the factor VIII-related antibody is believed to be due to the presence of contaminating immunoglobulins in the primary antiserum.

The significance of the transferrin detectable in low concentration in the different types of reticulum cells and immunocytes in this study is unknown. Transferrin has previously been detected in similar cells in reactive nodes,[25] and histiocytes.[40] There has recently been considerable interest in the transferrin receptors (TR) on cells. The TR appears to be expressed in much larger amounts on proliferating cells (compared to cells in the resting state) and on cells which have undergone malignant transformation.[41–44] The presence of TR on the surface of lymphocytes may be a useful marker for lymphocyte activation.[45] The occurrence of TR in normal and malignant tissue has recently been investigated with a panel of monoclonal antibodies.[46] Staining of the neoplastic cell population was seen in non-Hodgkin's lymphomas and Hodgkin's disease.[46] The presence of transferrin in immature immunocytes and its absence from mature plasma cells noted earlier in reactive nodes[25] may be a manifestation of increased metabolic functions of proliferating cells.[25]

Phenotypic analysis of cell suspensions in a case of giant lymph node hyperplasia (GLNH) revealed polyclonal sIg in 10 per cent of cells and immunofluorescence on ethanol-fixed smears from the cell suspensions and on frozen sections showed polyclonal cIg in 6 per cent of cells, and 52 per cent of fresh cells in suspensions formed E-rosettes.[5] The distribution of T cells, B cells and plasma cells as determined by cell surface marker and cIg studies did not differ from those observed in normal and reactive lymph nodes which in general display a predominance of T cells.[5]

The role of suppressor cell activity has been investigated in two children with GLNH.[6] These patients showed cell-mediated immunodeficiency as expressed in the low numbers of peripheral blood T cells and impairment of T cell function manifested by a negative graft versus host reaction.[6] Whether the suppressor T cells in these patients constitutes the aetiological factor inducing the condition or not remains to be clarified.[6]

In our two cases examined for the presence of T cells large numbers of suppressor T cells together with a few helper T cells were present within the interfollicular areas, a finding in contrast to reactive nodes where helper T cells predominate. Within the lymphocyte mantles of AFLNH a few scattered helper T cells were identified but none were present within the follicle centres unlike reactive nodes where many helper T cells are found mainly located in the light zone of the germinal centres.

Increased numbers of activated suppressor cells have been seen after viral infections including those caused by Epstein-Barr virus and cytomegalovirus.[47] In infectious mononucleosis the self-limiting increase in suppressor cells may account for transient impaired immunity but in patients with chronic graft versus host disease persistent circulating suppressor cells cause prolonged immunodeficiency.[48] The reversal of the ratio of helper to suppressor T cells normally seen in reactive nodes observed in two of our cases together with the much smaller numbers of Ig-containing cells suggests that AFLNH is a benign, non-lymphomatous, atypical hyperplastic condition possibly resulting from an abnormality of immunoregulatory T cell function secondary to a virus infection. The precise nature and pathogenesis of AFLNH however remains to be confirmed and although there are some morphological and clinical features that resemble a form of lymphoid hamartoma our immunohistochemical findings are not consistent with this view.

ACKNOWLEDGEMENTS

Our thanks are due to Miss G. L. Parkinson for typing the manuscript. Financial costs were met by a generous grant from the Endowment Fund Research Committee of the Central Birmingham Health District.

REFERENCES

1. Castleman B, Iverson L, Menendez V. Localised mediastinal lymph node hyperplasia resembling thymomas. *Cancer* 1956; **9:** 822–830.
2. Anagnostou D, Harrison CV. Angiofollicular lymph node hyperplasia (Castleman). *J Clin Pathol* 1972; **25:** 306–311.
3. Dorfman RF, Cibull M. Castleman's disease. *Recent Results in Cancer Research* 1978; **64:** 284–287.
4. Keller AR, Hochholzer L, Castleman B. Hyaline-vascular and plasma cell types of giant lymph node hyperplasia of the mediastinum and other locations. *Cancer* 1972; **29:** 670–683.
5. Diamond LW, Braylan RC. Immunologic markers and DNA content in a case of giant lymph node hyperplasia (Castleman's disease). *Cancer* 1980; **46:** 730–735.
6. Shohat B, Cohen I, Fogel R, Zaigov R. Suppressor mononuclear cells in giant lymph node hyperplasia and thymoma. *Cancer* 1981; **48:** 923–926.
7. Mufarriz A, Fazzini E, Feiner HD. Giant lymph node hyperplasia an immunopathologic and ultrastructural study of a case of the multicentric plasma cell variant. *Arch Pathol Lab Med* 1982; **106:** 92–95.
8. Frizzera G, Massarelli G, Banks PM, Rosai J. A systemic lymphoproliferative disorder with morphological features of Castleman's disease: pathologic findings in 15 patients. *Amer J Surg Pathol.* 1983; **7:** 211–231.
9. Marshall AHE. A method for the demonstration of reticuloendothelial cells in paraffin sections. *J Pathol Bacteriol* 1948; **60:** 515–517.
10. Curran RC, Gregory J. Effects of fixation and processing on immunohistochemical demonstration of immunoglobulin in paraffin sections of tonsil and bone marrow. *J Clin Pathol* 1980; **33:** 1047–1057.
11. Curran RC, Gregory J. The unmasking of antigens in paraffin sections of tissue by trypsin. *Experientia* 1977; **33:** 1400–1401.
12. Crocker J. The enzyme histochemistry of lymphoid and non-lymphoid cells of the human palatine tonsil: a basis for the study of lymphomas. *J Pathol* 1981; **134:** 81–95.
13. Crocker J, Jones EL, Curran RC. A quantitative study of α-naphthyl acetate esterase-positive cells in non-Hodgkin's lymphomas and reactive lymph nodes. *J Clin Pathol* 1982; **35:** 1066–1068.
14. Nanba K, Jaffe ES, Braylan RC, Soban EJ, Berard CW. Alkaline phosphatase-positive malignant lymphoma: a subtype of B-cell lymphomas. *Amer J Clin Pathol* 1977; **68:** 535–542.
15. Chayen J, Bitensky L, Butcher RG. Practical Histochemistry. London: Wiley, 1973.
16. Abel MR. Lymph node hamartoma versus chronic choristoma of pulmonary hilum. *Arch Pathol* 1957; **64:** 584–588.
17. Harrison EG, Bernatz PE. Angiofollicular mediastinal lymph node hyperplasia resembling thymoma. *Arch Pathol* 1963; **75:** 284–292.
18. Lattes R, Patcher MR. Benign lymphoid masses of probable hamartomatous nature. *Cancer* 1962; **15;** 197–214.
19. Fisher ER, Sieracki JC, Goldberg DM. Identity and nature of isolated lymphoid tissue (so called nodal hyperplasia, hamartoma, and angiomatous hamartoma) as revealed by histologic, electron microscopic and heterotransplantation studies. *Cancer* 1970; **25:** 1286–1300.
20. Gaba AR, Stein RS, Sweet DL, Daina Variakojis. Multicentric giant lymph node hyperplasia. *Amer J Clin Pathol* 1978; **69:** 86–90.
21. Cohen H. Tumor-like proliferations of lymphoid tissue. Occurrence in deltoid muscle and mediastinum. *Journal of Mount Sinai Hospital* 1957; **24:** 750–760.
22. Tamaddon K. Angiomatous lymphoid choristoma with bone formation: a case report and review of the literature. *Pathol Res Prac* 1980; **169:** 101–105.
23. Tung KSK, McCormack LJ. Angiomatous lymphoid hamartoma. *Cancer* 1967; **20:** 525–536.
24. Garneau R, Fournier M. Hamartomas et choristomes lymphovasculaires (hyperplasie pseudotumorale des ganglions medistinaux). *Ann Anat Pathol* 1964; **9:** 223–230.
25. Curran RC, Gregory J, Jones EL. The distribution of immunoglobulins and other plasma proteins in human reactive lymph nodes. *J Pathol* 1982; **136:** 307–332.
26. Curran RC, Jones EL. Immunoglobulin-containing cells in human tonsils as demonstrated by immunohistochemistry. *Clin Exper Immunol* 1977; **28:** 103–115.
27. Curran RC, Jones EL. The lymphoid follicles of the human palatine tonsil. *Clin Exper Immunol* 1978; **31:** 251–259.
28. Lennert K. Malignant Lymphomas other than Hodgkin's Disease. Berlin: Springer-Verlag, 1978.
29. Mueller J, Brun DEL RE G, Buerki H, Keller H-U, Hess MW, Cottier H. Nonspecific acid esterase activity: a criterion for differentiation of T and B lymphocytes in mouse lymph nodes. *Euro J Immunol* 1975; **5:** 270–274.
30. Knowles DM, Hoffman HT, Ferrarini, M, Kunkel HG. The demonstration of acid α-naphthyl acetate

esterase activity in human lymphocytes usefulness as a T-cell marker. *Cell Immunol* 1978; **35:** 112–123.

31. Seymour GJ, Dockrell HM, Greenspan JS. Enzyme differentiation of lymphocyte subpopulation in sections of human lymph nodes, tonsils and periodontal disease. *Clin Exper Immunol* 1978; **32:** 169–178.
32. Zicca A, Leprini A, Cadoni A, Franzi AT, Ferrarini M, Grossi CE. Ultrastructural localisation of alpha-naphthyl acid esterase in human T_M lymphocytes. *Amer J Pathol* 1981; **105:** 40–60.
33. Crocker J, Williams M. An enzyme histochemical study of the sinuses of reactive lymph nodes. *J Pathol* 1984; **142:** 31–38.
34. Freemont AJ, Jones CJP. Light microscopic, histochemical and ultrastructural studies of human lymph node paracortical venules. *J Anat* 1983; **136:** 349–362.
35. Muller-Hermelink HK. Characterisation of the B-cell and T-cell regions of human lymphatic tissue through enzyme histochemical demonstration of ATPase and 5′-nucleotidase. *Virchow Arch B* 1974; **16:** 371–378.
36. Jaffe EA. Synthesis of factor VIII antigen by cultured human endothelial cells. *Ann NY Acad Sci* 1975; **240:** 62–69.
37. Jaffe EA. Endothelial cells and the biology of factor VIII. *New Engl J Med* 1977; **296:** 377–383.
38. Sixma JJ, Kater L, Bourna BN, Schmitz DU, Moulin F, DeGraffe S, Tuit G. Immunofluorescent localisation of factor VIII-related antigen, fibrinogen and several other plasma proteins in hemostatic plugs in humans. *J Lab Clin Med* 1976; **87:** 112–119.
39. Shearn SAM, Peake IR, Giddings JC, Humphrys J, Bloom AL. The characterisation and synthesis of antigens related to factor VIII in vascular endothelium. *Thromb Res* 1977; **11:** 43–56.
40. Mason DY, Taylor CR. Distribution of transferrin, ferritin, and lactoferritin in human tissues. *J Clin Pathol* 1978; **31:** 316–327.
41. Judd W, Poodry CA, Strominger JL. Novel surface antigen expressed on dividing cells but absent from non-dividing cells. *J Exp Med* 1980; **152:** 1430–1435.
42. Trowbridge IS, Omary MB. Human cell surface glycoprotein related to cell proliferation is the receptor for transferrin. *Proc Natl Acad Sci USA* 1981; **78:** 3039–3043.
43. Sutherland R, Delia D, Schneider C, Newman R, Kemshead J, Greaves M. Ubiquitous cell surface glycoproteins on tumor cells is proliferation associated receptor for transferrin. *Proc Natl Acad Sci USA* 1981; **78:** 4515–4519.
44. Brown JP, Hewick RM, Hellström I, Hellström KE, Doolittle RF, Dreyer WJ. Human melanoma-associated antigen p97 is structurally and functionally related to transferrin. *Nature* 1982; **296:** 171–173.
45. Goding JW, Burns GF. Monoclonal antibody OKT-9 recognizes the receptors for transferrin on human acute lymphocytic leukemia cells. *J Immunol* 1981; **127:** 1256–1258.
46. Gatter KC, Brown G, Trowbridge IS, Woolston R-E, Mason DY. Transferrin receptors in human tissues: their distribution and possible clinical relevance. *J Clin Pathol* 1983; **36:** 539–545.
47. Reinherz EL, O'Brien C, Rostenthal P, Schlossman SF. The cellular basis for viral-induced immunodeficiency: analysis by monoclonal antibodies. *J Immunol* 1980; **125:** 1269–1274.
48. Reinherz EL, Parkman R, Rappeport J, Rosen FS, Schlossman SF. Aberrations of suppressor T cells in human graft-versus host disease. *New Engl J Med* 1979; **300:** 1061–1068.

PUBLISHING AGREEMENT

1. It is our custom to request authors to vest the worldwide copyright of their papers in John Wiley & Sons Limited for the full term of copyright and we would be grateful if you would confirm your acceptance of these terms by signing and returning the agreement below. We will not withhold permission for any reasonable request from you to publish any part of this paper in connection with any other work by you, provided the usual acknowledgements are given regarding copyright notice and reference to the original publication.
2. If it is appropriate, the author's employer may sign this agreement, and in any event the employer may reserve the right to use the paper internally or for promotional purposes only, by so indicating on this agreement. It is understood that proprietary rights other than copyright (including patent rights) are reserved.
3. If the author is a U.S. Government employee and this work was done in that capacity the assignment applies only to the extent allowable by U.S. law. If at least one co-author is *not* a government employee, said author should sign the agreement.
4. If the author is an employee of the British Government then HMSO will grant a non-exclusive licence to publish this paper in the Journal in any form or media provided British crown copyright and user rights (including patent rights) are reserved.
5. The author warrants that the manuscript is the author's original work, and has not been published before. (If excerpts from copyrighted works are included, the author will obtain written permission from the copyright owners and show credit to the sources in the manuscript.) The author also warrants that the article contains no libellous or unlawful statements, and does not infringe on the rights of others.
6. If the work was prepared jointly the author agrees to inform co-authors of the terms of the agreement, and to sign on their behalf.

With the qualifications listed above I assign to John Wiley & Sons Limited, the copyright of my paper entitled ______________________________

____

for publication in ______________________________

______________________ Signed

______________________ Date

If the paper is rejected this assignment is null and void.

JOURNAL OF PATHOLOGY, VOL. **144**: 149–161 (1984)

THE ROLE OF CELL INJURY AND THE CONTINUING INFLAMMATORY RESPONSE IN THE GENERATION OF SILICOTIC PULMONARY FIBROSIS

D. H. BOWDEN AND I. Y. R. ADAMSON

Pathology Department, University of Manitoba, Winnipeg, Canada

Received 17 February 1984
Accepted 30 April 1984

SUMMARY

The pathogenesis of silicosis involves interaction between pulmonary macrophages and fibroblasts. The consequences of direct injury to pulmonary cells and the role of inflammatory cells other than the macrophage have received little attention. These were studied over a 20 week period after instilling silica to mice by correlating the changing inflammatory response, as revealed by bronchoalveolar lavage and lung sections, with the cellular location of silica particles and the development and resolution of granulomatous lesions. Within 24 h, a massive concentration of particles and PMN was seen in centrilobular locations with acute focal necrosis of type 1 epithelial cells. Rapid epithelial repair occurred but PMN were recovered from the lung up to 20 weeks. In the alveoli, silica was ingested by PMN and AM, resulting in the death of some cells; free particles crossed the epithelium and were found predominantly in peribronchial macrophages. Silicotic granulomas formed within a week and consisted mainly of fibroblasts macrophages and some PMN. It is suggested that the necrosis of type 1 epithelium and the continuing efflux with serial destruction of PMN may be important factors in the generation of silicotic fibrosis.

KEY WORDS—Silica, lung injury, fibrosis, alveolar macrophages.

INTRODUCTION

Serial interactions between silica particles, macrophages and fibroblasts form the basis of prevailing theories regarding the genesis of silicotic fibrosis.[1] Killing of pulmonary macrophages, a major component of the chain reaction, is followed by the release of silica crystals and their rephagocytosis by a fresh crop of cells. These events are complemented by a mechanism which ensures the continuing availability of new alveolar phagocytes. When macrophages ingest silica they release chemical attractants thereby inducing the required amplification of macrophagic production and release, a process that is perpetuated by serial ingestion, cell killing, release of crystals and rephagocytosis.[2] This accounts for the continuing high output of pulmonary macrophages following even a brief exposure to silica.

The coincident appearance of granulocytes (PMN) in response to silica has also been described.[3–5] The mechanisms of PMN recruitment appears to be nonspecific since an acute outpouring of these cells is seen within a few hours of the administration of non-toxic particles such as carbon and polystyrene.[6,7] The response in these instances is brief and self-limited, but with the continuing cycle of phagocytosis and cell death observed with silica one might expect to see recurring waves of PMN efflux. In a recent paper we described the serial cytokinetic and biochemical events that follow a single pulmonary instillation of silica to mice.[8] The results suggested that both macro-phages and polymorphonuclear leukocytes contribute to the development of the fibroblastic response.

In the present paper we extend these observations

Addressee for correspondence Dr D. H. Bowden, Pathology Department, 770 Bannatyne Avenue, Winnipeg, Manitoba R3E OW3, Canada.

This research was supported by the Medical Research Council of Canada.

0022–3417/84/110149–13$01.30

by describing the morphological characteristics of the pulmonary response over a 20 week period following the administration of silica. In addition to the changing inflammatory response, as revealed in lavaged material and in sections of the lung, we examine the necrobiotic effect of silica on cells other than the macrophage, the relationship of such injury to transepithelial passage of particles into the interstitium and the role of the PMN in the genesis and development of the silicotic lesions.

Previous studies on the pathogenesis of silicosis have concentrated on either the early events related to macrophage–silica interactions[5,9] or the late stages when fibrosis is already established. The time span of the present serial study permits an overall view of the pathologic changes from initial cell efflux and cell injury through the development and regression of the silicotic nodules to the residuum of peribronchiolar fibrosis.

MATERIALS AND METHODS

Crystalline silica (2 mg), particle diameter 0·3 μm (Dowson and Dobson, South Africa) in 0·1 ml sterile water was instilled intratracheally to 70 male Swiss Webster mice under mild anaesthesia. The animals, in groups of four, were killed at days 1, 2, 3, 5, 7, 10 and weeks 2, 4, 6, 8, 10, 12, 16, 20; each animal received 2 μCi/g tritiated thymidine 1 h before death. Control animals were injected with 0·1 ml sterile water and were sacrificed less frequently after the first week since a previous study showed no changes in the lung at 1 week when compared with non-injected controls.[7]

At sacrifice, a tracheotomy was performed and the lungs were washed four times with 1·0 ml saline, the lavage fluid was pooled for each animal, the cell suspension was centrifuged to a pellet, which was fixed in osmic acid and prepared for embedding in

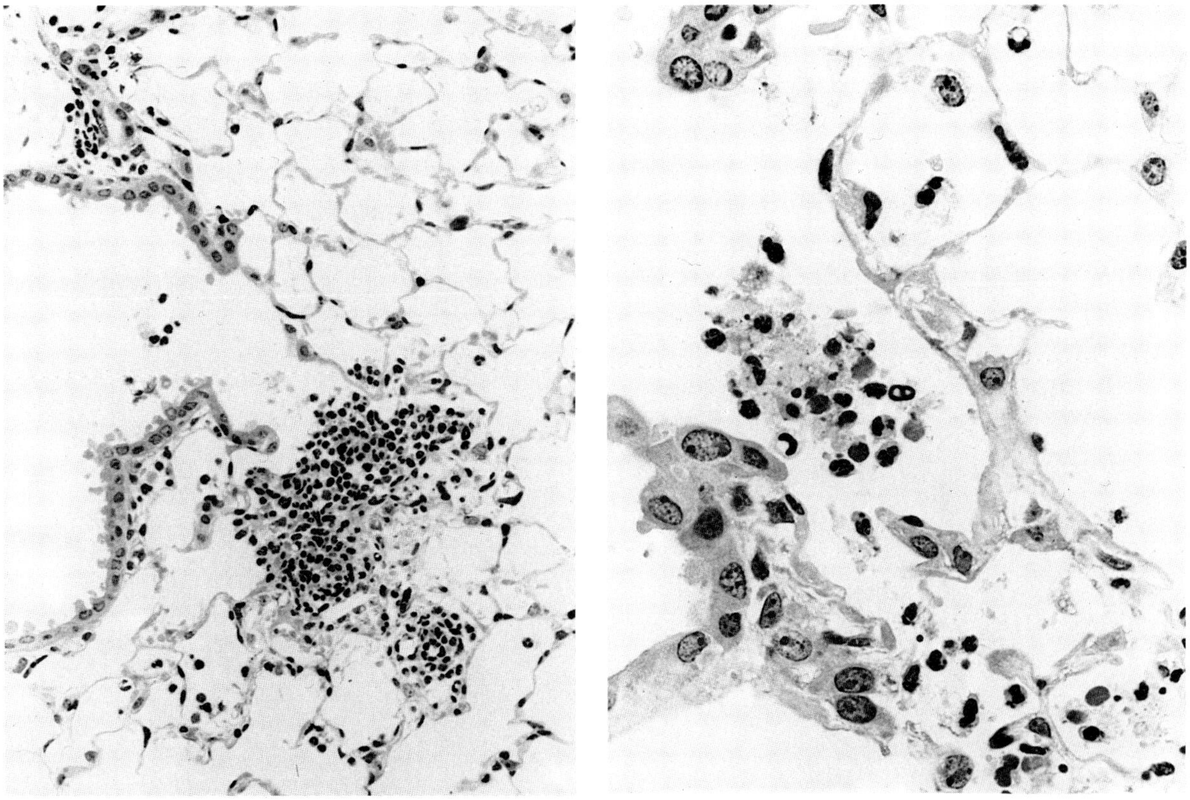

(a) (b)

Fig. 1—One day after silica. (a) Inflammatory cells are clustered at the bronchiolar opening. H & E, × 162. (b) Higher magnification shows that the exudate is composed of PMN and macrophages. H & E, × 675

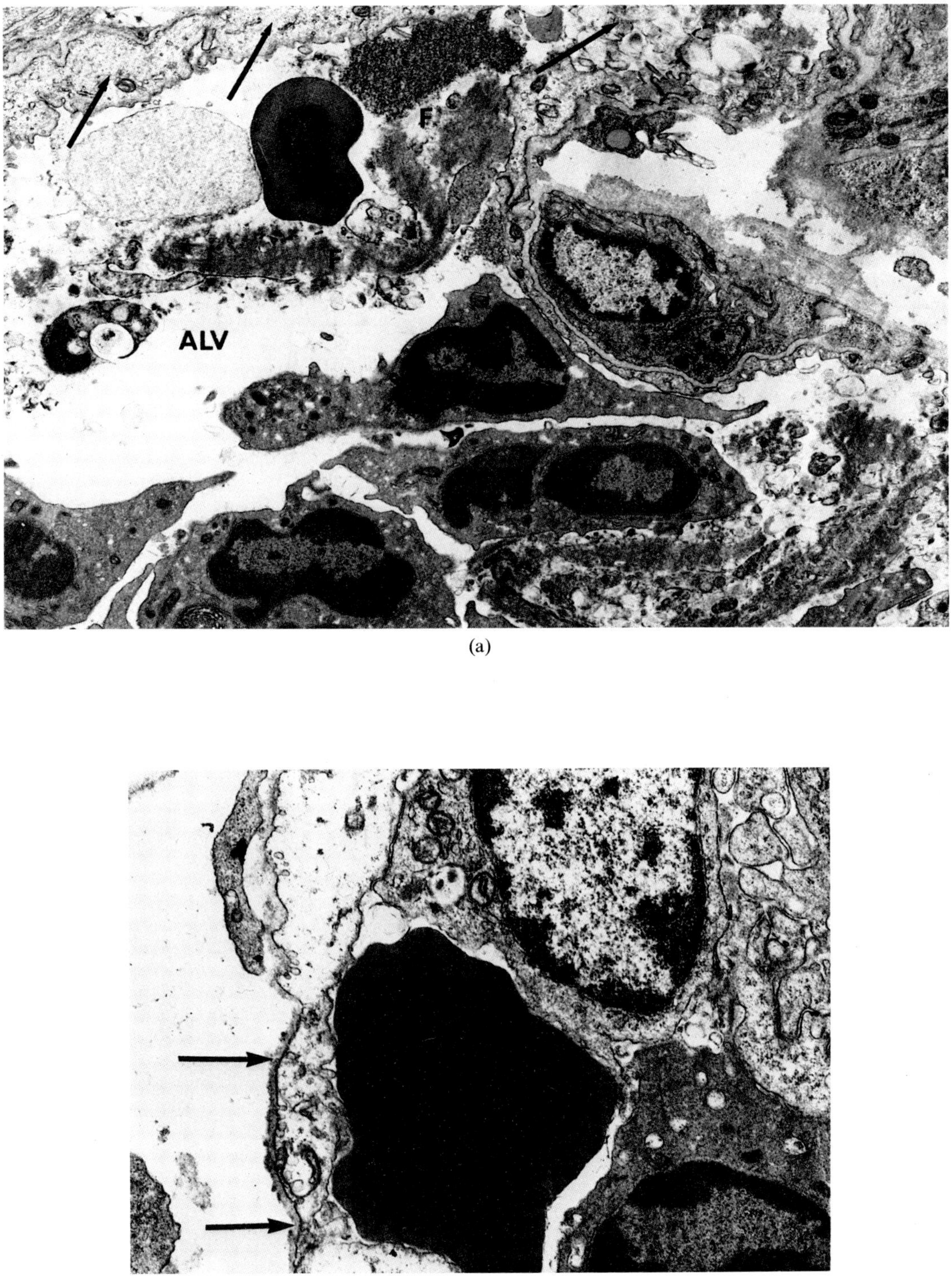

(a)

(b)

Fig. 2—Electron micrographs, 1 day after silica. (a) The alveolus (ALV) is filled with PMN and fibrin (F) lying on a degenerating type 1 epithelial cell (arrows) × 11475. (b) Type 1 cell necrosis has left a denuded basement membrane (arrows) × 13500

Spurr resin. Both 0·5 μm and ultrathin sections were examined.

After lavage, the bronchus leading to the right lung was clamped; this lung was removed, weighed and frozen for biochemical analysis.[8] The left lung was inflated with 2 per cent buffered glutaraldehyde, removed, and most of the tissue was processed for embedding in glycol methacrylate. Sections (0·75 μm thick) were prepared for autoradiography with the use of Kodak NTB2 emulsion. The remaining tissue sample was postfixed in osmic acid, dehydrated through alcohols before embedding in Spurr resin. Thin sections were examined by electron microscopy.

RESULTS

The early changes

The morphologic changes observed 24 h after the administration of silica are predominantly centrilobular. At the openings to the terminal bronchioles silica crystals are surrounded by polymorphonuclear leukocytes (PMN) intermingled with a lesser number of alveolar macrophages (AM) (Fig. 1). The junctions of terminal bronchioles and alveolar ducts are lined with fibrin and electron micrographs reveal focal necrosis of type 1 epithelial cells beneath the exudate (Fig. 2). Viewed at low magnifications the pathologic changes are best described as peribronchiolar exudative alveolitis with the PMN as the predominant cell. The cellular components observed in pellets prepared from lung washings are a reflection of the pulmonary inflammatory exudates; the pellets contain a mixture of PMNs and AMs with free and phagocytosed silica (Fig. 3).

The heavy concentration of silica in the alveolar ducts and the peribronchial alveoli persists for about 2 days. Although clearance of particles was not measured, the massive concentration of PMN and AM at these sites and the amount of silica

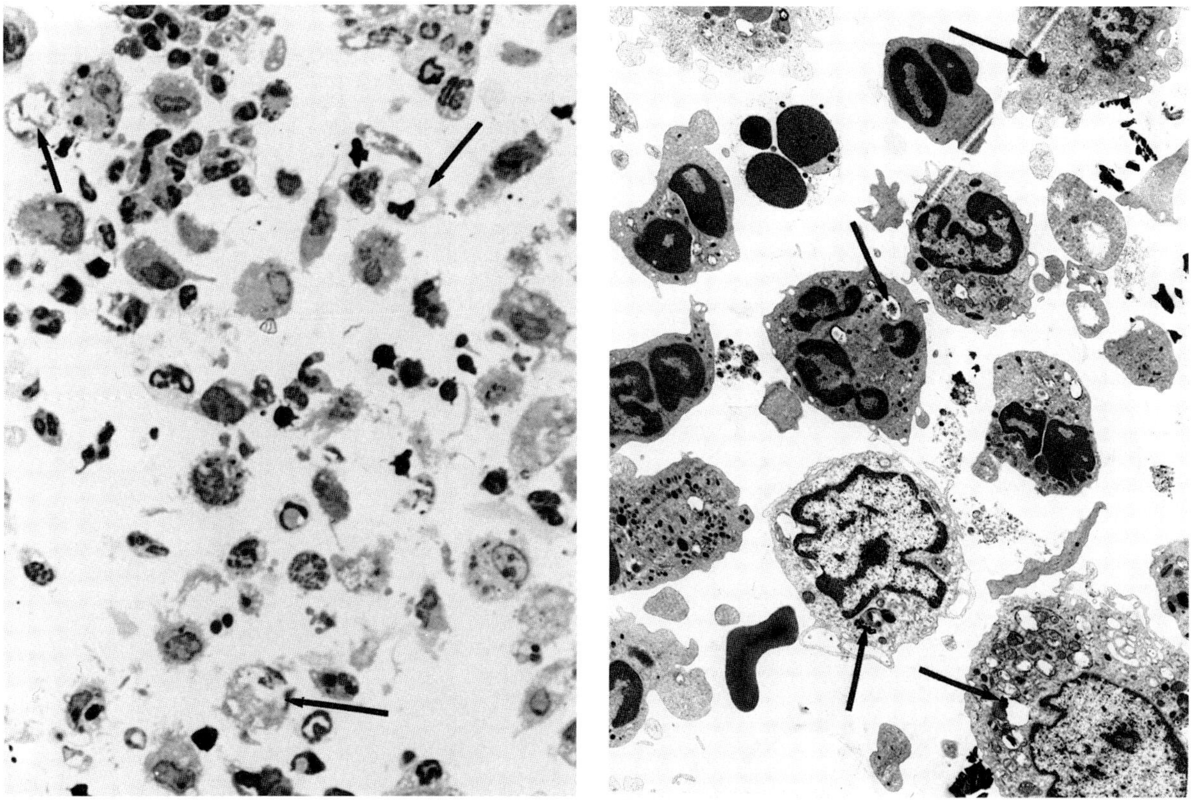

(a) (b)

Fig. 3—Pellet of lavaged cells showing a mixture of PMN and AM. (a) Some cells show damage from phagocytosed silica (arrows). 1 day, 0·5 μm section, toluidine blue × 720. (b) Electron micrograph of same pellet shows PMN and AM, both cell types containing ingested particles (arrows); some free particles are also shown. × 5400 observed within these cells suggest rapid clearance via the tracheobronchial pathway. The peribronchiolar and perivascular distribution of the early lesions induced by silica is demonstrated particularly well in autoradiographs (Fig. 4). The presence of labelled monocytes in blood vessels and in perivascular spaces suggests a pathway for these cells en route to the airways and air sacs; nuclear labelling and mitotic activity in type 2 epithelial cells in the centrilobular zones at 3 days indicates the prompt reparative response of these cells to injury of neighbouring type 1 cells (Fig. 4, 5). Regeneration of epithelial cells and subsequent differentiation results in total restitution of the normal alveolar lining; mitotic activity of type 2 cells, maximal at 48 h, subsides rapidly and thereafter no evidence of epithelial injury is observed.

Within the alveoli, crystals of silica, phagocytosed by alveolar macrophages, appear to induce injury in many of these cells (Fig. 3a). The sequential changes from early engulfment through lysosomal dissolution and destruction of the cell are illustrated in Fig. 6. Similar changes are observed in the PMN, suggesting a common sequence of phagocytosis followed by lysosomal rupture and release of proteolytic enzymes (Fig. 7). The presence of silica particles within the cytoplasm of type 1 cells, indicates the inability of alveolar phagocytes to cope with the acute load (Fig. 8). Within 24 h, particles are found lying free in the interstitium and within phagosomes of interstitial macrophages (Fig. 9); by 3 days, these macrophages are aggregated into nodular collections adjacent to terminal bronchioles and perivascular spaces.

Whereas the sharp demarcation of the centrilobular lesions from the normal appearing distal respiratory units persists for the duration of the experiment, the cellular components of the lesions change progressively as the initial avalanche of PMN subsides. By the third day the macrophage appears as the dominant cell in the inflammatory foci although PMN continue to be found in the free

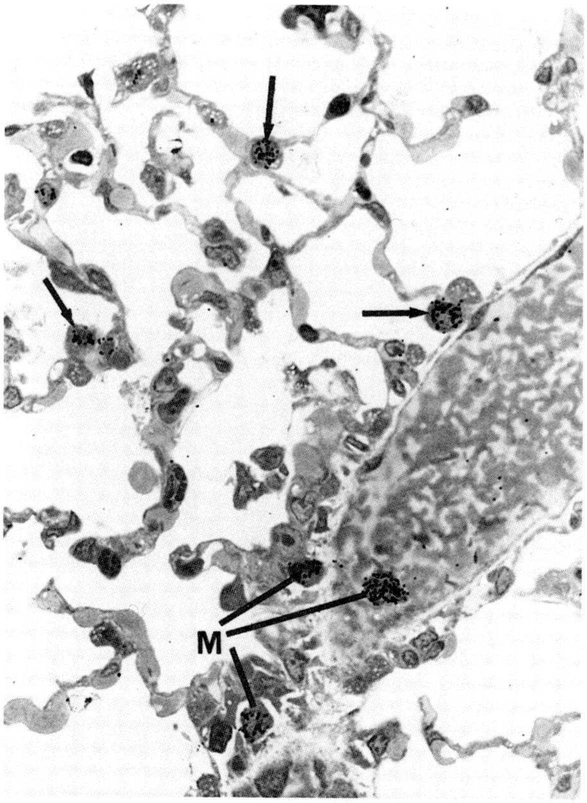

Fig. 4—Autoradiograph, 2 days after silica. Cells of the mononuclear phagocyte series (M) are labelled in addition to labelling of type 2 cuboidal epithelial cells (arrows). H & E, ×675

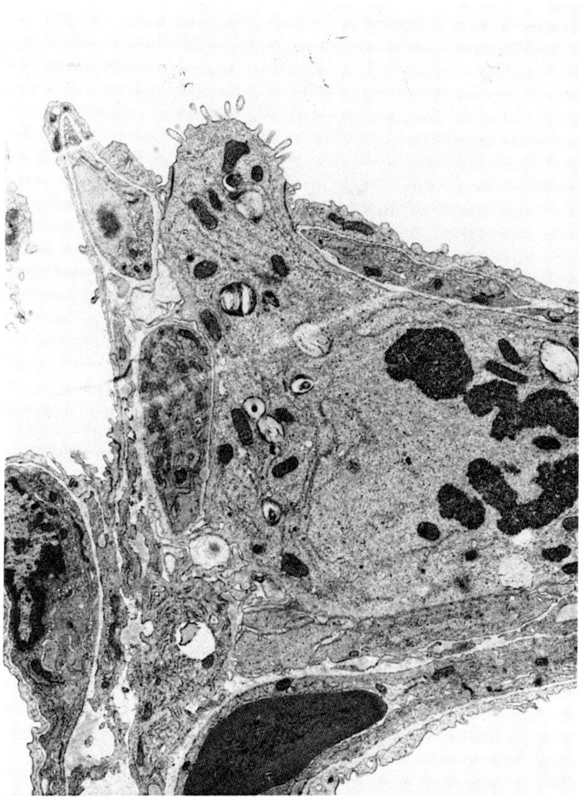

Fig. 5—Two days after silica, a mitotic figure is seen in a type 2 epithelial cell, recognized by its microvilli and cytoplasmic lamellar bodies. EM, ×8100

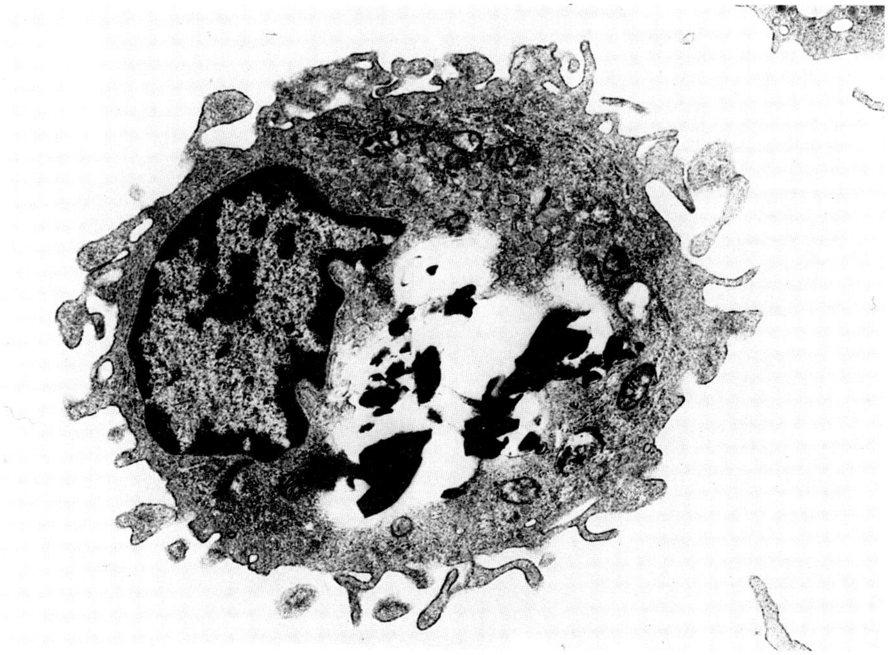

Fig. 6—(a) Electron micrographs of lavaged alveolar macrophages after silica. At 2 days, cell contains silica but shows little cytoplasmic change. × 17000

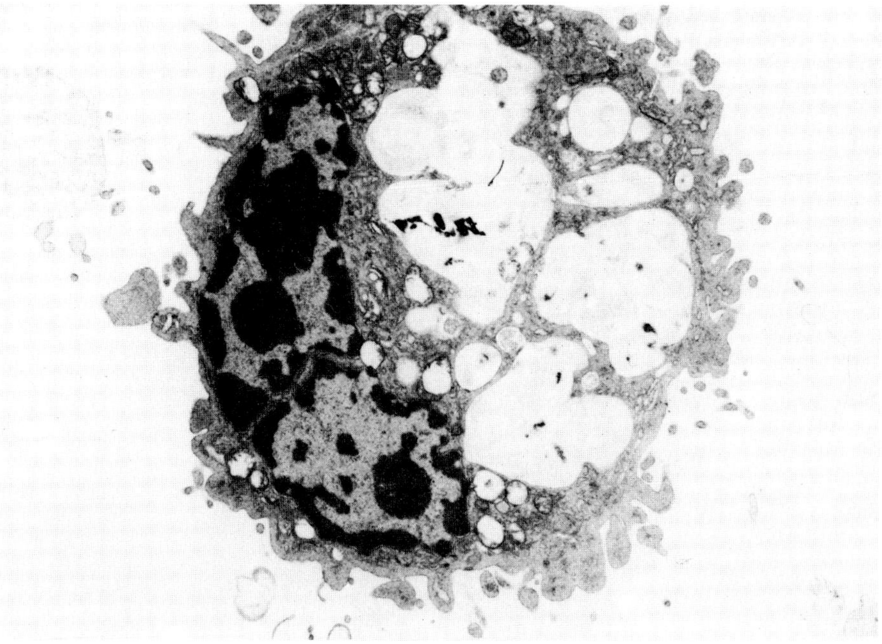

Fig. 6—(b) Electron micrograph of lavaged alveolar macrophage after silica. At 5 days the cell containing silica is larger and shows swelling of lysosomes. × 10000

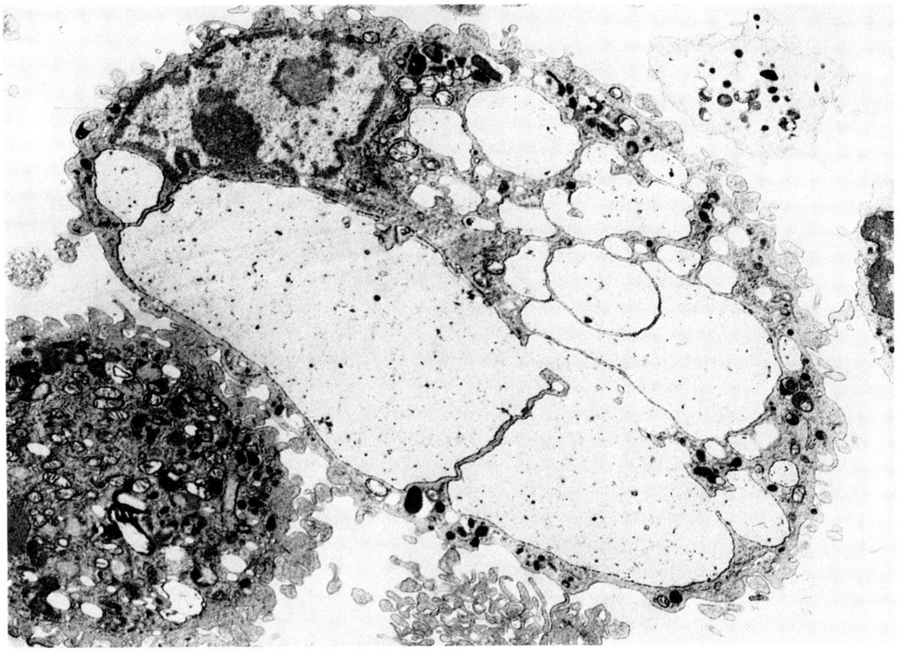

Fig. 6—(c) Electron micrograph of lavaged alveolar macrophage after silica. At 5 days this cell is considerably swollen an shows evidence of lysosomal membrane disruption. × 8300

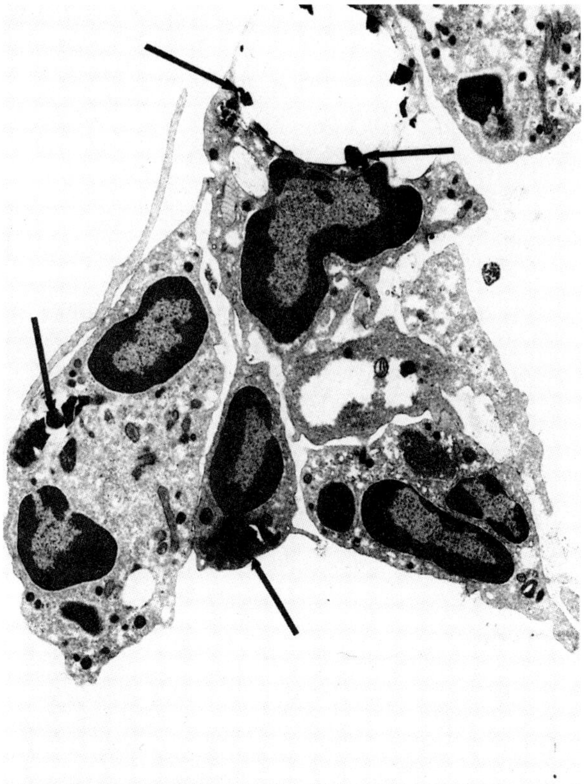

Fig. 7—Three days after silica, many PMN have ingested particles (arrows) and show lysosomal disruption. EM, × 15300

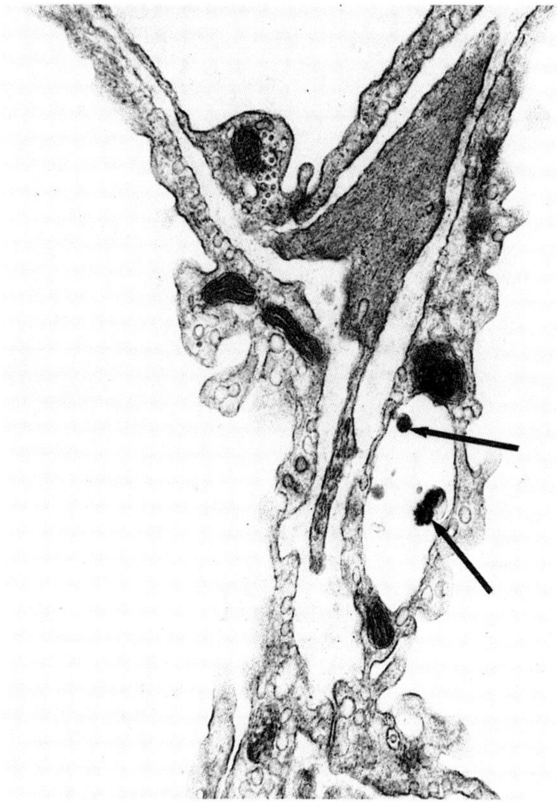

Fig. 8—Electron micrograph of alveolar wall, 2 days after silica. Small particles are found in vacuoles of the type 1 epithelial cell cytoplasm (arrows). × 34200

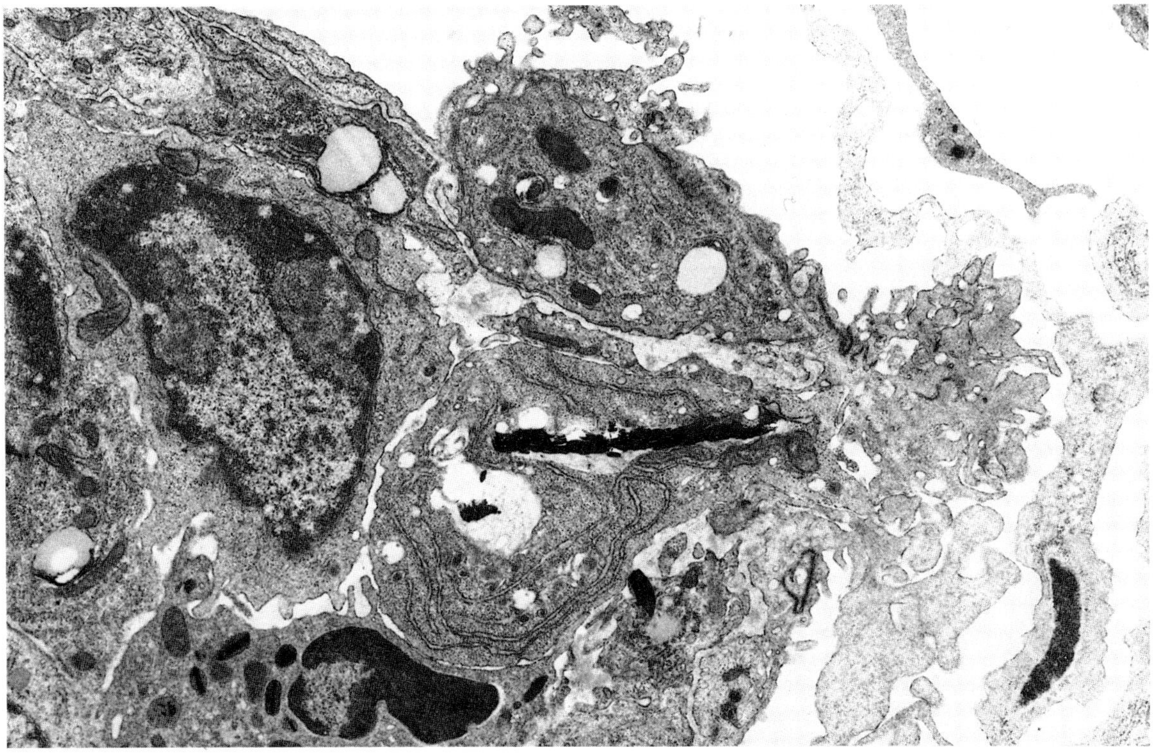

Fig. 9—Two days after silica, particles are found in cells located within the pulmonary interstitium. EM, × 13 500

exudates and within the interstitium. At this time the first recognizable peribronchiolar aggregates of cells are seen. Some of the macrophages within these nodular granulomas contain silica, some are labelled with tritiated thymidine and a few mitotic figures are observed (Fig. 10). By the fifth day, fibroblasts are seen in the peribronchiolar nodules; some of these calls are labelled with tritiated thymidine and the electron micrographs confirm the mixture of fibroblasts and macrophages containing silica (Fig. 11).

The later changes

The inflammatory response persists in the lung over the 20 week duration of the experiment. Although the macrophage continues to be the most prominent cell in the air sacs and within the interstitium, PMN persist as a significant component; these cells are observed in lung washings several months following the instillation of silica (Figs 12, 13). Coincident with epithelial regeneration described above, some of the luminal inflammatory exudates undergo organization; by 1 week fibroblasts produce a loose framework of collagen and these deposits may occlude most of the bronchiolar lumen (Fig. 14). Progression of these lesions is not observed and later in the experiment intraluminal bronchiolar obstruction could not be demonstrated.

The silicotic granulomas are clearly demarcated within the pulmonary interstitium by one week when the predominant macrophages and fibroblasts show some cell division. Granulocytes, though not numerous, are seen in most of the nodules. Subsequent development of the granulomas is not synchronous, some subside rapidly while others remain cellular with a low level of mitotic activity persisting for many weeks. In the majority of granulomas, proliferative activity subsides after 28 days and, as the nodules shrink in size, the newly formed collagen assumes a linear configuration, merging with the pre-existing peribronchiolar connective tissue. In some animals, fresh crops of siliceous granulomas appear later in the experiment. After 20 weeks, macrophages and PMN bearing silica crystals are recovered from the lungs by lavage and are still observed in lung sec-

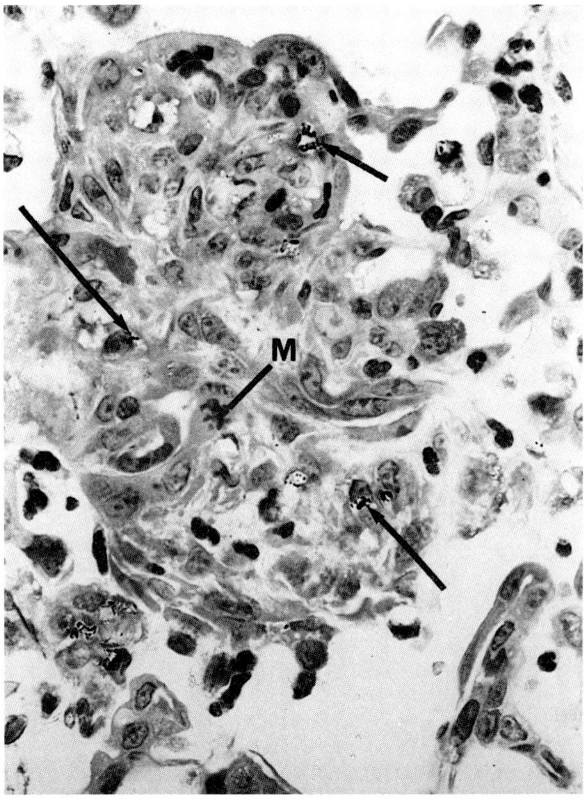

Fig. 10—Nodular granuloma 5 days after silica showing a mixture of fibroblasts, macrophages and some small dark PMN. Silica particles are seen (arrows) and a cell in mitosis (M) can be recognized. H & E, × 675

tions (Fig. 15) but, apart from some shrunken granulomas and peribronchial scarring, it is difficult to demonstrate a significant degree of alveolar fibrosis using morphologic techniques. Biochemical analysis, however, revealed that there was a 100 per cent increase in total hydroxyproline in these lungs after silica when compared with age-matched controls.[8]

DISCUSSION

The fibrogenic activity of silica has been attributed to toxic interactions with cell membranes and the release of fibroblast stimulating factors by macrophages.[1,13,14] The predominant macrophage response to silica observed in long term inhalation experiments has diverted attention from the acute effects of silica and from the interactions of the crystals with pulmonary cells and with inflammatory cells other than the macrophage. The events described in the present experiment extend from a few hours to 20 weeks following the instillation of a single bolus of silicon dioxide. This procedure was used in preference to inhalation to facilitate the precise timing of events from instillation to fibrosis. In previous studies we have shown that the overall distribution of cells remaining in the lung after lavage is similar to that observed in non-lavaged lung fixed *in situ*.[15,16]

The rapid movement of particles from the periphery of the lung to the bronchioles and their adjacent air sacs effectively clears most of the alveoli within 24 h. In this phase, clearance of silica is not different from inert particles such as carbon or polystyrene.[7,17] Similarly the initial efflux of macrophages and PMN is comparable for various particles, the critical factor being the number of particles reaching the alveoli.[17] At this point the similarities cease. The reaction to carbon and polystyrene is limited to the exudation of inflammatory cells with transient focal oedema and no evidence of epithelial necrosis. With silica, there is focal centrilobular necrosis of type 1 epithelial cells accompanied by a fibrinous exudate. These focal necroses are rapidly repaired by proliferation of type 2 cells. An increase in cuboidal cells after silica was first described by Policard *et al.*[18] and type 2 cell hyperplasia is now generally regarded as the standard reparative reaction after type 1 cell injury.

The proximity of the epithelial injury to the exudate of PMN and macrophages suggests that the phagocytosis of particles and the subsequent release of proteolytic enzymes may be responsible for the injury. The relationship is unlikely to be direct since the instillation of particles, such as carbon or polystyrene, induces an equivalent inflammatory cell exudate with no evidence of accompanying cell injury.[15,17] In the case of silica, however, injury to lysosomal membranes has been demonstrated in macrophages and an examination of the electron micrographs in this experiment indicates a similar process occurring in the PMN which is quantitatively, a more potent donor of proteases than the macrophage.[3] Furthermore, whereas the PMN response to carbon is brief, the persistence of these cells for many weeks after the instillation of silica, introduces the possibility of continuing protease-induced injury to pulmonary cells. A second possibility also needs to be considered. The centripetal movement of silica crystals during the first 24 h brings a high concentration of particles into close contact with the epithelium of

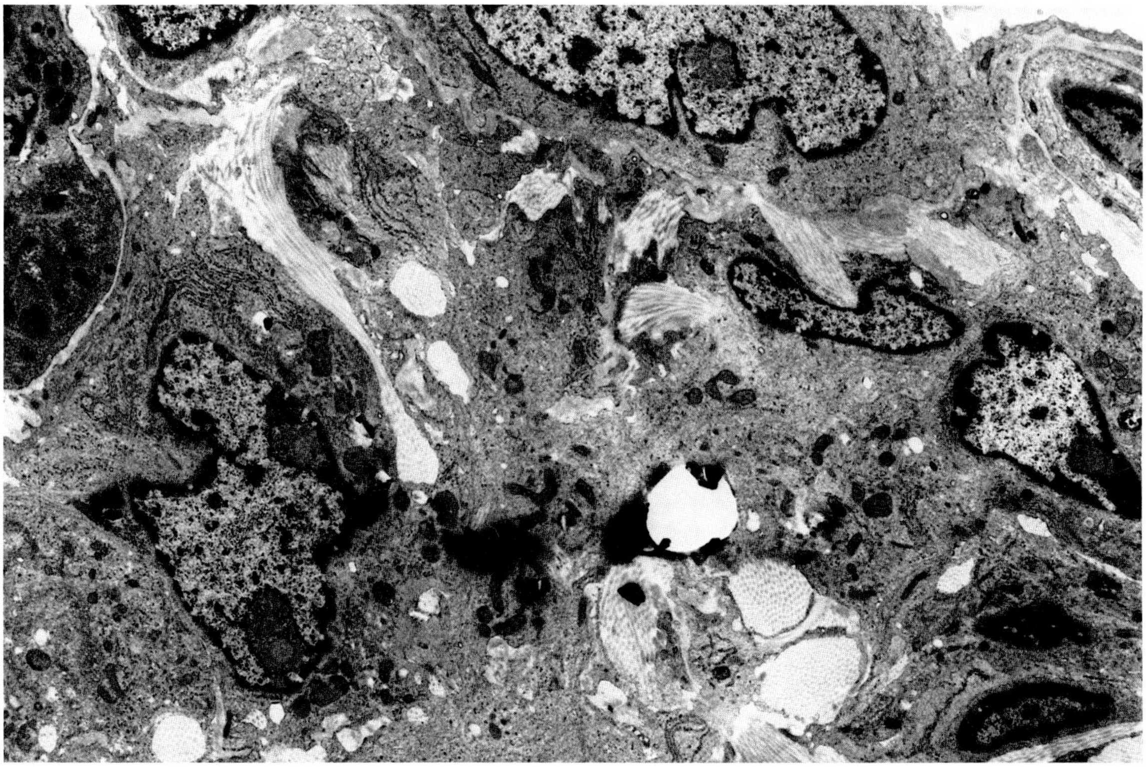

Fig. 11—Electron micrograph of granuloma showing fibroblasts, collagen and macrographs containing silica in the pulmonary interstitium. × 7650

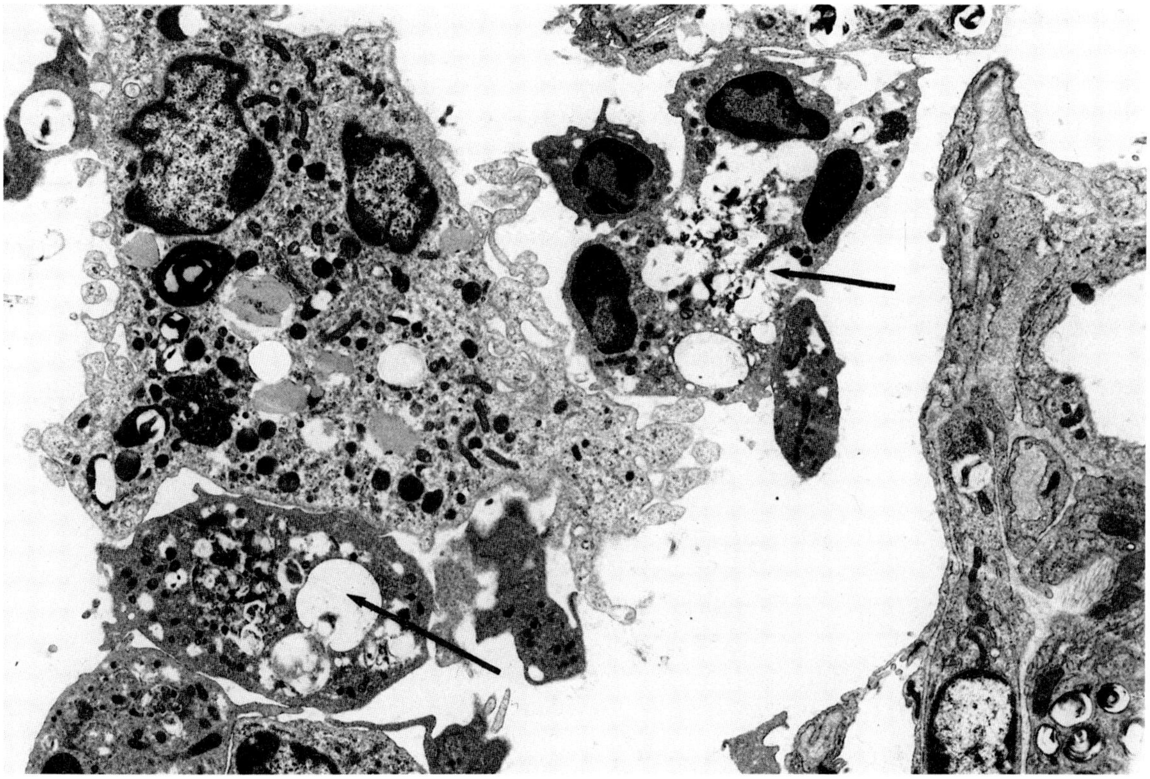

Fig. 12—Lung 16 weeks after silica. PMN and AM are found in the alveoli. Evidence of lysosomal disruption is seen (arrows). EM, × 7650

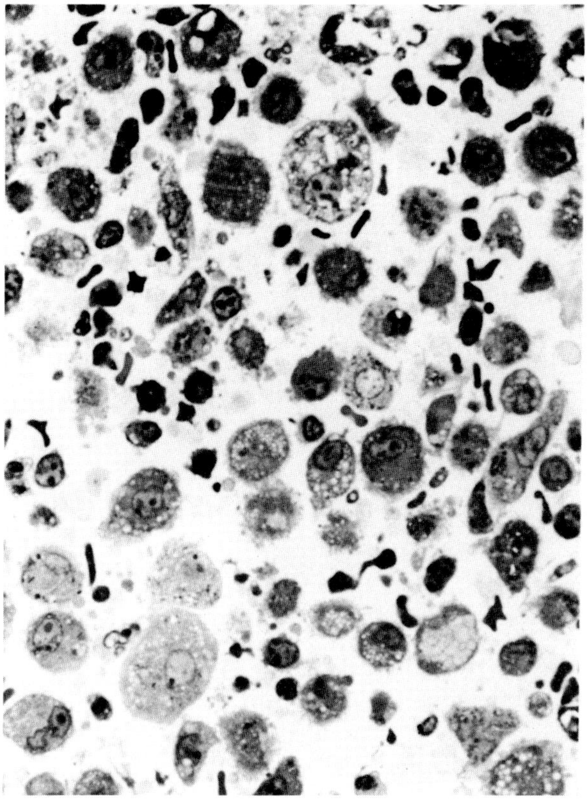

Fig. 13—Pellet of lavaged cells, 16 weeks after silica shows predominantly macrographs but PMN are still present. Toluidine blue stain, × 720

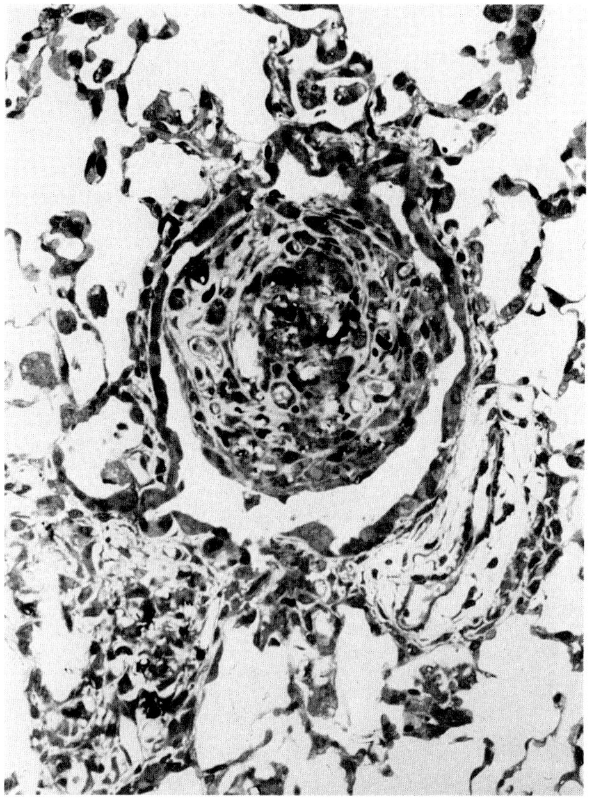

Fig. 14—One week after silica, an area of nodular fibrosis obstructs the bronchiolar lumen. The nodule has cells containing silica in the centre. H & E, × 162

centrilobular ducts and air sacs. Direct membrane toxicity has been demonstrated, [13,19] and it is not unlikely that the concentrated silica crystals directly change the surface membranes of the alveolar cells. Such particle–membrane interaction can alter membrane permeability and increase calcium influx to the cell[20]. Whether the progression of cell injury to cell death involves excess calcium levels or proteolytic enzymes, damage to the epithelial barrier would be expected to increase the likelihood of free particles passing from the air sacs to the interstitium, where they are ingested by phagocytes.

In most of the standard classifications of interstitial pulmonary fibrosis, silica is listed as an aetiologic agent. This is somewhat misleading since restrictive lung disease with diffuse alveolar fibrosis is not a feature of uncomplicated silicosis.[21] The reason for this is apparent when one considers how the pathways of dust clearance predispose the focal aggregations of particles in the peribronchial and perivascular connective tissues leaving the peripheral air sacs relatively unaffected.

Within the peribronchial granulomas the predominant cells are macrophages and fibroblasts which, according to the classical theory propounded by Heppleston,[1] are exclusively involved in the generation of the fibrous nodules. The demonstration of the continuing presence of PMN combined with the known action of the macrophage in releasing chemoattractants for PMN[4,7] suggests the matter may not be so straightforward. Several additional possibilities exist; PMN through the release of enzymes may amplify tissue injury and the fibrous response; on the other hand, production of collagenase by these cells may modulate or terminate the fibrogenic process.

The progressive nature of silicosis is thought to be dependent upon successive waves of phagocytosis, cell destruction and release of particles, a process that continues long after exposure to silica ceases. The observations presented in this paper suggest that silicotic fibrogenesis may be to some extent self-limiting. The peribronchial granulomas heal and the peribronchial scars that remain after

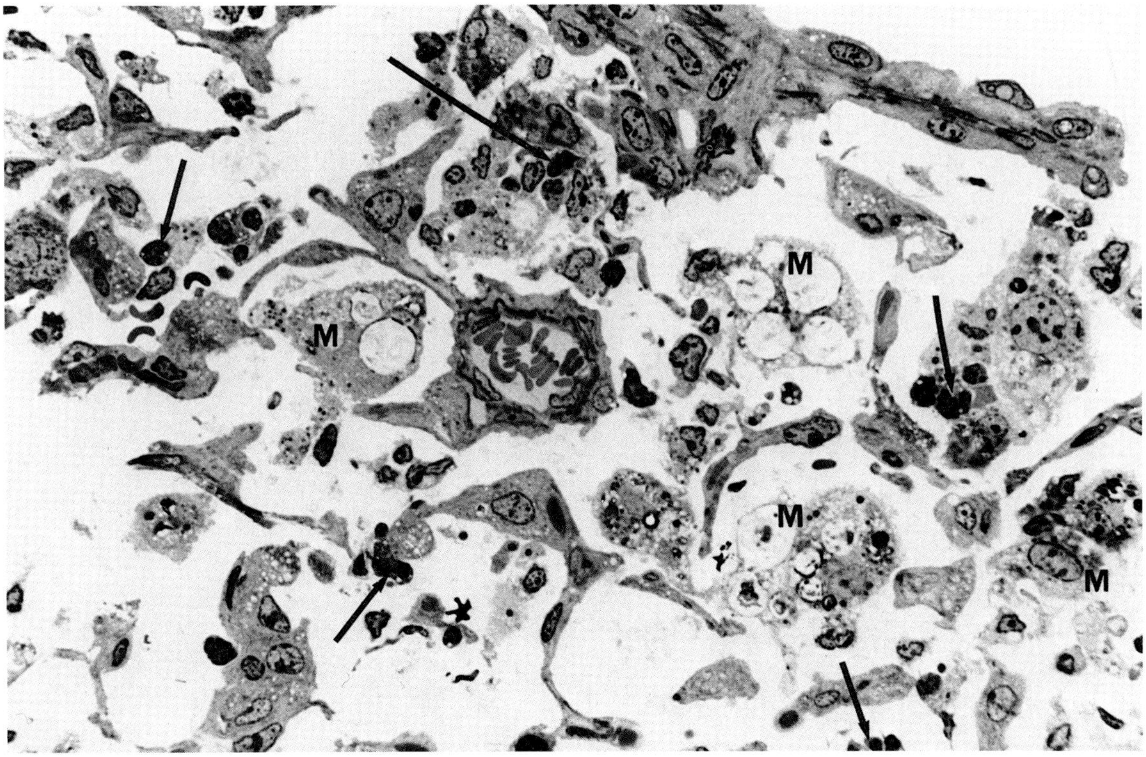

Fig. 15—Lung 20 weeks after silica. Though little fibrosis is seen, the alveoli contain a mixture of large, some vacuolated macrophages (M) and PMN (arrows). Toluidine blue stain, ×765

20 weeks are not easily discerned by conventional morphologic techniques. Biochemical determinations of hydroxyproline in these lungs demonstrate a significant increase in collagen from 4 weeks onward, levels that remain elevated until 20 weeks when the experiment was terminated.[8] Taken in conjunction with the morphological data it is reasonable to conclude that as the cellular granulomas subside, the residuum of collagen becomes incorporated into the peribronchiolar connective tissue. The location of this excess collagen, and the absence of significant scarring on the walls of peripheral air sacs may account for the remarkable paucity of symptoms in many of the people who are exposed to silica, and for the poor correlation between the radiologic demonstration of peribronchial scars and the lack of significant impairment of lung function.[21]

REFERENCES

1. Heppleston AG. Cellular reactions with silica. In: Bendz G, Lidquist I, eds. Biochemistry of Silicon and Related Problems. New York: Plenum Publishing Corp., 1978: 357–379.
2. Privalova LI, Katsnelson BA, Osipenko AB, Yushkov BN, Babushkina LG. Response of phagocyte cell system to products of macrophage breakdown as a probable mechanism of alveolar phagocytosis adaptation to deposition of particles of different cytotoxicity. *Environ Health Perspec* 1980; **35:** 205–218.
3. Sykes SE, Morgan A, Moores SR, Jones ST, Holmes A, Davison W. Evidence for a dose-dependent inflammatory response to quartz in the rat lung and its significance in early changes in collagen metabolism. *Environ Health Perspec* 1983; **51:** 141–146.
4. Lugano EM, Dauber JH, Daniele RP. Silica stimulation of chemotactic factor release by guinea pig alveolar macrophages. *J Reticuloendothel Soc* 1981; **30:** 381–390.
5. Lugano EM, Dauber JH, Daniele RP. Acute experimental silicosis. Lung morphology, histology and macrophage chemotaxin secretion. *Am J Pathol* 1982; **109:** 27–36.
6. Bowden DH, Adamson IYR. Adapative responses of the pulmonary macrophagic system to carbon. I. Kinetic studies. *Lab Invest* 1978; **38:** 422–429.
7. Adamson IYR, Bowden DH. Chemotactic and mitogenic components of the alveolar macrophage

response to particles and neutrophil chemoattractant. *Am J Pathol* 1982; **109:** 71–77.
8. Adamson IYR, Bowden DH. Role of polymorphonuclear leukocytes in silica-induced pulmonary fibrosis. *Am J Pathol* 1984; in press.
9. Morgan A, Moores SR, Holmes A, Evans JC, Evans NH, Black A. The effect of quartz, administered by intratracheal instillation, on rat lung. I. The cellular response. *Environ Res* 1980; **22:** 1–12.
10. Reiser KM, Haschek WM, Hesterberg TW, Last JA. Experimental silicosis. II. Long term effects of intratracheally instilled quartz on collagen metabolism and morphologic characteristics of rat lungs. *Am J Pathol* 1983; **110:** 30–41.
11. Dale K. Late effects of moderate doses of quartz dust on pulmonary function and tissue. *Scand J Resp Dis* 1973; **54:** 231–243.
12. Dale K. Late effects of large doses of quartz dust on pulmonary function and tissue. An experimental study on rabbits. *Scand J Resp Dis* 1973; **54:** 244–254.
13. Kane AB, Stanton RP, Raymond EG, Dobson ME, Knafele ME, Farber JL. Dissociation of intracellular lysosomal rupture from the cell death caused by silica. *J Cell Biol* 1980; **87:** 643–651.
14. Allison AC, Harington JS, Birbeck M. An examination of the cytotoxic effects of silica on macrophages. *J Exp Med* 1966; **124:** 141–153.
15. Adamson IYR, Bowden DH. Adaptive responses of the pulmonary macrophagic system to carbon. II. Morphologic studies. *Lab Invest* 1978; **38:** 430–438.
16. Bowden DH, Adamson IYR. Pathways of cellular efflux and particulate clearance after carbon instillation to the lung. *J Pathol* 1984; **143:** 117–125.
17. Adamson IYR, Bowden DH. Dose response of the pulmonary macrophagic system to various particulates and its relationship to transepithelial passage of free particles. *Exp Lung Res* 1981; **2:** 165–175.
18. Policard A, Collet A, Pregermain S. Etude au microscope electronique du granulome pulmonaire silicotique experimental. *Presse Med* 1957; **65:** 121–124.
19. Nash T, Allison AC, Harington JS. Physico-chemical properties of silica in relation to its toxicity. *Nature* 1966; **210:** 259–261.
20. Farber JL. How do mineral dusts cause lung injury? *Lab Invest* 1983; **49:** 379–380.
21. Parkes WR. Occupational Lung Disorders, 2nd edn. London: Butterworth's, 1982: 143–151.

JOURNAL OF PATHOLOGY, VOL. **144**: 163–169 (1984)

HISTOMORPHOMETRIC ANALYSIS OF SCLEROTIC BONE FROM IDIOPATHIC MYELOID METAPLASIA (NINE CASES)

J. M. COINDRE

Laboratoire d'Anatomie Pathologique, UER II, Université de Bordeaux II, 33076 Bordeaux, France and Laboratoire d'Anatomie Pathologique, Fondation Bergonié, 180 rue de Saint-Genès, 33076 Bordeaux Cedex, France

J. REIFFERS

Service d'Hématologie, Hôpital du Haut-Lévèque, 33600 Pessac, France

J. F. GOUSSOT AND A. DE MASCAREL

Laboratoire d'Anatomie Pathologique, UER II, Université de Bordeaux II, 33076 Bordeaux, France

AND

A. BROUSTET

Service d'Hématologie, Hôpital du Haut-Lévèque, 33600 Pessac, France

Received 27 March 1984
Accepted 14 May 1984

SUMMARY

The osteosclerosis of idiopathic myeloid metaplasia was investigated by a histodynamic study of undecalcified bone from nine patients. In all cases osteosclerosis resulted from woven bone formation. In moderate osteosclerosis only intrabecular woven bone was observed, with osteoclastic hyperresorption, hyperosteoidosis with many osteoblasts, and an increased calcification rate. This may represent an early stage of the disease, osteosclerosis resulting from increased bone remodelling, with woven bone formation by osteoblasts. However, in extensive osteosclerosis both intratrabecular and medullary woven bone was observed, with moderate osteoclastic hyperresorption, hyperosteoidosis without osteoblasts and a very low calcification rate. The latter pattern could correspond to an advanced stage, and could result from stromal bone formation without osteoblasts. The classical histodynamic profile of osteomalacia was sometimes observed. The link between bone pain and possible osteomalacia remains vague.

KEY WORDS—Idiopathic myeloid metaplasia, sclerotic bone, histomorphometry.

INTRODUCTION

Although bone lesions are constant in idiopathic myeloid metaplasia, histological studies relative to the subject are very few and relatively out of date.[1–3] Moreover, to our knowledge, no histomorphometric study on undecalcified bone with measurement of calcification rate exists. This technique, which has been applied to other osteosclerotic diseases such as Paget's disease[4] and bone metastases from prostatic carcinoma,[5] allows a very detailed examination of the dynamics of bone lesions.

Addressee for reprints: Dr J. M. Coindre, Laboratoire d'Anatomie Pathologique, UER II, Université de Bordeaux II, 33076 Bordeaux, France.

0022–3417/84/110163–07$01.00

MATERIAL AND METHODS

Patients

Nine patients (six males and three females) with confirmed idiopathic myeloid metaplasia were included in this study. The patients ranged in age from 56 to 71 years (mean 64). None of these patients had a history of fractures but two of them complained of bone pains situated mainly in the lower part of the body. x-Rays of the skull, pelvis, lumbar spine and dorsal spine were taken; these showed obvious bone sclerosis in patients 1, 3 and 7, moderate bone sclerosis in patients 4, 6 and 8, and no abnormality at all in patients 2, 5 and 9.

Biochemistry

The following were determined: haemaglobin and full blood count, serum urea nitrogen, serum creatinine, serum bilirubin, prothrombin time, serum albumin, calcium, phosphate and alkaline phosphatase; and urinary calcium, phosphorus and hydroxyproline excretion. Serum immunoreactive parathyroid hormone (iPTH) was performed by radioimmunoassay using an antibovine PTH C-terminal antibody.

Serum calcium and phosphorus levels and the mean urinary calcium and phosphorus excretion rate was normal. The mean serum alkaline phosphatase (135 ± 36 IU/l, normal range = 20–95 IU/l) and urinary hydroxyproline excretion (367 ± 194 μmol/24 h, normal range = 232 ± 148 μmol/l 24 h) were moderately, but not significantly, increased. The iPTH concentration was also normal.

Histodynamic study

An iliac bone biopsy was taken with an 8 mm inner diameter trephine, after a double labelling of the calcification front with tetracycline. The following schedule was used: dimethylchlortetracycline (600 mg/day, orally) for 2 days, 12 days without the drug and then a further 4 days with the same dose of tetracycline. Two fragments were taken from each patient. One was decalcified and stained with haematoxylin–eosin–safranin, by silver impregnation (Gomori) and Masson's stain for general histological assessment. The other sample was embedded in methyl methacrylate without prior decalcification. Eleven undecalcified 8 μm sections were cut with a Jung K microtome. Five sections were stained with solochrome cyanin R, four with Goldner's method and two with toluidine blue at pH 4·3. Four additional 15 μm thick unstained sections were used for tetracycline double labelling analysis under fluorescence.

Histomorphometric parameters were quantified using an integrating eyepiece: areas were measured by point counting and surfaces by intersection counting.

The following parameters were measured: (a) the trabecular bone volume (TBV) (the percentage of trabecular bone tissue in the total spongy bone space), the proportion of woven bone in the trabecular bone tissue, and the lamellar and woven TBV (under polarized light);

(b) bone resorption parameters: (i) the total resorption surface (TRS) (which represents the percentage of the total trabecular bone surface scalloped, with or without osteoclasts); (ii) the number of osteoclasts per square mm of bone section (Ocl/mm^2);

(c) Bone apposition parameters: (i) the trabecular osteoid surfaces (TOS) (which represents the percentage of the total trabecular surface covered by osteoid); (ii) the trabecular osteoid volume (TOV) represents the percentage of total trabecular bone tissue occupied by osteoid; (iii) the thickness index of the osteoid seams (T10) represents the ratio (TOV/TOS) $\times$ 100, and estimates the true thickness of the osteoid seams; (iv) the calcification rate (CR): determined by dividing the average distance between the two tetracycline labels by the time interval between the labelling period, CR being expressed in μm/day.

The results were compared with normal values obtained by Courpron *et al.*[6] and Meunier *et al.*[7] Our own control values (18 patients, mean age: 62 years) are similar to these normal values (see Table I).

Statistical analysis

Wilcoxon's test was used for statistical comparisons. The mean values are quoted with one standard deviation.

RESULTS

Above and beyond the customary histological examination, performed after decalcification, the present study dealt with a histodynamic analysis on undecalcified bone (see Table I).

Increased bone density

Trabecular bone volume was always higher, generally twice that of control values ($39·8 \pm 11·1$ per cent). Normal value in age and sex—matched controls: $17·4 \pm 1·6$ per cent[6] $p < 0·01$).

Table I—Individual histomorphometric parameters in patients with sclerotic bone from idiopathic myeloid metaplasia

Patient number	Age (years) at biopsy/sex	TBV (%)	%of woven bone	Woven TBV (%)	Lamellar TBV (%)	TRS (%)	Ocl/mm² (%)	TOS (%)	TOV	TIO	CR (μm/day)
1‡	57/M	34·8	83·3	29·0	5·8	6·0	0·16	26·1	4·5	17·2	0·69
2	63/M	30·8	11·0	3·4	27·4	12·8	0·57	35·8	7·2	20·1	0·84
3‡	67/F	47·0	55·1	25·9	21·1	2·9	0·15	83·4	33·6	40·3	<0·20
4†	67/M	42·6	45·5	19·4	23·2	8·1	1·11	82·7	15·7	19·0	0·67
5	71/M	23·8	27·3	6·5	17·3	10·0	0·71	36·4	7·5	20·6	0·89
6†	63/M	42·9	27·0	11·6	31·3	11·1	0·31	20·8	3·3	15·9	0·56
7*‡	56/F	61·2	63·9	39·1	22·1	6·6	0·19	56·3	9·9	17·6	<0·20
8*†	70/F	44·3	58·2	25·8	18·5	6·8	0·43	45·3	9·5	21·0	<0·20
9	60/M	31·0	25·5	7·9	23·1	22·9	2·72	68·2	11·0	15·1	1·02
Mean values		39·8±11·1§	44·1±23·1§	18·7±12·1§	21·1±7·1	9·7±5·8§	0·71±0·82	50·6±23·4§	11·4±9·1§	20·8±7·6	0·59±0·32
Normal values[6,7]		17·4± 1·6	0	0	17·4±1·6	3·6±1·1	<0·20	13·6±3·0	2·4±0·5	18·0±0·7	0·72±0·12
Control values (from our laboratory)		18·4± 6·2	0	0	18·4±6·2	3·7±1·2	<0·20	15·4±7·0	2·5±1·2	17·0±3·4	0·67±0·14

* Bone pain.
† Moderate bone sclerosis.
‡ Obvious bone sclerosis.
§ Different from normal value = $p < 0{\cdot}01$.

Woven bone constituted 44·1 ± 23·1 per cent of the trabecular bone and the lamellar TBV was nearly normal (22·1 ± 7·1 per cent). The new woven bone either adhered to pre-existing lamellar trabeculae, or was isolated in the medullary tissue. In three cases (patients 2, 5 and 9), it was found only in the trabeculae, and in small quantities. In these cases, TBV was moderately higher, with normal trabecular architecture.

Bone resorption

Total resorption surfaces were greater in eight cases (9·7 ± 5·8 per cent. Normal value: 3·6 ± 1·1 per cent[6]) ($p < 0{\cdot}01$).

The number of osteoclasts per square millimetre was increased but without statistical significance (0·71 ± 0·82 Ocl/mm^2. Normal value: 0·20/mm^2).

The three patients with moderately increased bone density and only intratrabecular woven bone showed marked hyperresorption with hyperosteoclastosis (Fig. 1).

Bone formation

Hyperosteoidosis was constant. Trabecular osteoid volume (11·4 ± 9·1 per cent. Normal value in age and sex-matched controls: 2·4 ± 0·5 per cent[7] $p < 0{\cdot}01$) and trabecular osteoid surfaces (50·6 ± 23·4 per cent. Normal value in age and sex-matched controls: 13·6 ± 3·0 per cent[7] $p < 0{\cdot}01$) were markedly increased. The thickness index of the osteoid seams was normal (20·8 ± 7·6 per cent. Normal value: 18·0 ± 0·7 per cent[7], but was distinctly increased in patient 3 (Fig. 2).

The calcification rate in trabecular bone was not significantly different from normal (0·59 ± 0·32 μm/day. Normal value: 0·72 ± 0·12 μm/day). Patients with a markedly increased bone density (patients 3, 7 and 8) showed a drastic drop of their calcification rate (Fig. 3), while patients with a moderately increased bone density and only intratrabecular woven bone (patients 2, 5 and 9) showed an increased calcification rate (Fig. 4).

On the whole, two clearly separate histodynamic profiles were apparent. First, there was moderately increased bone density accounted for entirely by intratrabecular woven bone, marked hyperresorption, hyperosteoidosis with a normal thickness of osteoid seams and an increased calcification rate (patients 2, 5 and 9). Second, there was markedly increased bone density with profuse trabecular and medullary woven bone, with moderate hyperresorption, hyperosteoidosis with a normal or increased thickness of osteoid seams and a very low calcification rate (patients 3, 7 and 8).

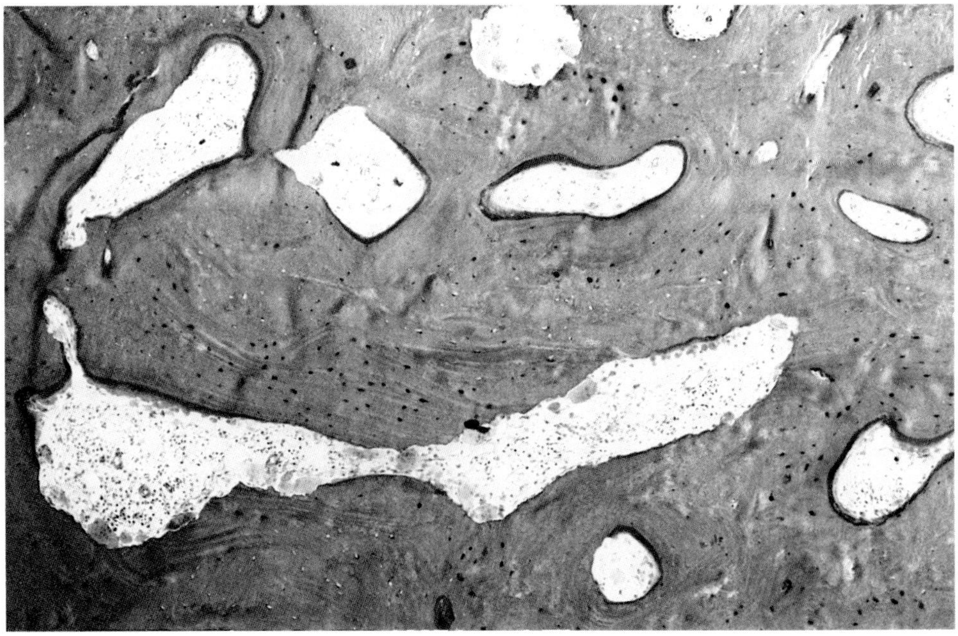

Fig. 1—Numerous foci of osteoclastic resorption in cortical bone. Goldner stain, × 25 (case 9)

DISCUSSION

Two points will be discussed: increased bone density, and the hyperosteoidosis with lack of mineralization which was observed in three patients.

Increased bone density

Increased bone density is a characteristic feature in idiopathic myeloid metaplasia. Radiologically, it varies from 25[8] to 66 per cent.[9] It has often been noted on bone biopsies but trabecular bone volume

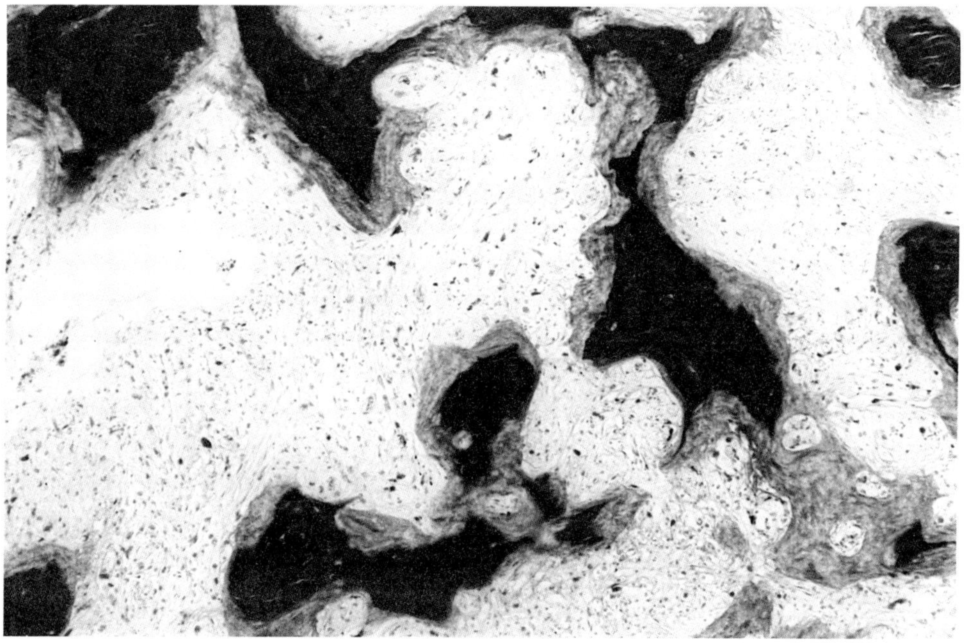

Fig. 2—Osteoid seams are widespread and thickened. Solochrome cyanin stain, × 64 (case 3)

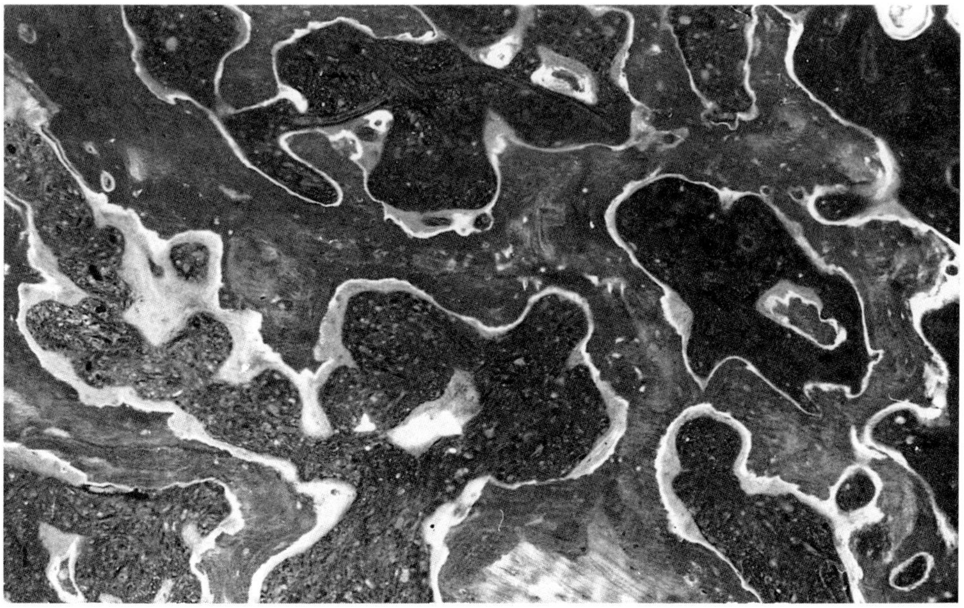

Fig. 3—Unstained section under fluorescence after a double labelling with tetracycline. There is only a single thin fluorescent label demonstrating an extremely low calcification rate. × 25 (case 3)

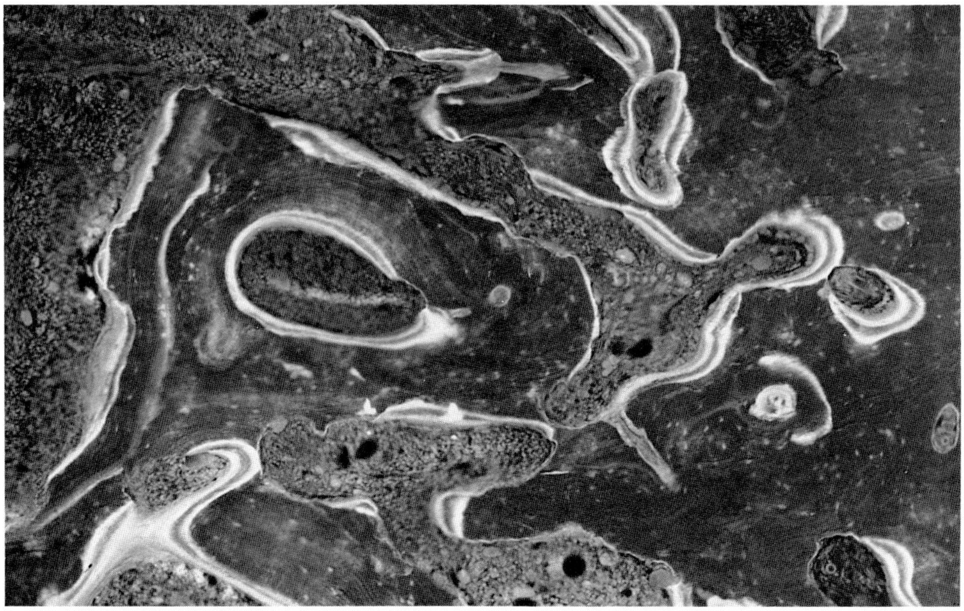

Fig. 4—Unstained section under fluorescence after a double labelling with tetracycline. Tetracycline doubly labelled surfaces are extended and the distance separating the two labels is wide demonstrating an increased calcification rate. × 25 (case 9)

has never been formally quantified. TBV of our patients was always increased and generally exceeded twice that of normal values. On average, 44·1 per cent of trabecular bone was made up of woven bone, with the result that lamellar TBV was close to normal, where the bone is entirely lamellar. The increased bone density can thus be explained by the formation of woven bone.

The bone biopsies showed two kinds of woven bone: woven bone laid down on pre-existing lamellar trabeculae, and woven bone isolated in the fibrous medullary tissue. The latter has been termed stromal bone.[10] In three patients (patients 2, 5 and 9), there was no stromal bone, and TBV was lower than that in the other patients (28·5 per cent as opposed to 45·5 per cent) with a lesser quantity of woven bone (21·3 per cent as opposed to 55·5 per cent of the trabecular bone). These patients showed increased total resorption surfaces, with many osteoclasts and an increased calcification rate. Moreover, osteoid seams of normal thickness were often edged with osteoblasts. These three patients had an increased osteoblastic appositional rate because they showed an increased calcification rate and osteoid seams of normal thickness.[7] This increased formation of woven bone by osteoblasts may be linked to the osteoclastic hyperresorption, as seen in Paget's disease.[4] This kind of bone lesion could correspond to an early stage as Oechslin has suggested.[11] Stromal bone may then appear due to transformation of intra-medullary and juxtatrabecular collagen tissue, without the action of osteoblasts.

Paget's disease and sclerotic bone metastases are the most frequent causes of acquired increased bone density. In Paget's disease osteosclerosis results from an over-production by osteoblasts of woven bone, which is the consequence of osteoclastic hyperresorption.[4] This latter could be caused by a viral agent.[12] The bone lesions of the early stage of idiopathic myeloid metaplasia may appear similar, but the medullary lesions are the key to the correct diagnosis. Patients 2, 5 and especially 9, show this feature. However, the advanced lesions are very different from those observed in Paget's disease. There are but few osteoclasts and osteoblasts, the stromal bone is present and the calcification rate is normal or slowed down. The osteosclerosis of bone metastases usually prostatic, results from bone formation by osteoblasts without preliminary resorption,[5] and also from stromal bone formation.[10] The advanced stage of idiopathic myeloid metaplasia may appear similar and the proportion of woven bone is also similar in these two kinds of osteosclerosis ($40{\cdot}3 \pm 21{\cdot}27$ per cent in the sclerotic bone metastases by Galasko[10]). The presence of metastatic epithelial cells in the fibrosis allows the diagnosis to be made.

Hyperosteoidosis with lack of mineralization

All our patients showed hyperosteoidosis, and three showed reduced mineralization (patients 3, 7 and 8). The features of their bone lesions were: extensive osteosclerosis (TBV = 50·8 per cent) increased intratrabecular and stromal woven bone (59·1 per cent of trabecular bone), considerable hyperosteoidosis (TOV = 17·7 per cent) and a dramatically low calcification rate ($< 0{\cdot}20\ \mu$m/day). This description suggests an advanced stage with lack of mineralization. Moreover, one of our three patients (patient 3) showed a very high thickness index of the osteoid seams, which constitutes the classical histodynamic picture of osteomalacia.[7] Two of these patients (patients 7 and 8) experienced bone pain; however calcium-phosphorus homeostasis was normal. This hyperosteoidosis, with lack of mineralization, could correspond to true osteomalacia, but this possibility remains to be verified. This bone lesion could be a result either of a negative calcium balance due to the high calcium requirement of the bone tissue, or of a relative lack of vitamin D; this would resemble the osteomalacia sometimes seen in sclerotic bone metastases from carcinoma of the prostate.[5]

ACKNOWLEDGEMENT

We wish to thank Professor P. J. Meunier for his many valuable suggestions.

REFERENCES

1. Kerneis JP, Savoie JC. L'ostéomyélosclérose et les réactions de la substance osseuse dans la splénomégalie myéloide de l'adulte. *Sang* 1954; **24:** 833–849.
2. Chomette G, Laumonier R, Taylot J. Anatomie pathologique des lésions osseuses des hémopathies malignes. *Sang* 1960; **31:** 183–205.
3. Roberts BE, Woods CG, Miles DW, Paterson CR. Bone changes in polycythaemia vera and myelosclerosis. *J Clin Path* 1969; **22:** 696–700.
4. Meunier PJ, Coindre JM, Edouard CM, Arlot ME. Bone histomorphometry in Paget's disease. Quantitative and dynamic analysis of pagetic and nonpagetic bone tissue. *Arthr Rheum* 1980; **23:** 1095–1103.
5. Valentin-Opran A, Edouard C, Charhon S, Meunier PJ. Histomorphometric analysis of iliac bone metastases of prostatic origin. In: Donath A, Courvoisier B, eds. Bone and Tumors. Symposium CEMO III, Genève: Médicine et hygiène 1980: 24–28.
6. Courpron P, Meunier PJ, Edouard C, Bernard J, Bringuier JP, Vignon G. Données histologiques quantitatives sur le vieillissement osseux humain. *Rev Rhum* 1973; **40:** 469–483.
7. Meunier PJ, Edouard C, Richard D, Laurent J. Histomorphometry of osteroid tissue. The hyperosteoidoses. In Meunier PJ, ed. Bone Histomorphometry. Paris: Armour Montagu, 1977: 249–261.
8. Linman JM, Bethell FH. Agnogenic myeloid metaplasia. Its natural history and present day management. *Am J Med* 1957; **22:** 107–122.
9. Croizat P, Revol L, Morel P, Mouriquand C, Drapier P. A propos de 42 cas cliniques de réticulomyélose aleucémique essentielle (ostéofibroréticulomyélose). *Sang* 1958; **29:** 346–383.
10. Galasko CSB. Bone metastases studied in experimental animals. *Clin Orthop Related Res* 1981; **155:** 269–285.
11. Oechslin RJ. Osteomyelo-sklerose und skelett. *Acta Haemat (Basel)* 1956; **16:** 214–234.
12. Rebel A, Malkani K, Basle M. Anomalies nucléaires des ostéoclastes de la maladie osseuse de Paget. *Nouv Presse Méd* 1974; **20:** 1299–1301.

ENDOCRINE CELLS IN INTESTINAL METAPLASIA OF THE STOMACH

P. MINGAZZINI

Dipartimento di Biopatologia Umana, Sezione di Anatomie Patalogica, Universitá di Roma, La Sapienza, Italy

F. CARLEI

6º Clinica Chirurgica, Universitá di Roma, La Sapienza, Italy

F. MALCHIODI-ALBEDI

Dipartimento di Biopatologia Umana, Sezione di Anatomie Patalogica, Universitá di Roma, La Sapienza, Italy

E. LEZOCHE

6º Clinica Chirurgica, Universitá di Roma, La Sapienza, Italy

A. COVOTTA

IV Semeiotica Chirurgica, Universitá di Roma, La Sapienza, Italy

V. SPERANZA

6º Clinica Chirurgica, Universitá di Roma, La Sapienza, Italy

AND

J. M. POLAK

Royal Postgraduate Medical School, Hammersmith Hospital, London W12 0HS, U.K.

Received 20 January 1984
Accepted 14 May 1984

SUMMARY

In this study we have investigated the mucin profile and the endocrine cell population in gastric endoscopic biopsies from 22 patients affected by chronic gastritis and intestinal metaplasia and in five surgical specimens of stomachs removed because of intestinal-type carcinoma (4) or peptic ulcer (1). High iron diamine-Alcian blue (HID-Ab) staining and peptide immunocytochemistry (peroxidase anti-peroxidase technique) were used. Forty-one foci of intestinal metaplasia were detected, 15 produced sulphomucins and 26 sialomucins. Of the endocrine cells investigated, gastrin and somatostatin cells were the most frequently observed, while cholecystokinin, glucose-dependent insulinotropic peptide-, secretin- and enteroglucagon-containing cells were also found in the metaplastic areas, but less frequently. No significant correlation was found between the type of mucin and the types of endocrine cells present, the latter usually resembling those normally found in the small intestine. On the basis of these results we conclude that intestinal metaplasia involves mucin- and peptide-producing cells of the stomach in a variable manner, with no correlation between the two.

KEY WORDS—CCK, chronic gastritis, endocrine cells, enteroglucagon, gastrin, GIP, intestinal metaplasia, precancerous lesions, secretin, somatostatin.

INTRODUCTION

Different types of intestinal metaplasia of gastric mucosa have been distinguished according to different histological and histochemical patterns. Special attention has been given to the so-called colonic type of intestinal metaplasia,[1,2] which is characterized by the presence of sulphomucins similar to those found in the large intestine. An incomplete type of intestinal metaplasia, where mucus-secreting columnar cells, resembling gastric foveolar cells, replace the absorptive cells, has also

Addressee for correspondence: Dr J. M. Polak, Department of Histochemistry, Hammersmith Hospital, London W12 0HS, U.K.

0022–3417/84/110171–08$01.00

been described.[3] It has been demonstrated that the incomplete type of intestinal metaplasia with production of sulphomucins is significantly more frequent in patients with the intestinal type of gastric carcinoma than in benign cases.[2,4]

Endocrine cell population in intestinal metaplasia has also been the subject of a number of investigations and the presence of Grimelius'-positive argyrophil cells and other endocrine cells has been clearly demonstrated.[5,6]

This study was undertaken to assess whether there is any correlation between the type of mucus produced (sulphomucins versus sialomucins) and the types of endocrine cell detected in metaplastic areas.

MATERIALS AND METHODS

Twenty-two endoscopic biopsies of gastric mucosa showing chronic gastritis only and five resected stomachs (four for gastric carcinoma and one for prepyloric peptic ulcer) were selected for this study. The age of the patients ranged from 43 to 59 (mean 54) years. Specimens from small and large intestine showing no histological abnormalities were included as controls for mucin studies.

The samples were fixed in Bouin's solution for 24 h, dehydrated, embedded in paraffin and serially sectioned at 4 μm thickness. In addition to the conventional haematoxylin and eosin staining, the high iron diamine/Alcian blue (HID AB)[7] procedure was performed to evaluate the production of sulpho- and sialomucins as well as the PAS-AB at pH 2·5 techniquc to dctect areas of incomplete metaplasia. Further sections were used for immunocytochemistry (peroxidase anti-peroxidase method).[8]

Immunocytochemistry

The sections were deparaffinized and brought to water. The primary antiserum was applied and the sections were left overnight at 4°C in a moist chamber. The properties of the antisera used are summarized in Table I. They were then washed in phosphate buffer (0·02 M pH 7·25) and incubated for 1 h in the second antibody (goat anti-rabbit IgG, Miles Laboratories, diluted $\frac{1}{100}$). After rinsing, rabbit peroxidase anti-peroxidase (UCB, diluted $\frac{1}{300}$) was applied to the sections for a further hour. The specific sites of immunoreactivity were visualized by hydrogen peroxide and 3,3-diaminobenzidine (SIGMA 25 mg/100 ml). The sections were mounted in permanent medium and semiquantitative analysis was performed, evaluating the number of positive cells over five glandular structures in the foci of intestinal metaplasia.

Controls

The specificity of the immunostaining was verified by absorption tests with a variety of homologous (0·5 nmol/ml) and heterologous peptides (greater than 10 nmol/ml of diluted antiserum). Incubation with pre-immune primary serum alone was also performed.

Histochemical reactions for mucins were carried out on normal intestine.

RESULTS

Mucin studies (Table II)

In the 27 specimens, 41 foci of intestinal metaplasia (29 localized in the antrum and 12 in the body-fundus) were identified. The HIB Ab stain

Table I—Characteristics of antibodies

	Ref. No.	Specificity	Dilution	Raised in
Gastrin	144	C term	1/2000	Rabbit
Somatostatin 14	744	Whole molecule	1/10000	Rabbit
Cholecystokinin	280	9–20	1/5000	Rabbit
Secretin	53	whole	1/5000	Rabbit
Glucose dependent (GIP) insulin-releasing peptide	378	whole	1/15000	Rabbit
Glucagon	499	N term	1/5000	Rabbit
2nd layer (Miles Lab)		Rabbit IgG	1/100	Goat
PAP complex (UCB peptides)		Peroxidase molecule	1/300	Rabbit

Table II—Mean number of cells per five glands

	No. of specimens		No. of foci	GAS	SOM	CCK	SEC	GIP	EG
Atrophic gastritis	22	Sulphated	0	—	—	—	—	—	—
		Sialilated	22	5–6	2–3	1	0–1	0–1	2
Carcinoma	4	Sulphated	15	4–6	2	1	0–1	1	2–3
		Sialilated	2	5–6	2–3	0–1	—	0–1	2
Peptic ulcer (pre-pyloric)	1	Sulphated	0	—	—	—	—	—	—
		Sialilated	2	5–6	2	1	—	1	1–2

showed a predominance of sulphomucins in 15 of these foci and of sialomucins in 26 (Fig. 1). All the foci of intestinal metaplasia with predominance of sulphomucins were found in the specimens of the mucosa surrounding carcinomas and none in the endoscopic biopsies or in the stomach resected for peptic ulcer.

No difference in mucin production was detected

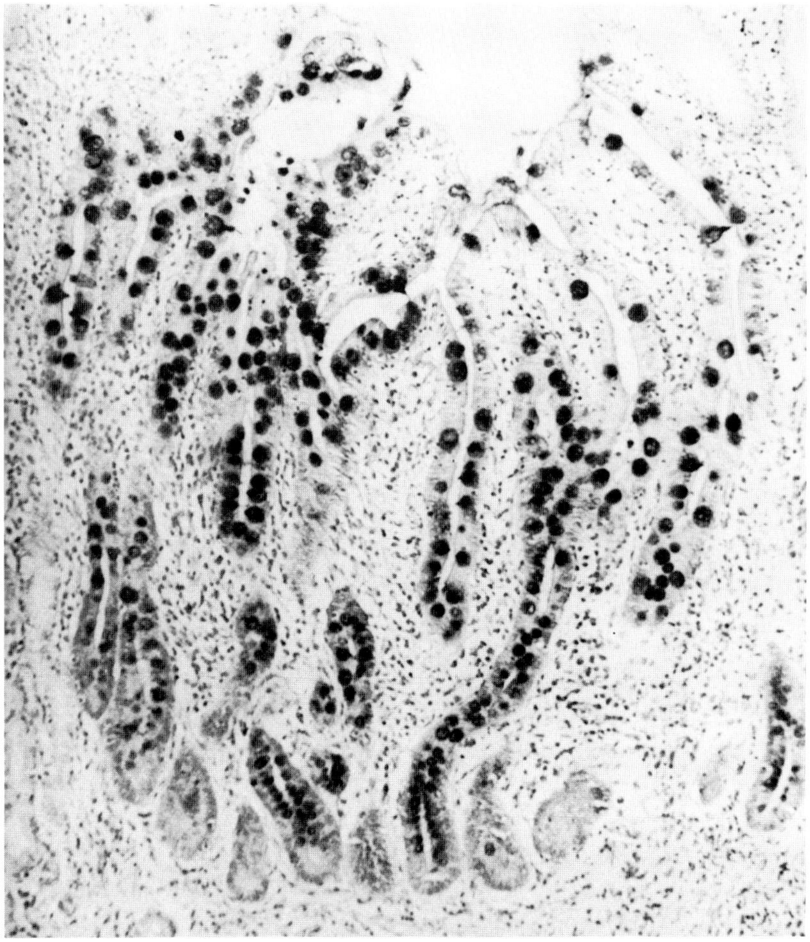

Fig. 1—Focus of intestinal metaplasia complete-type clearly showing a predominance of sulphated mucins (black) in the goblet cells. Antral mucosa surrounding a carcinoma. Bouin's fixation, 5 μm paraffin section. HID-Ab technique, ×80

among foci located in the gastric body and those in the antrum; moreover, sulphated and sialilated mucins were always detected in different proportion in all 27 specimens. Finally, few foci producing sialomucins were also present in the mucosa surrounding carcinomas.

The PAS-AB technique allowed detection of several, but very limited, areas of incomplete intestinal metaplasia. Only in one focus was this pattern generalized (Fig. 2). It was localized in the mucosa surrounding the carcinoma and was characterized by large amounts of sulphomucins.

Immunocytochemistry (Table II)

Immunocytochemistry revealed that gastrin and somatostatin cells were the most frequent endocrine cells (Figs. 3, 4). They were present in nearly all the foci both in sulphomucin- and in sialomucin-producing types of intestinal metaplasia; in 18 foci gastrin cells were remarkably abundant (more than five cells for five glandular spaces), while the somatostatin cells never exceeded three for five glandular spaces. Again, no significant differences in mucous production were detected in the areas where gastrin and somatostatin cells were most abundant. Enteroglucagon cells were rarely seen (absent in 16 cases, present in 21). Usually no more than two cells for five glandular spaces were counted (Fig. 5) but in four foci from two gastrectomy specimens for carcinoma there were 2–3 enteroglucagon cells for five glandular spaces. In these foci (one of them being the only focus of incomplete intestinal metaplasia detected) a predominance of sulphomucins was also found.

Glucose-dependent insulinotropic peptide (GIP) cells and cholecystokinin (CCK) cells were rarely present since only single cells of each type could be identified in a minority of foci (12 over 41 for GIP cells and nine for CCK cells) variably containing sulphated and/or sialilated mucins.

Secretin cells were nearly always absent, single positive cells being observed only in three foci (one with sulphated, two with sialilated mucins).

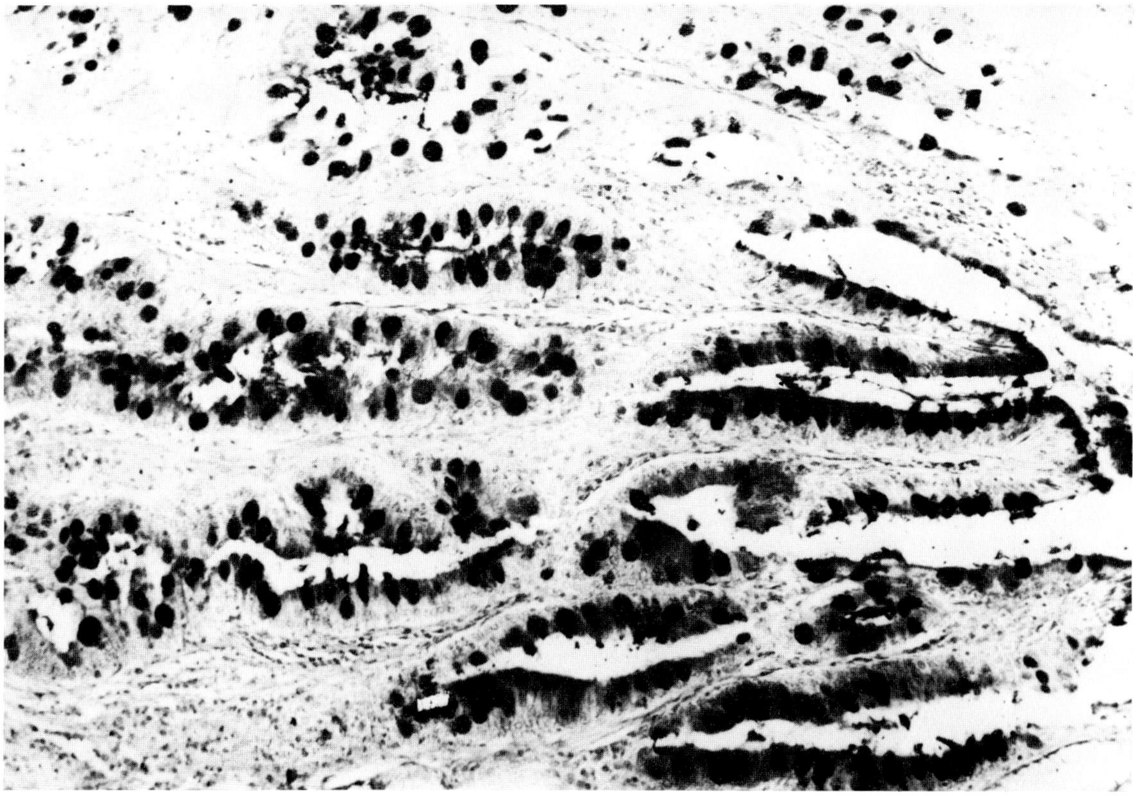

Fig. 2—Incomplete type of intestinal metaplasia showing numerous mucous-secreting columnar cells present among the goblet cells. Gastric antrum—surgical specimen. Bouin's fixation, 5 μm paraffin section. HID-Ab technique, ×90

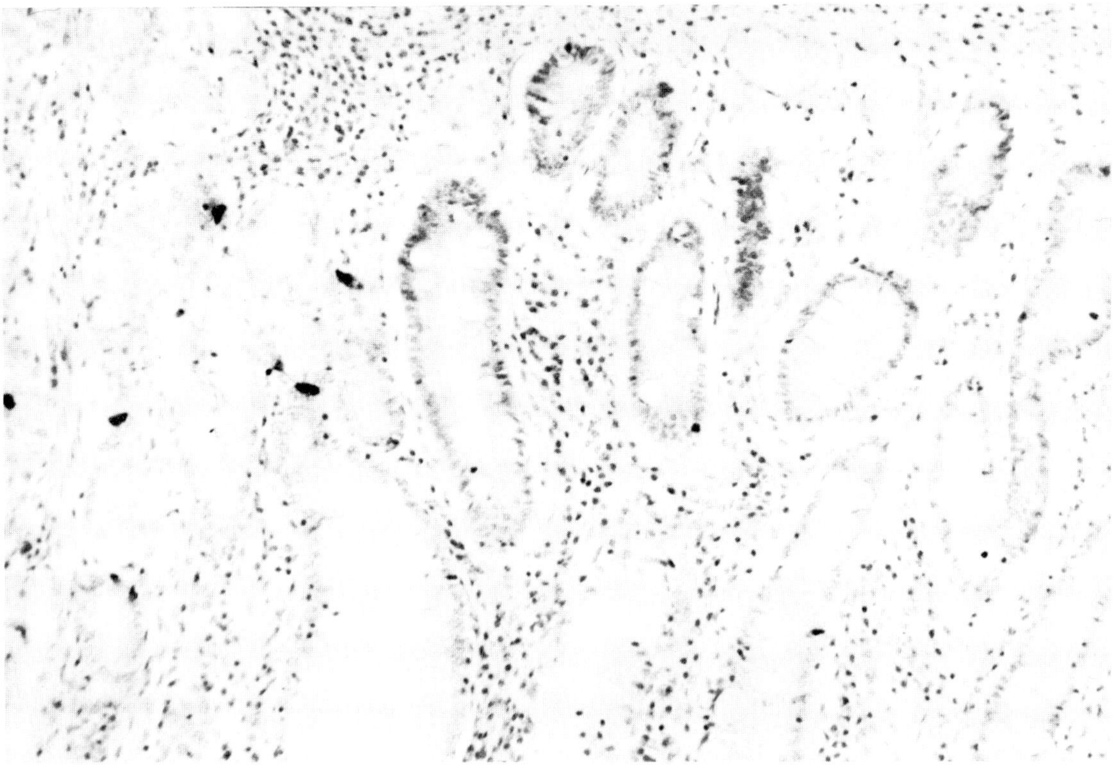

Fig. 3—Scattered gastrin-immunoreactive cells in intestinal metaplasia producing sialilated as well as sulphated mucins. Gastric antrum. Bouin's fixation, 5 μm paraffin section. PAP technique, $\times 200$

Controls

Immunocytochemistry—Disappearance of the immunocytochemical staining was obtained only using antisera pre-absorbed with the corresponding peptide (0·5 nmol/ml of diluted antisera) and with pre-immune primary serum, while absorptions with heterologous peptides had no effect.

HID-Ab controls—In normal small intestine, nearly all the goblet cells appeared blue after the HID Ab reaction (sialomucins), while in large intestine the majority of cells showed a brown stain, demonstrating the presence of sulphomucins.

DISCUSSION

In the comparative histochemical and immunohistochemical investigation which we carried out on intestinal metaplasia of gastric mucosa, our results suggest that the sulphomucin-producing foci of intestinal metaplasia (so-called 'colonic type') and the sialomucin-producing foci ('small intestinal type') do not differ significantly from each other as far as the endocrine cell population is concerned. Despite the fact that the endocrine cells of the intestine are differently distributed, secretin and CCK cells being absent from the large intestine,[9] all the endocrine cell types which were present in the sialomucin-producing type of intestinal metaplasia could also be identified in similar numbers in the sulphomucin-secreting type.

Our observations suggest that the unknown factors which determine the modifications in mucus production (i.e. the shift from predominantly sialilated mucins typical of the small intestine to those rich in sulphated groups, characteristic of the colon) do not correlate with the endocrine cell differentiation which always resembles that characteristic of the small intestine.[5,9]

In normal stomach, gastrin cells are confined to the antrum; in conditions such as type A atrophic gastritis they may increase in number and even reach overt hyperplasia;[10] in two samples from the mucosa surrounding a carcinoma arising from the

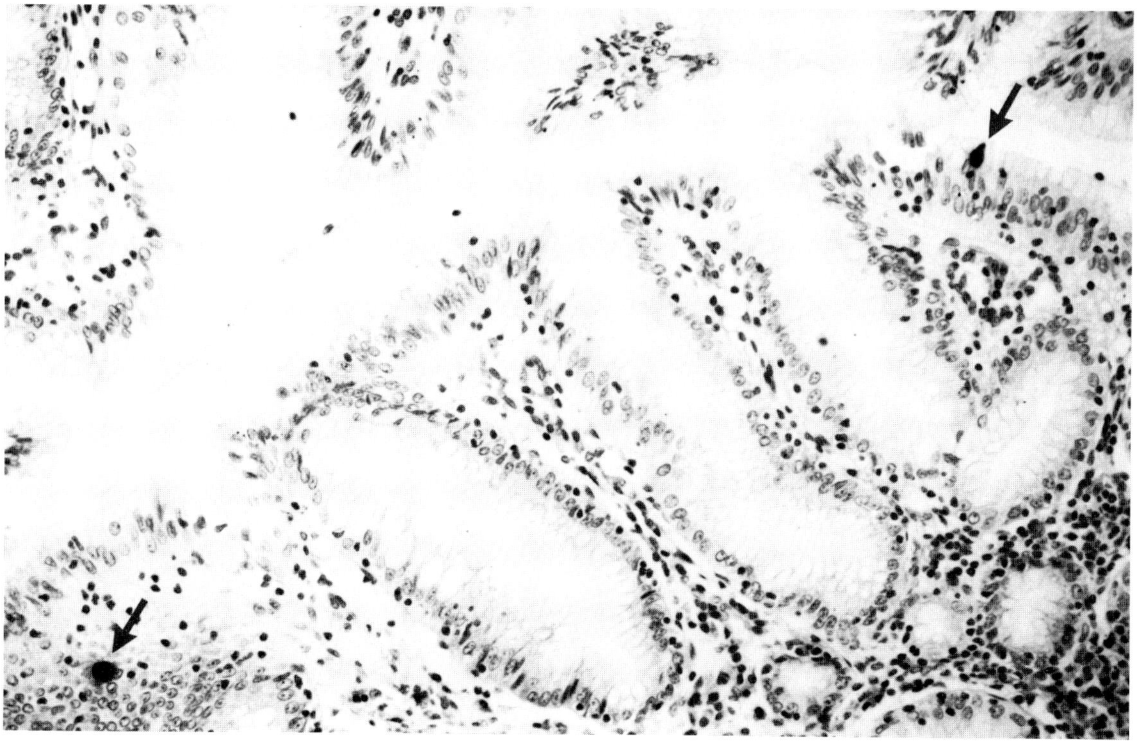

Fig. 4—Scattered somatostatin-containing endocrine cells (arrows) in an area of sialomucins producing intestinal metaplasia. Gastric antrum. Bouin's fixation, 5 μm paraffin section. PAP technique, $\times 270$

gastric body we found an unusually high number of gastrin cells in the oxyntic mucosa which also showed atrophic gastritis (Fig. 6); this may be related to the occurrence of pseudopyloric metaplasia which is a common finding in group A atrophic gastritis.

Although we found a relatively frequent occurrence of enteroglucagon cells in four foci with the sulphated (colonic) type of mucin including the one showing the incomplete type of intestinal metaplasia, we cannot strictly correlate the presence of enteroglucagon cells with these types of metaplasia since these cells were also present in 17 other foci (seven sulphated- and 10 with sialilated-mucins). Nevertheless, the occurrence of enteroglucagon cells in intestinal metaplasia associated with gastric carcinoma certainly deserves further investigation.

An increase of gastrointestinal endocrine cells has been observed in intestinal metaplasia when some features of intestinal differentiation (expression of enzymes, presence of Paneth cells) were absent.[6] Since in this type of metaplasia a closer relationship to gastric cancer has also been postulated,[11] it would be worth studying the endocrine cell population in those conditions of gastric mucosa in which dedifferentiation takes places, such as the various degrees of gastric dysplasia.

In conclusion, we believe that metaplasia of the gastric mucosa affects both mucous cells and endocrine cells in a variable manner, although there is no apparent correlation between the changes induced.

REFERENCES

1. Tegelbjaerg PS, Nielsen HO. Small intestinal type and 'colonic type' intestinal metaplasia of the stomach and their relationship to the histogenetic types of gastric adenocarcinoma. *Acta Path Microbiol Scand Sect A* 1978; **86:** 351–355.
2. Segura DI, Montero C. Histochemical characterisation of different types of intestinal metaplasia in gastric mucosa. *Cancer* 1983; **52:** 498–503.
3. Ming SC, Goldman H, Freiman DG. Intestinal metaplasia and histogenesis of carcinoma of the human stomach. *Cancer* 1967; **20:** 1418–1425.
4. Jass JR, Filipe MI. Variants of intestinal metaplasia

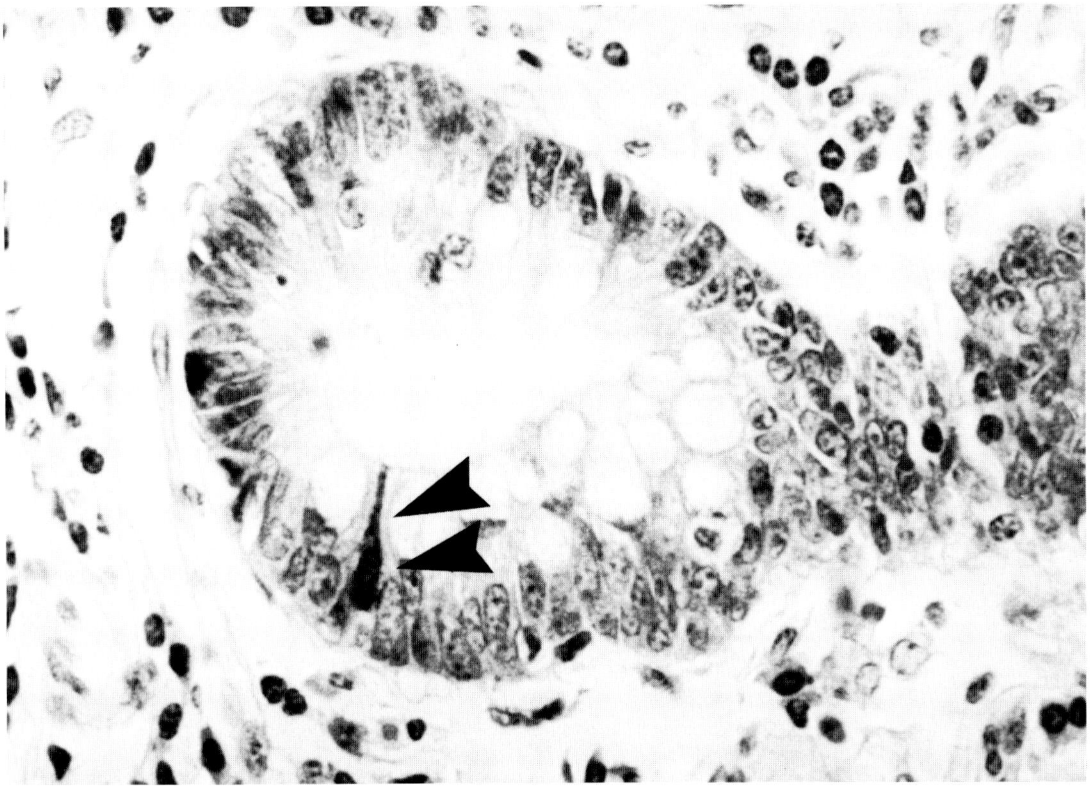

Fig. 5—Enteroglucagon-containing cell (arrow) with a cytoplasmic process extended to the lumen in an intestinal type gland from a focus of sialomucin-containing intestinal metaplasia. Gastric body. Bouin's fixation, 5 μm paraffin section. PAP technique, × 500

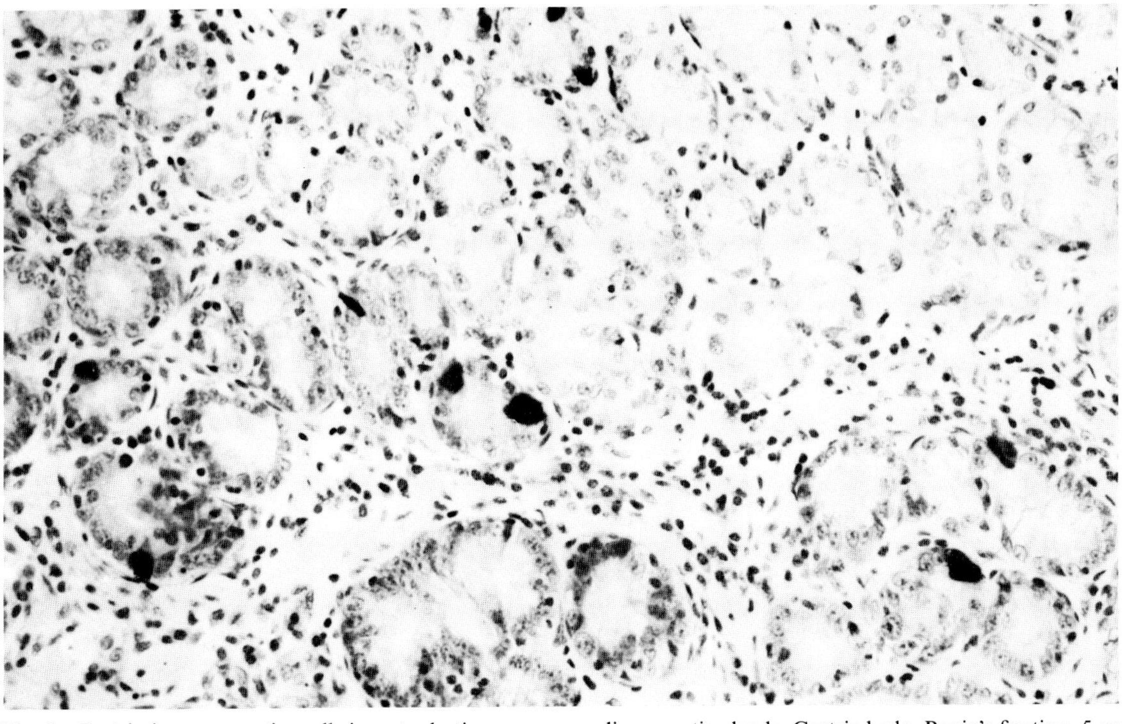

Fig. 6—Gastrin immunoreactive cells in metaplastic area surrounding oxyntic glands. Gastric body. Bouin's fixation. 5 μm paraffin sections. PAP technique, × 255

associated with gastric carcinoma. *Histopathology* 1979; **3:** 191–199.

5. Bordi C, Ravazzola M. Endocrine cells in the intestinal metaplasia of gastric mucosa. *Am J Pathol* 1979; **96:** 391–398.
6. Tsutsumi Y, Nagura H, Watanabe K, Yanaihara N. A novel subtyping of intestinal metaplasia of the stomach, with special reference to the histochemical characterizations of endocrine cells. *Virchows Arch (Pathol Anat)* 1983; **401:** 73–88.
7. Spicer SS. Diamine methods for differentiating mucosubstances histochemically. *J Histochem-Cytochem* 1965; **13**(3): 211–234.
8. Sternberger LA. Immunocytochemistry. 2nd edn. New York: John Wiley, 1979.
9. Pearse AGE, Polak JM. The diffuse neuroendocrine system and the APUD concept. In: Bloom SR, ed. Gut Hormones. Edinburgh, London, New York: Churchill Livingstone, 1978: 33–38.
10. Walsh JH, Grossman MI. Gastrin. *N Engl J Med* 1975; **292;** 1324–1332, 1333–1384.
11. Matsukura N, Suzuki K, Kawachi T, Aoyagi M, Sugimura T, Kitaoka H, Numajiri H, Shirota A, Itabashi M, Hirota T. Distribution of marker enzymes and mucins in intestinal metaplasia in human stomach and relation of complete and incomplete types of intestinal metaplasia to minute gastric carcinomas. *J Natl Cancer Inst* 1980; **65:** 231–240.

JOURNAL OF PATHOLOGY, VOL. **144**: 179–187 (1984)

PERSISTENCE OF INERT MACROMOLECULES (IMPOSIL) IN THE RAT MESANGIUM AND GLOMERULAR FUNCTIONAL DISTURBANCE

N. P. GOODE

Renal Research Unit, St. James's University Hospital, Leeds, U.K.

A.M. DAVISON

Department of Renal Medicine, St. James's University Hospital, Leeds, U.K.

G. GOWLAND

University Department of Immunology, The General Infirmary, Leeds, U.K.

S. R. APARICIO

Electron Microscopy Unit, St. James's University Hospital, Leeds, U.K.

AND

M. SHIRES

Renal Research Unit, St. James's University Hospital, Leeds, U.K.

Received 5 November 1983
Accepted 17 May 1984

SUMMARY

Imposil iron–dextran is an inert tracer that has been used to study mesangial uptake and clearance of macromolecular material from the glomerular circulation. Such a tracer may be a useful marker of altered mesangial function in animals with some forms of glomerulonephritis. We have studied mesangial handling of intravenously injected Imposil (50 mg/100 g body weight) in normal rats by light, immunofluorescence and electron microscopy for up to 3 months. Mesangial cell uptake was maximal at 48–54 h. Extrusion and drainage of tracer to the vascular pole and distal tubule was evident at 3 days but iron was still present in mesangial cells at 3 months. Possible functional renal impairment resulting from persistent mesangially sequestered tracer was examined by measuring daily urine protein and iron excretion. A possible relationship between failure of mesangial cells to eliminate inert tracer and increasing glomerular permeability is demonstrated, suggesting that Imposil and similar inert macromolecules cannot be used for long-term studies of mesangial function.

KEY WORDS—Rat, mesangium, glomerulus, iron–dextran.

INTRODUCTION

Numerous investigators have examined mesangial uptake of macromolecules from the glomerular circulation[1] using a variety of inert tracers including colloidal carbon,[2,3] thorotrast, [4,5] ferritin, [6,7] iron–dextran[8,9] and more physiological tracers, including aggregated proteins[10–14] and immune complexes.[15–17] These studies demonstrate persistence of inert tracers in the mesangium for prolonged periods,[3] whereas biodegradable tracers readily enter the mesangium but rapidly disappear.[12] Kinetic studies[2,8,14] have delineated a clearance pathway from the glomerular capillary lumen through the mesangium to the glomerular hilum.

Addressee for correspondence: Dr A. M. Davison, Department of Renal Medicine, St. James's University Hospital, Leeds, U.K.

0022–3417/84/110179–09$01.00

The present study examines the consequences of uptake and retention of the iron–dextran complex Imposil by the rat mesangium and follows the clearance of the tracer from this site over 3 months, to assess the potential of Imposil as a kinetic marker of mesangial clearance function in healthy and glomerulonephritic rats.

MATERIAL AND METHODS

Experimental design

Male Wistar rats, 5–8 weeks old, maintained on a standard laboratory diet, received a single intravenous injection (0·5 ml/100 g body weight) of the iron–dextran complex, Imposil 200, containing 10 per cent elemental iron (1·79 mol/l), (Fisons Pharmaceuticals Ltd.).

Groups of three or four animals were studied at 5 min, 30 min, 2 h, 8 h, 48 h, 54 h, 65 h, 3 days, 6 days and 2 weeks after injection. Thirteen experimental and seven control animals were examined at 3 months, four from each of these groups being maintained in metabolic cages throughout the 3-month period.

Tissue examination

Tissue for light microscopy, fixed in 10 per cent buffered formal saline, was stained with haematoxylin and eosin, periodic acid–Schiff and Perl's Prussian blue reaction, using standard procedures.

Tissue for electron microscopy was fixed in 3 per cent glutaraldehyde in 0·1 M phosphate buffer, post-fixed in 2 per cent osmium tetroxide in cacodylate buffer, dehydrated through graded alcohols and embedded in Araldite. Five blocks were examined from each animal, thin sections being mounted on 200 μm single hole grids, as described previously.[18] Sections were examined and photographed unstained at 40 kV using a Jeol-100S electron microscope.

Snap-frozen tissue for immunofluorescence microscopy, sectioned at 5 μm and fixed in ethanol/ether (1 : 1) for 10 min and 95 per cent ethanol for 20 min was examined by direct and indirect immunofluorescence for the detection of rat IgG, IgA, IgM, complement C3 and rat serum albumin (RSA), using fluorescein isothiocyanate (FITC)-conjugated rabbit anti-rat IgG (Miles), FITC-conjugated rabbit anti-RSA antiserum (Nordic) and anti-rat IgA, IgM and C3 antisera (Nordic) followed by FITC-conjugated rabbit anti-goat IgG (Miles). Immunofluorescence was viewed and photographed under incident light on a Leitz Dialux 20 microscope.

Urine analysis

Daily 24 h urine volumes from animals kept in metabolic cages were measured and stored at −20°C until required.

Urinary protein was measured by a benzethonium chloride turbidometric assay[19] using bovine serum albumin as protein standard (Armour).

Urinary iron excretion was measured by a bathophenanthroline colorimetric assay according to the method of Thompson *et al.*[20]

Statistical methods

Urinary protein excretion results were evaluated by the Mann–Whitney U-test for the analysis of non-parametric data.

RESULTS

Intravenous injection of 50 mg of Imposil per 100 g body weight, produced transient wheezing and twitching which subsided within 5–10 min. All animals appeared to recover within 30–60 min.

Light microscopy did not reveal any obvious glomerular abnormality. The ferric iron component of Imposil was demonstrated as the blue reaction product of Perl's Prussian blue reaction (PBR). Figure 1 illustrates the intensity and relative distribution of PBR-stained material in different renal compartments in paraffin-embedded sections from groups of animals killed at various time intervals. The distribution was highly reproducible amongst animals in each experimental group.

Electron microscopically, Imposil was identified as highly electron-dense, rod-shaped particles (22·0 nm × 3·7 nm) which were easily distinguished against the lighter, less granular background of unstained sections.

Vascular distribution

Imposil in the glomerular circulation was maximal 5 min after injection, falling sharply at 30 min and 2 h when some glomeruli contained no tracer. Circulating Imposil was again demonstrated in glomerular capillaries at 8 h, coinciding with large

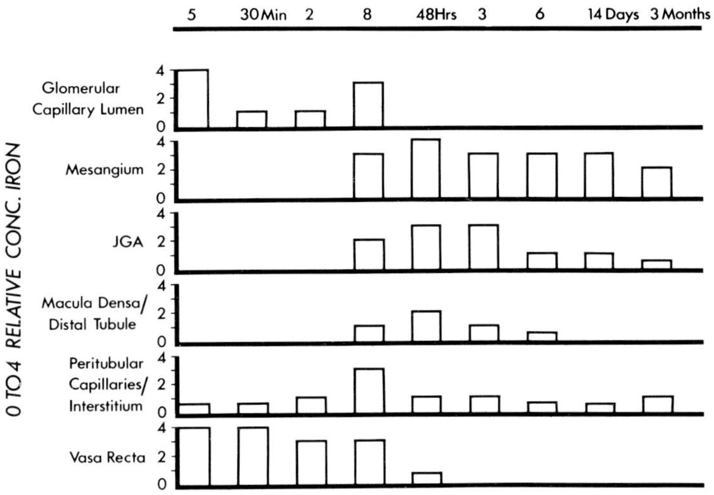

Fig. 1—Relative intensity and distribution of Perl's Prussian blue staining in different renal compartments at various time intervals, based on examination of 5 μm kidney sections. Staining: 0 = no staining; $\frac{1}{2}$ = trace; 1 = weak, limited; 2 = moderate, limited; 3 = moderate, extensive; 4 = heavy, extensive

amounts of tracer in peritubular capillaries and interstitium. At later time intervals tracer was almost entirely intracellular.

Mesangium

Imposil particles present in mesangial intercellular spaces and matrix at 30 min reached a maximal concentration at 8 h. At later time intervals extracellular tracer was only occasionally seen, notably in the axial mesangial and JGA matrix at 3 days and 6 days, when particles were observed both in a free and aggregated form.

Maximal mesangial cell uptake was seen at 48 h to 54 h, when aggregates occupied the mesangium from the peripheral capillary loops down to the hilum. There was considerable variation in the amount of Imposil contained in different mesangial cells. Intracellular particles were seen both in membrane-bound secondary lysosomes and lying free with the cytoplasm of mesangial cells either as discrete particles or as loose aggregates which lacked any demonstrable limiting membrane (Fig. 2).

Secondary lysosomes occupied an eccentric position in the cell cytoplasm at 65 h and by day 3, cells were seen to be releasing the contents of their secondary lysosomes into intercellular spaces (Fig. 3). The size and number of secondary lysosomes in mesangial cells was reduced between 3 and 6 days. Electronlucent rings and holes were evident in remaining secondary lysosomes, whilst in others tracer was less densely aggregated than previously noted.

Significant PBR-staining was evident around the macula densa and distal tubule in 5 per cent of glomeruli at 8 h increasing to a maximal incidence of 30 per cent at 54 h (Fig. 4). Despite this drainage of tracer from the mesangium, tracer aggregates were still detectable in mesangial cells at 3 months, appearing similar in concentration and distribution to those seen at 2 weeks. Some experimental and control animals showed paramesangial electron-dense deposits in a distribution similar to that demonstrated by immunofluorescence.

Other renal compartments

Tracer particles were not detected in the glomerular basement membrane and were only rarely sighted in the urinary space. Glomerular epithelial and proximal tubular cells contained small amounts of tracer at 8 h and 48 h. At 3 months a varied distribution of PBR-stained material was seen in segments of proximal tubules and heavier deposition was noted in distal tubular cells, although no staining was evident at the level of the macula densa.

Immunofluorescence

The 3 month immunofluorescence findings are summarized in Table I. Granular mesangial and

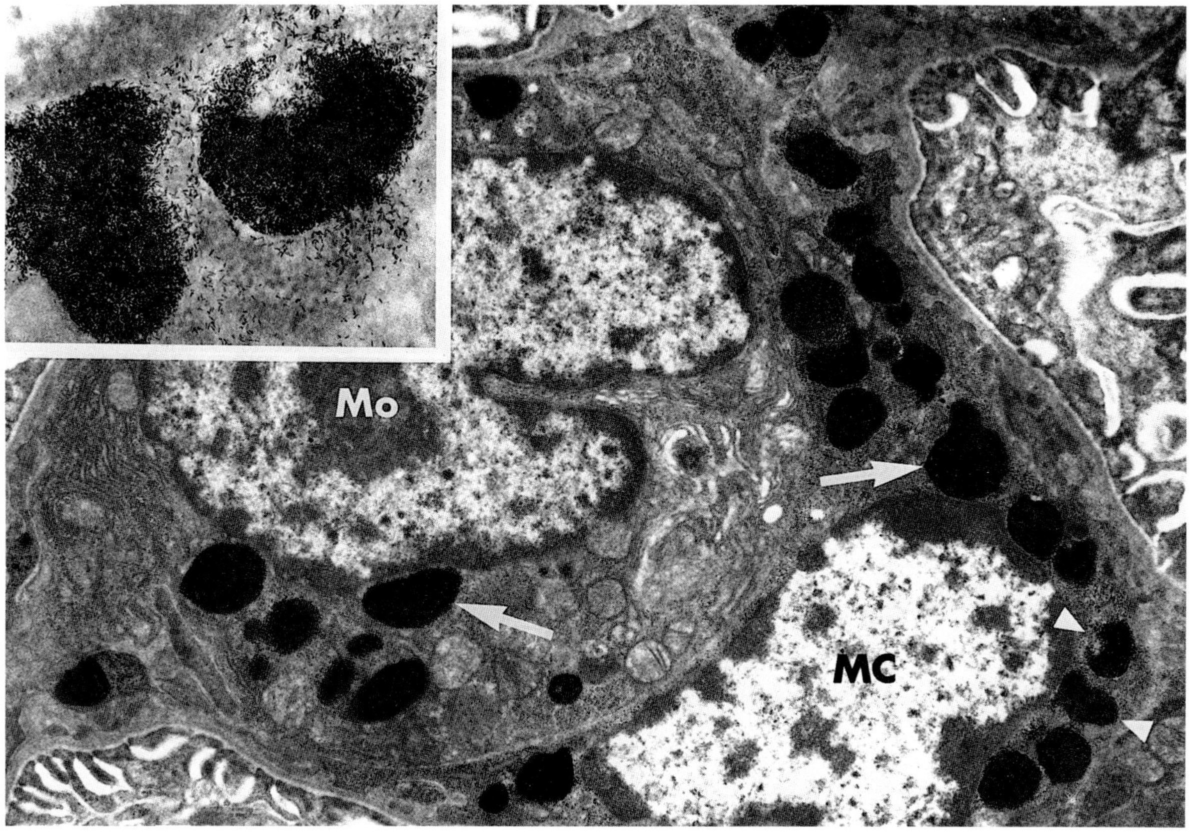

Fig. 2—Electron micrograph of a mesangial cell (MC) and a rare infiltrating monocyte (Mo) at 48 h following Imposil injection shows tracer aggregates in numerous secondary lysosomes of both cells (arrowed). Inset—Higher magnification of the area indicated by arrowheads demonstrates both free intracellular particles and tracer contained within secondary lysosomes. Unstained × 12350; inset × 57000

glomerular capillary wall IgM deposition was noted in 4/7 control rats, either alone or associated with a similar deposition of IgA 2/7 or IgG 1/7. One control animal (metabolic caged) showed deposits of all three classes of immunoglobulins, (G > A > M), and moderate deposits of C3 in a predominantly mesangial distribution, similar to IgG. Glomerular epithelial cell droplets containing RSA were present in two control rats; scanty droplets were seen in limited tubular segments of one of these animals.

Glomerular immunoglobulin deposition was essentially similar in experimental and control rats. RSA droplets were seen in glomerular epithelial cells of all Imposil-treated rats. Tubular cells contained RSA droplets in 11 experimental animals, associated with IgG in seven animals. Tubular C3, associated with RSA, but in only one case associated with IgG droplets, was restricted to three Imposil-treated rats maintained in metabolic cages.

Urinary protein excretion

Urinary protein excretion is summarized in Fig. 5. Results are plotted as the Imposil and control group weekly mean 24 h urinary protein and range. Considerable overlap in the amount of protein excreted by experimental and control groups was seen up to the second week. However, by the fifth week the urinary protein excreted by the Imposil group was significantly greater than that excreted by control animals ($P < 0{\cdot}05$). Three Imposil-treated rats continued to excrete relatively large amounts of protein throughout the 3 months whilst in one there was a steady reduction towards normal from the seventh week.

Ultrastructural examination of tissue from animals at 3 months did not reveal any differences in the epithelial foot processes or glomerular basement membrane thickness of proteinuric and con-

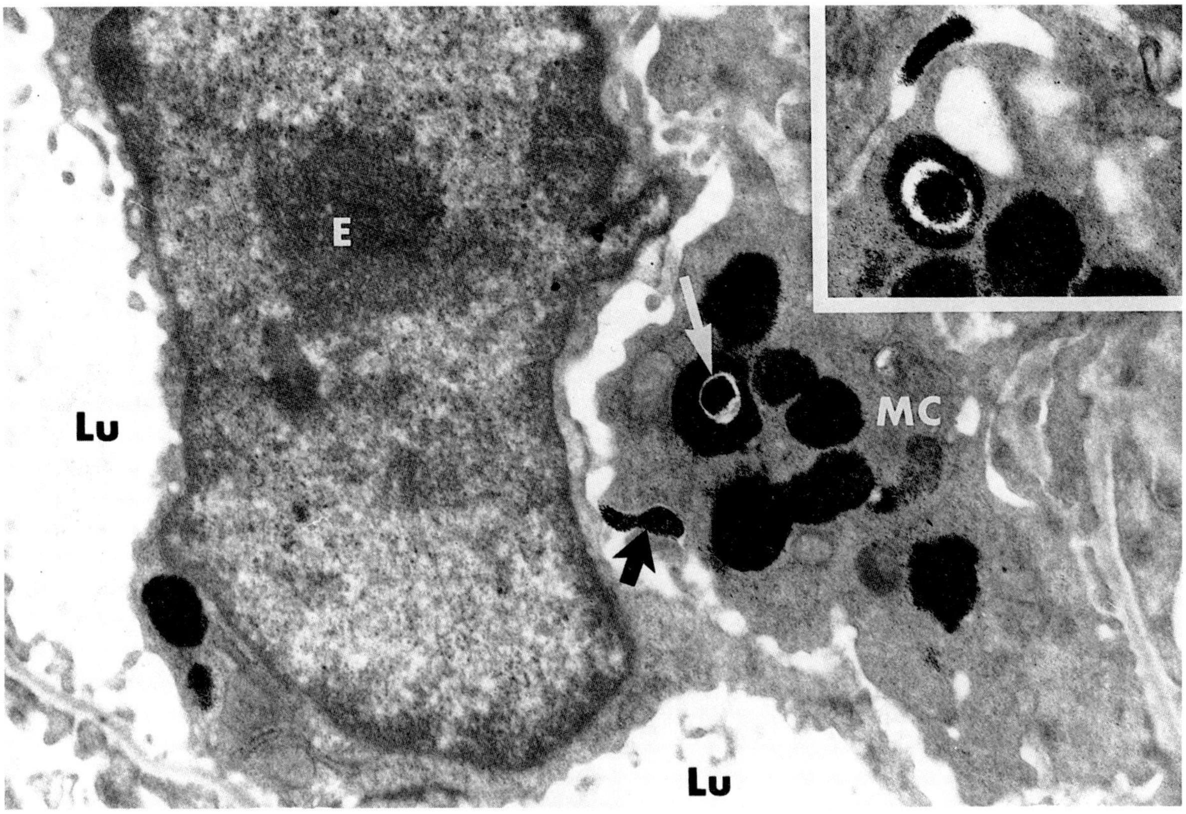

Fig. 3—Electron micrograph of an endothelial cell (E) and part of a mesangial cell (MC) at day 3. An electronlucent ring is seen in a mesangial cell lysosome (long arrow) and aggregated tracer is seen in a vacuole (short arrow) opening into the subendothelial space. Capillary lumen (Lu). Inset—An adjacent area showing aggregated tracer in the intercellular space and another secondary lysosome with an electronlucent ring. Unstained, × 22800; inset, × 30400

trol rats (mean thickness: 154 ± 16 nm and 159 ± 15 nm ($\pm$SD), respectively).

Urinary iron excretion

Urinary iron excretion over the first 27 days is summarized in Fig. 6. Imposil rats displayed a wide range in iron excretion and individual animals showed a marked day-to-day variation in their rates of excretion. A marked drop in urinary iron excretion was evident in all Imposil rats 2 days after injection, coinciding with maximal cellular uptake of the tracer. The mean total iron excreted by control and Imposil rats over 27 days was 1·83 μmoles and 3·84 μmoles, respectively. This increased excretion by Imposil rats, however, only represents <0·3 per cent of the total dose of iron injected.

DISCUSSION

Imposil iron–dextran complex was investigated in this study as a marker of mesangial phagocytic function because of the inert nature of the tracer and the ease with which it can be histochemically and ultrastructurally located. The study examines the sequential changes in the mesangium and possible renal disturbances associated with the long-term retention of tracer which may preclude the use of Imposil and similar tracers as markers of mesangial function. The kinetics of mesangial uptake and clearance of Imposil has been examined in a short-term study (48 h) in mice by Leiper *et al.*[8] and in a limited 3-week study in mice and rats by Suurmeijer *et al.*[9] However, except for the monitoring of circulating serum iron levels,[9] no metabolic investigations were performed in these studies and no examination was made of the possibility of endo-

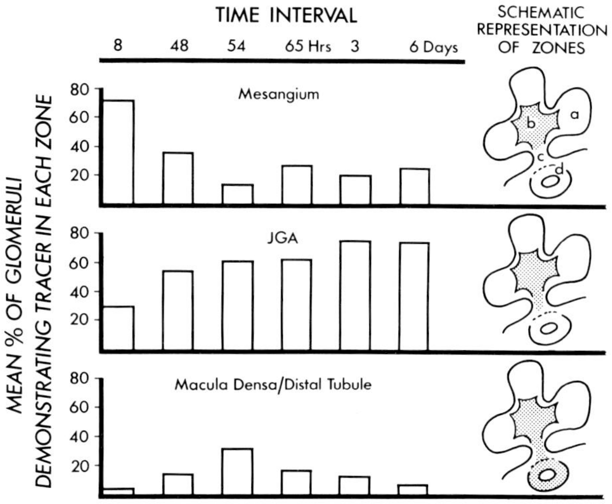

Fig. 4—Relative incidence of iron in different compartments at various time intervals. A minimum of 10 glomeruli per animal in each group, which included the mesangium, JGA and distal tubule, were scored depending upon where tracer was restricted to the mesangium or was present also in the JGA or distal tubule. (a) Glomerular capillary loop; (b) mesangium; (c) JGA; (d) macula densa/distal tubule

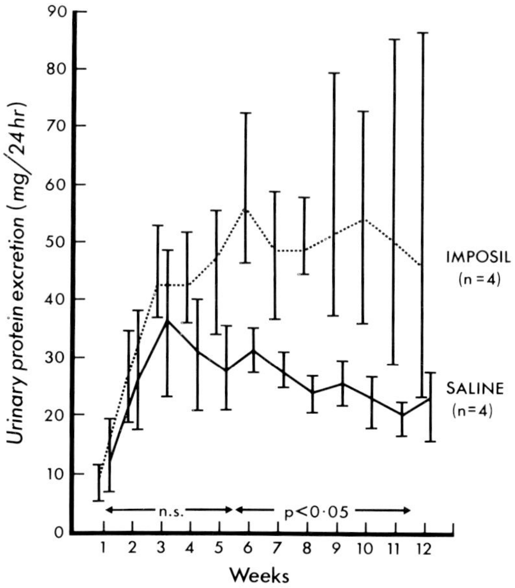

Fig. 5—Urinary protein excreted by four Imposil-treated and four saline control rats maintained in metabolic cages for 12 weeks. Mean 24 h urinary protein and range for each week of the experiment is shown

genous immune complex deposition associated with mesangial tracer ingestion.

Several investigators have demonstrated that a high blood level of tracer is required to saturate the systemic mononuclear phagocytic system before significant uptake by the mesangium is observed.[2,21,22] The large intravenous dose of Imposil required to produce significant mesangial uptake in this study produced a toxic reaction which may have been associated with a redistribution of renal blood flow, resulting in disappearance of tracer from some glomerular capillaries whilst it was still visible in vasa rectae (Fig. 1). The reappearance of tracer in glomerular capillaries at 8 h could have resulted from restoration of the glomerular microcirculation or release of material from other organ systems. Liver and spleen contained large amounts of iron throughout the experiment. This apparent disturbance of renal blood flow may limit the use of Imposil in short-term studies.

We confirm avid uptake of tracer by mesangial cells and limited deposition of iron around the distal tubule at the level of the macula densa.[8] However, we suggest that tracer within macula densa and distal tubular cells represents an overflow phenomenon resulting from the accumulation of unusually large amounts of tracer in the JGA region of some glomeruli.

Table I—Incidence of immunofluorescent deposits in Imposil and saline control rats at 3 months

	No. in group	Site of deposits	Immunofluorescence RSA	G	A	M	C3
Imposil	13	Glomeruli	13(100)	4(31)	3(23)	9(69)	3(23)
		Tubules	11(85)	7(54)	0	0	3(23)
Saline	7	Glomeruli	2(29)	2(29)	2(29)	4(57)	1(14)
		Tubules	1(14)	0	0	0	1(14)

Figures in parentheses indicate percentage of animals in each group with positive staining.

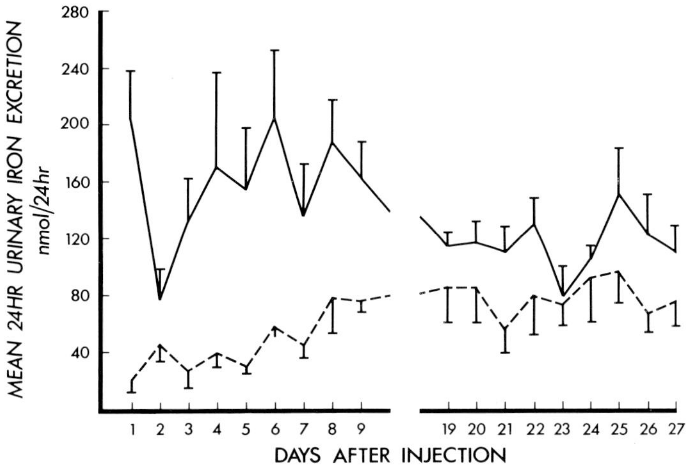

Fig. 6—Urinary iron excreted by four Imposil-treated (——) and four saline control rats (------) over the first 27 days following Imposil injection. Mean values ±1 SEM are shown

The small amounts of iron detected in the urine do not suggest any major release of iron into the distal tubular lumen ($<0\cdot3$ per cent of the total dose of iron excreted in 1 month). However, this may be expected since uptake of tracer by the mesangium represents only a very small proportion of that taken up by the mononuclear phagocytic system and subsequent release of mesangial intracellular tracer appears to be a slow, insidious process.

Following mesangial cell uptake (maximal at 48 h–54 h) limited release and drainage of intracellular tracer between 3 and 6 days appears to result from extrusion of mesangial secondary lysosomes. Electronlucent rings and holes, frequently seen in mesangial lysosomal aggregates at this time, probably result from loss of extruded material. Little evidence of tracer extrusion was noted after 6 days. The presence of free tracer particles in mesangial cells may reflect cellular overload and lysosomal breakdown or the release of tracer from endosomes following receptor-mediated endocytosis.[23]

Large amounts of iron in the interstitium at 8 h may have reached this site by passage of circulating tracer across the wall of peritubular capillaries.[24] Alternatively, tracer aggregates draining through the mesangium to the JGA region may be released into the interstitium,[2,14] as suggested by the presence of aggregates in interstitial spaces and in interstitial phagocytic cells at 3 months, when circulating tracer was no longer present.

The presence of RSA and IgG droplets in podocytes and some tubular segments in Imposil-treated rats at 3 months is highly suggestive of proteinuria. However, there was no clear relationship between the amount or type of glomerular immunoglobin deposition and the degree of proteinuria, as Imposil and control animals demonstrated similar patterns of immune complex deposits. Measurement of urinary protein excretion confirmed a gradual onset of proteinuria in Imposil-treated rats, which was significantly greater than in control animals from the fifth week of the study ($p<0\cdot05$) and this difference persisted to the 12th week in three of the four animals.

The development of proteinuria would appear to be related to the iron–dextran injection. It is possible that the proteinuria develops following mesangial cell compromise arising as a result of a failure of these cells to eliminate iron–dextran aggregates. A deficiency in the glomerular basement membrane may result, due to an interference in mesangial participation, in normal glomerular basement membrane turnover.[25] By comparison with the gradual increase in glomerular permeability seen in this study, transiently elevated urinary protein excretion has been documented in rats following injection with other inert tracers.[3,26,27] Daily subcutaneous injection of polyvinyl alcohol (PVA) has been associated with a mild but significant increase in urinary protein loss in Sprague-Dawley rats.[26,27] No other glomerular functional abnormalities were found in these animals and glomerular capillary loops and foot processes appeared intact despite the presence of large numbers of potentially harmful macrophages localized in the mesangium.[27] A transient increase in albuminuria has been reported in Wistar rats following a single intravenous injection of colloidal carbon which like Imposil has been shown to persist for weeks in the mesangium.[3] However, urine collections were only continued for 2 days before and 4 days after carbon injection so that the possible long-term functional disturbances associated with persistence of colloidal carbon in the mesangium are not established. Although the mechanism by which Imposil produces proteinuria is unclear, the association of the tracer with an alteration of glomerular function precludes its use as a marker of normal mesangial function in long-term studies.

ACKNOWLEDGEMENTS

This study was funded entirely by the Yorkshire Kidney Research Fund. Imposil was kindly supplied by Fisons Pharmaceutical Division, Animal Health, Loughborough, U.K. The authors wish to thank Mrs M. Smith for invaluable secretarial assistance in the preparation of the manuscript.

REFERENCES

1. Michael AF, Keane WF, Raij L, Vernier RL, Mauer SM. The glomerular mesangium. Editorial Review. *Kidney Int* 1980; **17:** 141–154.
2. Benacerraf B, McCluskey RT, Patres D. Localization of colloidal substances in vascular endothelium: A mechanism of tissue damage. *Am J Pathol* 1959; **35:** 75–84.
3. Elema JD, Hoyer J, Vernier RL. The glomerular mesangium: uptake and transport of intravenously injected colloidal carbon in the rat. *Kidney Int* 1976; **9:** 395–406.
4. Latta H, Maunsbach AB, Madden SC. The centrolobular region of the renal glomerulus studied by electron microscopy. *J Ultrastruct Res* 1960; **4:** 455–472.
5. Farquhar MG, Palade GE. Functional evidence of a third cell type in the renal glomerulus. *J Cell Biol* 1962; **13:** 55–87.
6. Farquhar MG, Wissig SL, Palade GE. Glomerular permeability. I. Ferritin transfer across the normal glomerular capillary wall. *J Exp Med* 1961; **113:** 47–65.
7. Takamiya H, Batsford S, Kluthe R, Vogt A. Comparison of the handling of ferritin and ferritin-protein conjugates by the glomerular mesangium. *Lab Invest* 1979; **40:** 18–24.
8. Leiper JM, Thomson D, Macdonald MK. Uptake and transport of Imposil by the glomerular mesangium in the mouse. *Lab Invest* 1977; **37:** 526–533.
9. Suurmeijer AJH, Grond J, Elema JD. The glomerular mesangium: a comparative study of mesangial handling of iron dextran complex and endogenous IgG in mice and rats. *Virchows Arch (Cell Pathol)* 1981; **37:** 357–368.
10. Menefee MG, Mueller CB, Bill A, Myers J. Transport of globin by the renal glomerulus. *J Exp Med* 1964; **120:** 1129–1138.
11. Michael AF, Fish AJ, Good RA. Glomerular localization and transport of aggregated protein in mice. *Lab Invest* 1967; **17:** 14–29.
12. Mauer SM, Fish AJ, Day N, Michael AF. The glomerular mesangium: I. Kinetic studies of macromolecular uptake in normal and nephrotic rats. *J Clin Invest* 1972; **51:** 1092–1101.
13. Mauer SM, Fish AJ, Day N, Michael AF. The glomerular mesangium. II. Studies of macromolecular uptake in normal and nephrotoxic nephritis in rats. *J Clin Invest* 1974; **53:** 431–439.
14. Lee S, Vernier RL. Immunoelectron microscopy of the glomerular mesangial uptake and transport of aggregated human albumin in the mouse. *Lab Invest* 1980; **42:** 44–58.
15. Haakenstad AO. Case JB, Mannik M. Effect of cortisone on the disappearance kinetics and tissue localization of soluble immune complexes. *J Immunol* 1975; **114:** 1153–1160.
16. Haakenstad AO, Mannik M. The disappearance kinetics of soluble immune complexes prepared with reduced and alkylated antibodies and with intact antibodies in mice. *Lab Invest* 1976; **35:** 283–292.
17. Haakenstad AO, Striker GE, Mannik M. The glomerular deposition of soluble immune complexes prepared with reduced and alkylated antibodies and with intact antibodies in mice. *Lab Invest* 1976; **35:** 293–301.
18. Aparicio SR, Wakefield C. An electron microscopy method for studying full cross-sections of human glomerulus. *J Clin Pathol* 1983; **36:** 1081–1082.
19. Iwata J, Nishikaze O. New turbidometric method for determination of protein in cerebrospinal fluid and urine. *Clin Chem* 1979; **25:** 1317–1319.
20. Thompson, Park, Payne. Personal communication 1983.
21. Wilson CB, Dixon FJ. Quantitation of acute and chronic serum sickness in the rabbit. *J Exp Med* 1971; **134:** 7s–18s.
22. Herbert LA, Stuart KA, Allhuser C, Rodey G. Measurement of the fractional uptake of macromolecules by the renal vascular bed compared to other vascular beds. *J Lab Clin Med* 1976; **88:** 716–724.
23. Richter GW. The iron-loaded cell—the cytopathology of iron storage. A review. *Am J Pathol* 1978; **91:** 362–404.
24. Venkatachalam MA, Karnovsky MJ. Extravascular protein in the kidney: an ultrastructural study of its

relation to renal peritubular capillary permeability using protein tracers. *Lab Invest* 1972; **27:** 435–444.

25. Walker F. The origin, turnover and removal of glomerular basement membrane. *J Pathol* 1973; **110:** 233–244.
26. Sterzel RB, Krause PH, Kregeler M. Experimental changes of the mesangial capacity to handle glomerular immune deposits in rats. *Contr Nephrol* 1976; **2:** 66–75.
27. Sterzel RB, Eisenbach GM, Seiler MW, Hoyer JR. Uptake of polyvinyl alcohol by macrophages in the glomerular mesangium of rats. Histologic and functional studies. *Am J Pathol* 1983; **111:** 247–257.

JOURNAL OF PATHOLOGY, VOL. **144**: 189–199 (1984)

SPINDLE CELL TUMOURS OF THE SKIN OF DEBATABLE ORIGIN. AN IMMUNOCYTOCHEMICAL STUDY

V. EUSEBI AND C. CECCARELLI

Istituto di Anatomia e Istologia Patologica, University of Bologna, Italy

F. PISCIOLI AND M. CRISTOFOLINI

Ospedale Civile, Trento, Italy

AND

J. G. AZZOPARDI

Department of Histopathology, The Royal Postgraduate Medical School, London, U.K.

Received 5 March 1984
Accepted 29 May 1984

SUMMARY

Twelve cases of malignant spindle-cell and sarcomatoid tumours of the skin of debatable nature were studied by immunocytochemical methods, using four antisera which might help contribute to resolution of the problems. The initial diagnosis made on structural grounds was confirmed by immunocytochemistry in six of eight cases in which a specific diagnosis had been made (one melanoma, three squamous carcinomas and two atypical fibroxanthomas). One case, initially regarded as AFX was reclassified as a squamous carcinoma, while a further case of possible AFX could not be confirmed by immunocytochemical study. Of the four cases in which structural examination was inconclusive, two were identified as squamous carcinomas and one as a melanoma by virtue of tumour markers. The fourth case was an intriguing actin-rich tumour of uncertain nature. Immunocytochemistry, despite certain limitations, has a valuable role to play in the analysis of the problematic spindle-cell malignant and pseudomalignant tumours of the skin.

KEY WORDS—Spindle-cell squamous carcinoma, atypical fibroxanthoma, desmoplastic malignant melanoma, immunocytochemistry.

INTRODUCTION

Spindle cell malignant tumours of the skin sometimes constitute a major diagnostic challenge to the histopathologist. There are certain tumours and tumour-like conditions which, while sharing similar histological appearances, vary as to histogenesis and biological behaviour. Spindle-cell squamous carcinoma, desmoplastic malignant melanoma and atypical fibroxanthoma must be differentiated from one another and from a variety of sarcomas. This is a notoriously difficult problem, not always solvable on morphological ground alone.

The nature and behaviour of the 'atypical fibroxanthoma' has been a topic of controversy in recent years.[1,2] The lesion was initially regarded as always benign,[3] but there have been a number of cases in which regional lymph node metastases developed unexpectedly.[4–6] This lesion is regarded by most workers as mesenchymal in nature,[3,7–10] but others have suggested that some, perhaps many, of them represent instances of spindle-cell metaplastic squamous carcinoma.[1,2]

In view of the diagnostic difficulties and the con-

Addressee for correspondence: Dr V. Eusebi, Istituto di Anatomia e Istologia Patologica, Policlinico S.Orsola, via Massarenti 9, I-40138 Bologna, Italy.

0022–3417/84/110189–11$01.10

flicting evidence we studied a series of spindle-cell tumours of the skin using immunocytochemical procedures.

MATERIALS AND METHODS

Twelve cases of spindle-cell or sarcomatoid tumours of the skin were selected for this study. They were all lesions referred to one of us (V.E.) for histopathological opinion. They were initially classified on the basis of haematoxylin-eosin (H & E) preparations as follows: one case of malignant melanoma, desmoplastic: three spindle-cell squamous carcinomas of sarcomatoid appearance: four atypical fibroxanthomas (AFX): and four malignant spindle-cell tumours which could not be identified further on morphological grounds.

All cases were studied using the immunoperoxidase anti-peroxidase (PAP)[11] and/or immuno β-galactosidase techniques.[12] The following primary antisera were employed: anti-actin antiserum diluted 1:500 (kindly given by Professor G. Bussolati, University of Turin); anti-epidermal keratin antiserum diluted 1:100 (kindly given by Professor D. J. Evans, R.P.M.S., London); anti-lysozyme antiserum diluted 1:2000 (DAKO Corporation); anti-S 100 protein diluted 1:5000 (kindly given by Dr G. L. Ferri, R.P.M.S., London).

Controls for the specificity of immunostaining were performed: (1) by using rabbit non-immune serum as the first layer; (2) by incubating adjacent sections with diluted antiserum preadsorbed with 1–50 mg/m of the respective antigen; (3) by omitting the first layer, (4) by including a section of known positivity for the different antisera.

RESULTS

Clinical data

Ten lesions were situated on the head, one on the arm and one on the leg. The mean age of the patients was 68·5 years, with a range of 55–79 years. There were ten male and two female patients. All 12 lesions were ulcerated. The mean follow-up to date is 23 months (range 6–33 months). None of the lesions has recurred after excision. Patient no. 1, aged 69 years, died of myocardial infarction.

Immunocytochemistry

The case diagnosed as desmoplastic malignant melanoma (Figs 1,2) was strongly positive for S 100 protein in most of the neoplastic cells, while all other antisera gave negative results (Fig. 3, Table I). The positivity was most marked in the invasive

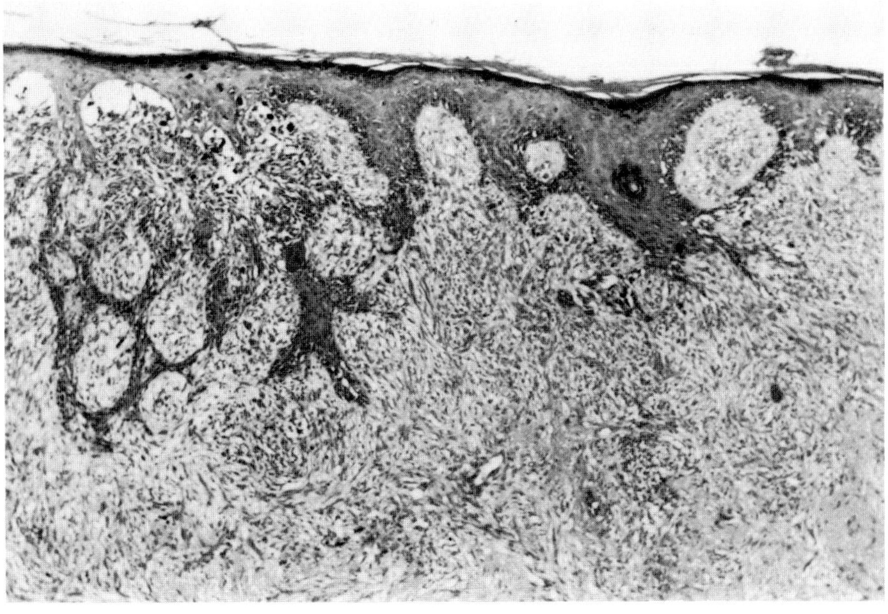

Fig. 1—Case 1: desmoplastic malignant melanoma. The junctional activity and the superficial pigmention are the diagnostic features of this spindle-cell tumour. H & E, × 75

component, less so in the areas of the junctional and intraepidermal components.

All three cases initially diagnosed as spindle-cell squamous carcinomas with sarcoma-like stroma (Fig. 4), according to Smith,[13] showed some areas at least which were positive with anti-keratin antisera, while there was no positive staining with the other antisera employed. This was expected since the diagnosis of squamous carcinoma was only made confidently on morphological grounds when

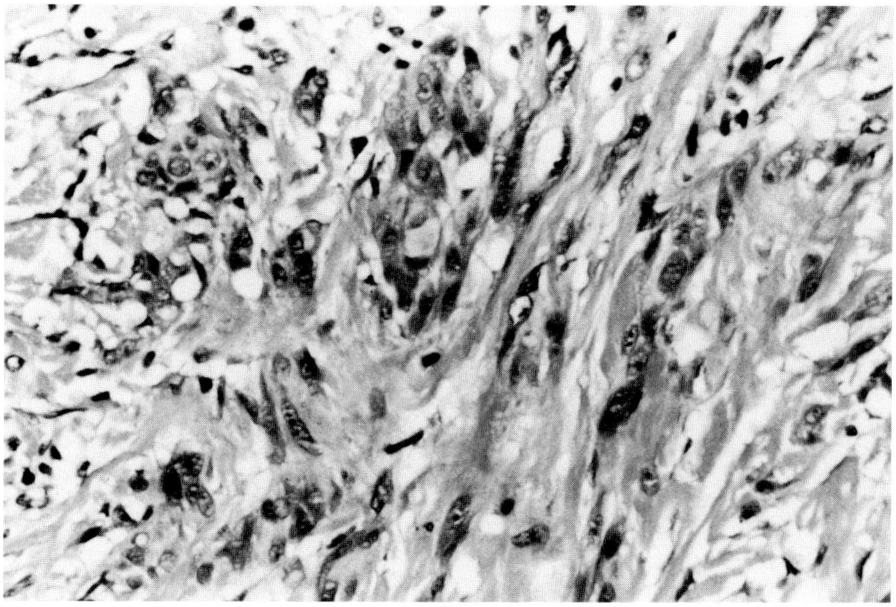

Fig. 2—Desmoplastic malignant melanoma (same case as Fig. 1): the deep part of the tumour shows elongated elements with occasional prominent nucleoli. H & E, × 350

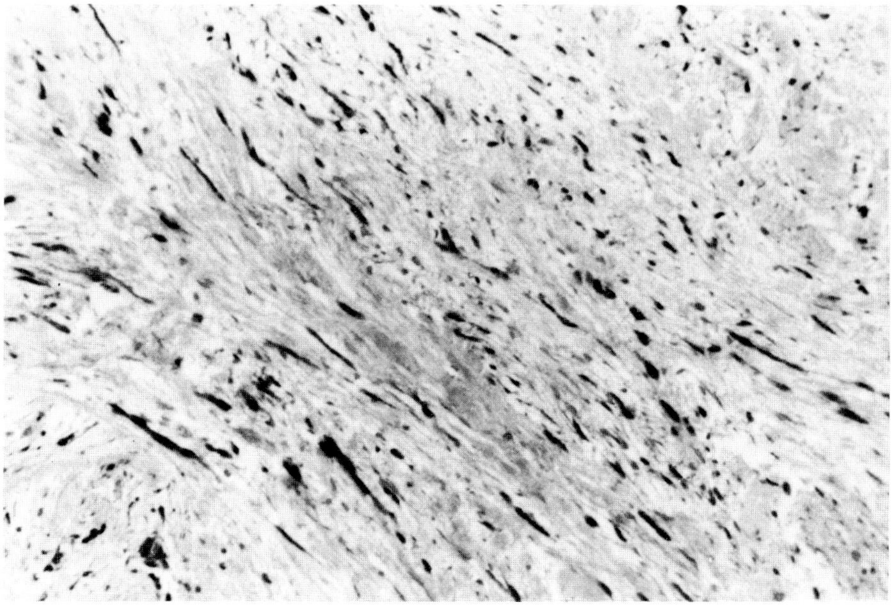

Fig. 3—Desmoplastic malignant melanoma (same case as Fig. 1): most of the spindle-cells are intensely stained. Anti-S 100 protein – PAP, × 125

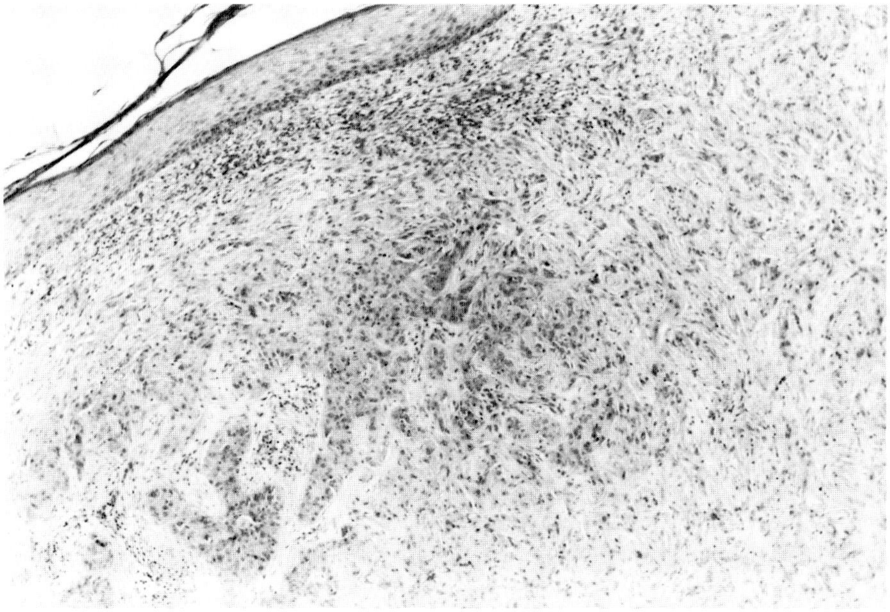

Fig. 4—Case 2: spindle-cell squamous carcinoma: the squamous component is self-evident. H & E, × 100

Table I

Case No.	Initial diagnosis	Age	Sex	Site	S-100	Keratin	Lysozyme	Actin	Revised diagnosis
1.	Desmoplastic malignant melanoma	69	M	Cheek	+	–	–	–	Confirmed
2.	Spindle-cell squamous carcinoma	55	M	Forearm	–	+	–	–	Confirmed
3.	Spindle-cell squamous carcinoma	67	F	Face	–	+	–	–	Confirmed
4.	Spindle-cell squamous carcinoma	79	M	Nose	–	+	–	–	Confirmed
5.	Atypical fibroxanthoma	71	F	Cheek	–	+	–	–	Spindle-cell squamous carcinoma
6.	Atypical fibroxanthoma	65	M	Leg	–	–	+	–	Confirmed
7.	Atypical fibroxanthoma	75	M	Cheek	–	–	+	–	Confirmed
8.	Atypical fibroxanthoma	71	M	Lip	–	–	–	–	Presumptive atypical fibroxanthoma
9.	Spindle-cell malignant tumour NOS	67	M	R.eyelid	+	–	–	–	Spindle-cell malignant melanoma
10.	Spindle-cell malignant tumour NOS	68	M	Nose	–	+	–	–	Spindle-cell squamous carcinoma
11.	Spindle-cell malignant tumour NOS	60	M	Cheek	–	+	–	–	Spindle-cell squamous carcinoma
12.	Spindle-cell malignant tumour NOS	75	M	Scalp	–	–	–	+	Actin-rich tumour

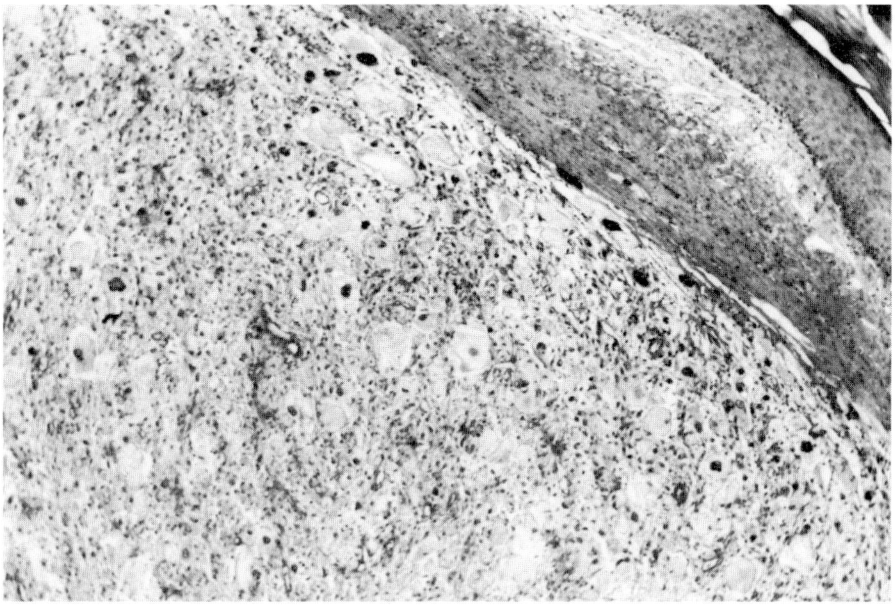

Fig. 5—Case 7: atypical fibroxanthoma: most of this tumour is composed of large cells with foamy cytoplasm. H & E, × 100

the evidence was strong, viz. when neoplastic cells were in continuity with the epidermis and when at least one focus of easily identifiable squamous tissue was present within the sarcoma-like elements. Positivity with the anti-keratin serum was very obvious in the morphologically squamous areas but, additionally, occasional single cells in the sarcoma-like component were also positive.

The four cases of atypical fibroxanthoma were diagnosed utilizing the criteria laid down by Fretzin and Helwig.[3] Two cases were mostly composed of spindle and foamy cells, intermingled with lymphocytes (Figs 5,6). The foamy cells stained positively for lysozyme. Negative reactions were obtained with all other antisera (Figs 7,8). A third case, consisting mainly of spindle cells intermingled with lymphoid elements, had a prominent well-defined storiform pattern in most of the lesion (Fig. 9). Despite this, the anti-keratin antiserum staining was positive, while all other antisera gave negative reactions (Fig. 10). The fourth case of AFX was negative with all antisera employed.

The most informative results were obtained with the tumours initially labelled 'malignant spindle-cell tumours', not identifiable further. Two of four cases stained positively with anti-keratin antiserum: one was strongly stained and one only weakly so. Of the other two cases, in one most of the cells were positive for S 100 protein (Fig. 11), in the other most cells stained with anti-actin antiserum (Fig. 12,13). No lysozyme-positive elements were found in this group of four tumours.

DISCUSSION

The choice of the antisera here employed was partly dictated by the exclusion of tumour forms, which although they can display a spindle cell pattern, are rarely found on the face and in the age group under consideration. Ten of our 12 patients presented with a lesion on the face and their mean age was 68 years. We, therefore, excluded from serious consideration tumours such as epithelioid sarcoma and rhabdomyosarcoma which are mainly found in young adult life and in childhood. The face is a very unlikely location for both fibrosarcoma and synovial sarcoma.[14] Actin has been detected most frequently in muscular cells, myoepithelial cells, and myofibroblasts.[15] Lysozyme has been found to be present in some histiocytic lesions of the skin, including atypical fibroxanthoma.[16] There are numerous reports on keratin as a marker of epithelial cells, noteworthy exceptions being the malignant synovioma and epithelioid sarcoma.[17,18] S 100 protein is widespread in several tissues; in the skin it is present, mainly in Langerhans cells, in naevi and in malignant melanomas.[19]

Because of the specificity and reliability of the tumour markers investigated, especially in the context of the cutaneous lesions in question, it is justifiable to draw certain conclusions from our results.

The case diagnosed as desmoplastic malignant melanoma was positive with S 100 protein antiserum, as was to be expected in conformity with the results obtained by Nakajima *et al.*[19] One of the four cases initially labelled 'malignant spindle-cell tumour NOS' was also positive for S 100 protein,

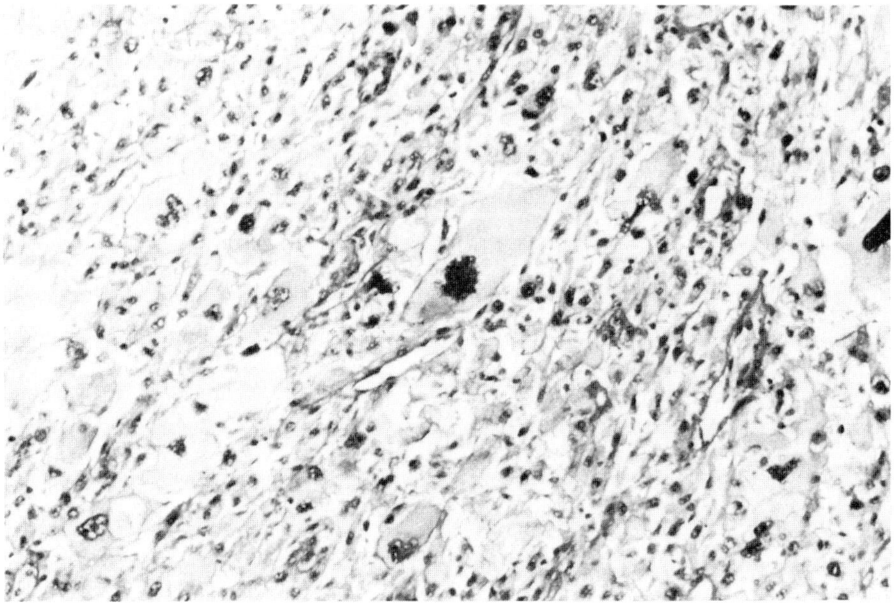

Fig. 6—Atypical fibroxanthoma (same case as Fig. 5): large cells with foamy cytoplasm at higher magnification. H & E, × 200

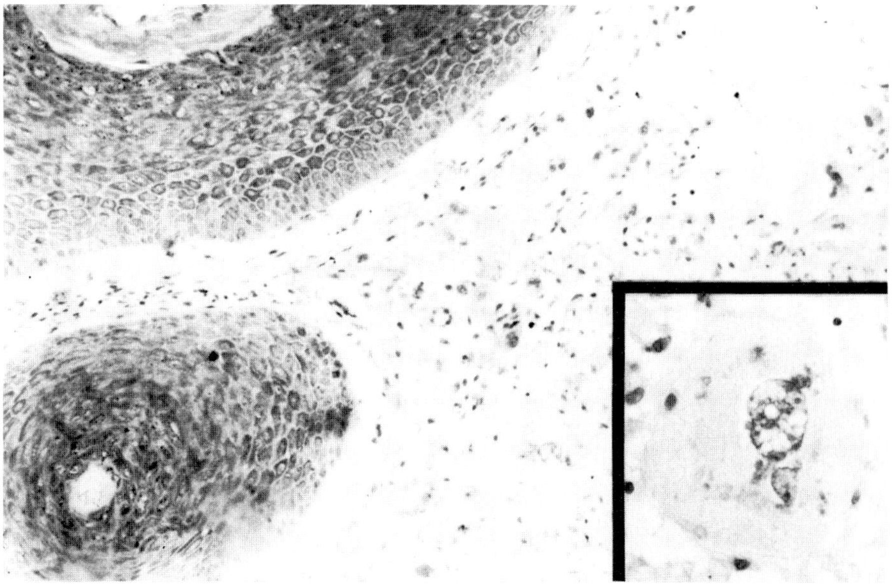

Fig. 7—Atypical fibroxanthoma (same case as Fig. 5): the epidermis appears positive with anti-keratin antiserum while the neoplastic elements are distinctively negative. PAP × 100; inset × 350

suggesting that this case probably also represents a spindle-cell malignant melanoma.

The three cases diagnosed as squamous carcinoma initially were positive for keratin, with isolated positive cells present even in the sarcomatoid parts. Three further cases, initially in other groups stained positively for keratin: two of these were spindle-cell tumours not identified further on structural grounds while one was initially categorized as an atypical fibroxanthoma. It appears

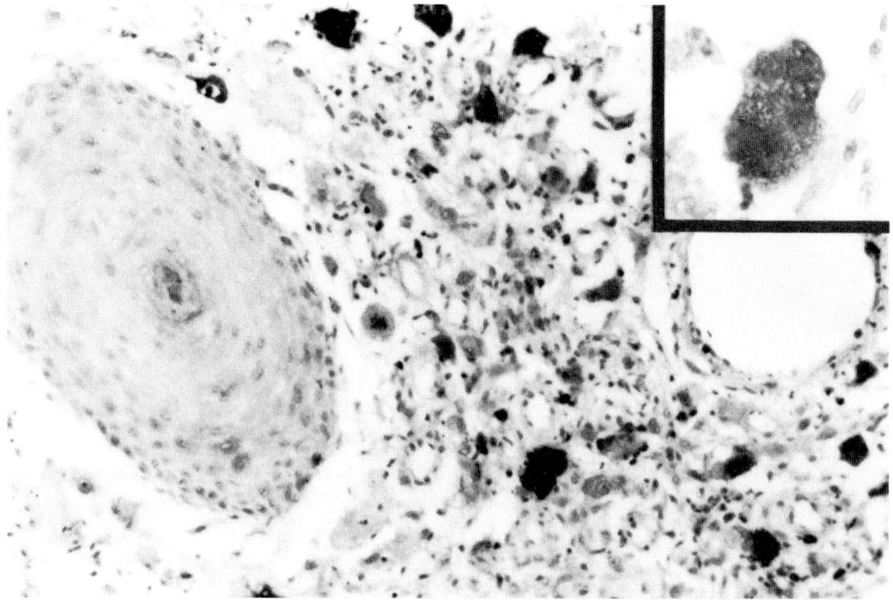

Fig. 8—Atypical fibroxanthoma (same case as Fig. 5): using anti-lysozyme antiserum several foamy cells as well as granulocytes appear strongly stained. PAP × 100; insert × 350

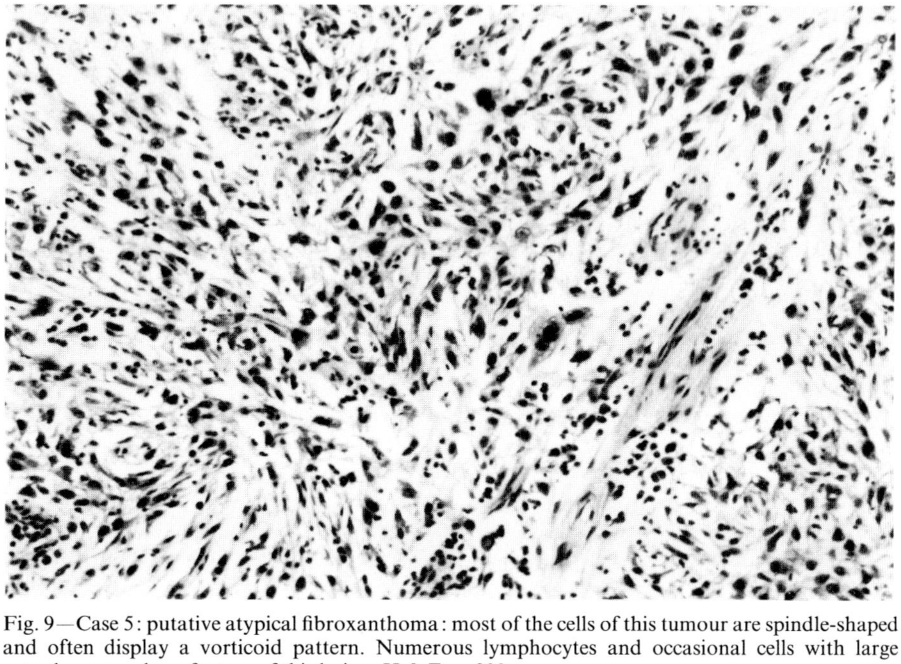

Fig. 9—Case 5: putative atypical fibroxanthoma: most of the cells of this tumour are spindle-shaped and often display a vorticoid pattern. Numerous lymphocytes and occasional cells with large cytoplasm are also a feature of this lesion. H & E, × 200

justifiable, on immunocytochemical grounds, to transfer these tumours to the spindle-cell squamous carcinoma group.

Of four cases of putative 'atypical fibroxanthoma', only two cases were positive with anti-lysozyme antiserum, one was positive with anti-keratin antiserum, while the fourth was negative with all antisera used. The lesion with cells containing keratin should be considered a spindle-cell squamous carcinoma. Two of the four were con-

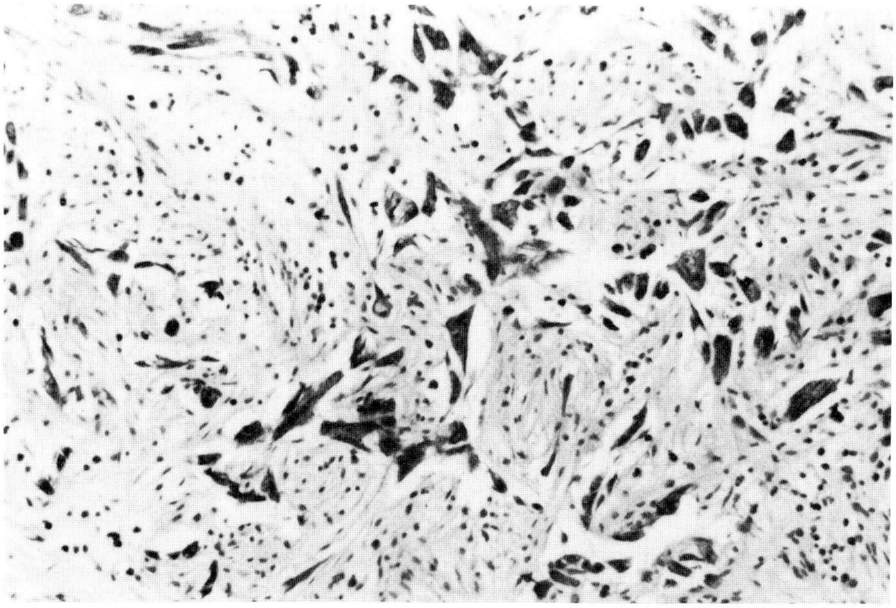

Fig. 10—Same case as Fig. 9: several cells express cytoplasmic epidermal keratin. Anti-epidermal keratin – PAP, ×200

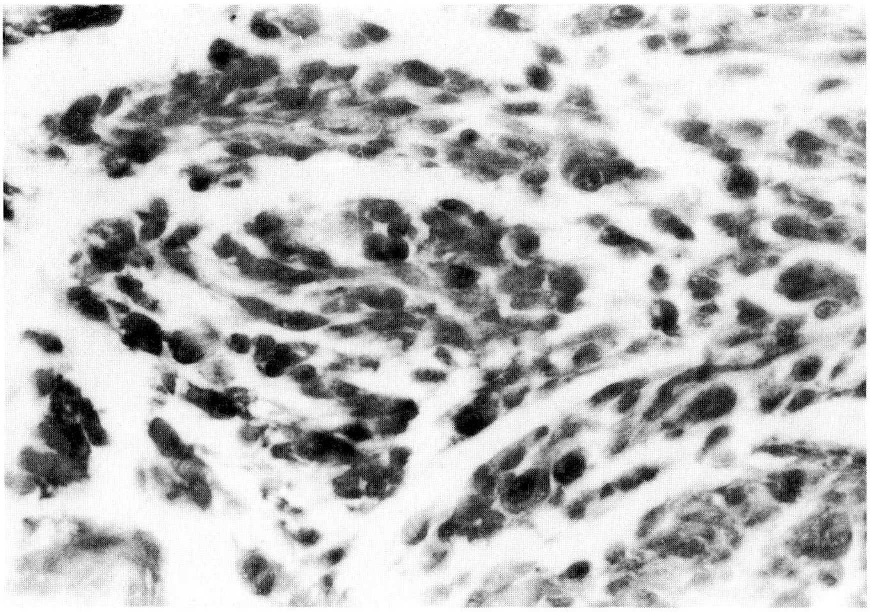

Fig. 11—Case 9: spindle-cell tumour: most of the cells appear positive using anti-S 100 protein antiserum. The nuclei have been counterstained with neutral red. Immuno-β-galactosidase, ×350

firmed as 'atypical fibroxanthoma', while a third is still provisionally regarded as such, but on evidence which is much less definitive. Doubts on the real nature of AFX were first mooted by Reed[1] and subsequently reaffirmed by Evans and Smith[2] who considered that most, if not all, 'atypical fibroxanthomas' are actually spindle-cell squamous carcinomas. This is probably a somewhat extreme view. One of the 10 cases of AFX in the series of Harmon[20] was weakly positive for keratin while

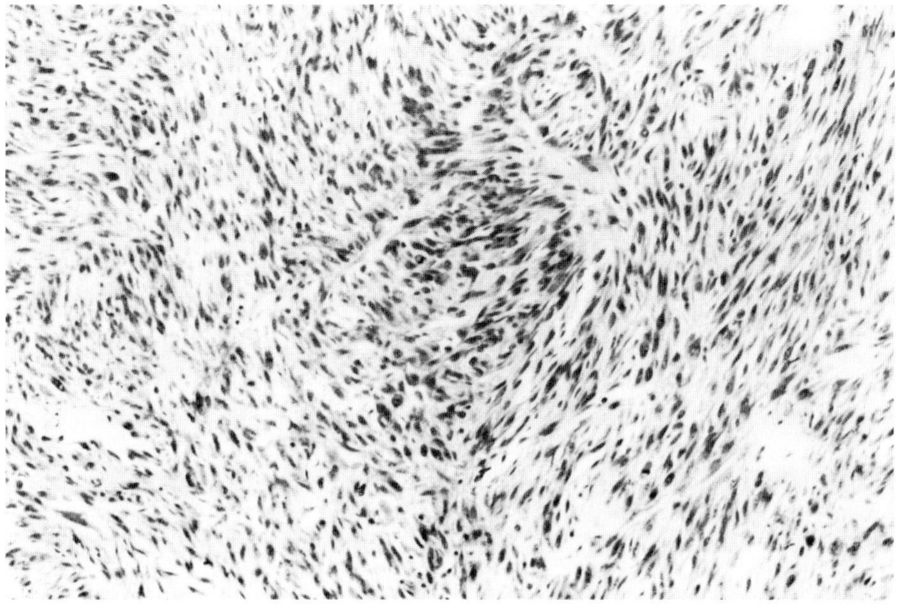

Fig. 12—Case 12: spindle-cell tumour: this tumour is mainly formed by spindle elements showing elongated hyperchromic nuclei. H & E, × 125

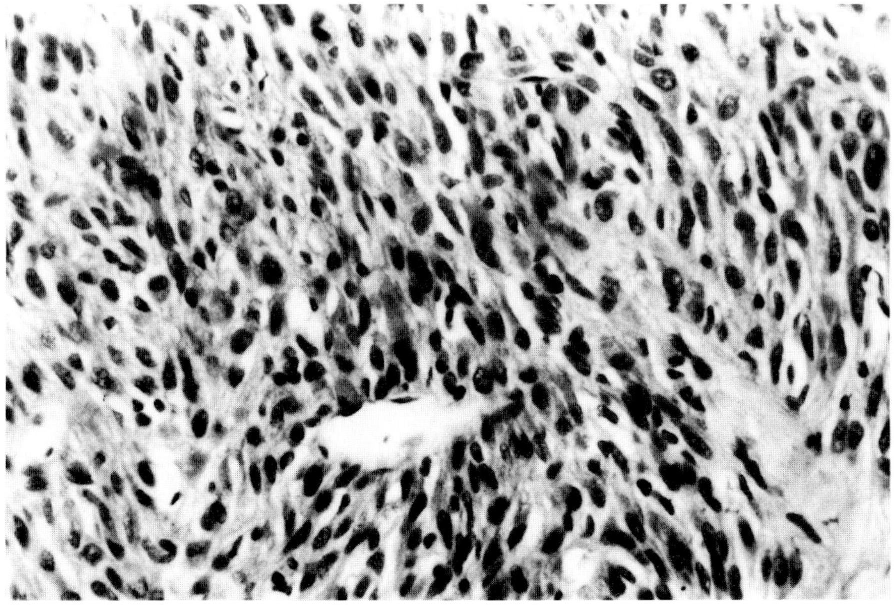

Fig. 13—Same case as Fig. 11: the neoplastic elements appear positive with anti-actin antiserum. The cytoplasm is strongly blue stained. The nuclei have been counterstained with neutral red. Immuno-β-galactosidase, × 250

three of the 10 were positive for lysozyme, findings which are rather similar to our own. It appears, therefore, that the condition of 'atypical fibroxanthoma', as currently defined, comprises a heterogeneous mixture of lesions, of which a true histiocytic benign lesion and a desmoplastic squamous carcinoma which stimulates a fibrohistiocytic lesion are the most common.

Immunocytochemistry proved most valuable in the group of tumours which could not be identified with any confidence on purely structural grounds. Of four such tumours, two are identifiable as squamous carcinomas and one as a malignant melanoma: we believe that the evidence warrants that they be transferred to these categories on histochemical grounds. Thus, of four tumours in this group, three can be placed in definite categories and only one remains enigmatic. This residual fourth case is an intriguing one since it was strongly positive with anti-actin antiserum but with no other antiserum.

On current evidence, we propose that this last tumour be identified merely as an 'actin-rich malignant spindle-cell tumour' of the skin. It cannot be identified more specifically at present. It may represent a mesenchymal neoplasm which differentiates into an actin-rich tumour, without exhibiting specific features of other distinct entities known to contain abundant actin in their cytoplasm, like the muscle sarcomas. It may represent a tumour of myofibroblasts. An alternative more remote possibility is that it represents a myoepithelial tumour, but this is unlikely since such a tumour would be expected to contain keratin. It is obviously necessary to study further examples of this unusual type of neoplasm before even tentative conclusions can be drawn about its precise nature. The anti-actin antiserum here employed was purified by affinity chromatography[15] and the staining was completely adsorbed by prior incubation with purified actin. Therefore we can reasonably exclude any cross reaction with intermediate filaments as recently suggested by Blewitt *et al.*[21]

In studying debatable spindle-cell lesions of the skin, immunocytochemistry is valuable in confirming the diagnosis of desmoplastic malignant melanoma and of spindle-cell squamous carcinoma. It attains its maximum value, perhaps, in its ability to identify specifically tumour types which are not identifiable objectively on structural grounds alone. It can, moreover, be useful in enabling one to recognize a potentially new entity like the actin-rich malignant spindle-cell neoplasm of the skin.

ACKNOWLEDGEMENTS

The authors wish to thank Professor G. Bussolati (Turin) for reading the manuscript and Dr A. Zina (Turin) and Dr R. Rosso (Pavia) for contributing two cases. Dr C. Ceccarelli is in receipt of a grant from Associazione Italiana per la Ricerca sul Cancro. This work was partially financed by Ministero Pubblica Istruzione.

REFERENCES

1. Reed RJ. New Concepts in Surgical Pathology of the Skin. New York: Wiley, 1976.
2. Evans HL, Smith JL. Spindle-cell squamous carcinomas and sarcoma-like tumors of the skin. *Cancer* 1980; **45:** 2687.
3. Fretzin DF, Helwig EB. Atypical fibroxanthomas of the skin: a clinicopathologic study of 140 cases. *Cancer* 1973; **31:** 1541.
4. Jacobs DS, Edwards WD, Ye RC. Metastatic atypical fibroxanthoma of skin. *Cancer* 1975; **53:** 457.
5. Dahl I. Atypical fibroxanthomas of the skin: a clinicopathological study of 57 cases. *Acta Pathol Microbiol Scand (A)* 1976; **84:** 183.
6. Kemp JD, Stenn KS, Arons M, Fisher J. Metastasizing atypical fibroxanthoma: coexistence with chronic lymphocytic leukemia. *Arch Dermatol* 1978; **114:** 1533.
7. Gordon HW. Pseudosarcomatous reticulohistiocytoma: a report of four cases. *Arch Dermatol* 1964; **90:** 319.
8. Kempson RL, McGavran MH. Atypical fibroxanthomas of the skin. *Cancer* 1964; **17:** 1463.
9. Hudson AW, Winkelman RK. Atypical fibroxanthoma of the skin: a reappraisal of 19 cases in which the original diagnosis was spindle-cell squamous carcinoma. *Cancer* 1972; **29:** 413.
10. Vargas-Cortes F, Winkelmann RK, Soule EH. Atypical fibroxanthomas of the skin: further observations with 19 additional cases. *Mayo Clin Proc* 1973; **48:** 211.
11. Sternberger LA. Immunohistochemistry. New York: Wiley, 1979.
12. Bondi A, Chieregatti G, Eusebi V, Fulcheri E, Bussolati G. The use of β-galactosidase as a tracer in immunocytochemistry. *Histochemistry* 1982; **76:** 153.
13. Smith JL. Spindle cell squamous carcinoma. In: Graham JH, Johnson WC, Helwig EB, eds. Dermal Pathology. New York: Harper and Row, 1972: Chapter 29.
14. Enzinger FM, Weiss SW. Soft Tissue Tumors. St. Louis: Mosby, 1983.
15. Bussolati G, Alfani V, Weber K, Osborn M. Immunocytochemical detection of actin on fixed and

embedded tissues: its potential use in routine pathology. *J Histochem Cytochem* 1980; **28:** 169.

16. Burgdorf WHC, Duray P, Rosai J. Immunohistochemical identification of lysozyme in cutaneus lesions of alleged histiocytic nature. *Am J Clin Pathol* 1981; **75:** 162.
17. Miettinen M, Lehto V-P, Virtanen I. Keratin in the epithelial-like cells of classical biphasic synovial sarcoma. *Virch Arch (Cell Pathol)* 1982; **40:** 157.
18. Chase D, Enzinger F, Weiss SW, Langloss JM. Keratin in epithelioid sarcoma: an immunohistochemical study. *Lab Invest* 1984; **50:** 9A.
19. Nakajima T, Watanabe S, Sato Y, Kameya T, Ishihara K. Immunohistochemical demonstration of S 100 protein in malignant melanoma and pigmented nevus and its diagnostic application. *Cancer* 1982; **50:** 912.
20. Harmon JB. Atypical fibroxanthoma and spindle cell squamous cell carcinomas of head and neck: an immunohistochemical study. *Lab Invest* 1983; **48:** 33A.
21. Blewitt RW, Aparicio SGR Bird CC. Epithelioid sarcoma: a tumour of myofibroblasts. *Histopathology* 1983; **7:** 573.

JOURNAL OF PATHOLOGY, VOL. **144**: 201–211 (1984)

ALTERATIONS IN THE BIOPHYSICAL PROPERTIES OF THE HUMAN ENDOTHELIAL CELL PLASMA MEMBRANE INDUCED BY A CHEMOTACTIC TRIPEPTIDE: CORRELATION WITH ENHANCED ADHERENCE OF GRANULOCYTES

CHARLES J. KIRKPATRICK* AND INGO MELZNER

Department of Pathology, University of Ulm, F.R.G.

Received 11 August 1983
Accepted 30 May 1984

SUMMARY

Human umbilical vein endothelial cells in monolayer culture were used to study the effects of the chemotactic tripeptide, *N*-formylmethionylleucylphenylalanine (FMLP), on structure and function of the endothelium. Endothelial cell morphology was unaffected by concentrations of 10^{-8}–10^{-4} M. No effect on endothelial cell proliferative capacity, as measured by the DNA content of cultures, was seen at the FMLP concentrations studied (10^{-8}–10^{-6} M). Using fluorescent molecular probes to investigate FMLP-induced alterations in membrane structure, it was shown using the monomer–excimer method with pyrene decanoic acid that FMLP caused a marked restructuring of the plasma membrane. This took the form of a restriction of the surface available to the lipophile reporter molecules, probably caused by a molecular reorganization of the membrane protein component. Experiments with diphenylhexatriene indicated that FMLP did not make the plasma membrane of the endothelial cell more fluid. Concomitant with these changes in the physical properties of the membrane, an FMLP-induced increase in granulocyte adherence to the endothelial cells was observed. A theoretical model is presented correlating granulocyte adherence with the lateral mobility of lipids in the endothelial cell membrane. The significance of the FMLP-induced increase in granulocyte adherence to endothelial cells for the pathogenesis of sepsis is discussed.

KEY WORDS—Chemotactic tripeptide, endothelial cell, fluorescent probes, membrane dynamics, granulocyte adherence.

INTRODUCTION

One of the characteristics of the acute inflammatory process is the presence of neutrophilic granulocytes at the focus of inflammation. The directed movement of these cells along a chemical gradient, chemotaxis, can be initiated and controlled by a variety of substances, including serum complement components[1] and leukotriene B_4, an oxygenation product of the cell membrane component arachidonic acid.[2] Synthetic peptides, such as *N*-formylmethionylleucylphenylalanine (FMLP), have been shown to possess not only chemotactic activity, but also chemical similarity to chemotactic peptides released from bacterial cell walls.[3,4]

Emigration of granulocytes from the circulatory system to the inflammatory focus is preceded by adherence of these cells to the endothelium. However, this phenomenon is still poorly understood.[5] This applies particularly to the cell membrane changes associated with adhesion. In the present investigation the interaction between the chemotactic tripeptide FMLP and human endothelial cells in monolayer culture was studied to establish whether endothelial cell morphology and proliferative capacity can be altered. In addition, biophysical

*Addressee for correspondence: C. J. Kirkpatrick, Ph.D. M.D. Department of Pathology, University of Ulm, Oberer Eselsberg, D-7900 Ulm, Federal Republic of Germany.

0022–3417/84/110201–11$01.10

methods using fluorescent reporter molecules were employed to obtain information on the dynamic changes in the endothelial cell membrane lipid component caused by FMLP. A correlation of membrane alterations with changes in the adherence of granulocytes to the endothelium was also attempted.

MATERIALS AND METHODS

Endothelial cell culture system

Endothelial cells were isolated from the human umbilical vein by the method of Jaffe *et al.*[6], details of which have been published elsewhere.[7] Briefly, the umbilical vein of an approximately 25 cm long piece of non-traumatized umbilical cord was cannulated at both ends and flushed twice with sterile 0·01 M HEPES-buffered saline (HBS; HEPES: *N*-2-hydroxyethylpiperazine-*N'*-2-ethanesulphonic acid, Sigma, Munich, F.R.G.). The endothelial cells were freed from the basement membrane using 10 ml of an 0·1 per cent collagenase solution in HBS (Worthington collagenase I, 132 U/mg, supplied by Interchem GmbH, Munich, F.R.G.) at 37°C for 10 min. The collagenase solution containing the isolated endothelial cells was flushed out with 30 ml HBS into a sterile 50 ml centrifuge tube containing 10 ml of Medium 199 with 20 per cent pooled human serum (Medium 199 with Earl's salts, L-glutamine and 25 mM HEPES; Gibco, supplied by Nunc GmbH, Wiesbaden, F.R.G.). After centrifuging for 7 min at 200 x*g*, the cells were plated in a 25 cm^2 culture flask (Falcon, supplied by Becton-Dickinson GmbH, Heidelberg, F.R.G.) containing 4 ml of Medium 199 with 20 per cent human serum and supplemented with penicillin, streptomycin and fungizone (100 U/ml, 100 μg/ml and 0·25 μg/ml respectively; Gibco). The monolayer cultures were incubated at 37°C in an atmosphere of 5 per cent CO_2 in air.

Cells were passaged by washing the cultures with HBS after removing the medium and incubating for 5 min at 37°C with a 1:1 (v/v) mixture of 0·2 per cent collagenase I in HBS and 0·02 per cent EDTA solution (ethylenediaminetetraacetic acid, tetrasodium salt, dihydrate, Sigma) in HBS containing 0·5 per cent bovine serum albumin (BSA, 35 per cent, Sigma). The collagenase solution containing the cells was then centrifuged for 3 min at 200 x*g* and the cells were resuspended in complete medium. Cultures were usually passaged using a splitting ratio of 1:3. All cultures were grown in plastic culture flasks which had been coated overnight at 4°C with a 0·2 per cent aqueous gelatin solution (gelatin, research grade, Serva, Heidelberg, F.R.G.). Cell viability was estimated using the trypan blue exclusion test. Only cells from subcultures up to passage VI were used for the experiments detailed below.

Isolation of granulocytes

Granulocytes were separated from heparinized venous blood of healthy human blood donors using density gradient separation on Ficoll–sodium diatrizoate solution (Ficoll-Paque, Pharmacia, Uppsala, Sweden) and dextran sedimentation as described by Bültmann *et al.*[8] The washed granulocytes were resuspended in Hanks'-HEPES buffer.

Preparation of chemotactic peptide and testing for biological activity

An aqueous solution of *N*-formyl-L-methionyl-L-leucyl-L-phenylalanine (FMLP; Sigma) was prepared by the method of Fehr and Dahinden.[9] FMLP (10 mg) was dissolved in 1 ml 0·1 N NaOH and 8 ml 0·1 M phosphate-buffered saline (PBS, pH 7·4) added. The pH of the solution was adjusted with 0·1 N HCl to 7·4 and the FMLP stock solution sterilized by filtration. In all experiments controls were treated with PBS *without* FMLP.

The biological activity of FMLP was tested by investigating uropod formation in granulocytes.[10] Thus, 50 μl of a granulocyte suspension (5×10^4 cells) in Hanks' balanced salt solution (BSS) or minimal essential medium (MEM, Gibco; total volume 1 ml) was incubated for 30 min at 37°C with 10^{-8} M FMLP. Glutaraldehyde (1 ml 3·5 per cent) (Serva, Heidelberg, F.R.G.) was then added and the suspension fixed for 30 min. The reaction mixture was centrifuged for 7 min at 450 x*g* and the cell sediment resuspended in 200 μl Gey's BSS (Gibco). The cells were examined on a glass slide under the microscope and the percentage of granulocytes with uropod formation determined.

Morphological studies

Endothelial cell subcultures were grown in gelatin-coated 60 mm Petri-style plastic culture dishes with or without a 24 × 40 mm glass coverslip. The effect of FMLP (10^{-8}—$^{-4}$ M) on endothelial cell morphology was studied over a period of 72 h from the beginning of subculture. Cultures were examined using phase-contrast and Nomarski differential interference contrast (DIC) microscopy.

Effect of FMLP on endothelial cell proliferation

The effect of FMLP (10^{-8}, 10^{-7} and 10^{-6} M) on endothelial cell proliferation was investigated using a modification[11,12] of the diphenylamine method of Burton[13], a spectrophotometric determination. In all experiments, control and test cultures were grown in 25 cm^2 plastic culture flasks coated with gelatin.

Effect of FMLP on physical properties of the endothelial plasma membrane

Use was made of the fluorescent reporter molecules (probes) 1,6-diphenyl-1,3,5-hexatriene (DPH; Fluka, Buchs, F.R.G.) and pyrene decanoic acid (PDA) to investigate the effects of FMLP on the physical state of the plasma membrane of the endothelial cell *in vitro*. The PDA probe was synthesized according to the method of Galla and Hartmann.[14]. The incorporation of the probes into the endothelial cell membranes was facilitated by the use of lipid vesicles as vehicle. PDA (150 μl) (10 mg/ml chloroform) were added to 450 μl L-dioleoyl-phosphatidylcholine (Sigma; 20 mg/ml chloroform) and vacuum dried at 50°C in a nitrogen stream. The lipid–probe mixture (3:1) was sonicated in 1 ml of Hanks' BSS until the suspension was no longer milky, indicating that the vesicles were smaller than the wavelength of blue light. The endothelial cells, grown on gelatin-covered glass coverslips (24 × 40 mm), were labelled by pipetting the PDA probe on to the cells and incubating for 30 min at 37°C. The DPH probe was prepared in the same way, although the lipid–probe ratio was increased to 9:1. Segments of coverslips with the labelled cells were transferred to the cuvette of the spectrofluorometer in Hanks' BSS.

Fluorescence depolarization with DPH[15,16] was measured using a Schoeffel RRS-Spectrofluorometer with two monochromators and photomultipliers on the emission side. The sample cuvette was kept at 37°C by a Peltier element. The DPH molecules were excited by linearly polarized light at 350 nm and the fluorescence intensity at 430 nm was simultaneously measured with two photomultipliers which were placed perpendicular to the exciting beam. In one photomultiplier the fluorescence intensity was measured in the same plane of polarization as the exciting beam $I_{\parallel}$), whereas in the other the plane of polarization was turned through 90° ($I_{\perp}$). The degree of polarization (P) where $P = \frac{I_{\parallel} - I_{\perp}}{I_{\parallel} + I_{\perp}}$ was calculated using an analog computer.

PDA fluorescence was determined using the monomer-excimer technique[17,18]. The PDA probe was excited at 348 nm and the fluorescence intensity measured and recorded over a 2 min period at slowly increasing wavelength (370–600 nm) in a Kontron spectrofluorometer.[7,19] The fluorescent signal caused by monomers represents sharp lines detected between 380 and 410 nm, whereas the signal due to excimers forms a broad band detected between 450 and 510 nm. The intensity of the fluorescent bands due to monomers (I) and excimers (I') was integrated in a digital computer and the parameter $\varphi = I'/I$ calculated. Observations were made at 24°C and 37°C.

Effect of FMLP on the adherence of granulocytes to endothelial cells

Endothelial cells were grown to confluence or subconfluence on gelatin-coated glass coverslips (24 × 40 mm) in 60 mm Petri-style culture dishes. The endothelial cells were then washed twice with Gey's BSS and the cultures treated with FMLP at concentrations of 10^{-8}, 10^{-7} and 10^{-6} M in Medium 199 without serum at 37°C. The time of FMLP treatment varied from 1·5 to 10 and 30 min. Following this the medium was removed and without washing the endothelial cells 2 ml of granulocyte suspension (10^6 cells/ml in Hanks'-HEPES buffer or in Medium 199 + 20 per cent pooled human serum) were added. After 10 min co-culture at 37°C the coverslips were removed and passed four times through an air-fluid interface (by dipping into a beaker containing Gey's BSS). Pilot experiments showed that this procedure was necessary to remove non-adherent granulocytes which were held in contact with the endothelial cell monolayer by surface tension forces. The coverslips with endothelial cells and adherent granulocytes were subsequently fixed for 30 min in 1·5–3 per cent glutaraldehyde in cacodylate buffer, pH 7·4 and washed with 0·1 M PBS. The 'adherence index' ($= A_T/A_0$) was taken as parameter of granulocyte adherence to the endothelial cells and was calculated from the mean value of the number of adherent granulocytes from seven microscopic fields (× 16 objective) in the test cultures (A_T) and the mean value determined under identical conditions in the control cultures (A_0).

Thus, the null hypothesis assumes that the adherence index in test systems is 1 (i.e. $A_T = A_0$). A statistical analysis was performed using analysis of variance with subsequent Welch test.

RESULTS

Endothelial cell culture system

Details of the characterization of the endothelial cell culture system have been presented elsewhere.[7,20] Briefly, the expression of the endothelial cell phenotype was monitored by the morphological appearance of the cells, as well as the presence of Factor VIII antigen and intracytoplasmic Weibel-Palade bodies.

Biological activity of FMLP

Uropod formation in isolated granulocytes served as proof of the biological activity of the FMLP used in the experiments. Figure 1 shows the difference between spontaneous and FMLP-induced uropod formation. Controls, which had been incubated with Hanks' BSS or MEM, gave a percentage of uropod-forming cells of 29 per cent and 32 per cent respectively. The corresponding values for FLMP-treated suspensions (10^{-8} M) were 93 and 95 per cent respectively.

Morphological studies

FMLP concentrations of 10^{-8}–10^{-4} M elicited no disturbance of endothelial cell adhesion to the growth substrate in subculture. The behaviour of the cells in culture and their morphology was not altered by the continuous presence of FMLP for 72 h (10^{-8}, 10^{-7} and 10^{-6} M) or 48 h (10^{-6}, 10^{-5} and 10^{-4} M). In all experiments FMLP-treated cultures were indistinguishable from control cultures when viewed with phase-contrast and Nomarski-DIC optics. In particular, no evidence of cytotoxicity was found (Fig. 2).

Effect of FMLP on endothelial cell proliferation

This parameter of endothelial cell function *in vitro* was measured indirectly by determining culture DNA content. FMLP concentrations of 10^{-8}, 10^{-7} and 10^{-6} M did not alter this parameter

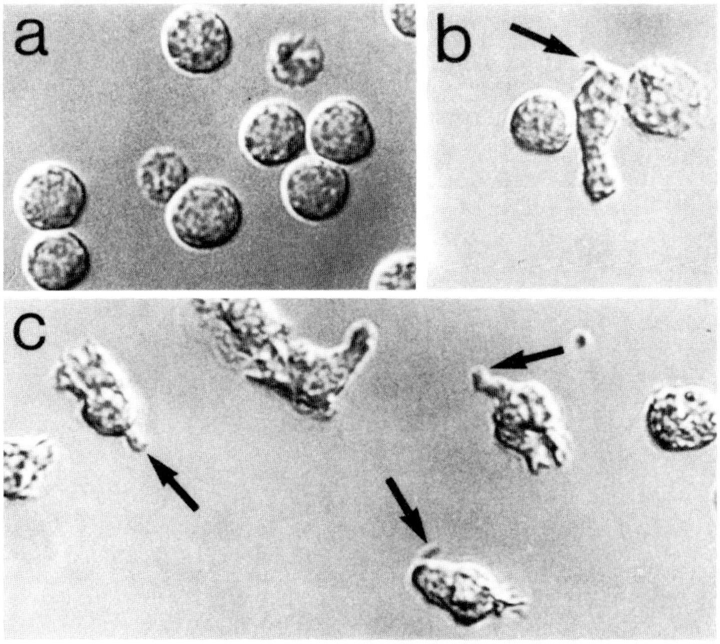

Fig. 1—Uropod formation in human peripheral blood granulocytes. Nomarski differential interference contrast optics. (a) Control, showing rounded granulocytes, × 830. (b) Control, with an elongated granulocyte demonstrating uropod formation (arrow) × 830. (c) Granulocytes treated with 10^{-8} M FMLP. The majority of cells is elongated and shows uropod formation (arrows), × 830

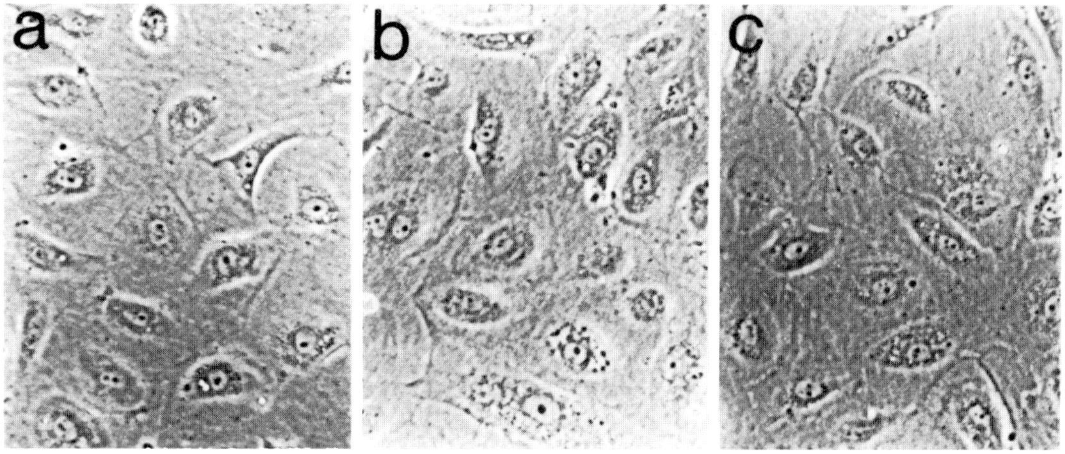

Fig. 2—Effect of FMLP on endothelial cell morphology. Endothelial cells (passage III) in gelatin-coated 60 mm Petri-style culture dishes. Medium 199+20 per cent FCS. (a) Control. Confluent polygonal-shaped cells after 40 h in subculture. Phase contrast, ×220. (b) 40 h-treatment of endothelial cell cultures with 10^{-6} M FMLP, present from beginning of subculture. No evidence of cytotoxicity. Phase contrast, ×220. (c) As in Fig. 2b, but in the presence of 10^{-4} M FMLP. No morphological differences compared with controls (see (a)). Phase contrast, ×220

in cultures grown to subconfluence over a period of 96 h (Fig. 3).

Effect of FMLP on physical properties of the endothelial plasma membrane

Morphological studies on endothelial cells after labelling with the fluorescent probes, DPH and PDA, as well as after measurement of the fluorescence depolarization (DPH probe) and PDA fluorescence in the monomer–excimer technique gave no evidence of endothelial cell damage.

Fluorescence depolarization

Concentrations of 10^{-8} and 10^{-7} M FMLP were used in these experiments. Measurement at 37°C of the degree of polarization, *P*, as a parameter of the membrane fluidity of the endothelial plasma membrane gave a value for *P* of 0·29 in control and test systems. Thus, FMLP caused no alteration of membrane fluidity.

Monomer–excimer technique (PDA probe)

This method enables lateral diffusion of molecules in the plane of the plasma membrane to be measured. The intensity ratio φ (=fluorescence intensity of excimers (I')/fluorescence intensity of monomers (I)) depends principally on the fluidity of the membrane and the local concentration of the fluorescent probe, which in turn reflects the molecular architecture of the membrane. The extent of excimer formation varied from culture to culture and depended on the degree of uptake of the PDA molecules from the lipid vesicles (as vehicle). Thus, in order to obtain comparable dose–response curves, the spectrum of FMLP concentrations was tested on a single pool of labelled endothelial cells,

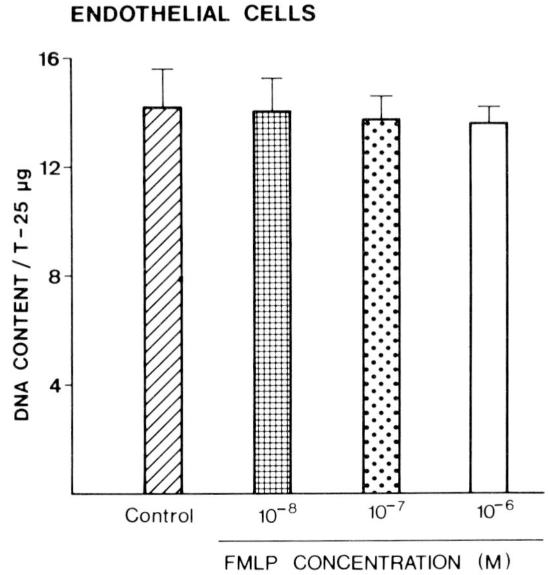

Fig. 3—Effect of FMLP (10^{-8}, 10^{-7} and 10^{-6} M) on the DNA content of endothelial cell cultures. FMLP present from beginning of subculture after 96 h treatment. Mean value±SD of mean—five observations per group. No statistically significant differences (analysis of variance)

and the procedure repeated on different cultures. The time-dependence of the intensity ratio φ was studied over a period of up to 15 min. During this time control endothelial cells (with PBS) showed a small gradual decrease in the percentage of excimers and thus a decrease in the parameter φ (Figs 4, 5). This was attributable to a bleaching effect.

The addition of FMLP (in PBS, volume 50 μl) to the endothelial cells in the cuvette (volume 500 μl) caused a shift in the fluorescence intensity in favour of excimer formation. This phenomenon was most marked at 24°C (compare Figs 4 and 5). Figure 4 shows that within 1 min after addition of FMLP (10^{-8}–10^{-5} M) the parameter φ was markedly elevated. In the case of 10^{-8} M this increase in φ was threefold. In most experiments the subsequent course of the curve showed a decrease in φ with time, although the base level, i.e. the value for φ at time zero, was not achieved. In one experiment a plateau phase was observed following initial elevation of φ (Fig. 4).

The ability of FMLP to increase excimer formation was also observed at 37°C, although the extent of the effect was clearly less than at 24°C and was not observed at all FMLP concentrations (Fig. 5). The elevation of the parameter φ was most apparent at the highest FMLP concentration studied (10^{-6} M).

Effect of FMLP on the adherence of granulocytes to endothelial cells

In addition to the biophysical studies, a functional parameter of the cell, namely the adherence of granulocytes to the endothelial cells was investigated. Three FMLP concentrations were investigated—10^{-8}, 10^{-7} and 10^{-6} M. At high FMLP concentrations a statistically significant increase in granulocyte adherence (60–290 per cent) was observed as rapidly as 1·5 min after exposure of the endothelial cells to the tripeptide (Figs 6, 7). Although the extent of the effect was different, the FMLP-induced elevation of granulocyte adherence was observed in medium with and without serum supplementation (Fig. 7). In the majority of experiments the 10^{-8} M concentration did not influence granulocyte adherence.

In experiments to investigate the dependence of granulocyte adherence on the length of FMLP treatment of the endothelial cells it was seen that the elevation of granulocyte adherence became evident early (1·5 min) after commencing treatment (Fig. 8). Longer treatment periods (10, 30 min) gave a less marked increase, if at all. In the particular experimental system illustrated in Fig. 8, the 10^{-8} M concentration did cause a statistically significant increase in granulocyte adherence after 1·5 min.

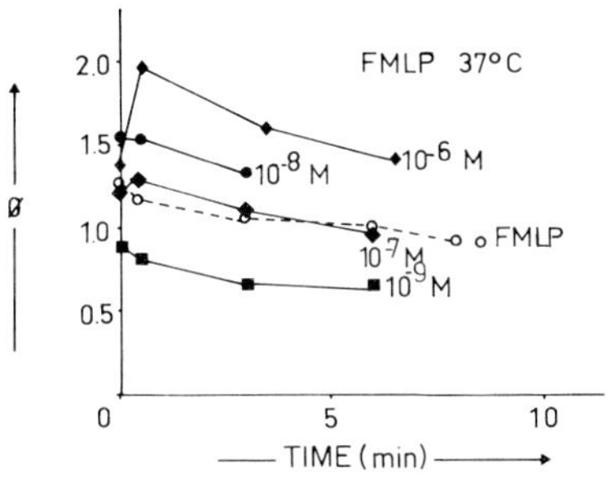

Fig. 5—Time-dependent effect of FMLP (10^{-9}–10^{-6} M) on the parameter φ in the monomer–excimer technique. Measurements at 37°C

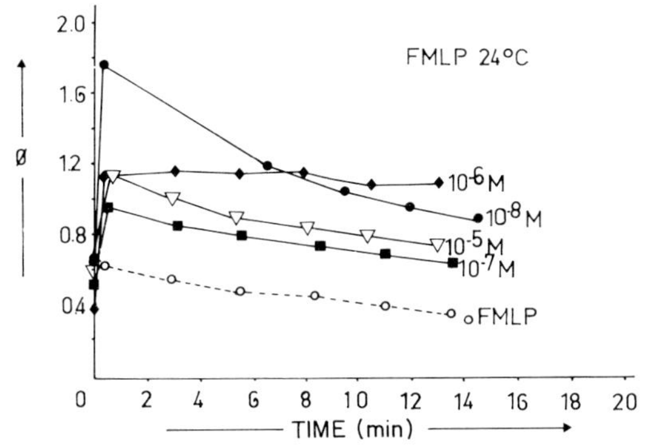

Fig. 4—Time-dependent effect of FMLP (10^{-8}–10^{-5} M) on the parameter φ ($=I'/I$), representing the ratio of the fluorescence intensity of excimers (I') to monomers (I). Measurements at room temperature (24°C)

DISCUSSION

In the present paper the interaction between the chemotactic tripeptide, FMLP, and human endothelial cells *in vitro* was investigated. Concentrations of 10^{-8}–10^{-4} M did not alter endothelial cell morphology or behaviour in subculture. No effect on endothelial cell proliferative capacity, as measured by the DNA content of cultures, was seen at the FMLP concentrations studied (10^{-8}–10^{-6} M). These results suggest that FMLP does not *directly* damage the endothelium. Despite the fact that FMLP is a synthetic tripeptide, it is generally accepted that its molecular structure resembles that of the chemotactic substances produced *in vivo*, for example, during bacterial inflammation.[3]

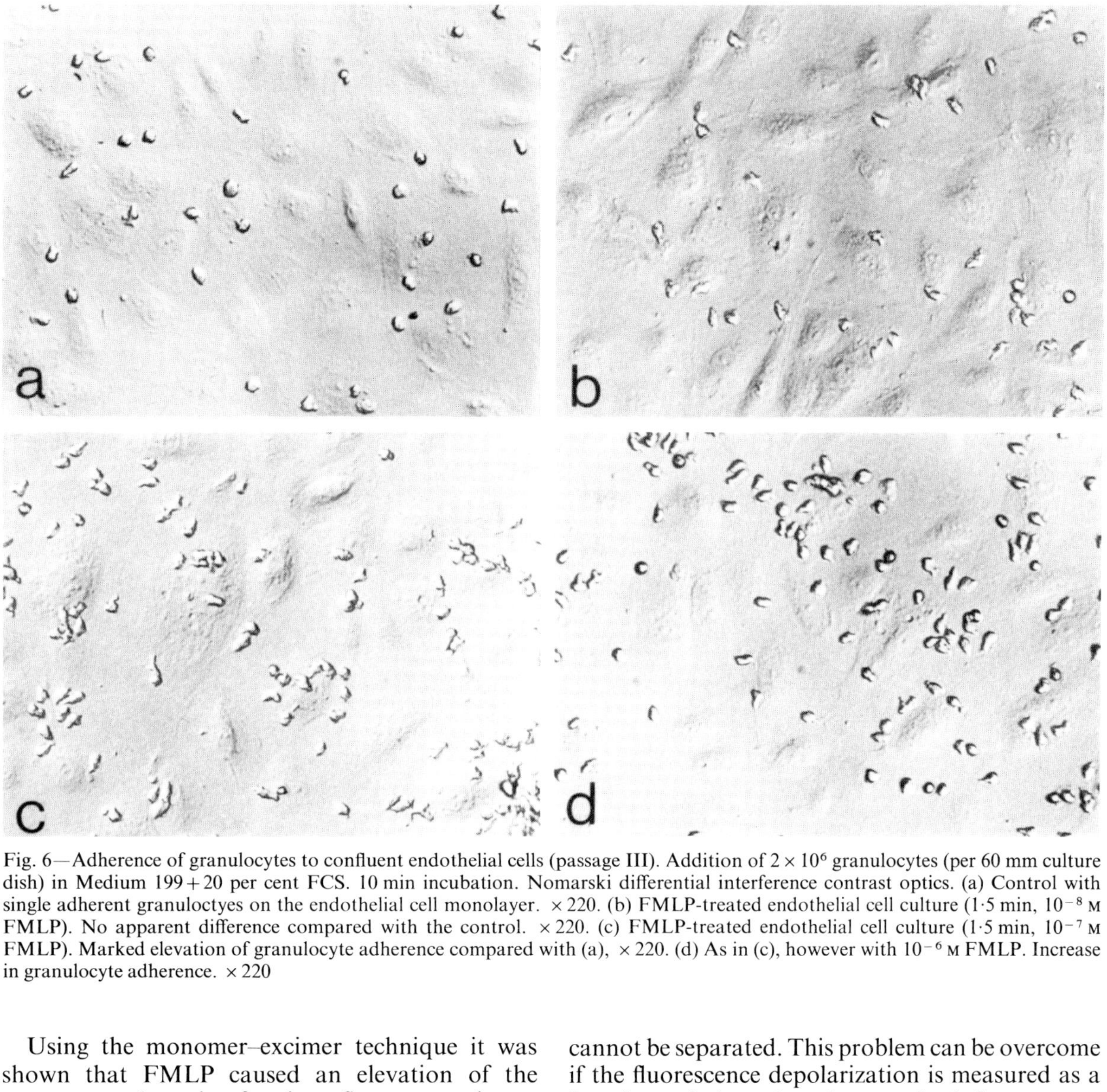

Fig. 6—Adherence of granulocytes to confluent endothelial cells (passage III). Addition of 2×10^6 granulocytes (per 60 mm culture dish) in Medium 199+20 per cent FCS. 10 min incubation. Nomarski differential interference contrast optics. (a) Control with single adherent granuloctyes on the endothelial cell monolayer. ×220. (b) FMLP-treated endothelial cell culture (1·5 min, 10^{-8} M FMLP). No apparent difference compared with the control. ×220. (c) FMLP-treated endothelial cell culture (1·5 min, 10^{-7} M FMLP). Marked elevation of granulocyte adherence compared with (a), ×220. (d) As in (c), however with 10^{-6} M FMLP. Increase in granulocyte adherence. ×220

Using the monomer–excimer technique it was shown that FMLP caused an elevation of the parameter φ (= ratio of excimer fluorescence intensity to monomer fluorescence intensity) in pyrene decanoic acid (PDA)-labelled endothelial cells. This increase in φ was due to increased formation of excimers. Experiments with the fluorescent probe, diphenylhexatriene (DPH), gave no evidence of an FMLP-induced alteration in membrane lipid rotation as measured by the degree of polarization. The latter is a measure of membrane fluidity.[21] Nevertheless, the steady state fluorescence depolarization applied in our experiments can only give information about trends in membrane architecture, because viscosity and order parameters cannot be separated. This problem can be overcome if the fluorescence depolarization is measured as a function of time, i.e. time-resolved fluorescence depolarization.[22] Unfortunately this facility was not available in our laboratory. With the above-mentioned reservation the elevation of the parameter φ may be interpreted as evidence of an increase in the local concentration of the reporter molecules.[7,23] To cause this increase in local concentration the surface area of the plasma membrane available for the reporter molecules must be decreased. Similar results from FMLP treatment of human granulocytes were interpreted by Bültmann *et al.*[24] as a biophysical indicator of the formation of 'functional units' (or receptors), probably as a

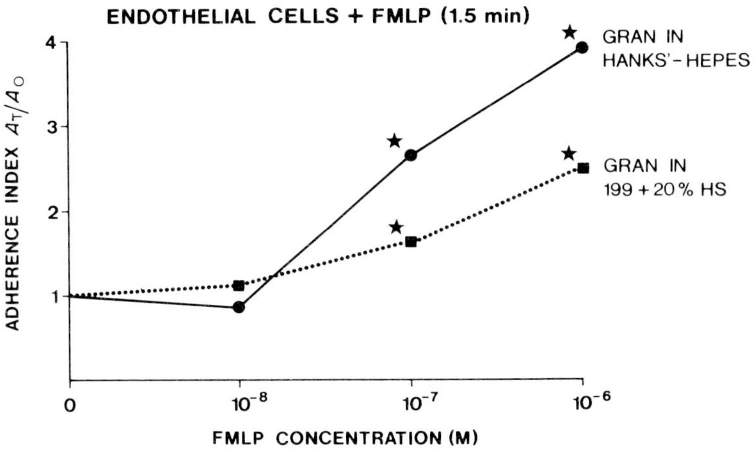

Fig. 7—Adherence index (A_T/A_0) under the influence of increasing concentrations of FMLP (10^{-8}–10^{-6} M). 1·5 min treatment of endothelial cell cultures. 10 min incubation with granulocytes (2×10^6 per 60 mm culture dish). Seven observations per group. ★ $P<0{\cdot}0001$; analysis of variance with Welch test

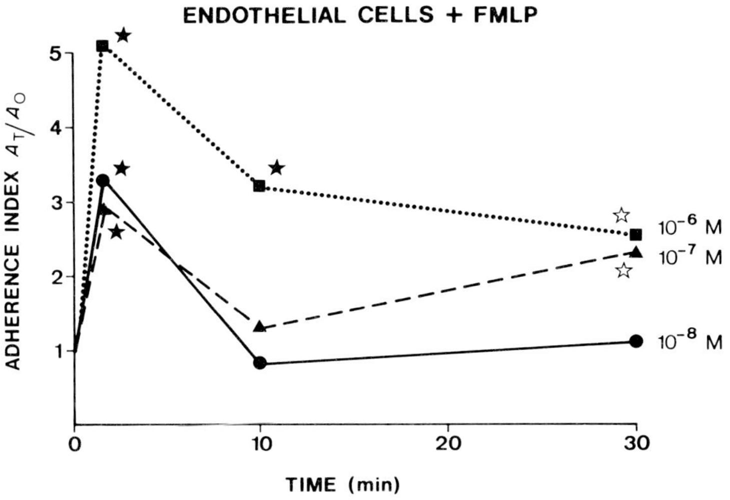

Fig. 8—Adherence index (A_T/A_0) as a function of duration of FMLP treatment at different concentrations. Adherence of granulocytes (2×10^6 in Hanks'-HEPES buffer per 60 mm culture dish) to FMLP-treated endothelial cells—10 min co-culture. Seven observations per group. ★ $P<0{\cdot}0001$; ☆ $P<0{\cdot}0002$; analysis of variance with Welch test

result of restriction of the lipid domains in the membrane caused by a molecular restructuring of the membrane protein component. This hypothesis may also hold true for the present study.

Support for the hypothesis is provided by a number of publications describing the induction of receptors in granulocytes by FMLP.[25–27] Although not so well documented, it has been suggested by Hoover *et al.*[28] that endothelial cells also possess high affinity surface receptors for FMLP.

Although the molecular events responsible for the FMLP-induced membrane modulation detected by biophysical methods remain unclear, possible mechanisms involved may be proposed from the detailed studies already performed on the interaction between chemotactic peptides and granulocytes. Thus, O'Dea *et al.*[29] showed that treatment of rabbit neutrophil granulocytes with FMLP was followed by a carboxymethylation of proteins in the membrane. This methylation process was interpreted by these authors as a means of neutralizing the negative charge on the carboxyl groups of membrane proteins and thereby resulting in conformational changes. However, this reaction could not be confirmed in human granulocytes.[30]

Snyderman *et al.*[30] described a quite different form of methylation of membrane components. These authors showed that 1 min after FMLP treatment of guinea-pig macrophages the methylation of phosphatidylethanolamine was inhibited. They postulated that the interaction between FMLP and surface receptors was followed by an inhibition of phospholipid methylation in the adjacent membrane components. If such processes are operative in the endothelial cell membrane under FMLP treatment, it is conceivable from a biophysical point of view that the physical properties of the membrane may be modulated, which in turn could explain the altered cellular function such as increased granulocyte adhesion.

The present paper also describes the ability of FMLP at concentrations of 10^{-7} and 10^{-6} M to increase the adherence of granulocytes to endothelial cells. In only one experiment was this effect seen by 10^{-8} M FMLP, the optimal dose required to elicit a chemotactic reaction.[9] Furthermore, it has been shown that the maximal elevation of granulocyte adherence occured 1·5 min following treatment of the endothelial cell monolayer with FMLP. The ability of FMLP to enhance the adherence of granulocytes to artificial substrates and to endothelial cells has been described by other authors.[28,31,32]

One of the important findings in the present investigation is the fact that the physical changes in the endothelial cell membrane induced by FMLP were detected over a time period in which the elevation of granulocyte adherence to the endothelial cells was observed. This concordance between the two events suggests that they may be causally related to one another. This view receives support from the consideration that the cell membranes of the interacting cells are intimately involved in granulocyte adherence to the endothelium. It is thus possible, if only tentative, that the FMLP-induced restructuring of the endothelial plasma membrane may lead to increased granulocyte adherence.

It is also instructive to compare this biophysical and functional correlation under FMLP treatment with results obtained from similar experiments on virus treatment of endothelial cells *in vitro*. In our laboratory it has been shown that the enteroviruses, Echo 9, Echo 12 and Coxsackie B3 virus, caused an elevation of granulocyte adherence to cultured endothelial cells.[7,23] Concomitant with these alterations in the functional parameter, i.e. granulocyte adherence, marked changes occurred in the physical properties of the endothelial plasma membrane, however in a way diametrically opposed to the FMLP-induced alterations. Thus, after virus treatment of the endothelial cells the excimer formation by the pyrene decanoic acid fluorescent probe *decreased*, whereas following FMLP treatment excimer formation *increased*. This apparent paradox may be resolved by postulating a 'ground state' for the membrane, in which, under physiological conditions, granulocyte adherence is minimal (Fig. 9). A modulation of surface membrane architecture, represented by the physical parameter φ (in the monomer–excimer technique), whether it be a reduction or elevation of membrane domains (virus- or FMLP-induced effect respectively), elicits the same functional response, namely an elevated adherence of granulocytes to the endothelial cells.

The FMLP-induced elevation of granulocyte adherence to endothelial cells may be relevant to the

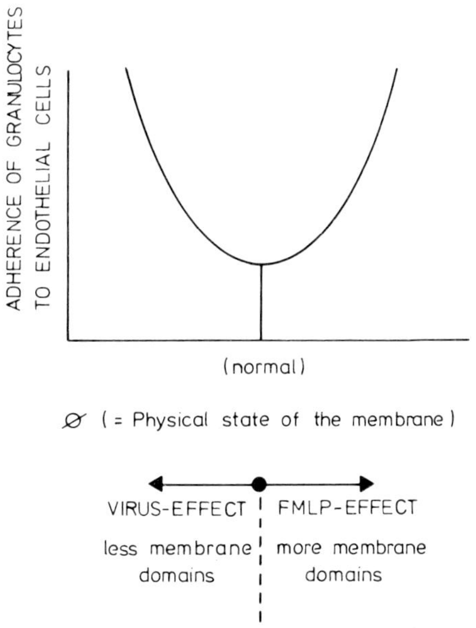

Fig. 9—Schematic representation of the relationship between the adherence of granulocytes to endothelial cells and changes in membrane architecture (measured as the parameter (φ) in the monomer–excimer technique), caused by viruses or FMLP

clinical course of sepsis. Ward and Becker[33] reported a complete and irreversible loss of the chemotactic response of neutrophilic granulocytes following prolonged exposure to activated complement components. The process was termed 'deactivation'. Fehr and Dahinden[9] investigated this phenomenon in FMLP-treated granulocytes. The maximal chemotactic response was achieved with 10^{-9}–10^{-8} M FMLP, whereas concentrations $>10^{-7}$ M caused not only an inhibition of chemotaxis but also a reduction of chemokinesis.

It may be postulated that if the above mechanisms are operative in the circulatory system *in vivo*, high intravascular concentrations of chemotactic factors, as may occur in sepsis, may indirectly promote the further development of infection by causing intravascular sequestration of granulocytes and preventing their emigration. The results presented in this paper, showing that FMLP concentrations $>10^{-7}$ M cause increased granulocyte adherence to endothelial cells *in vitro* add support to this hypothesis.

ACKNOWLEDGEMENTS

We thank Professor H. Gruler (Department of Biophysics, University of Ulm) for his invaluable help with the biophysical studies and Miss Waltraud Riedel and Miss Sylvia Braun for their excellent technical assistance. We gratefully acknowledge the expert help of Mr Klaus Feilen (Computer Centre, University of Ulm) with the statistical analysis.

REFERENCES

1. Wissler, JH, Stecher VJ, Sorkin E. Chemistry and biology of the anaphylatoxin-related serum peptide system. III. Evaluation of leucotactic activity as a property of a new peptide system with classical anaphylatoxin and cocytotaxin as components. *Eur J Immunol* 1972; **2:** 90.
2. Ford-Hutchinson AW. Leukotriene B4 and neutrophil function: a review. *J Roy Soc Med* 1981; **74:** 831.
3. Schiffmann E, Corcoran BA, Wahl SM. *N*-Formyl methionyl peptides as chemoattractants for leukocytes. *Proc Natl Acad Sci USA* 1975; **72:** 1059.
4. Showell HJ, Freer RJ, Zigmond SH *et al.* The structure activity relations of synthetic peptides as chemotactic factors and inducers of lysosomal enzyme secretion for neutrophils. *J Exp Med* 1976; **143:** 1154.
5. Jones G, Hurley JV. The effect of prostacyclin on the adhesion of leucocytes to injured vascular endothelium. *J Pathol* 1984; **142:** 51.
6. Jaffe EA, Nachman RL, Becker CG, Minick CR. Culture of human endothelial cells derived from umbilical veins. Identification by morphologic and immunologic criteria. *J Clin Invest* 1973; **52:** 2745.
7. Kirkpatrick CJ. Endothelzellkulturen—ein Modell zur Untersuchung der Pathogenese der Entzündung. Morphologische, biochemische und biophysikalische Beobachtungen. Habilitation-Thesis, The University of Ulm 1984.
8. Bültmann B, Eggers HJ, Haferkamp O. Selective inhibition of human neutrophil chemotaxis by Echovirus, type 9. *Klin Wochenschr* 1981; **59:** 571.
9. Fehr J, Dahinden C. Modulating influence of chemotactic factor-induced cell adhesiveness on granulocyte function. *J Clin Invest* 1979; **64:** 8.
10. Davis BH, Walter RJ, Pearson CB, Becker EL, Oliver JM. Membrane activity and topography of f-Met-Leu-Phe-treated polymorphonuclear leukocytes. Acute and sustained responses to chemotactic peptide. *Amer J Pathol* 1982; **108:** 206.
11. Corvol M-T, Malemud CJ, Sokoloff L. A pituitary growth-promoting factor for articular chondrocytes in monolayer culture. *Endocrinology* 1972; **90:** 262.
12. Kirkpatrick CJ. The articular chondrocyte monolayer as an experimental model in the study of cartilage growth and destruction. MD Thesis, The Queen's University of Belfast, 1982.
13. Burton K. A study of the conditions and mechanism of the diphenylamine reaction for the colorimetric estimation of deoxyribonucleic acid. *J Biochem* 1956; **62:** 315.
14. Galla H-J, Hartmann W. Excimer-forming lipids in membrane research. *Chem Phys Lipids* 1980; **27:** 199.
15. Jähnig F. Structural order of lipids and proteins in membranes: evaluation of fluorescence anisotropy data. *Proc Natl Acad Sci USA* 1979; **76:** 6361.
16. Heyn MP. Determination of lipid order parameters and rotational-correlation times from fluorescence depolarization experiments. *FEBS Lett* 1979; **108:** 359.
17. Galla H-J, Sackmann E. Lateral diffusion in the hydrophobic region of membranes: use of pyrene excimers as optical probes. *Biochim Biophys Acta* 1974; **339:** 103.
18. Sackmann E. On the application of excimers as optical probes in membrane research. *Z Phys Chem* 1976; **101:** 391.
19. Bültmann B, Melzner I, Haferkamp O, Gruler H. Selective inhibition of human neutrophilic chemotaxis by Echo virus, type 9. Virus-induced changes in membrane fluidity. *Path Res Pract* 1982; **175:** 308.
20. Kirkpatrick CJ. Interaction between enteroviruses and human endothelial cells *in vitro*: virus-induced alterations of endothelial cell proliferation and morphology. Submitted for publication.

21. Shinitzky M, Barenholz Y. Fluidity parameters of lipid regions determined by fluorescence polarization. *Biochim Biophys Acta* 1978; **515:** 367.
22. Karnovsky MJ, Kleinfeld AM, Hoover RL, Klausner RD. The concept of lipid domains in membrane. *J Cell Biol* 1982; **94:** 1.
23. Kirkpatrick CJ, Bültmann BD, Gruler H. Interaction between enteroviruses and human endothelial cells *in vitro*: alterations in the physical properties of the endothelial cell plasma membrane and adhesion of human granulocytes. *Amer J Pathol*, in press.
24. Bültmann BD, Allmendinger P, Raus RU *et al.* F-Met-Leu-Phe- and Echo 9 virus-interaction with human granulocytes. Changes of cell membrane structure. *Amer J Pathol* 1984; **116:** 46.
25. Aswanikumar S, Corcoran B, Schiffmann E *et al.* Demonstration of a receptor on rabbit neutrophils for chemotactic peptides. *Biochem Biophys Res Commun* 1977; **74:** 810.
26. Niedel J, Wilkinson S, Cuatrecasas P. Receptor-mediated uptake and degradation of ^{125}I-chemotactic peptide by human neutrophils. *J Biol Chem* 1979; **254:** 10 700.
27. Mackin WM, Huang C-K, Becker EL. The formylpeptide chemotactic receptor on rabbit peritoneal neutrophils. I. Evidence for two binding sites with different affinities. *J Immunol* 1982; **129:** 1608.
28. Hoover RL, Folger R, Haering WA, Ware BR, Karnovsky MJ. Adhesion of leukocytes to endothelium: roles of divalent cations, surface charge, chemotactic agents and substrate. *J Cell Sci* 1980; **45:** 73.
29. O'Dea RF, Viveros OH, Axelrod J, Aswanikumar S, Schiffmann E, Corcoran BA. Rapid stimulation of protein carboxymethylation in leukocytes by a chemotactic peptide. *Nature* 1978; **272:** 462.
30. Snyderman R, Pike MC, Kredich NM. Role of transmethylation reactions in cellular motility and phagocytosis. *Molec Immunol* 1980; **17:** 209.
31. Boxer LA, Yoder M, Bonsib S *et al.* Effects of a chemotactic factor, *N*-formylmethionyl peptide, on adherence, superoxide anion generation, phagocytosis, and microtubule assembly of human polymorphonuclear leukocytes. *J Lab Clin Med* 1979; **93:** 506.
32. Oseas RS, Allen J, Yang H-H, Baehner RL, Boxer LA. Mechanism of dexamethasone inhibition of chemotactic factor induced granulocyte aggregation. *Blood* 1982; **59:** 265.
33. Ward PA, Becker EL. The deactivation of rabbit neutrophils by chemotactic factor and the nature of the activatable esterase. *J Exp Med* 1968; **127:** 693.

JOURNAL OF PATHOLOGY, VOL. **144**: 213–220 (1984)

ENDOTHELIAL CELL CHANGES IN ACUTE HEPATITIS. A LIGHT AND ELECTRON MICROSCOPIC STUDY

K. A. BARDADIN* AND P. J. SCHEUER

Department of Histopathology, Royal Free Hospital and School of Medicine, London, U.K.

Received 27 April 1984
Accepted 24 July 1984

SUMMARY

Hepatic endothelial cells were studied by light and electron microscopy in 48 patients with acute hepatitis due to virus infection or drug idiosyncrasy. Light microscopy revealed cell swelling and appearance of dense refractile intracytoplasmic granules staining with the amylase PAS reaction and for iron by Perls' method. They were orcein-negative. These cells, regarded as 'activated' endothelial cells, were found throughout the parenchyma, especially in the classical form of acute hepatitis. In acute hepatitis with bridging, panacinar or periportal necrosis, activated endothelial cells were prominent in the necrotic areas. They were constantly seen lining newly formed capillaries in these sites. By electron microscopy, the intracytoplasmic granules had the characteristics of primary or secondary siderosomes. In areas of capillarization, basement membrane material was seen on the aspect of the activated cells facing the space of Disse. Activated endothelial cells may play a part in protecting hepatocytes from injury.

KEY WORDS—Acute hepatitis, endothelial cells, ultrastructure.

INTRODUCTION

Acute hepatitis, whether caused by virus infection or drugs, is characterized morphologically by a combination of liver cell damage, cholestasis, regeneration, infiltration by inflammatory cells and a sinusoidal cell reaction. Sinusoidal cells contain abundant amylase (diastase) PAS-positive (DPAS) and orcein-positive material. This is considered to be a manifestation of phagocytosis of hepatocellular and other remnants.[1,2] The cells also commonly contain stainable iron, probably derived partly from damaged liver cells.[3]

Sinusoidal cells probably play a part in the complicated immune reactions which form an essential aspect of the hepatitic process. However, most morphological studies of hepatitis have dealt principally with changes in the liver cells and there has been little attempt to analyse the reactions of the sinusoidal cell population in detail.

In a previous study, one of us described changes in endothelial cells in the livers of patients with chronic active hepatitis.[4] The cells bulged into the sinusoidal lumens. They contained increased numbers of dense bodies and micropinocytotic vesicles. Golgi complexes were enlarged. Amorphous material accumulated at the cell surfaces facing the space of Disse. Cells showing these changes were designated 'active' endothelial cells. In addition, there were endothelial cells with hemidesmosomes, to which reticulin fibres were attached. These contained less dense bodies than other cells, but rough endoplasmic reticulum (RER) was increased. The cells resembled the fibroblastic reticulum cells previously described in lymph nodes.[5] Bardadin and Desmet[4] suggested that activation of endothelial cells, formation of fibroblastic reticulum cells and subsequent transformation of sinusoids into capil-

Addressee for correspondence: Professor Peter J. Scheuer, Department of Histopathology, Royal Free Hospital, Pond Street, London NW3 2QG, U.K.

*Present address: Postgraduate Medical Centre, Warsaw, Poland.

0022–3417/84/110213–08$01.00

laries constituted a mechanism for the protection of liver cells against potentially harmful foreign antigens.

In the course of studying sinusoidal cells in acute hepatitis, we observed changes in endothelial cells similar to those in chronic hepatitis. The observations form the subject of this paper.

MATERIALS AND METHODS

Forty-eight liver biopsy specimens were studied, all from patients with acute hepatitis seen at the Royal Free Hospital, London from 1977 to 1983. The diagnosis was based on a combination of clinical and histological features. There were four aetiological groups (types A, B, non-A, non-B and drug hepatitis), based on the clinical history and on testing of serum for IgM anti-HAV and markers of hepatitis B virus infection. On the basis of the histological appearances, the groups were further subdivided into classical acute hepatitis with spotty (focal) necrosis, acute hepatitis with bridging necrosis, acute hepatitis with panacinar necrosis and acute hepatitis with periportal necrosis. The latter pattern refers to cases with substantial piecemeal necrosis, sometimes designated 'acute hepatitis with possible transition to chronic hepatitis'.[6] Numbers of biopsies in each category, together with numbers studied by electron as well as light microscopy, are given in Table I. Biopsies were designated as showing 'fully developed' or 'late' acute hepatitis, according to previously stated criteria.[7] The fully developed stage was characterized by extensive liver cell damage and inflammation, whereas in the late stage cell damage was less prominent. The fully developed stage was rarely seen more than 3 months after onset.

Paraffin sections were prepared by standard methods and stained with haematoxylin and eosin, PAS after amylase (diastase) digestion (DPAS), Perls' method for iron and Shikata's orcein method. Reticulin fibres were demonstrated by Gordon and Sweets' method. Samples for electron microscopy were obtained in 41 of the 48 cases. Small pieces (2–6) were immediately fixed in 3·0 per cent glutaraldehyde in cacodylate buffer at 4°C, dehydrated and embedded in Lemix resin. Semithin and thin sections were cut on a Reichert OMU 4 ultramicrotome. Semithin (1 μm thick) sections were stained with toluidine blue for light microscopy. Ultrathin sections for electron microscopy were stained with uranyl acetate and lead citrate, and examined in a Phillips 201 transmission electron microscope. Approximately 2000 photographs were prepared for analysis of sinusoidal cell populations.

RESULTS

General cytological features

Light microscopy—A wide variety of changes was seen among the sinusoidal cell population. A constant and striking feature was the increase, as compared with normal liver, of cells positive with the DPAS stain. On the basis of this stain and of general morphological differences, two main groups of sinusoidal cells could be distinguished.

Macrophage-like cells

These were of irregular, often amoeboid shape, and typically occupied the sinusoidal lumens or lay within portal tracts. Their cytoplasm contained DPAS-positive granules and brown clumps of ceroid pigment, sometimes within the same cell. The granules varied greatly in size. Orcein staining showed similar granules irrespective of the cause of the hepatitis, but the remaining cytoplasm was unstained. The Perls' stain for iron, when positive, gave a diffuse cytoplasmic reaction (Fig. 1). Similar but bigger phagocytic cells were seen in areas of perivenular necrosis and in necrotic bridges.

Table I—Liver biopsies (no. studied by electron microscopy in parentheses)

Cause	Morphological pattern of hepatitis				
	Classical	Bridging	Panacinar	Periportal	Total
A	14 (8)	3 (3)	2 (1)	1 (1)	20 (13)
B	3 (3)	3 (3)	1 (1)	0	7 (7)
NANB	5 (5)	1 (1)	0	0	6 (6)
Drugs	5 (5)	4 (4)	2 (2)	4 (4)	15 (15)
Total	27 (21)	11 (11)	5 (4)	5 (5)	48 (41)

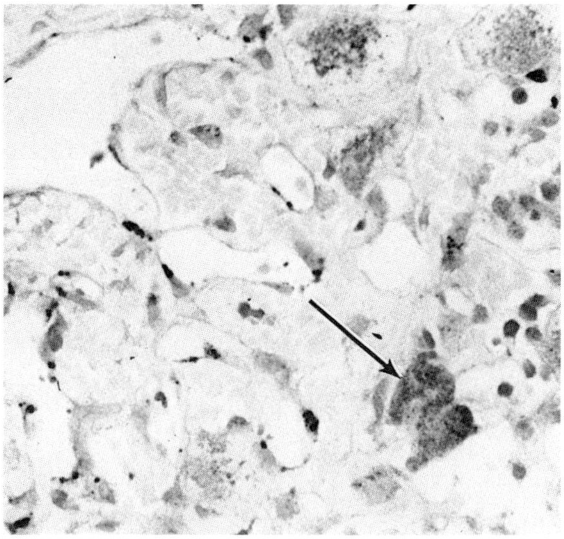

Fig. 1—Iron-rich granules are seen in endothelial cells lining sinusoids. Macrophages (arrow) also contain stainable iron. Perls' stain

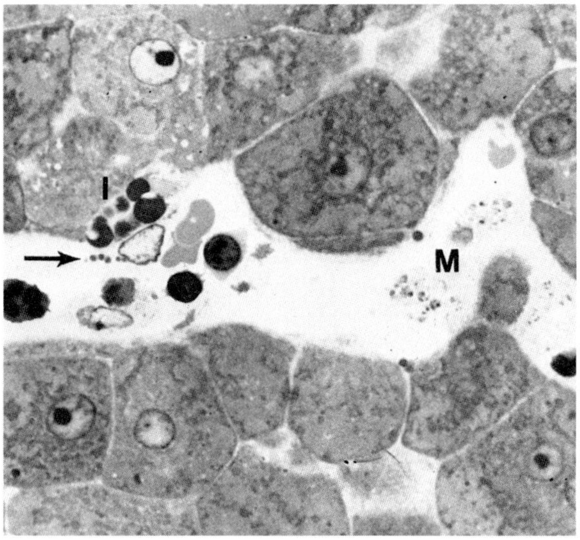

Fig. 2—Semithin resin section showing endothelial-cell granules (arrow), macrophages (M) and an Ito cell (I) filled with lipid droplets. Toluidine blue

Endothelium-like cells

These were elongated cells of regular, smooth outline, lining the sinusoids and also seen among inflammatory cells within portal tracts and in areas of bridging necrosis. In the perinuclear region of the cytoplasm there were small refractile, often brown pigmented granules, arranged in single file. Some of these granules were DPAS-positive. Perls' method gave strong positive staining in the granules, but left the cytoplasm unstained (Fig. 1). This fine granular reaction for iron was also seen in the endothelium of terminal hepatic venules ('centrilobular' veins), and in venules and capillaries of the portal tracts. Arterial endothelium was unstained. The orcein stain gave negative results in all endothelial cells. The small refractile granules sometimes identified cell processes in sinusoidal walls as being of endothelial origin, even when the nucleus and remainder of the cell body were not seen.

Semithin sections stained with toluidine blue and examined by light microscopy showed a similar division into macrophage-like and endothelium-like cells (Fig. 2). The small granules of the latter stained deep blue. The granule-containing cells were observed lining sinusoids, often in inflamed areas. Their cytoplasm tended to bulge into the lumen of the sinusoid. They were easily distinguished from the Ito cells (lipocytes) which were rich in lipid droplets, and from macrophages, which showed great variation in cell shape and size and which contained granular inclusions of variable size and staining, usually yellow or green in colour.

Electron microscopy—Under the electron microscope, it was possible to identify the endothelium-like cells described above as definite endothelial cells by means of their position, shape, granule content and pinocytotic vesicles. Their exact appearance differed from area to area.

Most often, endothelial cells were seen lining the sinusoids. However, they were sometimes displaced towards the centre of the sinusoidal lumen by accumulation of other cells within the space of Disse. Endothelial cells were seen to bulge into the lumen, and could even span the sinusoid to form a bridge. Occasionally, small granuloma-like accumulations of different cells including endothelial cells filled the lumen (Fig. 3). These cell accumulations were common in the early weeks of acute hepatitis. They were also seen to a smaller extent and in isolated foci in the later stages. The presence of the distinctive dense granules made recognition of endothelial cells easy within the cell accumulations in spite of changes in their position and shape.

Endothelial cells were often swollen and oedematous, and thus different in shape from similar cells in normal liver (Fig. 4). With the electron

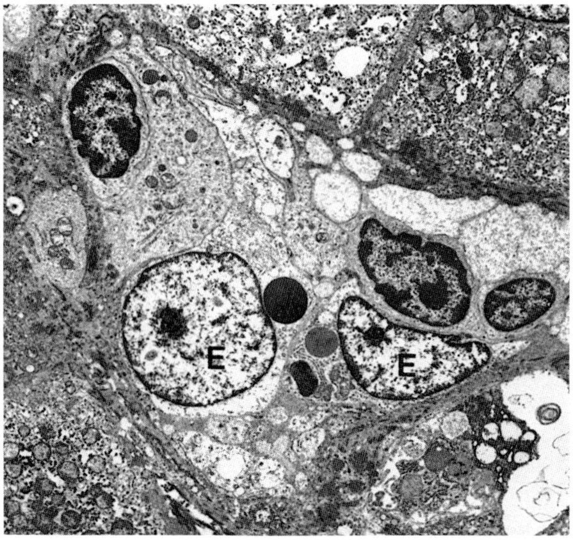

Fig. 3—Electron micrograph of a granuloma-like accumulation of cells within a sinusoid. Two endothelial cells (E) have dense granules in their cytoplasm. ×3515

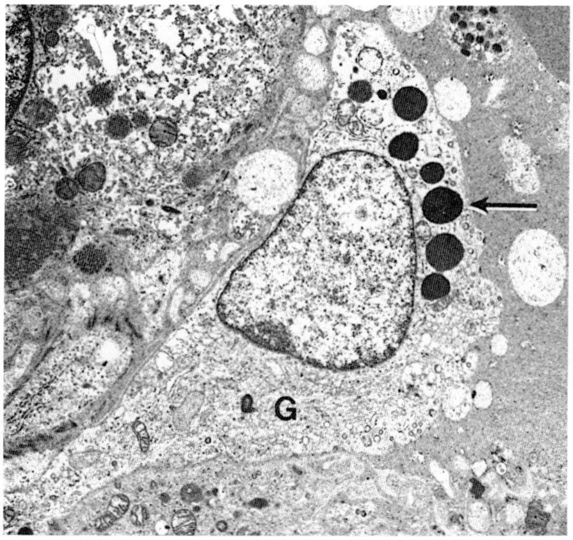

Fig. 4—An activated endothelial cell with abundant cytoplasm in which there are several dense bodies (arrow) and a prominent Golgi zone (G). ×5415

microscope, the granules observed by light microscopy were round or ovoid, 1–2 μm in diameter and located near the nucleus and in the long cytoplasmic processes. In some instances they were seen to be surrounded by a single membrane, but often the details of the periphery were obscured by the high electron density of the granules. They were usually homogeneous, but occasionally had a core of greater electron density. Compound bodies apparently formed by fusion of several granules were common in the late stage of acute hepatitis. Macropinocytotic vesicles filled with flocculent material were seen among the granules, and there was an impression of transitional forms between the two types of structure. We did not observe fusion between the granules and macro- or micropinocytotic vesicles. The granules and pinocytotic vesicles were in close proximity to mitochondria and endoplasmic reticulum.

The endothelial cells differed in a number of respects from macrophages. The latter were irregular in shape, with abundant cytoplasm containing many primary and secondary lysosomes; these were not seen in endothelial cells (Fig. 5). Occasionally, there were scanty granules within the cytoplasm of macrophages which resembled the endothelial cell granules described above. The nuclei of the two cell types varied considerably in shape and appearance, and were often unhelpful in differentiation. The surface of the endothelial cells was smooth and straight or undulating in outline, and never had microvilli. Macrophages, on the other hand, had irregular processes and microvilli. Incomplete basement membranes composed of amorphous, moderately electron-dense material were sometimes seen on the surfaces of endothelial cells facing the space of Disse (Fig. 6).

Endothelial cells in different forms of hepatitis

No fundamental differences were seen in endothelial cells from the various aetiological categories of hepatitis, though there was considerable variation from one case to another in the same category.

In the fully-developed stage of the classical form of acute hepatitis, activated endothelial cells as described above were numerous in all biopsies studied. They were iron-positive in 11 out of 13 biopsies, and were evenly scattered throughout the parenchyma. By electron microscopy, the granules were mostly rounded and discrete, and irregular compound granules were scanty. In the late stage of classical acute hepatitis, granules were mostly iron-negative, but still present throughout the acini. On electron microscopy they were mainly seen as compound granules. Amorphous material was often present on the aspect of the endothelial cells facing the space of Disse, but formed basement membranes were rare, both in the fully-developed and late stages.

Appearances were substantially different in acute

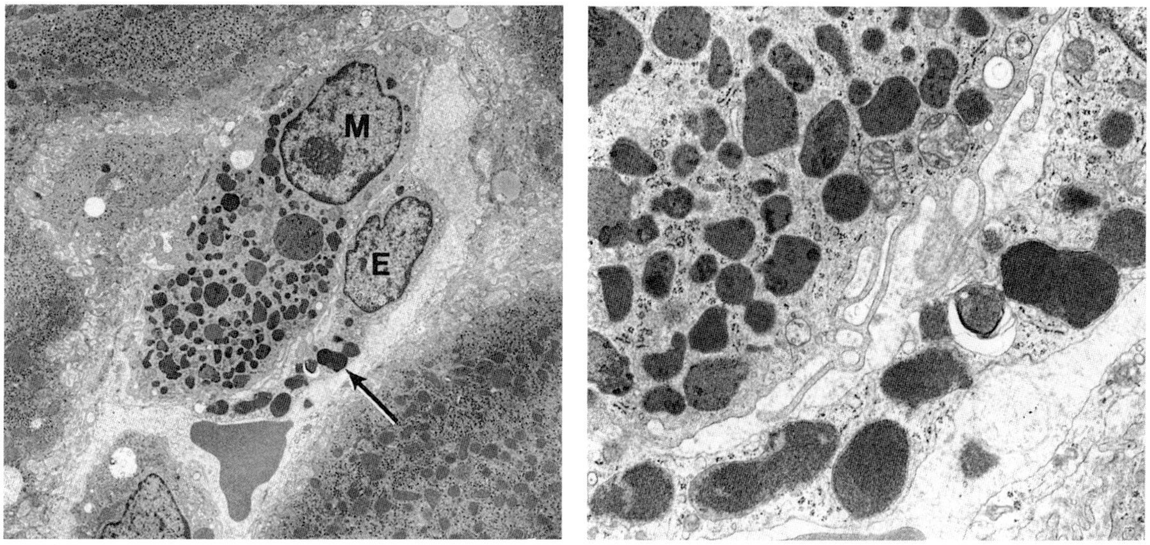

(a) (b)

Fig. 5—(a) A macrophage (M) and endothelial cell (E) are seen in a sinusoid. Note the heterogeneity of lysosomes in the macrophage, and formation of compound dense bodies (arrow) in the endothelial cell. These are also seen at higher magnification in (b). × 3610 (Fig. 5a); × 11 685 (Fig. 5b)

hepatitis with bridging, panacinar or periportal necrosis. Activated endothelial cells were mainly seen in and around necrotic areas where liver-cell plates were completely disrupted, but vascular channels were easily recognized. They often took the form of true capillaries rather than sinusoids

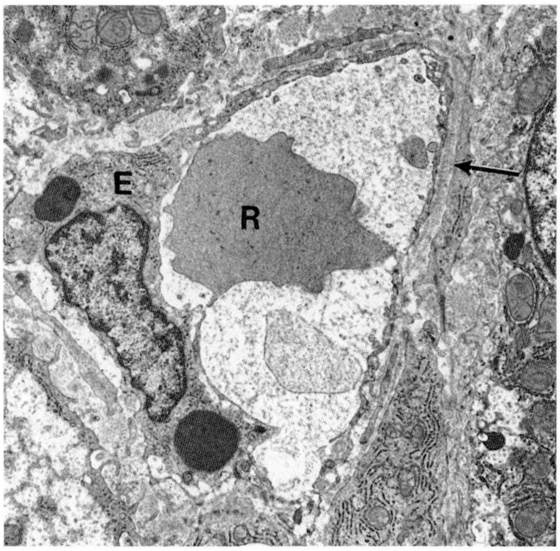

Fig. 6—A sinusoid containing a red blood cell (R) is lined by a continuous endothelium (E). The latter has an incomplete basement membrane (arrow). × 5890

(Fig. 7), with continuous endothelial lining and basement membranes. These were interposed between the capillary endothelium and perisinusoidal cells. The endothelial cells lining the capillaries contained granules, less numerous than in classical acute hepatitis. Macrophages were never observed in the lumens of the capillaries. In the parenchyma immediately adjacent to the necrotic areas vascular structures of capillary type were sometimes present; however, here they were less abundant, and basement membrane material was only seen in the form of incomplete layers of amorphous material. Macrophages were sometimes present, but were less numerous than in sinusoids. Perisinusoidal cells of various types were only inconstantly seen between endothelium and hepatocytes. Reticulin fibres, when present, were closely apposed to perisinusoidal cells, lying between these and the endothelium.

DISCUSSION

The results of this study indicate that there are substantial alterations in the appearance and arrangement of endothelial cells in all forms of acute hepatitis. The main changes observed were cell swelling, accumulation of cytoplasmic granules, and transformation of sinusoids into true capil-

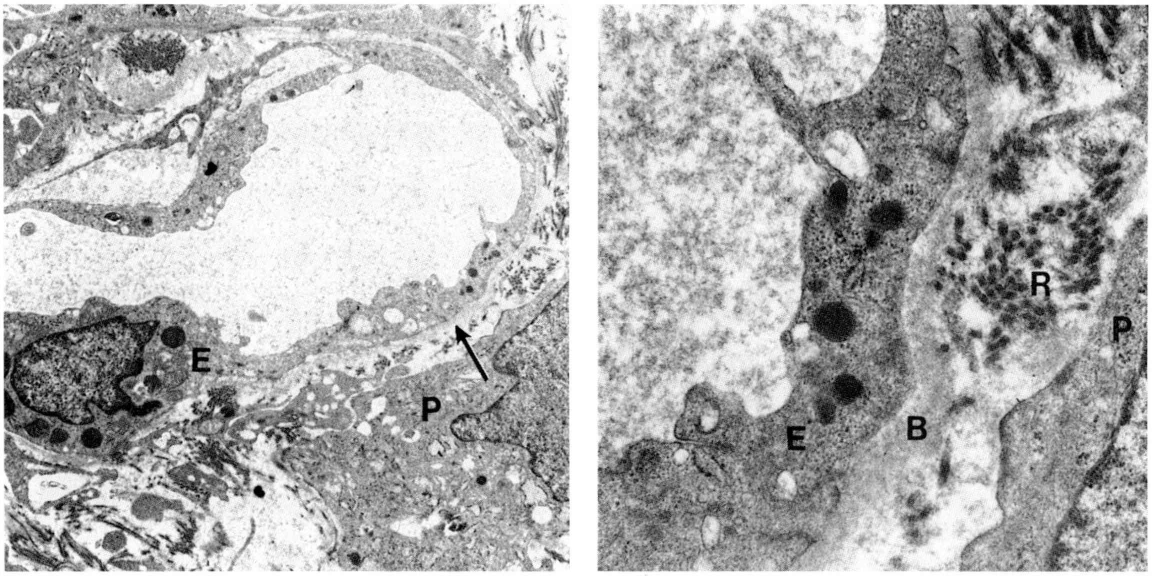

(a) (b)

Fig. 7—(a) Electron micrograph of a capillary in an area of necrosis. The complete endothelial layer (E) is surrounded by a basement membrane (arrow). A perisinusoidal cell (P) is of uncertain type, but is probably a fibroblastic reticulum cell. Part (b) shows a higher magnification of the area near the arrow; the basement membrane (B) lies close to the endothelial cell (E), whereas reticulin fibres (R) are closely related to the perisinusoidal cell (P). × 6300 (Fig. 7a); × 22000 (Fig. 7b)

laries. The granules often stained for iron with Perls' method, and could easily be distinguished from the diffuse iron-positive material in macrophages.

Düllman *et al.*[8] also found different morphological forms of iron-positive material in sinusoidal cells following intravenous administration of iron. In iron-deficient patients receiving intravenous saccharated iron oxide, a finely granular Prussian-blue reaction was seen in Kupffer cells and sinusoidal endothelial cells soon after administration. In the Kupffer cells the reaction was both granular and diffuse, whereas endothelial cells showed only granular iron-positive material. Hengeveld *et al.*,[3] in their study of iron metabolism in acute hepatitis, also observed two types of iron-positive material in sinusoidal cells and found ferritin particles within dense bodies in endothelial cells by electron microscopy.

Dense bodies are constantly found in small numbers within the sinusoidal endothelium of normal liver,[9] as well as in endothelial cells of capillaries, post-capillary venules and small veins in other organs.[10] Inclusions have also been demonstrated in cells lining lymphatics, but these were paracrystalline in appearance.[11] The dense granules found in the present study are similar in appearance to primary and compound siderosomes,[12] being rich in iron and lined by a single membrane. The origin and formation of siderosomes is not well understood. A possible origin from lysosomes or mitochondria has been suggested,[12] but our observations do not support either of these for hepatic endothelial cells. We observed an increased number of macropinocytotic vesicles at the luminal aspect of activated endothelial cells, these vesicles containing flocculent material of variable, often high electron density. Such vesicles sometimes resembled the dense bodies. It is likely that protein and iron are taken up by endothelial cells from the blood, and form the basis of endothelial cell granules. A similar sequence was observed by Wisse[13] when Thorotrast was administered to rats; particles of Thorotrast were immediately taken up into macropinocytotic vesicles and dense bodies and it often proved difficult to distinguish these structures. On the basis of his findings, Wisse[13] suggested that the dense bodies were derived from macropinocytotic vesicles rich in Thorotrast. Transformation to compound bodies was also observed. The findings differed from ours in that Thorotrast remained unchanged in the period of observation. However, this is not unexpected, since protein and iron are natural substances which take part in normal metabolic processes. Close proximity of endothelial granules to endoplasmic reticulum and mitochondria suggests that their content might form the substrate for metabolic reactions leading to the formation of materials essential to the functions of activated endothelial cells. We suggest that in acute hepatitis this function might be the synthesis of basement membrane material. Capillarization of sinusoids[14] and the accumulation of glycoproteins in the space of Disse[15] may represent an important reaction of the liver in disease, protecting the hepatocytes from injurious agents. Although found in chronic as well as acute hepatitis, capillarization does not appear to be a marker of impending chronicity since we found it in biopsies from patients with type A hepatitis, which does not become chronic.

We suggest that the process of capillarization of sinusoids can be subdivided into a number of different but interrelated stages.

(1) Sinusoidal reaction. The normal structure of the sinusoids is preserved, but amorphous material accumulates in the space of Disse, adjacent to activated endothelial cells. Macrophages are usually present. This type of reaction is prominent in all forms of acute hepatitis.

(2) Formation of pseudocapillaries. In addition to the sinusoidal reaction, continuous endothelial lining and fragments of basement membrane are found. Macrophages may or may not be seen in the lumen. This reaction is focal, and is especially seen near zones of necrosis.

(3) Formation of true capillaries. Vessels are lined by a continuous layer of endothelial cells surrounded by a complete basement membrane. Reticulin fibres are interposed between this membrane and the perisinusoidal cells. Macrophages are absent. True capillaries are typically seen within areas of liver cell necrosis, especially in bridging necrosis and periportal necrosis.

True capillarization is characterized not only by changes in the endothelial cells themselves, but also by the presence of perisinusoidal cells. In their absence, only amorphous basement membrane material is found. The close proximity of reticulin fibres to perisinusoidal cells around true capillaries suggests that these fibres are likely to be synthesized by perisinusoidal rather than activated endothelial cells. The nature of these perisinusoidal cells has not been analysed in detail in the present study. Some of them might correspond to the fibroblastic reticulum cells typical of lymph nodes,[5] and found in human liver in chronic active hepatitis.[4] Such cells, common in chronic active hepatitis, were, however, uncommon in our material. There are thus differences in the host cellular reaction in acute and chronic phases of hepatitis.

ACKNOWLEDGEMENTS

The authors are grateful to Miss J. Lewin and Mrs L. Boxer for technical help with electron microscopy, to the staff of the Histopathology laboratory of the Royal Free Hospital for material for light microscopy, and to clinical colleagues for access to clinical data. Mr F Moll kindly helped in the preparation of figures. The work was supported by a grant from the Medical Research Council.

REFERENCES

1. Peters RL. Viral hepatitis: a pathologic spectrum. *Am J Med Sci* 1975; **270:** 17–31.
2. Ishak KG. Light microscopic morphology of viral hepatitis. *Am J Clin Pathol* 1976; **65:** 787–827.
3. Hengeveld P, Zuyderhoudt FMJ, Jöbsis AC, van Gool J. Some aspects of iron metabolism during acute viral hepatitis. *Hepato-gastroenterologia* 1982; **29:** 138–141.
4. Bardadin K, Desmet VJ. Ultrastructural observations on sinusoidal endothelial cells in chronic active hepatitis. *Histopathology*, in press.
5. Tykocinski M, Schinella RA, Alba Greco M. Fibroblastic reticulum cells in human lymph nodes. An ultrastructural study. *Arch Pathol Lab Med* 1983; **107:** 418–422.
6. Bianchi L, De Groote J, Desmet VJ *et al.* Acute and chronic hepatitis revisited. *Lancet* 1977; **ii:** 914–919.
7. Scheuer PJ. Acute hepatitis. In: Scheuer PJ. Liver Biopsy Interpretation. 3rd ed. London: Bailliere Tindall, 1980; 60–74.
8. Düllman J, Wulfhekel U, Hausmann K. Differences between Kupffer cells and endothelial cells of human liver in iron storage and release under normal conditions, after i.v. iron administration and in iron overload. In: Wisse E, Knook DL, eds. Kupffer Cells and Other Liver Sinusoidal Cells. Amsterdam: Elsevier/North Holland Biomedical Press, 1977; 233–241.
9. Wisse E. An electron microscopic study of the fenestrated endothelial lining of rat liver sinusoids. *J Ultrastr Res* 1970; **31:** 125–150.
10. Rhodin JAG. Ultrastructure of mammalian venous capillaries, venules and small collecting veins. *J Ultrastr Res* 1968; **25:** 452–500.

11. Albertine KH, Fox LM, O'Morchoe CCC. Lymphatic endothelial cell inclusion bodies. *J Ultrastr Res* 1980; **73:** 199–210.
12. Ghadially FN. Siderosomes, haemosiderin and ferritin. In: Ghadially FN, ed. Ultrastructural Pathology of the Cell and Matrix. 2nd ed. Boston: Butterworths, 1981; 474–481.
13. Wisse E. An ultrastructural characterization of the endothelial cell in the liver sinusoid under normal and various experimental conditions, as a contribution to the distinction between endothelial and Kupffer cells. *J Ultrastr Res* 1972; **38:** 528–562.
14. Schaffner F, Popper H. Capillarization of hepatic sinusoids in man. *Gastroenterology* 1963; **41:** 239–242.
15. Popper H, Paronetto F, Barka T. PAS positive structures of non-glycogenic character in normal and abnormal liver. *Arch Pathol* 1960; **70:** 300–313.

BOOK REVIEWS

Pathology of Glomerular Disease. Edited by SEYMOUR ROSEN. Contemporary Issues in Surgical Pathology Volume 1. Series Editor LAWRENCE M. ROTH. Churchill Livingstone, Edinburgh, 1983. No. of pages: xii + 274. Price: £35.00 (clothbound). ISBN: 0 443 08198 0.

This book contains a worthwhile collection of review articles concerning many aspects of glomerular pathology likely to concern the diagnostic histopathologist. Two of the chapters are on general topics—one on classification of glomerular disorders and the second on immmunoperoxidase procedures. Four chapters discuss histologically defined forms of glomerulonephritis viz: crescentic, membranous, membranoproliferative and the minimal change/focal and segmental glomerulosclerosis group. Then there are two chapters on the immunologically defined IgA nephropathies and anti-GBM glomerulonephritis. The remaining chapters discuss glomerular lesions etiologically associated with plasma cell dyscrasias, transplantation, hereditary states, the haemolytic uraemic syndrome, SLE and prior infections.

The editor and most of the authors (10) are from the U.S.A. but the international aspirations of the book are backed with five authors from France and one each from Finland, West Germany and the U.K. The series claims to present a "state of the art assessment .... of the surgical pathology of a particular anatomic site" and to do this by selective reviews rather than by a systematic textbook approach. This aim is achieved admirably by some of these chapters. For example Magda Stilment on crescentic glomerulonephritis not only gives a thoughtful account of this subject but contributes many pertinent remarks on the interpretation of immunohistological observations, which are not to be found in the chapter on immunoperoxidase studies.

Curtis B. Wilson on anti-GBM nephritis is similarly outstanding, being informative and authoritative though not dogmatic. Morel-Maroger, Veroust and Preud-'homme give an excellent account of the glomerular lesions associated with plasma cell dyscrasias, summarizing usefully a vast amount of literature and making their experience accessible to those who have seen much less. Not all of the chapters are successful. In his own chapter, the editor has disciplined himself more than some of his contributors with regard to space. This results in his contribution on classification of glomerular disease being tightly written but perhaps not sufficiently explanatory to be very useful to its intended readers.

The book does not claim to be comprehensive so one cannot really be disappointed in not finding an up to date account of normal glomerular structure. Similarly, important glomerular pathology, such as that associated with Diabetes mellitus, hypertension and ischaemia, is mentioned only in passing. The wilder shores of immunopathologic speculation are avoided as is most of the post Dixon experimental work.

Clearly, the ideal reader of this book is a diagnostic histopathologist interested in and familiar with renal pathology who wishes to have a collection of review articles on the disease groups generally diagnosed by needle biopsy. Such a reader will enjoy this book but will probably find that he is already familiar with much of its content.

D. R. DAVIES
St. Thomas' Hospital
London

The Determinants of Viral and Bacterial Pathogenicity Edited by H. SMITH, J. P. ARBUTHNOTT and C. A. MIMS. The Royal Society, London, 1983. No. of pages: viii + 163. Price: £24.75 (clothbound). ISBN: 0 85403 216 9.

Understanding of microbial pathogenicity is now moving from 'observation' to molecular 'explanation'. This book is the proceedings of a 2 day discussion meeting held in London at the Royal Society in February, 1983. The meeting aimed to contrast common problems posed by both bacterial and viral pathogenicity in the hope that gaps might be revealed which might indicate directions for future research. Thus, contributors were asked to consider microbial pathogenicity in 15 different papers in terms of the common problems of mucous membrane interactions, entry to the host, multiplication *in vivo*, evasion and modulation of host defences and damage to the host. Inevitably in a book based on a meeting the coverage of topics depends primarily on the individual interests of participants and there are some notable omissions. Thus, the problem of how viruses invade mucous surfaces is reviewed without reference to the fast expanding area of knowledge concerning how influenza, vesicular stomatitis and other viruses enter mucosal cells. The book contains some notable reviews of interest to both pathologists and microbiologists covering such topics as immunopathological mechanisms in streptococcal disease, immunosuppressive effects of virus infection, immunomodulation by bacteria and host damage by bacterial toxins. Many of the reviews are currently useful as background material for undergraduate teaching but, at £24.75, it is unlikely to be bought by many undergraduates and the reviews will inevitably rapidly become out of date. This is a book which can be recommended for purchase by Medical School libraries, departments of microbiology or pathology and the more affluent postgraduate researcher.

M. E. WARD
Southampton General Hospital

JOURNAL OF PATHOLOGY, VOL. 144: 222–223 (1984)

ANNOUNCEMENTS

THE JOHNS HOPKINS MEDICAL INSTITUTIONS

CLINICAL CYTOPATHOLOGY FOR PATHOLOGISTS 1985 POSTGRADUATE INSTITUTE

The Twenty-sixth Postgraduate Institute for Pathologists in Clinical Cytopathology given by The Johns Hopkins University School of Medicine, consists of two courses, both of which must be taken:

—March–May 1985, Home Study Course A is provided each registrant for intensive personal study; and

—6–17 May 1985, In-residence Course B at the Johns Hopkins Medical Institutions, Baltimore, Maryland, U.S.A.

This Institute is designed solely for pathologists who are Certified (or qualified for certification) by the American Board of Pathology or its international equivalent. It provides an intensive refresher in all aspects of the field of clinical cytopathology with time devoted to newer developments and techniques, special problems and recent applications including immunodiagnosis and needle aspiration. Topics are covered in lectures, explored in small informal conferences and discussed over the microscope with the Faculty. Abundant self-instructional material is available to augment at individual pace. A loan set of slides with texts (Course A) will be sent to each participant within the United States and Canada for home-study during March and April before Course B in Baltimore. Prior special arrangements to study Course A must be made by participants outside of the United States and Canada. Credit hours 152 in AMA Category I. Application and completed pre-registration is advised before 30 November 1984; however, completed pre-registration must be accomplished before 5 April 1985, unless by special arrangement.

Further information from: John K. Frost, M.D., 604 Pathology Building, The Johns Hopkins Hospital, Baltimore, Maryland 21205, U.S.A.
The entire Course is given in English.

THE ANNUAL MEETING OF THE UNITED STATES–CANADIAN DIVISION OF THE INTERNATIONAL ACADEMY OF PATHOLOGY

11–15 March 1985

SHERATON CENTRE
Toronto, Ontario, Canada

Scientific papers, poster sessions, 13 specialty conferences, and 45 short courses are scheduled. Two special courses will be offered on 'Advances in the Application of Immunocytochemistry to Diagnostic Surgical Pathology' with Dr Cecilia Fenoglio as Course Director and 'Diagnostic Cellular and Molecular Pathology' with Dr Benjamin Trump as Course Director. The long course will be on 'The Pathogenesis of Liver Diseases' with Drs Emmanuel Farber and M. J. Phillips as Course Directors. The Maude Abbott Lecture will be delivered by Dr Kenneth M. Brinkhous on Tuesday 12 March. Timely Topics in Pathology will feature a session on the 'Pathogenesis and Lesions of Acid Rain' presented by Dr Robert Leader.

Further information from: Dr Nathan Kaufman, Secretary–Treasurer, United States–Canadian Division of the International Academy of Pathology, 1003 Chafee Avenue, Augusta, Georgia 30904, U.S.A. Telephone (404) 724 2973.

THE 36TH ANNUAL MEETING OF THE HISTOCHEMICAL SOCIETY (NORTH AMERICA)

3–5 May 1985

SHERATON HOTEL
Crystal City, VA (Washington DC area)

Symposia will include: 'Cellular and Molecular Mechanisms of Generating Polarity in Epithelial and Neuronal Cells'; '*In Situ* Hybridization with Nucleolide Probes—a Histochemical Tool'; 'Advances in New Technology (Presidential Symposium)'; and 'Basement Membrane Function and Morphogenesis'. Two workshops will be offered: 'Quantitative Electron Microscopy' and 'Clinical Quantitative Hematology Cytochemistry'. With the exception of selected papers related to symposia, all submitted papers will be presented in a poster session. Abstract forms are published in the November issue of the *Journal of Histochemistry and Cytochemistry*, Abstract deadline: 15 January 1985. The Washington Area Electron Microscopy Society is sponsoring a symposium on 'Ultrastructural Enzyme Histochemistry' and combined participation in the two meetings is encouraged.

Further information from: Dr Ronald R. Cowden, Program Chairman, Department of Biophysics, Quillen-Dishner College of Medicine, Box 15130A, East Tennessee State University, Johnson City, Tennessee 37614, U.S.A. or Dr Constance Oliver, Secretary, Laboratory of Oral Biology/Physiology, Building 30, Room 21, National Institute of Dental Research, NIH, Bethesda, Maryland 20205, U.S.A.

PUBLISHING AGREEMENT

1. It is our custom to request authors to vest the worldwide copyright of their papers in John Wiley & Sons Limited for the full term of copyright and we would be grateful if you would confirm your acceptance of these terms by signing and returning the agreement below. We will not withold permission for any reasonable request from you to publish any part of this paper in connection with any other work by you, provided the usual acknowledgements are given regarding copyright notice and reference to the original publication.
2. If it is appropriate, the author's employer may sign this agreement, and in any event the employer may reserve the right to use the paper internally or for promotional purposes only, by so indicating on this agreement. It is understood that proprietary rights other than copyright (including patent rights) are reserved.
3. If the author is a U.S. Government employee and his work was done in that capacity the assignment applies only to the extent allowable by U.S. law. If at least one co-author is *not* a government employee, said author should sign the agreement.
4. If the author is an employee of the British Government then HMSO will grant a non-exclusive licence to publish this paper in the Journal in any form or media provided British crown copyright and user rights (including patent rights) are reserved.
5. The author warrants that the manuscript is the author's original work, and has not been published before. (If excerpts from copyrighted works are included, the author will obtain written permission from the copyright owners and show credit to the sources in the manuscript.) The author also warrants that the article contains no libellous or unlawful statements, and does not infringe on the rights of others.
6. If the work was prepared jointly the author agrees to inform co-authors of the terms of the agreement, and to sign on their behalf.

With the qualifications listed above I assign to John Wiley & Sons Limited, the copyright of my paper entitled ______________________________

____

for publication in ______________________________

______________________________ Signed

______________________________ Date

If the paper is rejected this assignment is null and void.

JOURNAL OF PATHOLOGY, VOL. 144: 225–226 (1984)

EDITORIAL

FROM WHERE COMES THE OSTEOCLAST?

Our interest in the provenance of the human osteoclast is justified by the important role of these cells in the responses of bone to metabolic disturbances, their implication in the pathogenesis of Paget's disease,[1] and their assumed presence in giant cell tumours.

Three possible origins for the osteoclast have been suggested: (i) from an osteoprogenitor stem cell differentiating into osteocytes, osteoblasts and osteoclasts; (ii) from the mononuclear phagocyte system; (iii) from an as yet unidentified circulating mononuclear cell (the preosteoclast).

Early views on the origin of osteoclasts were based on the idea that bone cells (osteocytes, osteoblasts and osteoclasts) were derived from a common progenitor cell. This hypothesis was refined by the autoradiographic studies of Tonna and Cronkite[2] which led to the conclusion that osteoclasts were formed by the fusion of osteoblasts. Recent observations have, however, resurrected the notion, first expounded by Jordan in 1925,[3] that osteoclasts are of haemopoietic origin.[4]

Persuasive evidence that osteoclasts originate from a remotely-derived circulating precursor cell rather than from a local marrow-derived precursor comes from a series of elegant experiments on regenerating newt limbs, grafted quail limb buds, parabiotic rats, and osteopetrotic mice.[5]

Because it is well known that macrophages can fuse to form phagocytic multinucleate cells many investigators have tentatively assumed that the multinucleate osteoclasts form similarly.[6] There is other evidence: macrophages possess calcitonin receptors[7] and can resorb bone directly.[8] But compelling evidence against an origin from macrophages includes: macrophages in contact with bone are devoid of a ruffled border at the apposing surface; macrophages and the giant cells derived from them do not show a morphological response to calcitonin; osteoclasts lack the Fc and C3 receptors borne by macrophages; and macrophages do not restore the resorption defect of osteopetrosis.[9] Differences between macrophage and osteoclast-mediated bone resorption also include discrepant responses to endotoxin and cortisol.[8] However, macrophages are themselves a heterogeneous population and attempts to confirm or refute any kinship between macrophages and osteoclasts must employ a wide range of phenotypic and functional markers.

Investigators of osteoclast ontogeny and function have employed cells from various sources: (i) authentic osteoclasts from normal bone; (ii) surrogate osteoclasts prepared by forming macrophage polykaryons *in vitro*; (iii) putative osteoclasts from giant-cell lesions.

Authentic osteoclasts from bone would be ideal and have now been fractionated from non-human sources. While macrophage polykaryons are certainly capable of resorbing bone, their lack of calcitonin responsiveness and their histochemical profile question their status as surrogate osteoclasts. Giant cells from human giant-cell tumours are technically easier to work with though their osteoclastic pedigree demands careful validation.

Before assessing the phenotypic similarities between osteoclasts and other cells, the putative osteoclast population must first be defined. Marks' recent definition that an osteoclast is a 'multinucleated cell next to a bone surface'[9] may exclude many oligonuclear cells that behave like osteoclasts.[10] Alternatively, cells bearing a morphological resemblance to osteoclasts, but in pathological lesions of bone (e.g. tumours), may be studied as paradigms of normal osteoclasts. Because uncertainties still surround the precise histogenesis of giant-cell tumours ('osteoclastomas')—and in particular of polykaryons within them—the identity of the giant cell must be rigourously established before conclusions can be reached about the ontogeny of osteoclasts.

Burmester *et al.*[11] recently defined a total of four cell types in giant-cell tumours on the basis of reactivity with immune probes: the giant cells themselves were heterogeneous; about 50 per cent expressed Ia antigens and Møu-50 reactivity shared by a monoblastoid cell line. Burmester *et al.* postulated that the cell types in giant-cell tumours may represent a recapitulation of osteoclast differentiation.

The study by Horton *et al.*[12] published in this issue of *The Journal of Pathology* is of considerable relevance to the debated histogenesis of 'osteoclastoma' giant cells and the ontogeny of osteoclasts. In tumours, however, it may be unwise to assume that the phenotypic integrity of cells is wholly preserved or otherwise escapes unsullied: some markers may be unexpectedly lost or acquired or be expressed at a lower density than on the parent cell. The multinucleated osteoclasts commonly encountered in pathological circumstances may give misleading false-negative results for surface markers even though their resorptive capacity is enhanced: for example, macrophage polykaryons—more effective at resorbing bone than their mononuclear precursors[13]—show diminished surface binding sites for IgG.[14] Osteoclasts may require the microenvironment of bone for full phenotypic expression, though it might be expected that even in some pathological situation their ancestry may be betrayed by the retention of at least a few markers.

Now that such a wide range of exquisitely specific monoclonal reagents is available to investigators in this field, we must anticipate a study of the phenotype of osteoclasts in or eluted from the more natural microenvironment of bone before firm conclusions can be drawn about their origin.

J. C. E. Underwood
University of Sheffield Medical School

REFERENCES

1. Harvey L, Gray T, Beneton MN, Douglas DL, Kanis JA, Russell RGG. Ultrastructural features of the osteoclasts from Paget's disease of bone in relation to a viral aetiology. *J Clin Pathol* 1982; **35:** 771–779.
2. Tonna EA, Cronkite EP. Use of tritiated thymidine for the study of the origin of the osteoclast. *Nature* 1961; **190:** 459–460.
3. Jordan HE. The experimental production of osteoclasts in the frog, *Rana pipiens. Anat Rec* 1925; **30:** 107–121.
4. Bonucci E. New knowledge on the origin, function and fate of osteoclasts. *Clin Orthop* 1981; **158:** 252–269.
5. Loutit JF, Nisbet NW. The origin of osteoclasts. *Immunobiology* 1982; **161:** 193–203.
6. Teitelbaum SL, Kahn AJ. Mononuclear phagocytes, osteoclasts and bone resorption. *Mineral Electrol Metabol* 1980; **3:** 2–9.
7. Minkin C, Blackman L, Newbrey J, Pokress S, Posek R, Walling M. Effects of parathyroid hormone and calcitonin on adenylate cyclase in murine mononuclear phagocytes. *Biochem Biophys Res Commun* 1977; **76:** 875–881.
8. Mundy GR. Monocyte-macrophage system and bone resorption. *Lab Invest* 1983; **49:** 119–121.
9. Marks SC. The origin of osteoclasts. *J Oral Pathol* 1983; **12:** 226–256.
10. Kaye M. When is it an osteoclast? *J Clin Pathol* 1984; **37:** 398–400.
11. Burmester GR, Winchester RJ, Dimitrin-Bona A, Klein M, Steiner G, Sissons HA. Delineation of four cell types comprising the giant cell tumor of bone: expression of Ia and monocyte–macrophage lineage antigens. *J Clin Invest* 1983; **71:** 1633–1648.
12. Horton MA, Rimmer EF, Lewis D, Pringle JAS, Fuller K, Chambers TJ. Cell surface characterization of the human osteoclast: phenotypic relationship to other bone marrow-derived cell types. *J Pathol* 1984; **144:** 281–294.
13. Fallon MD, Teitelbaum SL, Kahn AJ. Multinucleation enhanced macrophage-mediated bone resorption. *Lab Invest* 1983; **49:** 159–164.
14. Mariano M, Nikitin T, Malucelli BE. Immunological and non-immunological phagocytosis by inflammatory macrophages, epithelioid cells and macrophage polykaryons from foreign-body granuloma. *J Pathol* 1976; **120:** 151–159.

JOURNAL OF PATHOLOGY, VOL. **144**: 227–232 (1984)

RETICULUM CELLS: CHARACTERIZATION AND IMMUNE FUNCTIONS AND THE NATURE OF HODGKIN AND REED–STERNBERG CELLS

E. L. JONES

Department of Pathology, Medical School, University of Birmingham, Birmingham B15 2TJ, U.K.

Received 9 May 1984
Accepted 10 May 1984

KEY WORDS—Reticulum cells, Hodgkin's disease, Reed–Sternberg cells.

INTRODUCTION

The term 'reticulum cell' although controversial is still in common use even though there is no general agreement on its precise definition. In simple morphological terms 'reticulum cells' have been considered in the past, to be stellate-shaped cells with pale, non-basophilic, slender cell processes and a light, oval or polymorphic, leptochromatic nucleus with a distinct nuclear membrane and a small or medium-sized nucleolus. It is clear, however, that this purely morphological description can be applied to a variety of cells with different functions. The different types of 'reticulum cells' can now be distinguished by special techniques such as electron microscopy, enzyme histochemistry, immunohistochemistry, and functional studies. In addition, the silver impregnation method of Marshall[1] is a useful and relatively inexpensive technique for the demonstration of 'reticulum cells' in paraffin sections, although experience has shown that the metalophil impregnation may be difficult to perform and somewhat unpredictable in its results. Here the results of the metalophil impregnation of histiocytes in a range of reactive and neoplastic lymphoid tissues are presented.[2,3]

In practise four main types of 'reticulum cell' are recognized, histiocytic (HRC), fibroblastic (FRC), dendritic (DRC) and interdigitating (IDRC).[4] The structure, staining characteristics and immune functions of these cells is discussed and the possible nature and origin of Hodgkin (H) and Reed–Sternberg (RS) cells reviewed.

0022–3417/84/120227–06$01.00

HISTIOCYTIC RETICULUM CELL

The HRC is a large, rounded, phagocytic cell widely distributed throughout all areas of lymph nodes, although they are particularly numerous within the lymph sinuses and germinal centres. Ultrastructurally HRC have a round or oval nucleus with a central nucleolus. The broad cytoplasm extends into elongated cell processes lying between the lymphoid cells. Within the cytoplasm, well-formed Golgi zones, profiles of smooth and rough endoplasmic reticulum and many large phagolysozomes, containing recognizable cell and membrane remnants are seen. Small electron dense lysozomes are present and mitochondria are often numerous indicative of a high metabolic activity. Within the basal zones of the germinal centres of secondary lymphoid follicles the HRC often contain phagocytosed cells and nuclear fragments ('tingible-body' macrophages) resembling a 'starry-sky' pattern. Enzyme histochemically the HRC are strongly positive for acid phosphatase and nonspecific esterase and are weakly positive for 5′-nucleotidase, aminopeptidase and adenosine triphosphatase. They show a variable degree of metalophilia.

The function of the HRC is unclear although they appear to be actively phagocytic cells of the mononuclear-phagocyte system derived from bone marrow monocytes.

In follicular lymphomas HRC are present in smaller numbers and show less phagocytic activity than in reactive follicles.[5]

Surface marker studies have shown that HRC express Fcγ and C3b receptors and a proportion are Ia-positive.[6]

The HRC may be implicated in histiocytic sarcomas.[4,7]

FIBROBLASTIC RETICULUM CELL

The FRC are found in relation to blood vessels in all regions of the lymph node but especially in germinal centres and the lymphocyte coronas. They cannot be specifically identified on light microscopy.

Ultrastructurally FRC are often electron dense, although others of lower electron density frequently show a dilated rough endoplasmic reticulum reminiscent of fibroblasts. The nucleus is oblong and indented with a central nucleolus. The cytoplasm usually contains a few free ribosomes, scanty smooth endoplasmic reticulum and occasionally a small Golgi apparatus. These cells are closely related to reticulin fibres through hemidesmosomes and the cytoplasm may contain bundles of tonofibrils. The FRC are not actively phagocytic and they are thought to form the reticulin fibres of the lymph node. Cytochemically they show large amounts of surface enzyme alkaline phosphatase but only small amounts of nonspecific esterase and acid phosphatase. They are only weakly metalophil. It is now thought likely, at least in the rabbit, that DRC develop from transformation of FRC during the development of germinal centres.[8] Electron microscopical investigations revealed transitional forms between typical FDC, which formed the framework of the splenic white pulp, and typical DRC. During this transformation, the enzyme histochemical pattern of alkaline phosphatase disappeared and a positive α-naphthyl acetate esterase reaction appeared in the transformed cells. The number of DRC increases during enlargement of the germinal centres by transformation of FDC present in the adjoining lymphocyte corona.[8]

DENDRITIC RETICULUM CELL

According to current concepts the DRC is a specific structural cell of B cell regions of lymphoreticular tissue. They are present in large numbers in the upper light zone of germinal centres and lymphocyte coronas, where their long branching processes form a delicate three dimensional network within which germinal centre cells are enmeshed. They may be difficult to recognize from the HRC on light microscopy.

They are strongly metalophilic with long branching dendritic processes. Ultrastructurally they have an oval nucleus with a central solitary nucleolus and coarse condensed chromatin along the nuclear membrane. The cytoplasmic rim is often narrow and contains profiles of smooth endoplasmic reticulum but no lysozomes or phagosomes. A distinctive feature is the fine interwoven network of cytoplasmic processes lying between the centrocytes and centroblasts. Desmosomal projections between adjacent dendritic cell processes are seen. Between these cell processes, electron-dense granular material is present which corresponds to antigen–antibody complexes.

Cytochemically they contain a moderate amount of nonspecific esterase, generally less than HRC, although they are negative for acid phosphatase. They are strongly positive for 5′-nucleotidase.

DRC have been shown by autoradiographic and immunohistochemical techniques to have a high affinity for immune complexes. Thus they appear to play a primary role in the trapping of antigen within germinal centres. DRC are present in smaller numbers and are functionally less active in follicular lymphomas compared to reactive follicles.[5] They may also be involved in B cell homing since neoplastic germinal centre cells in cases of follicular lymphoma can be shown by light and electron microscopy to accumulate within a meshwork of DRC. Human DRC can now be delineated in cryostat sections with a mouse monoclonal antibody.[9] It is probable that the DRC are derived from the stroma-forming FRC, at least in the rabbit,[8] although this remains to be determined for other species. The follicular DRC express the C3b receptor, are HLA-DR positive and stain with an anti-human monocyte antibody.[10]

The DRC may give rise to a sarcoma of these cells. Recently van der Valk *et al.*[11] using the results of light microscopical, ultrastructural, immunohistochemical and enzyme histochemical investigations described four tumours of the follicular compartment of the lymph node, in which the proliferating cell appeared to be the DRC.

INTERDIGITATING RETICULUM CELL

This name was applied because of the interlocking appearance of the cell membranes and the finger-like protrusions into their cytoplasm, extruding from lymphocytes, which are trapped between their cytoplasmic extensions. They are found in the thymus-dependent inner portion of the periarticular lymphoid sheaths of the spleen, in the medulla of the thymus and in the thymus-dependent paracortical areas of lymph nodes.[12] The nuclei are often indented with small nucleoli which lie either centrally or along the nuclear membrane. The rim of cytoplasm is broad with elongated processes.

Ultrastructurally the nucleus is markedly indented and lobed, with dispersed chromatin. The cytoplasm contains numerous short narrow vesicles, profiles of rough and smooth endoplasmic reticulum, a medium or large Golgi apparatus and often large membrane bound vesicles. The cell surface is especially characteristic with numerous processes forming an interdigitating system and membrane invaginations with neighbouring IDRC and lymphocytes. The cytoplasm contains a moderate number of ribosomes and abundant mitochondria. Birbeck granules typical of Langerhans cells (LC) are not usually present. In contrast to the HRC, the non-specific esterase reaction and acid phosphatase activity are weakly positive. Characteristically the IDRC show a moderate to strong adenosine triphosphatase reaction. The cells are moderately metalophilic with long branching processes.

The IDRC appear to be closely related to LC.[6] The LC may be a highly differentiated end-stage of a bone-marrow derived cell line similar to, but separate from, the known phagocytic macrophage cell line. On the basis of the similarity of LC and IDRC it is postulated that the LC may function in antigen presentation, lymphokine production, provision of a micro-environment for T lymphocytes, and prostaglandin secretion.[6] There have been several recent reviews of the origin, function and immunobiology of LC.[6,13–15] It is also probable that the veiled cells observed in lymph draining the skin are related to the IDRC and LC based on similarities in enzyme histochemistry, ultrastructure and contact sensitization studies.[16] Epidermal LC expresses Fcγ and C3 receptors and are Ia-positive. The IDRC, like LC, bear Ia antigens but are probably Fcγ and C3 receptor negative.[17] The S-100 antigen, an acidic Ca^{2+}-binding protein has recently been identified in IDRC of peripheral lymphoid tissue, human thymic medulla[18,19] and in thymomas.[20] It is now likely with antibody probes that tumours derived from the IDRC will be increasingly recognized. Histiocytosis X is now believed to be a LC granuloma and there are reports of monocytic leukaemias with cells containing LC granules.

SINUS ENDOTHELIAL CELL

The lymphatic sinuses are lined by flat elongated endothelial-type 'littoral' cells. Within the sinuses there are phagocytic 'reticular' cells (intrasinusoidal reticulum cells). The metalophil method is particularly valuable in demonstrating these cells.

Macrophages and lymphocytes alter not only morphological and physiological characteristics of endothelial cells but also their antigenic expression.[21] The sinus lining cells may be involved in antigen-uptake and sampling and could interact with lymphoid and antigen-handling cells which pass through them. The 'littoral' cells but not the 'reticular' cells have been shown to contain IgA and J chain.[22] Recently, the 'littoral' and 'reticular' cells have also been shown to be strongly positive for acid phosphatase and β-glucuronidase, weakly positive for 5′-nucleotidase and negative for alkaline phosphatase.[23] These cells also contain cathepsin B, a marker for histiocytes.[24] Although there remain many gaps in our understanding of the interactions between immunocompetent cells and endothelial cells, it is now clear that these cells can significantly influence each others' development, growth, differentiation and function.[21]

ORIGIN OF HODGKIN AND REED–STERNBERG CELLS

Despite a considerable interest in the pathogenesis of Hodgkin's disease (HD) the true origin of H and RS cells is still unknown. Many different theories have been proposed. The more recent ones have related H and RS cells to B cells,[25–27] macrophages[28–32], dendritic reticulum cells,[33] interdigitating reticulum cells[34] or myelomonocytic precursor cells.[35] These conflicting theories of the origin of H and RS cells are further complicated by the suggestion that these cells may vary in type between one category of HD and another.[34,36,37] Moreover, Hansmann and Kaiserling[34] concluded from electron microscopic findings that H and RS cells might be derived from either immunoblasts, macrophages, or IDRC, and that it may be possible for H and RS cells of more than one derivation to be present in the same case.

Lymphoid cells

The concept of a lymphoid origin was based mainly on the detection of IgG in the cytoplasm of RS cells.[25–27] Additional studies have shown, however, that these cells contain both κ and λ chains,[38,39] whereas normal and neoplastic B cells contain either κ or λ but not both. Furthermore, H and RS cells consistently lack J chains.[30,32] It seems likely, therefore, that the intracytoplasmic immunoglobulin has been acquired from an exogenous source.[29,40] Ultrastructural studies have not confirmed this however, since electron microscope immunoperoxidase preparations have shown a cytoplasmic granular product not related to endocytic structures. This distribution has been interpreted as indicating both specific ribosomal synthesis[41,42] and non-specific leakage into the cell.[40] Stuart *et al.*[43] have recently reported positive staining of RS cells at the light and ultrastructural level with three monoclonal B cell antisera using the biotin-avidin immunochemical procedure. In addition the RS cells failed to react with a monoclonal anti-monocyte serum.

Macrophage cell

An origin from histiocytes for H and RS cells was based on morphological data and the finding that fluorescein-labelled IgG can be internalized by RS cells from the extracellular environment.[29] Other findings supporting a histiocytic origin were the trace production of lysozyme in long-term cultures of H and RS cells,[28] and uptake of Indian ink particles[28] and the detection of αl-antitrypsin.[31,32,44]

Dendritic reticulum cell

Curran and Jones[33] on the basis of the silver impregnation of H and RS cells proposed an origin from DRC of germinal centres, at least for the lymphocyte predominant nodular subtype of HD. Payne *et al.*[32] suggested that the uptake of immune complexes by RS cells may be considered as a deranged function of a particular macrophage subset that is involved in the uptake or handling of immune complex, a finding that is in keeping with the suggestion that RS cells are related to DRC. The results of Van Unnik[2] also point to a relation with DRC, although in the study of Naiem *et al.*[9] the H and RS cells failed to stain with a monoclonal antibody directed against follicular DRC.

Granulocytic cell

Of recent interest is the finding of a granulocytic cell-specific antigen on H and RS cells.[45] The presence of these antigens on H and RS cells in most cases of HD suggest that these cells are not heterogeneous, but homogeneous in origin and nature, at least in the majority of cases and the H and RS cells may be more closely related to cells of the granulocytic cell lineage than any other type of cell of the lymphoid system. Stein and his colleagues[46,47] have investigated this hypothesis with a panel of monoclonal antibodies reactive with cells of lymphoid and granulopoietic tissue. Their results showed that H and RS cells are devoid of markers specific or characteristic of B cells, macrophages, DRC, IDRC, or cells of erythropoietic or thrombopoietic origin. The vast majority of H and RS cells contain granulocyte-related antigens detectable with the monoclonal antibodies TÜ9 and 3C4 but consistently lack other granulocytic cell markers such as peroxidase and chloroacetate esterase.

Ki-1 cell

Monoclonal antibodies raised against a HD-derived cell line included one, Ki-1, that was found to be selectively reactive with H and RS cells and a small but distinct cell population in normal lymphoid tissue and bone marrow.[46,47] The latter, as yet unidentified, cell population appears to be the normal equivalent of H and RS cells.[46,47] These Ki-1 positive cells are located at the outer rim of the lymphocyte corona in reactive follicles and differed from that of all other known cell types. Ki-1 positive cells were also detected in smaller numbers in the B cell areas of the spleen, thymic medulla and bone marrow. These recent important antibody probes with the Ki-1 antibody have shed new light on the nature and origin of the elusive RS cell and will inevitably lead to a new era of research in unravelling the Hodgkin maze.

REFERENCES

1. Marshall AHE. A method for the demonstration of reticulo-endothelial cells in paraffin sections. *J Path Bact* 1948; **60:** 515–517.
2. Van Unnik JAM. The application of the metalophil method for the demonstration of histiocytes. *J Pathol* 1984; **144:** 233–239.
3. Van Unnik JAM, de Weger RA. Metalophil histiocytes in non-Hodgkin lymphomas particularly in

malignant proliferations of B-lymphocytes. *J Pathol* 1984; **144:** 241–251.

4. Lennert K. Malignant Lymphomas other than Hodgkin's Disease. Histology, Cytology, Ultrastructure, Immunology. Vol. 52. Berlin: Springer-Verlag, 1978 456–467.
5. Rademakers LHPM, Peters JPJ, Van Unnik JAM. Histiocytic and dendritic reticulum cells in follicular structures of follicular lymphoma and reactive hyperplasia: a quantitative electron microscopical analysis. *Virchows Arch B (Cell Path)* 1983; **44:** 85–98.
6. Thorbeck EGJ, Silberberg-Sinakin I, Flotte TJ. Langerhans cells as macrophages in skin and lymphoid organs. *J Invest Dermatol* 1980; **75:** 32–43.
7. Van Der Valk P, Te Velde J, Jansen J, Ruiter DJ, Spaander PJ, Cornelisse CJ, Meijer CJLM. Malignant lymphoma of true histiocytic origin: histiocytic sarcoma. A morphological, ultrastructural, immunological, cytochemical and clinical study of 10 cases. *Virchows Arch A (Pathol Anat)* 1981; **391:** 249–265.
8. Heusermann U, Zurborn K-H, Schroeder L, Stutte HJ. The origin of the dendritic reticulum cell. An experimental enzyme-histochemical and electron microscope study on the rabbit spleen. *Cell Tissue Res* 1980; **209:** 279–294.
9. Naiem M, Gerdes J, Abdulaziz Z, Stein H, Mason DY. Production of a monoclonal antibody reactive with human dendritic reticulum cells and its use in the immunohistochemical analysis of lymphoid tissue. *J Clin Pathol* 1983; **36:** 167–175.
10. Van Der Valk P, Van Der Loo EM, Jansen J, Daha MR, Meijer CJLM. Analysis of lymphoid and dendritic cells in human lymph node, tonsil and spleen. *Virchows Arch B (Cell Pathol)* 1984; **45:** 169–185.
11. Van Der Valk P, Ruiter DJ, Den Ottolander GJ, Te Velde J, Spaander PJ, Meijer CJLM. Dendritic reticulum cell sarcoma? Four cases of a lymphoma probably derived from dendritic reticulum cells of the follicular compartment. *Histopathology* 1982; **6:** 269–287.
12. Eikelenboom P. Characterization of non-lymphoid cells in the white pulp of the mouse spleen, an *in vivo* and *in vitro* study. *Cell Tiss Res* 1978; **195;** 445–460.
13. Stingl G, Tamaki K, Katz SI. Origin and function of epidermal Langerhans cells. *Immunol Rev* 1980; **53:** 149–174.
14. Silberberg-Sinakin I, Gigli I, Baer RL, Thorbecke GJ. Langerhans cells: role in contact hypersensitivity and relationship to lymphoid dendritic cells and to macrophages. *Immunol Rev* 1980; **53:** 203–232.
15. Friedman PS. The immunobiology of Langerhans cells. *Immonology Today* 1981; **2:** 124–128.
16. Drexhage HA, Mullink H, De Groot J, Clarke J, Balfour BM. A study of cells present in peripheral lymph of pigs with special reference to a type of cell resembling the Langerhans cell. *Cell Tiss Res* 1979; **202:** 407–430.
17. Dukor P, Bianco C, Nussenzweig V. Tissue localization of lymphocytes bearing a membrane receptor for antigen–antibody complement complexes. *Proc Natl Acad Sci* 1970; **67:** 991–997.
18. Takahashi K, Yamaguchi H. Ishizechi J, Nakajima T, Nakazato J. Immunohistochemical and immunoelectron microscopic locations of S-100 protein in the interdigitating reticulum cells of the human lymph node. *Virchows Arch B (Cell Pathol)* 1981; **37:** 125–135.
19. Nakajima T, Watanabe S, Sato Y, Shimosato Y, Motoi M, Lennert K. S-100 protein in Langerhans cells, interdigitating reticulum cells and histiocytosis cells. *Gann* 1982; **73:** 429–432.
20. Lauriola L, Michetti F, Stolfi VM, Tallini G, Cocchia D. Detection by S-100 immunolabelling of interdigitating reticulum cells in human thymomas. *Vichow Arch B (Cell Path)* 1984; **45:** 187–195.
21. Baldwin WM. The symbiosis of immunocompetent cells and endothelial cells. *Immunology Today* 1982; **3:** 267–269.
22. Curran RC, Jones EL. Intrasinusoidal cells in reactive lymph nodes. In: Levy E, ed. Advances in Pathology. Vol 1. Oxford: Pergamon, 1982: 349–352.
23. Crocker J, Williams M. An enzyme histochemical study of the sinuses of reactive lymph nodes. *J. Pathol* 1984; **142:** 31–38.
24. Crocker J, Burnett D, Jones EL. Immunohistochemical demonstration of Cathepsin B in the macrophages of benign and malignant lymphoid tissues. *J. Pathol* 1984; **142:** 87–94.
25. Kadin ME, Newcombe SR, Gold SB, Stites DP. Origin of Hodgkin's cells. *Lancet* 1974; **ii:** 167–168.
26. Boecker WR, Hossfeld DK, Gallmeiner WM, Schmidt CG. Clonal growth of Hodgkin's cells. *Nature* 1975; **258:** 235–236.
27. Taylor CR. An immunohistological study of follicular lymphoma, reticulum cell sarcoma and Hodgkin's disease. *Eur J Cancer* 1976; **12:** 61–75.
28. Kaplan HS, Gartner S. 'Sternberg–Reed' giant cells of Hodgkin's disease: cultivation *in vitro*, heterotransplantation, and characterization as neoplastic macrophages. *Int J Cancer* 1977; **19:** 511–525.
29. Kadin ME, Stites DP, Levy R, Warnke R. Exogenous immunoglobulin and the macrophage origin of Reed–Sternberg cells in Hodgkin's disease. *New England J Med* 1978; **299:** 1208–1214.
30. Isaacson P. Immunochemical demonstration of J chain: a marker of B-cell malignancy. *J Clin Pathol* 1979; **32:** 802–807.
31. Isaacson P, Wright DH. Anomolous staining patterns in immunohistologic studies of malignant lymphoma. *J Histochem Cytochem* 1979; **27:** 1197–1199.
32. Payne SV, Wright DH, Jones KJM, Judd MA. Macrophage origin of Reed–Sternberg cells: an immunohistochemical study. *J Clin Pathol* 1982; **35:** 159–166.

33. Curran RC, Jones EL. Hodgkin's disease: an immunohistochemical and histological study. *J Pathol* 1978; **125:** 39–51.
34. Hansmann ML, Kaiserling E. Electron microscpic aspects of Hodgkin's disease. *J Cancer Res Clin Oncol* 1981; **101:** 135–148.
35. Diehl V, Kirchner HH, Burrichter H, Stein H, Fonatsch C, Gerdes J, Schaadt M, Heit W, Uchanska-Ziegler B, Ziegler A, Heintz F, Suenko K. Characteristics of Hodgkins disease-derived cell lines. *Cancer Treat Rep* 1982; **66:** 615–632.
36. Poppema S, Kaiserling E, Lennert K. Hodgkins disease with lymphocyte predominance, nodular type (nodular paragranuloma) and progressively transformed centres, a cytochemical study. *Histopathology* 1979; **3:** 295–308.
37. Poppema S, Kaiserling E, Lennert K. Nodular paragranuloma and progressively transformed germinal centres, ultrastructural and immunohistologic findings. *Virchows Arch B (Cell Pathol)* 1979; **31:** 211–225.
38. Landaas TØ, Godal T, Halvorsen TB, Characterization of immunoglobulins in Hodgkin cells. *Int J Cancer* 1977; **20:** 717–722.
39. Mason DY, Stein H, Naiem M, Abdulaziz Z. Immunohistological analysis of human lymphoid tissue by double immunoenzymatic labelling. *J Cancer Res Clin Oncol* 1981; **101:** 13–22.
40. Poppema S, Elema JD, Hailie MR. The significance of intracytoplasmic proteins in Reed–Sternberg cells. *Cancer* 1978: **42:** 1793–1803.
41. Bernau D, Feldmann G, Vorhauer W. Hodgkin's disease: ultrastructural localization of intracytoplasmic immunoglobulins with malignant cells. *Br J Haematol* 1978; **40:** 51–57.
42. Reynes M, Paczynski V, Galtier M, Diebold J. Ultrastructural synthesis in tumour cells in Hodgkin's disease. *Int J Cancer* 1979; **23:** 474–481.
43. Stuart AE, Volsen SG, Zola H. The reactivity of Reed–Sternberg cells and monoclonal antisera at thin section and ultrastructural levels. *J Pathol* 1983; **141:** 71–82.
44. Poppema S. The diversity of immunohistological staining pattern of Sternberg–Reed cells. *J Histochem Cytochem* 1980; **28:** 788–791.
45. Stein H, Uchanska-Ziegler B, Gerdes J, Ziegler J, Wernet P. Hodgkin and Sternberg–Reed cells contain antigens specific to late cells of granulopoiesis. *Int J Cancer* 1982; **29:** 283–290.
46. Stein H, Gerdes J, Schwab U, Lemke H, Mason DY, Ziegler A, Schienle W, Diehl V. Identification of Hodgkin and Sternberg–Reed cells as a unique cell type derived from a newly-detected small cell population. *Int J Cancer* 1982; **30:** 445–459.
47. Stein H, Gerde SJ, Schwab H, Lemke H, Diehl V, Mason DY, Bartels H, Ziegler A. Evidence for the detection of the normal counterpart of Hodgkin and Sternberg–Reed cells. *Haematol Oncol* 1983; **1:** 21–29.

JOURNAL OF PATHOLOGY, VOL. **144**: 233–239 (1984)

THE APPLICATION OF THE METALOPHIL METHOD FOR THE DEMONSTRATION OF HISTIOCYTES

J. A. M. VAN UNNIK

Institute of Pathology, State University, Pasteurstraat 2, 3511 HX Utrecht, The Netherlands

Received 5 March 1984
Accepted 27 July 1984

SUMMARY

The metalophil method has been performed on 250 sections of a wide variety of inflammatory and neoplastic lesions in which different types of histiocytes might be encountered. In lymph nodes, dendritic histiocytes related to the B-lymphocyte system were consistently metalophil. They appeared as small cells with slender extensions in lymph nodes with follicular hyperplasia and/or sinus histiocytosis and in some cases of Hodgkin's lymphomas or as larger pleomorphic cells in primary or secondary malignancies of lymph nodes. Small, rounded cells were seen in some cases of marked paracortical reaction, in dermatopathic lymphadenitis and in some cases of mycosis fungoides. These cells most probably represented Langerhans cells and interdigitating reticulum cells, which are related to the T-lymphocyte system. Interdigitating cells become metalophil when they are activated or proliferating. Epithelioid cells in different benign and malignant lesions were metalophil like the sinus histiocytes of the lymph nodes, the Kupffer cells of the liver and the alveolar histiocytes in the lung. Foreign-body giant cells in lymph nodes after lymphography were also metalophil. The sinus lining cells lymph nodes were also well-delineated. Histiocytes of malignant histiocytic proliferations were sometimes metalophil as were the so-called histiocytes in malignant fibrous histiocytomas. Epithelial cells, particularly the basal cells of squamous epithelium often take up the silver. Carcinoma cells were sometimes metalophil and the method appeared not to be of value in the differentiation between metastatic carcinomas and lymphomas. The most promising application seems to be the study of the distribution of dendritic histiocytes in malignant proliferations of B-lymphocytes.

KEY WORDS—Metalophil method, histiocytes, dendritic reticulum cells, malignant lymphoma, Hodgkin's disease.

INTRODUCTION

The studies on the monocyte–macrophage system have recently expanded our knowledge of the different functional capabilities and morphological appearances of the cells commonly designated as histiocytes. It is shown that cells widely different in localization, function and morphology may be considered as different expressions of histiocytes. These cells have in all probability a common bone marrow derived precursor. There is strong evidence pointing to the same monocytic origin for Kupffer cells in the liver, alveolar histiocytes in lungs, Langerhans cells in the skin, sinus histiocytes in lymph nodes and at least a part of the variety of so-called reticulum cells of the lymph nodes.[1]

The concept of the histiocyte as a typical phagocytic scavenger cell is complemented by its role as an intermediate for capturing and preparing antigens at the initiation of the lymphocyte immune reaction. The intimate connections between histiocytes and lymphocytes are now well-established both functionally and morphologically.[2,3]

In 1948 Marshall described a metalophil method for 'the demonstration of reticuloendothelial cells in paraffin sections.'[4] Curran and Jones[5,6] demonstrated with the aid of this method the presence of different kinds of metalophil cells in Hodgkins and non-Hodgkins lymphomas.

The aim of this study is to explore the staining properties of different types of histiocytes with the metalophil method and the possible staining of other tissue components which might interfere with the interpretation of the results with this method.

0022–3417/84/120233–07$01.00

MATERIAL AND METHODS

Paraplast-embedded material of 250 cases of a great variety of reactive and malignant lymphoid and nonlymphoid lesions was available. These cases were obtained from different sources. Thirty-eight cases were obtained from the trials on non-Hodgkin lymphomas of the European Organization for Reseärch on Treatment of Cancer (EORTC), 29 cases were referred to the author for consultation and 183 cases originated from the Academic Hospital in Utrecht. According to the different origins of this material the fixation and embedding procedures varied. The specimens from the Academic Hospital were fixed in buffered formalin or in a mixture of acetic acid 5 per cent, alcohol 75 per cent, concentrated formaldehyde solution 20 per cent. For the metalophil method some specimens were fixed in a mixture consisting of 6 per cent macrodex dissolved in 0·9 per cent sodium chloride solution: 8 parts, concentrated formaldehyde solution: 1 part, 1 per cent calcium chloride solution: 1 part.

All cases were routinely stained with haematoxylin and eosin, Giemsa, methyl green pyronin, PAS, and Gordon and Sweet's method for reticulin. The staining for metalophil cells was performed according to Katsura *et al.*[7] After completion of this study we employed the original method of Marshall[4], which gave identical results and is less cumbersome. The following diagnostic categories were studied.

Normal reactive lymph nodes often with some degree of follicular hyperplasia and/or sinus histiocytosis 55; lymph nodes with a marked paracortical reaction 3; lymph nodes showing the effect of lymphography 3; lymph nodes with sarcoidosis 7; lymph nodes with tuberculosis 2; lymph nodes with cat scratch disease 2; lymph nodes with toxoplasmosis 2; dermatopathic lymphadenitis 7; metastatic carcinoma in lymph nodes 12; Hodgkin's disease 15; non-Hodgkin lymphomas 125; angioimmunoblastic lymphadenopathy 1; malignant histiocytosis 5; thymoma 3; encephalomalacia with mast cells 1; malignant fibrous histiocytoma 4; liver tissue 2; seminoma 1.

RESULTS

Different types of histiocytes

In normal reactive lymph nodes with follicular hyperplasia and/or sinus histiocytosis, small metalophil cells with slender branching extensions were typically seen in the germinal centre and at the periphery of the follicles (Fig. 1). Sometimes these dendritic histiocytes, as they were termed by Curran and Jones[5] were more numerous at the periphery of the follicles, and sometimes more numerous in the centre. In the interfollicular tissue some of these dendritic histiocytes were present in varying numbers.

'Starry sky' macrophages in the follicles took up the stain inconsistently. Especially when they had a large amount of pale cytoplasm, they were hardly impregnated. In those cases they could often be recognized by the chromatin particles in their cytoplasm (*vide infra*). Smaller histiocytic reticulum cells in the follicles could be differentiated from the dendritic histiocytes by their more rounded form and lack of dendritic processes.

The cytoplasm of sinus histiocytes was readily stained by this method (Fig. 1) and the sinuses clearly delineated. The same degree of cytoplasmic staining was shown by foreign-body giant cells seen in lymph nodes following lymphography (Fig. 2). The nuclei of these multinucleated cells appeared as clear holes in the dark-stained cytoplasm. Mast cells in the neighbourhood of encephalomalacia took up the silver particles in the same way. Kupffer cells in the liver were strongly metalophil (Fig. 3).

Epithelioid cells were equally well seen. This held true for the different types of these cells seen in close proximity to the necrosis in cat scratch disease and tuberculosis, in toxoplasmosis, sarcoidosis (Fig. 4) and in the diffuse infiltrations of these cells as seen in a case of angioimmunoblastic lymphadenopathy and in non-Hodgkins lymphomas.

Langerhans cells of the skin were not well demonstrated as especially the lower layers of squamous epithelium were prone to be stained by the metalophil method (*vide infra*). The histiocytes present in dermatopathic lymphadenitis[8,9] were visible as dark staining rounded cells in 4 of the 7 cases of this lesion (Fig. 5). As distinct from dendritic histiocytes these cells had only very short cytoplasmic extensions or lacked them altogether. Besides some widely dispersed dendritic histiocytes no other metalophil cells were commonly present in the paracortical areas. However, in one case of marked paracortical reaction representing increased T-cell activity many rounded positive cells were seen in the enlarged paracortical areas.

Three cases of mycosis fungoides were examined, two occurring in the skin and one on a lymph node. In these lesions rounded dark-staining cells were seen resembling the cells in marked paracortical

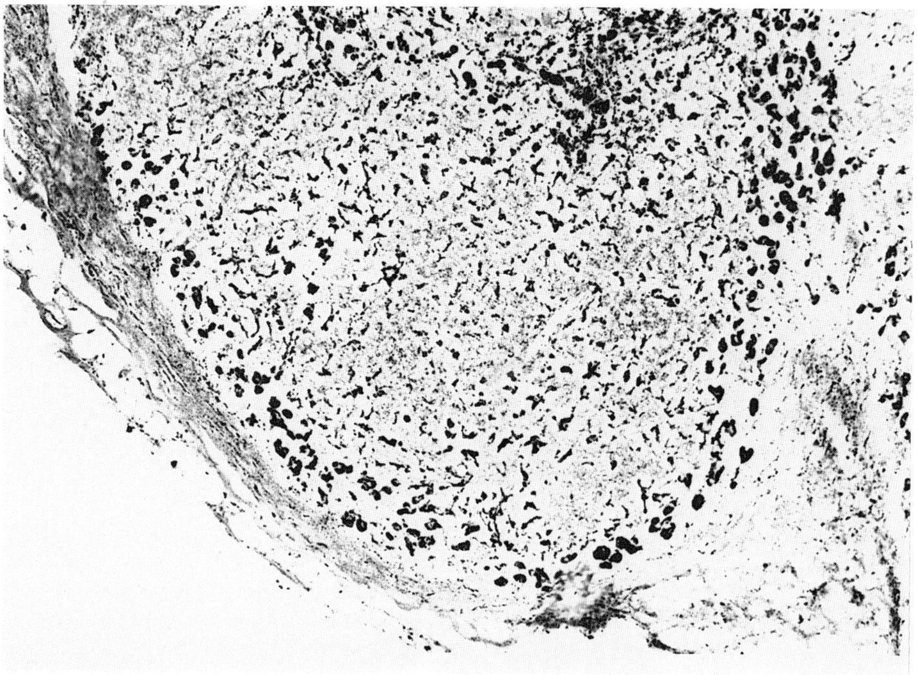

Fig. 1—Reactive lymph node showing a follicle and marginal sinus. The slender dendritic histiocytes contrast with the more rounded sinus histiocytes. The fibrous capsule is slightly impregnated by this method. × 125

reactions and dermatopathic lymphadenitis (Fig. 6). The same type of histiocyte was seen in a Lennert lymphoma which proved to be a T-cell lymphoma. One unclassifiable lymphoma consisted of small T-lymphocytes intermingled with histiocytes which electron microscopically were like the rather ill-defined 'dark reticulum cells'.[10,11] This type of histiocyte was clearly metalophil.

Dendritic histiocytes in varying shape and number were present in other non-Hodgkin lymphomas. Their relation with the different entities of the Kiel classification is described elsewhere.[12]

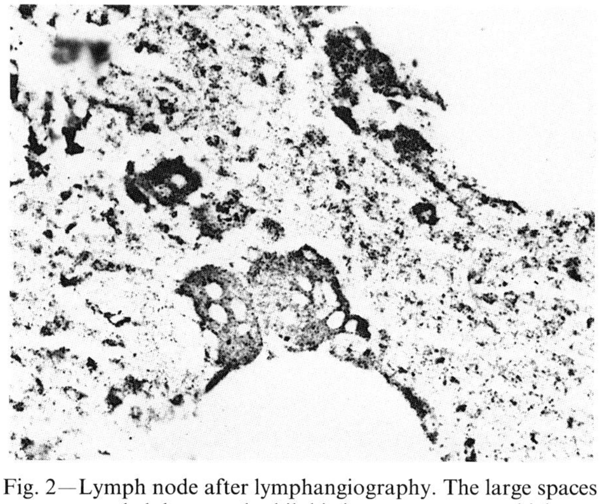

Fig. 2—Lymph node after lymphangiography. The large spaces are surrounded by metalophil histiocytes, among which are multinucleated giant cells. × 300

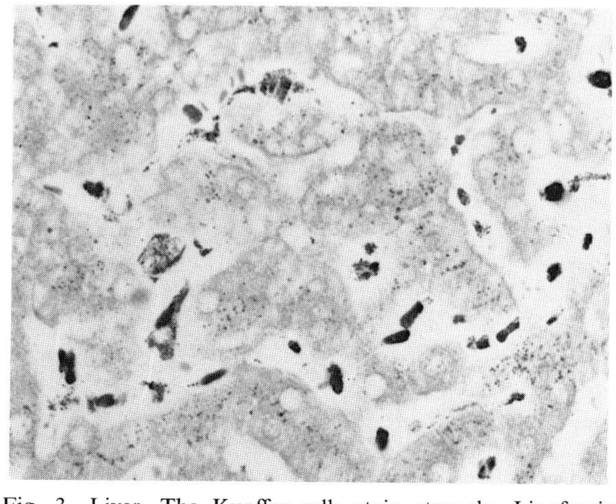

Fig. 3—Liver. The Kupffer cells stain strongly. Lipofuscin granules also take up the silver precipitate. × 300

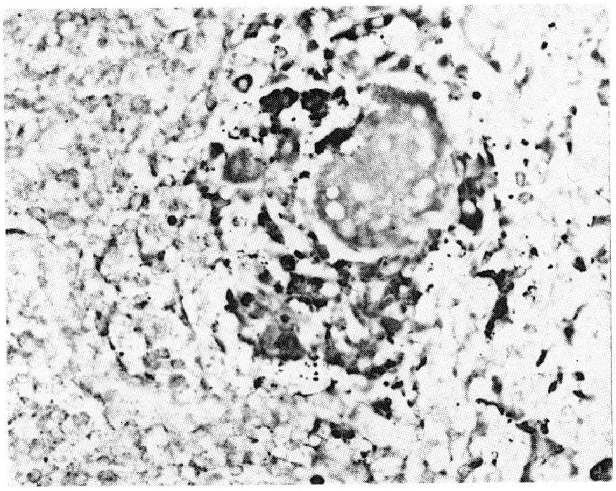

Fig. 4—Lymph node; sarcoidosis. Focus of metalophil epithelioid cells and a Langhans giant cell. × 300

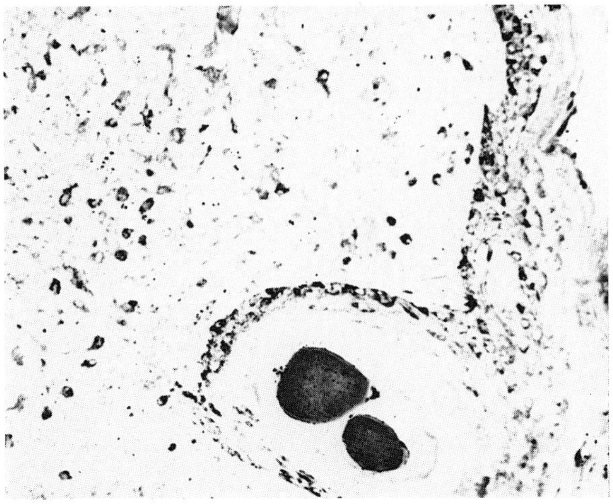

Fig. 6—Skin; mycosis fungoides. Scanty metalophil cells are present. These cells are rounded and generally devoid of dendrites. Note the clear holes in many of these cells, representing the nuclei. The basal layers of the squamous epithelium and keratin are metalophil. × 125

In all cases of Hodgkin's disease large and atypical branching metalophil cells were seen. These cells were present in the different Rye subtypes of Hodgkin's disease, i.e. lymphocyt predominance 4; nodular sclerosis 5; mixed cellularity 5; lymphocytic depletion 1. Some of these cells were very large and bizarre with short and plump dendritic metalophil cytoplasmic processes. Sometimes the dendrites were almost absent. Unstained nuclei appeared as holes in the dark stained cytoplasm, and some showed the typical mirror-image nucleus of Sternberg–Reed giant cells. Other pleomorphic metalophil cells with dendrites of varying length and number represented in all probability variants of Sternberg–Reed and Hodgkin cells. The large and very pleomorphic cells present in lymphocytic depletion type of Hodgkin's disease were clearly metalophil (Fig. 7).

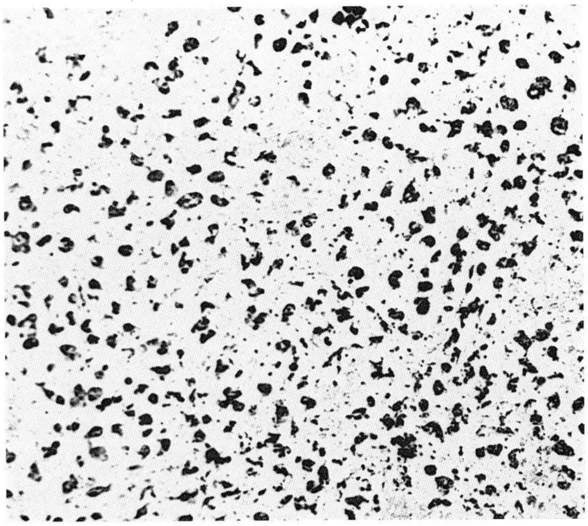

Fig. 5—Lymph node; dermatopathic lymphadenitis. In the interfollicular area many metalophil cells are visible resembling the metalophil cells in the skin in mycosis fungoides. × 125

Sections of malignant histiocytosis showed divergent results. Two of the five lesions examined presented strongly metalophil histiocytes, two other cases were negative in this respect. One case was repeatedly uninterpretable because of coarse silver deposition.

In five of the 12 cases of metastatic carcinoma in lymph nodes large atypical dendritic histiocytes were seen between the foci of carcinoma cells (Fig. 8). In seven cases no histiocytic reaction was found.

In three of the four soft tissue sarcomas diagnosed as malignant fibrous histiocytomas (MFH) the histiocyte-like cells were metalophil (Fig. 9). One of these cases, diagnosed as MFH with osteoclast-like giant cells, contained multinucleated giant cells with metalophil cytoplasm comparable to the cytoplasm of foreign-body giant cells.

Non-histiocytic cells and extra-cellular tissue components

In skin sections the cells of the squamous epithelium and in particular the cells of the basal layers took up the silver precipitate (Fig. 6). The same was seen in well-differentiated squamous cell car-

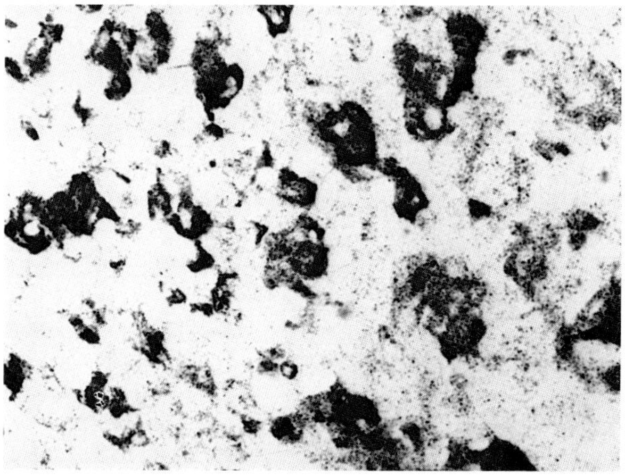

Fig. 7—Lymph node; Hodgkin's disease, lymphocytic depletion. The pleomorphic Sternberg–Reed cells and their variants are strongly metalophil. × 300

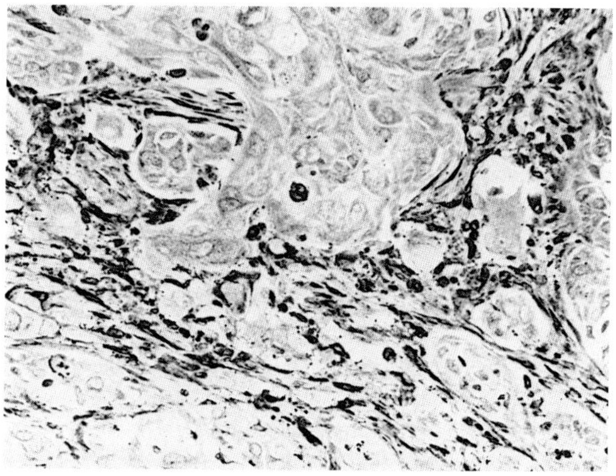

Fig. 8—Lymph node; metastatic squamous carcinoma. Between the carcinoma cells, elongated, pleomorphic and seemingly compressed dendritic histiocytes are present. × 125

cinoma. Adenocarcinoma and undifferentiated carcinoma cells were in some cases positive and in others completely negative. The tumour cells of a seminoma were negative.

In especially heavy stained sections condensed chromatin was impregnated, e.g. the nuclei of small lymphocytes and more often the chromatin particles in the cytoplasm of 'starry sky' macrophages. Reticulin and collagen fibres were occasionally impregnated in intensely-stained preparations and also the endothelial lining of blood- and lymph-vessels. Keratin present in the stratum corneum of the skin and in hairs took up the silver precipitate (Fig. 6).

DISCUSSION

Curran and Jones[5] stated that 'the metalophil method has a strong affinity for cells of the reticuloendothelial system'. Other cells and structures that may exhibit some metalophilia never give rise to serious difficulties in interpretation. In accordance with Curran and Jones two points merit special attention. Badly fixed preparations may give rise to a coarse granular precipitate that prevents proper interpretation. Thin sections are generally not satisfactory and if one wants to demonstrate dendritic structures sections of at least 10 μm are required. In addition, it is important that in the preparation of the sections the glasswork has to be cleaned with meticulous care. Sometimes despite all precautions and without reason the sections were uninterpretable because of unexpected silver precipitation.

Epithelioid cells in widely different lesions are consistently metalophil. Generally they are easily recognized by their relatively abundant cytoplasm and their affinity for the silver precipitate. Their cytoplasm is well-circumscribed and cytoplasmic extensions are usually not present but, in some cases of non-Hodgkin lymphoma with infiltration of epithelioid cells and in a case of tuberculous lymphadenitis, the epithelioid cells presented definite cytoplasmic dendrites of varying length. Curran and Jones[5] described dendritic extensions in epithelioid cells present in Hodgkin's disease.

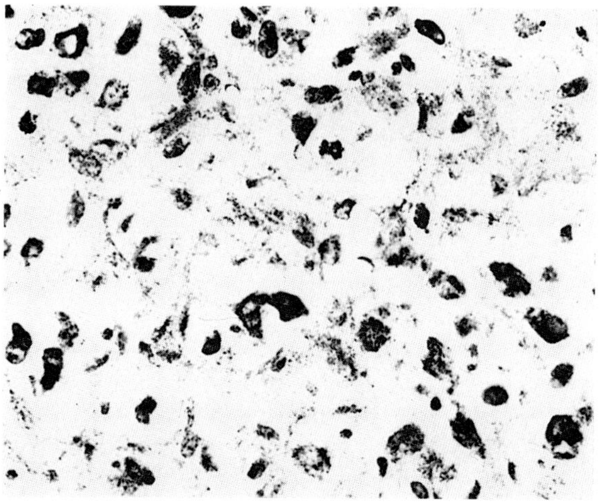

Fig. 9—Malignant fibrous histiocytoma. The histiocyte-like cells in this soft tissue sarcoma are strongly metalophil. × 300

The dendritic histiocytes make up a second group of consistently metalophil cells in lymph nodes. In all 55 reactive lymph nodes, often with some degree of follicular hyperplasia and/or sinus histiocytosis, conspicuous dendritic histiocytes were present in the follicles. In some reactive lymph nodes and some non-Hodgkin lymphomas they are small with slender dendrites. In other non-Hodgkin lymphomas and in metastatic lesions they may be large with coarse dendritic structures. As noted by Curran and Jones[5] the cells at the periphery of the follicles tend to be arranged with their long axes parallel to the circumference of the follicles. These dendritic histiocytes are confined to those areas of the lymph node which are predominantly populated by B-lymphocytes. It is tempting to hypothesize that they correspond with the dendritic reticulum cell or 'long-branching non-phagocytosing reticulum cell' which is a specific cell of the B-lymphocyte region and accordingly found in large numbers in germinal centres. On the ultrastructural level it can be seen that the cytoplasm of these cells interdigitates between the centroblasts and centrocytes as very fine interwoven processes[3]. Eikelenboom[13] studied the metalophil cells in rat spleen follicles with a combination of immunoenzyme histochemistry and enzyme histochemistry. He concluded that at least 'a number of branched metalophils are indeed dendritic cells'. Slender elongated metalophil cells at the periphery of follicles may represent fibroblastic reticulum cells as described by Curran *et al.*[14]

Interdigitating reticulum cells which are more rounded and lack cytoplasmic dendrites are typically found in the paracortical areas and are functionally connected with T-lymphocytes.[9] Metalophil cells are notably absent in these areas other than widely dispersed dendritic histiocytes. This is in agreement with Curran and Jones[5] who mention the absence of metalophil histiocytes in the T-region of the tonsil. The presence, however, of small rounded metalophil cells in the interfollicular tissue of a lymph node with a marked paracortical reaction makes it probable that under certain circumstances interdigitating cells may be demonstrated by the metalophil method.

Langerhans cells and interdigitating reticulum cells are closely related; they share many submicroscopic features[8] and the enzyme cytochemical patterns of both cell types are similar.[8,15,16] The metalophilia of Langerhans cells in the skin is difficult to evaluate because of the marked metalophilia of the basal layers. A characteristic finding in dermatopathic lymphadenitis is the expansion of the paracortical areas with a marked increase of interdigitating cells.[9] Langerhans cells are also regularly found in these lesions.[8] The accumulation of rather small rounded metalophil cells as seen in some of these lesions represent in all probability the increased numbers of interdigitating reticulum cells and possibly Langerhans cells.

According to Veldman and Kaiserling[9] interdigitating reticulum cells are an integral part of T-cell lymphomas of low grade malignancy such as mycosis fungoides. The presence of metalophil cells in two out of three cases of mycosis fungoides and in a case of a T-type Lennert lymphoma is in agreement with this view. These metalophil cells are morphologically similar to the cells found in the lymph node with marked paracortical reaction and in dermatopathic lymphadenitis. In all probability, interdigitating reticulum cells in an activated state may become metalophil.

The staining of the tumour cells in malignant histiocytosis is too inconsistent to be of diagnostic value. The metalophil cells in these lesions, if present, are rounded and rather well circumscribed without extensions.

Phagocytic cells such as foreign body giant cells, cells around foci of encephalomalacia and Kupffer cells are metalophil. However, not all phagocytic histiocytes take up the silver. The 'starry sky' macrophage, especially if it has a very pale cytoplasm, is definitely not metalophil in our hands. In agreement with the findings of Curran *et al.*[14] rounded metalophil histiocytic reticulum cells are often found in the basal part of the follicles. In the sinuses of lymph nodes, particularly in cases of sinus histiocytosis, numerous metalophil cells may be found. They have slender extensions and belong to the intrasinusoidal reticulum cells.[17] According to Curran *et al.* 'large and very actively phagocytic fixed macrophages' in the sinus are not metalophil.

The metalophilia of the histiocyte-like cells in malignant fibrous histiocytoma is noteworthy but the rather low degree of specificity of this method does not allow further conclusions about the nature of these cells.

This method did not prove to be of value in differentiating between anaplastic carcinoma and lymphoma. The cells of anaplastic carcinoma may be completely negative, sometimes they are metalophil like the large pleomorphic dendritic histiocytes which may be present between the carcinoma cells. The proliferation of these dendritic histiocytes as is seen in some lymph nodes with metastatic carcinoma, is in all probability a response to the malignant cells. Similar dendritic histiocytes are found in some categories of non-Hodgkin's lymphomas[12] and in Hodgkin's disease. In Hodgkin's disease even larger and more pleomorphic cells may be encountered. They appear to represent, at least partly, the Sternberg–Reed and Hodgkin cells[5] and they merge gradually with the pleomorphic large dendritic histiocytes which are also found as a reactive component.

The consistent metalophilia of dendritic histiocytes which are typically associated with the B-lymphocyte system provides the opportunity to study the presence and morphology of these histiocytes in malignant proliferations of B-lymphocytes.

ACKNOWLEDGEMENTS

This study was supported by the Netherlands Cancer Foundation (Koningin Wilhelmina Fonds, KWF). The author likes to thank Mrs Sri Tan-Ranoewisastro for the great care with which she developed the metalophil method; Mr E. Dumernit for preparing the photographs; and Mrs Christina Oprel for the efficient typing of the manuscript.

REFERENCES

1. Van Furth R. Cells of the mononuclear phagocyte system; nomenclature in terms of sites and conditions. In: van Furth R, ed. Mononuclear Phagocytes. Functional Aspects, Vol. 1. The Hague: Nijhoff Publishers, 1980; 1.
2. Carr I, Daems WT. The macrophage, a bird's-eye view. In: Carr I, Daems WT, eds. The Reticuloendothelial System, Vol. 1. Morphology. New York and London: Plenum Press, 1980; 8.
3. Müller-Hermelink HK, Lennert K. In: Lennert K, ed. Malignant Lymphomas other than Hodgkin's Disease. Berlin, Heidelberg, New York: Springer Verlag, 1978; 59–65.
4. Marshall AHE. A method for the demonstration of reticuloendothelial cells in paraffin sections. *J Path Bact* 1948; **60:** 513.
5. Curran RC, Jones EL. Hodgkin's disease: an immunohistochemical and histological study. *J Path* 1978; **125:** 39.
6. Curran RC, Jones EL. Non-Hodgkin's lymphomas: an immunohistochemical and histological study. *J Path* 1979; **129:** 179.
7. Katsura S, Satodate R, Fukuda Y, Terni Y. Morphological studies on the reticuloendothelial system in tumor-bearing hosts. 1. Silver impregnation for reticuloendothelial cells. *J Iwate Med Ass* 1964; **16,** 232.
8. Rausch E, Kaiserling E, Goos M. Langerhans cells and interdigitating reticulum cells in the thymus-dependent region in human dermatopathic lymphadenitis. *Virch Arch B* 1977; **25:** 327.
9. Veldman JE, Kaiserling E. In: Carr I, Daems WT, eds. The Reticulo-endothelial System, Vol. 1. Morphology. New York and London: Plenum Press, 1980; 381.
10. Izard J, De Harven E. Increased numbers of characteristic type of reticular cells in the thymus and lymph nodes of leukemic mice. An electron microscopic study. *Cancer Res* 1968; **28:** 421.
11. Mollo F, Monga G, Stramignoni A. Dark reticular cells in human lymphadenitis and lymphomas. *Virch Arch B* 1969; **3:** 117.
12. Van Unnik JAM, De Weger RA. Metalophilic histiocytes in non-Hodgkin lymphomas particularly in malignant proliferations of B-lymhpocytes. *J Path* 1984; **144:** 241–251.
13. Eikelenboom P. Dendritic cells in the rat spleen follicles. *Cell Tiss Res* 1978; **190:** 79.
14. Curran RC, Gregory J, Jones EL. The distribution of immunoglobulin and other plasma proteins in human reactive lymph nodes. *J Path* 1982; **136:** 307.
15. Kaiserling E, Lennert K. Die interdigiterende retikulumzelle im menslichen lymphknoten. Eine spezifische zelle der thymus-abhängigen region. *Virch Arch B* 1974; **16:** 51.
16. Elema JD, Poppema S. Infantile histiocytosis X (Letterer-Siwe disease). Investigations with enzyme-histochemical and sheep-erythrocyte rosetting techniques. *Cancer* 1978; **42:** 555.
17. Curran RC, Jones EL. Intrasinusoidal cells in reactive human lymph nodes. In: Levy F, ed. Advances in Pathology (Anatomic and Clinical). Oxford: Pergamon Press, Vol. 1, 1982; 349–352.

JOURNAL OF PATHOLOGY, VOL. **144**: 241–251 (1984)

METALOPHIL HISTIOCYTES IN NON-HODGKIN'S LYMPHOMAS PARTICULARLY IN MALIGNANT PROLIFERATIONS OF B-LYMPHOCYTES

J. A. M. VAN UNNIK AND R. A. DE WEGER

Institute of Pathology, State University, Pasteurstraat 2, 3511 HX Utrecht, The Netherlands

Received 5 March 1984
Accepted 27 July 1984

SUMMARY

The metalophil method for the demonstration of histiocytes was applied to 108 non-Hodgkin lymphomas diagnosed according to the Kiel classification. In 41 lymphomas the presence of histiocytes was assessed with the aid of the non-specific esterase reaction. The same procedures were performed on 12 lymph nodes with follicular hyperplasia and/or sinus histiocytosis. The number of histiocytes was estimated and graded from 0 to 3. A good correlation between the two methods was found. Dendritic histiocytes were typically absent in lymphocytic lymphomas (CLL type). The follicles were clearly delineated by the distribution of dendritic histiocytes in follicular centroblastic/centrocytic lymphomas. In diffuse centrocytic lymphomas a small to moderate number of slender dendritic histiocytes was seen (grades 1–2). In lymphoplasmacytic/lymphoplasmacytoid lymphomas and in diffuse centroblastic/centrocytic malignant lymphoma the majority showed a great number of pleomorphic dendritic histiocytes (grade 3). In high-grade malignant lymphomas (centroblastic, immunoblastic and lymphoblastic categories) either a high to moderate number of pleomorphic dendritic histiocytes was found or they were totally absent. The lack of histiocytes in centroblastic lymphomas was especially noteworthy. It is proposed that dendritic histiocytes proliferate or are attracted in malignant lymphomas by the presence of centrocytes, especially in combination with centroblasts and by the presence of plasmacytoid cells or their precursors. The frequent absence of dendritic histiocytes in high-grade malignant lymphomas may alternatively be explained by the loss of physiological properties in less differentiated cells.

KEY WORDS—Malignant lymphomas, metalophil histiocytes, dendritic histiocytes.

INTRODUCTION

With the development of immunological techniques the characterization of lymphoid cells in their different functional states has become possible. Based on the understanding of the different types of lymphocytes such as B- and T-lymphocytes and their morphological expressions during maturation and function, new concepts have evolved regarding the classification of non-Hodgkin lymphomas. They have in common the conception that neoplastic lymphoid cells are more or less fixed in a certain functional state. In this respect the Lukes and Collins classification[1–3] and the Kiel classification[4] have to be mentioned. In our opinion the cell types of the entities in the Kiel classification reflect more closely their physiological counterparts regarding terminology and definition.[5] In recent years it has become apparent that the lymphocytes in their different stages of modulation are intimately connected, structurally as well as functionally, to histiocytes. In this way, T-lymphocytes in the paracortical zone of the lymph node are related to a type of histiocyte designated as interdigitating reticulum cell[6] whereas B-lymphocytes in their stage of follicle centre cells are related to the so-called dendritic reticulum cells. The term 'microecology' reflects the mutual dependence of lymphocytes and histiocytes in the microenvironment of the lymph node.[7,8] If the con-

0022–3417/84/120241–11$01.10

cept of the functional classifications of non-Hodgkin lymphomas is valid, differences in type or pattern of histiocytes in these malignant lymphomas may be encountered.

The aim of this study is to explore the relations of dendritic histiocytes in the different entities of the Kiel classification with particular reference to the functional qualities of the lymphoma cells in the hope that this approach may be of help in defining these entities.

MATERIAL AND METHODS

The material consisted of 108 non-Hodgkin lymphomas and 12 reactive lymph nodes from a total of 250 cases in which the metalophil method was employed as described in a previous study.[9] In 49 non-Hodgkin lymphomas and 12 reactive nodes a histochemical method was used for the demonstration of histiocytes. Blocks of tissue from these cases were quenched in liquid nitrogen for the preparation of cryostat sections. The sections (6 μm thick) were reacted for non-specific esterase activity according to Yam *et al.*[10] Thirty-two of the 120 cases were available from the trials on non-Hodgkin lymphomas of the European Organization for Research on Treatment of Cancer (EORTC), 29 were referred for consultation and 59 originated from the Academic Hospital in Utrecht. Sections were routinely stained with haematoxylin and eosin, Giemsa, methyl green pyronin, PAS and Gordon and Sweet's method for reticulin.

The lymphomas were diagnosed according to the Kiel classification. The number of histiocytes revealed by the metalophil method was expressed by four grades: grade 0 no metalophil cells present, grade 1 a few cells visible, grade 2 a moderate number and grade 3 a large number present (Figs. 1–3). The sections stained for metalophil cells were studied without prior knowledge of the diagnosis. The same gradation was used for the number of non-specific esterase positive cells (Figs. 4–6).

RESULTS

In the non-Hodgkin lymphomas studied, two types of dendritic cells were found: small regular cells with delicate dendritic structures and large pleomorphic cells with irregular dendrites. As well as three dendritic histiocytes, in some cases a varying number of phagocytic histiocytes and epithelioid cells were seen. They were distinguishable from the dendritic cells by their abundant cytoplasm and lack of dendrites.

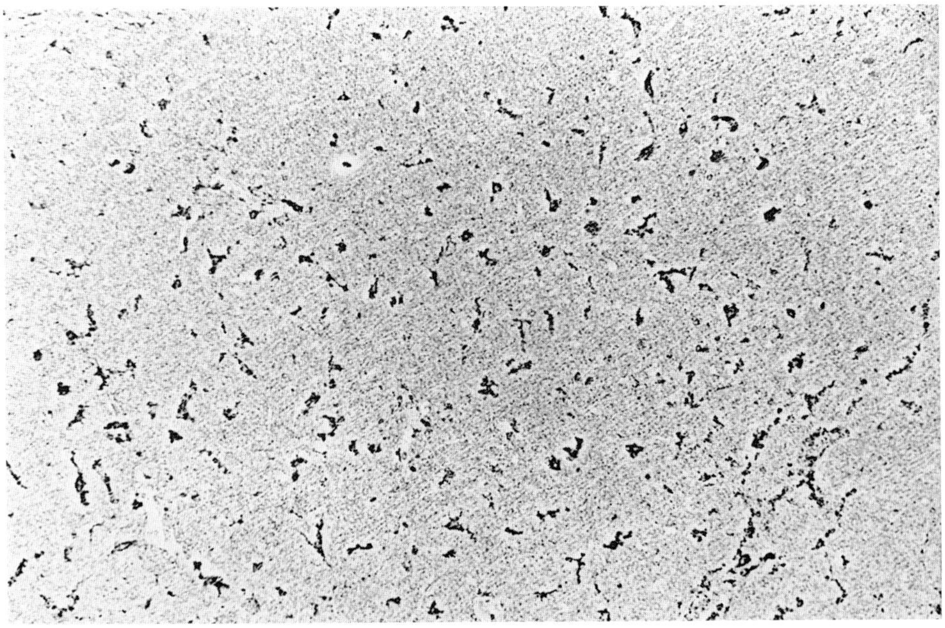

Fig. 1—Centrocytic lymphoma. Small numbers of metalophil dendritic histiocytes (grade 1) are present. These histiocytes are small with slender cytoplasmic dendrites. × 125

Malignant lymphoma: lymphocytic

Lymph nodes from 13 patients showed the appearances of lymphocytic lymphoma. They were composed of a monotonous infiltrate of small lymphocytes with round dark nuclei and granular karyoplasm. A small rim of cytoplasm surrounded the nuclei. A varying number of so-called 'para-

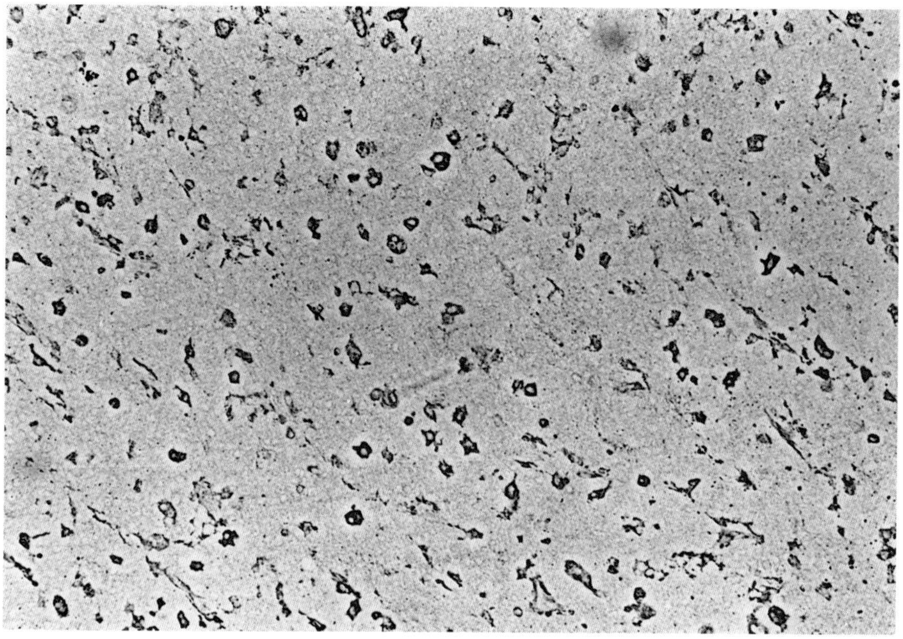

Fig. 2—Prolymphocytic lymphoma. Moderate numbers of metalophil dendritic histiocytes (grade 2) are present. × 125

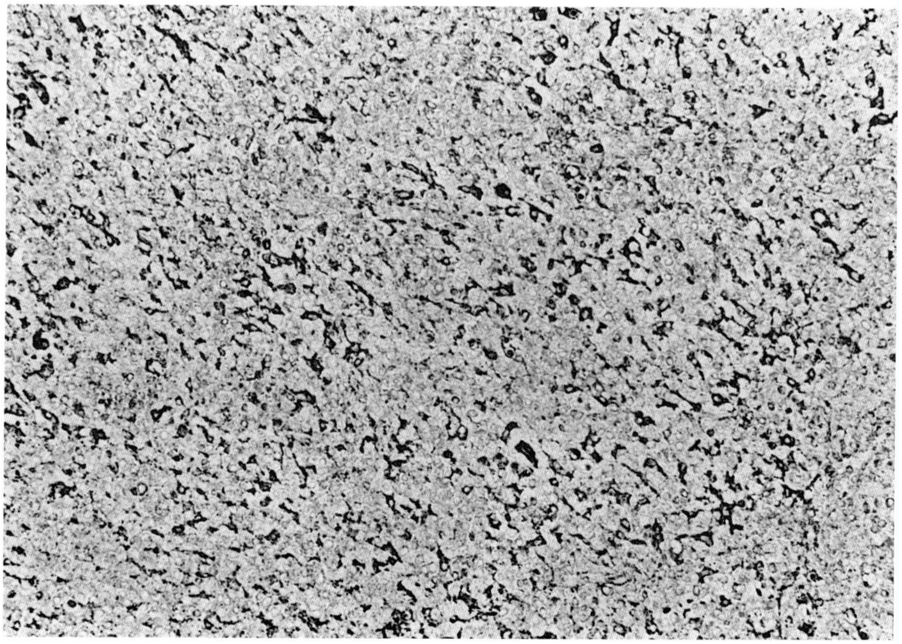

Fig. 3—Centrocytic lymphoma. Large numbers of metalophil dendritic histiocytes (grade 3) are seen. The histiocytes are not very pleomorphic. × 125

immunoblasts', with larger and paler nuclei and centrally placed nucleoli were regularly present. Clinically the diagnosis of chronic lymphocytic leukaemia was made in all cases. In 10 cases metalophil cells were not present. In one case a residual pattern was present with metalophil sinus histiocytes. A few small groups of dendritic histiocytes were visible in another case. The pattern sug-

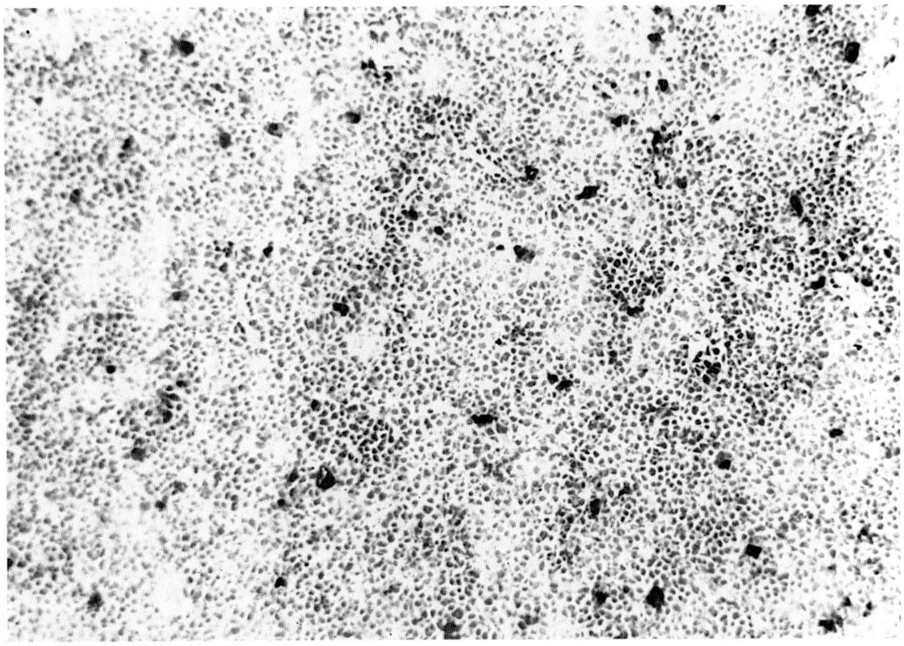

Fig. 4—Centrocytic lymphoma. Small numbers of non-specific esterase positive histiocytes (grade 1) are seen. × 125

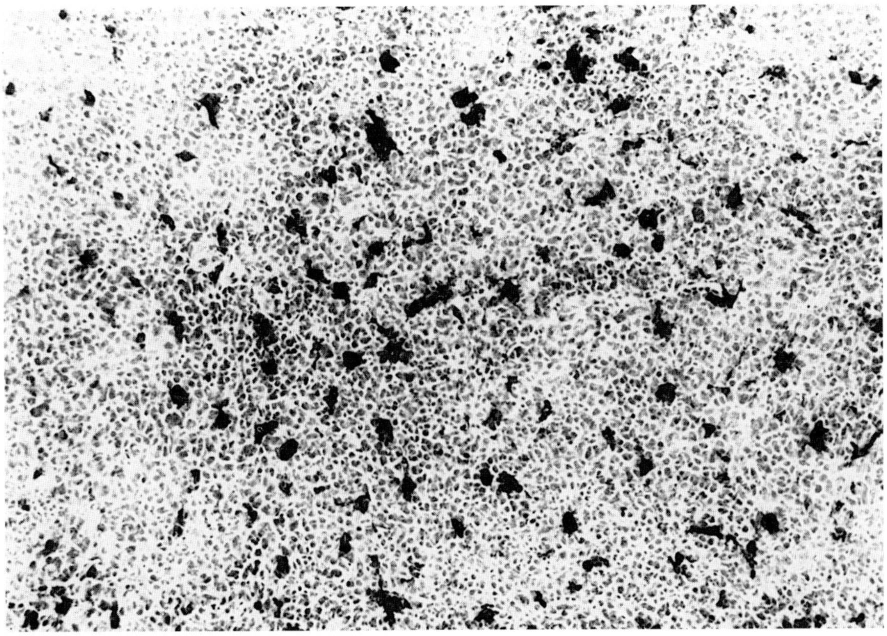

Fig. 5—Centroblastic/centrocytic lymphoma, diffuse. Moderate numbers of non-specific esterase positive histiocytes (grade 2) are seen. × 125

gested local remnants of pre-existing lymph node tissue. One section was interpreted as a lymph node with largely unimpaired architecture, locally infiltrated by a lymphocytic lymphoma. The metalophil staining revealed a normal pattern of sinus histiocytes and dendritic histiocytes outlining the intact follicles. Where the infiltration of the lymphoma cells was seen in the H and E and Giemsa stained sections, only some widely dispersed delicate dendritic histiocytes, noted as grade 1, were found.

In one patient a second lymph node was biopsied 2 years later, because of progressive generalized lymph node enlargement. The first node section was devoid of metalophil cells, the second biopsy section revealed in the H and E and Giemsa preparations a proliferation of large pleomorphic cells, typical of an evolution towards Richter's syndrome.[11] In the latter section a moderate number (grade 2) of metalophil dendritic histiocytes was found.

In contrast one lymphoma consisting of small lymphocytic cells with regular round nuclei containing one centrally placed tiny nucleolus surrounded by a narrow rim of cytoplasm was found. This was interpreted as the prolymphocytic variant of the lymphocytic type.[12] In this node a modest number of delicate dendritic histiocytes (grade 2) was found. Enzyme histochemistry was performed on 10 of these lymphomas. In seven no histiocytes were demonstrated, two contained a small number and one a moderate number of non-specific esterase positive histiocytes. The prolymphocytic lymphoma was classified as grade 1. It is noteworthy that the first lymph node biopsy of the patient who developed incipient Richter's syndrome after 2 years was the only one classified as grade 2, the second lymph node of this patient was classified as grade 1.

Malignant lymphoma: lymphoplasmacytic/ lymphoplasmacytoid (immunocytoma)

Fourteen lymphomas belonged to this category. The diagnosis was based on the presence of lymphocytes and plasmacytoid cells. In nine of these lesions a large number of dendritic histiocytes was seen (grade 3), in three cases a moderate number (grade 2) was present. The dendritic histiocytes were generally large and pleomorphic. In three the pattern of the dendritic histiocytes outlined follicular structures which were not evident in the H and E, Giemsa, or reticulin stained sections. In two no metalophil cells were found.

Eight of the 13 lymphomas of this category on which enzyme histochemical data were available contained many non-specific esterase positive cells,

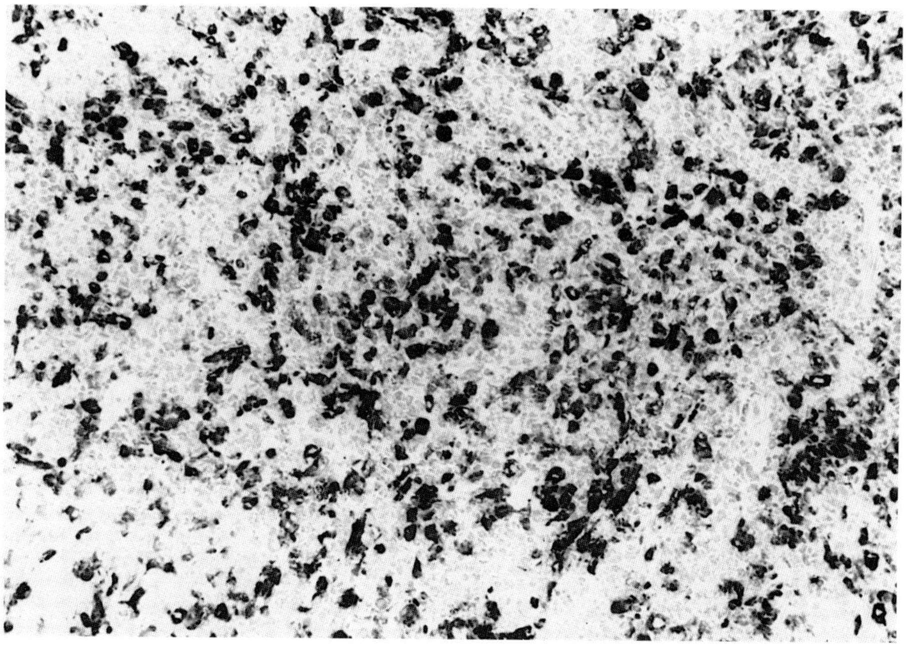

Fig. 6—Immunoblastic lymphoma. Large numbers of non-specific esterase positive histiocytes (grade 3) are seen. × 125

four contained a moderate number and one a few of these cells. In the cryostat preparations the pleomorphism of the histiocytes could be recognized, but less clearly than in the paraplast-embedded material on which the metalophil method was performed.

Malignant lymphoma: centrocytic

The diagnosis of centrocytic lymphoma was made in 15 cases. The cells were monomorphic, having irregular 'cleaved' nuclei. Nucleoli were not conspicuous. Generally a small amount of faintly basophil cytoplasm was present. One of these cases contained no dendritic histiocytes, six lymphomas contained a small number of dendritic histiocytes and seven a moderate number (grade 2). Only one case was classified as grade 3. The dendritic histiocytes were typically delicate with slender extensions even in the only lymphoma with many histiocytes (Fig. 3). In only one case containing a moderate number of dendritic histiocytes were these cells large and pleomorphic. Only three of these lymphomas were examined for the presence of non-specific esterase positive cells. In this respect one was classified as grade 1 (Fig. 4), and two as grade 2.

Malignant lymphoma: centroblastic/centrocytic, follicular

Fifteen lymphomas were centroblastic/centrocytic, follicular. The follicles were composed of centrocytes and centroblasts. The centrocytes corresponded with the description given of the cells of the centrocytic lymphomas. The centroblasts had a round nucleus with a distinct nuclear membrane and two or more conspicuous nucleoli often located at the periphery of the nucleus or at the nuclear membrane. The cytoplasm was basophilic. Between the follicles a dense infiltrate of small lymphocytes was seen. In all the cases, except one, the follicles could easily be recognized by the pattern of delicate histiocytes. In one case no metalophil cells were seen. Because of the structural distribution of the metalophil cells it was not possible to grade these cases. Cryostat sections from 12 cases were examined for the presence of non-specific esterase positive histiocytes. In all cases these histiocytes were present in the follicles mainly at the periphery of these structures. Dendritic extensions were visible but less pronounced than in the metalophil preparations. Grading was not possible with this method.

Malignant lymphoma: centroblastic/centrocytic, diffuse

The diagnosis of malignant lymphoma: centroblastic/centrocytic, diffuse was made on an intermingling of centroblasts and centrocytes without any follicular structure. The presence of a small number of centrocytes was considered sufficient to allow the separation of this entity from the purely centroblastic lymphomas.

The dendritic histiocytes were large, pleomorphic and numerous (Fig. 7). Ten of the 13 lymphomas were scored as grade 3, two as grade 2 and only one case exhibited a small number of dendritic histiocytes. In three lymphomas with many dendritic histiocytes, some areas were completely devoid of these cells (Fig. 8). In one case it was possible to correlate those areas with purely centroblastic regions in the Giemsa stained sections.

Five lymphomas were examined enzyme histochemically, four showed a large number (grade 3) and one a moderate number (grade 2) of rather pleomorphic histiocytes (Fig. 5). The section with a moderate number came from the same node in which areas devoid of metalophil cells were found. These areas could not be recognized in the cryostat sections.

Malignant lymphoma: centroblastic

Seven of the eight centroblastic lymphomas were totally devoid of dendritic histiocytes. One was negative in some parts, elsewhere many large and pleomorphic dendritic histiocytes were present. Enzyme histochemistry was performed on only one of these lymphomas and a moderate number of histiocytes was seen (grade 2). The same lymphoma was partially negative in the section stained for metalophil cells. These negative areas could not be recognized in the cryostat sections.

Malignant lymphoma: immunoblastic

Nineteen lymphomas were diagnosed as immunoblastic. They were predominantly composed of cells with round nuclei and large central nucleoli. The cytoplasm was basophilic, sometimes extending at one side of the cell, suggesting early plasmablastic differentiation. A great variability of pattern regarding the presence of metalophil cells was seen, in six no dendritic histiocytes were found, six showed a moderate number and seven a large number, three of the last group had negative areas. The histiocytes in all cases were large and pleomorphic. All four lymphomas which were examined enzyme histochemically revealed a large number of histiocytes (Fig. 6) including one lesion which was partially negative when stained for metalophil cells.

Malignant lymphoma: lymphoblastic

The lymphoma cells had predominantly rounded nuclei with fine chromatin and a narrow rim of

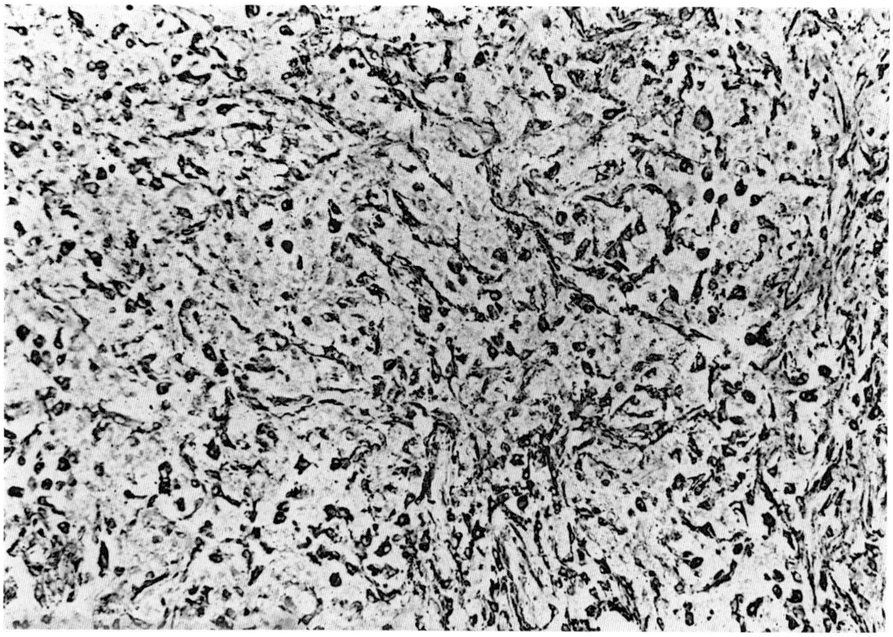

Fig. 7—Centroblastic/centrocytic lymphoma, diffuse. Dense infiltrate of metalophil cells. The histiocytes are pleomorphic with long, coarse and irregular dendrites. × 125

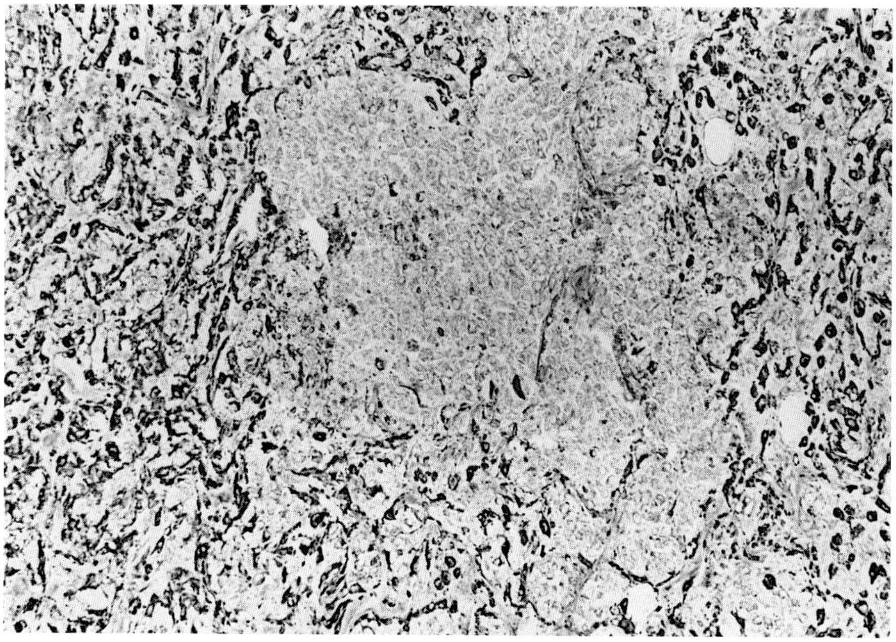

Fig. 8—Same case as Fig. 7. Grade 3 infiltrate of metalophil dendritic histiocytes with negative areas. × 125

strongly to moderately basophilic cytoplasm. In some lesions the nuclei had an infolded structure designated as gyrated or convoluted. Nucleoli were generally not conspicuous. Six of the 10 lymphomas in this category were devoid of metalophil cells, two were partially negative and two contained dendritic histiocytes in moderate numbers. In two of the negative lymphomas some residual compressed lymph node tissue was visible with a normal although deformed follicular pattern. Only one of the lymphomas of this category could be examined histochemically. 'Starry sky' histiocytes showed up which were not recognized in the sections stained for metalophil cells. Other histiocytes were not revealed by either method.

DISCUSSION

In the functionally orientated classifications of non-Hodgkin lymphomas a distinction is made between lymphomas of T-cell, B-cell and undefined or null-cell types.

Lymphomas of undefined or null-cell type

The best known category of the null-cell type is the null-lymphoblastic lymphoma. At least a part of this entity may be derived from stem cells of the bone-marrow.[13] *A priori* it seems unlikely that a particular histiocyte is related to this type of lymphoma. Appropriate material was not available to substantiate this supposition.

Lymphomas of T-cell type

A concomitant proliferation of interdigitating reticulum cells is described at the ultrastructural level in T-cell lymphomas of low grade malignancy.[8] In a previous study[9] it has been shown that the metalophil method does not satisfactorily demonstrate the interdigitating reticulum cells. From the same study it appears that in some cases of mycosis fungoides, a malignant T-cell lymphoma of low grade malignancy, metalophil cells in all probability representing interdigitating reticulum cells are present.

Lymphomas of B-cell type

The majority of the non-Hodgkin lymphomas are B-cell lymphomas.[3,14] Many of these lymphomas are derived from the cells of secondary follicles, these are the so-called follicle centre cell lymphomas of the Lukes and Collins classification[2] and the centroblastic and/or centrocytic lymphomas of the Kiel classification.[4] In this group the presence of the metalophil dendritic histiocytes may be expected especially if the centroblasts and centrocytes retain the capability to induce a proliferation or infiltration of this particular type of histiocyte.[9] Curran and Jones[15] with the aid of the metalophil method have demonstrated the presence of dendritic histiocytes in 18 of the 19 cases on non-Hodgkin lymphomas.

They showed the occurrence of small delicate and large pleomorphic dendritic histiocytes in the lesions. The classification of malignant lymphomas they used was primarily descriptive. For this reason and because the number of their cases was relatively small, their study did not allow conclusions about the relations between the dendritic histiocytes and the lymphoma cells in more functionally defined categories. In addition to the metalophil method, we have studied the presence and distribution of dendritic histiocytes by an enzyme histochemical method. Dendritic reticulum cells are positive for non-specific esterase and 5′-nucleotidase and negative for acid phosphatase.[6] The reaction for non-specific esterase was chosen because the colour of the reaction product allowed a more reliable interpretation.

One of the lymphomas included in the study of Curran and Jones[15] was diagnosed as lymphocytic, well-differentiated. No metalophil cells were seen. According to these authors their absence might signify a T-cell or at least a non-B-Cell origin for that particular lesion. In our series, however, 13 cases of lymphocytic lymphomas, corresponding to the lymphocytic well-differentiated type of Curran and Jones, metalophil cells were notably absent. In six of these 13 patients immunological examination of the leukaemic cells in peripheral blood disclosed a B-cell type lymphoma. In seven cases these data were not available. This type of B-cell lymphoma did not typically give rise to a concomitant proliferation or infiltration of dendritic histiocytes.

This is in agreement with data obtained with electron microscopy. Kaiserling[16] found in contrast to other malignant lymphomas in lymph nodes infiltrated by chronic lymphocytic leukaemia only a few reticulum cells. Mollo *et al.*[17] mentioned only the presence of some phagocytic histiocytes and dark reticulum cells in this type of malignant lymphoma. Veldman and Kaiserling[8] stated that dendritic reticulum cells never occur in lymphomas of chronic leukemia B-cell type. Only in less indolent forms of lymphocytic lymphoma, i.e. in one case of incipient Richter's syndrome and in one case diagnosed as prolymphocytic leukaemia, were a small to moderate number of delicate histiocytes seen in our material.

In the centrocytic lymphomas characteristically a small to moderate number of delicate dendritic histiocytes was found in all but one case. In all probability the diffuse lymphoma, lymphocytic, intermediate-differentiated of the National Lymphoma Investigation classification,[18] used in the study of Curran and Jones[15] corresponded to this category. One of the four lymphomas described by Curran and Jones showed pleomorphism of the metalophil dendritic histiocytes. In our series, pleomorphism was exceptional in this kind of lymphoma, and it was found in only one of the 15 lymphomas of this type. The small to moderate numbers of histiocytes detected enzyme histochemically in the three centrocytic lymphomas were in accordance with the data obtained by the metalophil method. Kaiserling[16] demonstrated the presence electron microscopically of dendritic reticulum cells in 12 out of 20 cases of centrocytic lymphoma. It may be that in these lymphomas where these cells are not particularly numerous they are more readily detected in the relatively thick sections used in the metalophil method.

Curran *et al.*[19] compared reactive follicles with those of follicular lymphomas. Besides the well-known difference regarding the presence of 'starry sky' macrophages in the follicles of reactive nodes, they showed a difference in distribution of histiocytic and dendritic cels in the follicles. In reactive nodes they observed a gradual transition from the rounded histiocytic cells in the basal zone to dendritic forms in the upper zone; whereas in follicular lymphomas 'cells of this (dendritic) type tend to be larger near the centre of the follicle and more slender towards its periphery'. In a quantitative electron microscopic study Rademakers *et al.*[20] showed that centroblastic/centrocytic, follicular lymphomas contained a variable number of dendritic reticulum cells. They were, however, significantly less in number as compared with reactive lymph nodes. In our material the distribution of metalophil cells in reactive and neoplastic follicles varied greatly and did not allow definitive conclusions to be made.

In M.L. centroblastic/centrocytic, diffuse, a large number of pleomorphic dendritic histiocytes was typically seen. These cells were nearly always absent in purely centroblastic lymphomas. An intermediate position is taken by lesions which are partly devoid of dendritic histiocytes, as was seen in some cases of centroblastic/centrocytic, diffuse lymphomas. In this study we restricted the diagnosis of centroblastic lymphoma to lesions in which centrocytes are practically absent. Only in this way the relation of dendritic histiocytes with the different cell types could be assessed.

Centroblastic/centrocytic, diffuse lymphomas were not mentioned as a separate entity in the ultrastructural survey of Kaiserling.[16] This author described reticulum cells in two of six cases of centroblastic lymphomas. In one of the centroblastic lymphomas with dendritic reticulum cells the presence of some 'anaplastic' centrocytes is mentioned explicitly. In the Kiel classification the presence of centrocytes to a certain degree is accepted in the diagnosis of centroblastic lymphoma.[13] Hence the material of Kaiserling is in all probability not entirely comparable to our cases.

It is concluded that dendritic histiocytes seem to be associated in particular with centrocytes or a combination of centrocytes with centroblasts. The absence of dendritic histiocytes in pure centroblastic lymphomas pointed to the specific relation of these histiocytes with centrocytes. This was in agreement with the observation that dendritic reticulum cells develop mainly in the light zone of the germinal centre where centrocytes are relatively most numerous.[19,21] On the other hand, a cellular dedifferentiation in the lymphomas of higher grade of malignancy with a concomitant loss of physiological properties might play a role in this respect.

The large number of pleomorphic dendritic histiocytes in lymphoplasmacytic/lymphoplasmacytoid lymphomas was noteworthy. Even the lymphoplasmacytic lymphomas typically connected with Waldenströms macroglobulinemia, which may resemble morphologically lymphocytic lymphoma, regularly contained many dendritic histiocytes. The completely negative findings in two immunocytomas might be due to the capricious nature of this method, especially as in one of these case many histiocytes were demonstrated by enzyme histochemistry.

Curran and Jones[15] observed a follicular pattern with this method. This is in agreement with the unexpected finding of indistinct follicular structures in some immunocytomas.

In immunoblastic lymphomas with respect to the presence of dendritic histiocytes, two groups seemed to exist, one without these cells present and the other with a moderate to large number of cells present. Judging from the descriptions given by Curran and Jones,[15] three of their lymphomas (cases 8, 12 and 14) might fit in with our conception of immunoblastic lymphoma. In these cases they found two cases with a moderate number and one case with a large number of dendritic histiocytes. Kaiserling[16] mentioned the presence of dendritic reticulum cells identified by electron microscopy in only one case. In his experience these cells are mostly absent. The association of dendritic histiocytes with plasmacytoid cells and their precursors is less obvious than their association with centrocytes although light microscopically[21] and ultrastructurally[16] transitional forms are described between centrocytes and plasmacytoid cells indicating a very close relationship between these two functional states of the B-lymphocyte. In recent years evidence has accumulated pointing to plasma cell differentiation in the follicle centre cell reaction.[21] In this sense at least, some plasma cell precursors belong to the follicle centre cell category and may be functionally related to dendritic histiocytes. A transformation has been described from follicular lymphoma to an immunoblastic Ig-producing lymphoma[22] and some composite lymphomas have also been reported consisting of centroblastic–centrocytic and lymphoplasmacytoid elements.[23]

With regard to the complete absence of dendritic histiocytes in a substantial proportion of the immunoblastic lymphomas, it has to be pointed out that morphological immunoblastic lymphomas may in fact be T-cell lymphomas. In our material only two cases were examined immunologically and found to be B-immunoblastic lymphomas, both contained many dendritic histiocytes. If those lesions without metalophil cells were T-immunoblastic lymphomas, they represent a third of the cases in this series. The data in the literature about the relative frequency of T- and B-immunoblastic lymphomas are contradictory. Our experience[5] is in agreement with Stein and Tollesdorf[24] pointing to a rarity of the T-cell immunoblastic lymphoma. Lukes *et al.*,[3] however, report an equal number of T- and B-immunoblastic lymphomas i.e. 15 in each category among 425 cases of malignant lymphoma. Foucar *et al.*[25] using the Lukes and Collins classification found in their series of 176 malignant lymphomas, four T-cell lymphomas and only one B-cell immunoblastic lymphoma. The differences between the American and European authors may be real or caused by a different immunological approach or more probably be due to a discrepancy in the morphological interpretation of immunoblastic lymphoma. The description given by Lukes *et al.*[3] for T-immunoblastic lymphoma is at variance with the histopathology of the cases of the immunoblastic lymphomas in this study. It seems most likely therefore that the absence of dendritic histiocytes is not related to the T-cell character of the immunoblastic lymphomas of this study. Dendritic reticulum cells may have an affinity for follicle centre cell-derived precursors of plasma-cells, a property which may be lost in immunoblasts in earlier stage of differentiation.

Lymphoblastic lymphomas belong to a heterogenous category. They may be of null-cell type, T- or B-cell type.[13] One of the varieties of the lymphoblastic lymphoma of the Kiel classification, termed 'small non-cleaved' in the Lukes and Collins classification is regarded as a follicle centre cell-derived lymphoma.[1,26,27] Two of the lymphoblastic lymphomas were found to be T-lymphoblastic and dendritic histiocytes were completely absent. Immunological data of the other lymphoblastic lymphomas were not available. So it can only be stated that some cases of morphologically defined lymphoblastic lymphomas contain a moderate or large number of pleomorphic dendritic histiocytes. In other lymphomas of this category they may be completely missing.

A marked degree of pleomorphism of the dendritic histiocytes was typically seen in immunocytoma, centroblastic/centrocytic, diffuse lymphoma and the lymphomas of high-grade malignancy, i.e. centroblastic, immunoblastic and lymphoblastic lymphomas. In centrocytic lymphoma, follicular centroblastic/centrocytic lymphoma and in the few cases of (pro) lymphocytic lymphoma containing dendritic histiocytes, these cells were small with slender extensions. The pleomorphism may be related to a higher degree of malignancy, as the same kind of pleomorphic histiocytes may be encountered in lymph nodes with metastatic carcinoma.[9]

ACKNOWLEDGEMENTS

This study was supported by the Netherlands Cancer Foundation (Koningin Wilhelmina Fonds, KWF). The authors like to thank Mrs Sri Tan-Ranoewisastro for the great care with which she developed the metalophil method; Mr Chris Van Basten for the histochemical preparations; Mr E. Dumernit for preparing the photographs and Mrs

Christina Oprel for the efficient typing of the manuscript.

REFERENCES

1. Lukes RJ, Collins RD. Immunologic characterization of human malignant lymphomas. *Cancer* 1974; **234:** 1488.
2. Lukes RJ, Collins RD. New approaches to the classification of the lymphomata. Symposium on non-Hodgkin's lymphomas. *Br J Cancer* 1975; **31,** suppl. II: 1.
3. Lukes RJ, Parker JW, Taylor CR, Tindle BH, Cramer AD, Lincoln TL. Immunologic approach to non-Hodgkin lymphomas. Analysis of the results of multiparameter studies of 425 cases. *Seminars in Hematology* 1978; **15:** 322.
4. Lennert K. Malignant Lymphomas Other Than Hodgkin's Disease. Berlin, Heidelberg, New York: Springer Verlag, 1978; 83–110.
5. Van Heerde P, Feltkamp A, Feltkamp-Vroom TM, Koudstaal J, Van Unnik JAM. Non-Hodgkin's lymphoma. Immunohistochemical and electron microscopical findings in relation to light microscopy. *Cancer* 1980; **46:** 2210.
6. Müller-Hermelink HK, Lennert K. The cytologic, histologic and functional bases for a modern classification of lymphomas. In: Lennert K, ed. Malignant Lymphomas Other Than Hodgkin's Disease. Berlin, Heidelberg, New York: Springer Verlag, 1978; 45–50.
7. Müller-Hermelink HK, Kaiserling E. Different reticulum cells of the lymph node: microecological concept of lymphoid tissue organization. In: Van den Tweel JG, Taylor CR, Bosman FT, eds. Malignant Lymphoproliferatic Diseases. Boerhaave Series, Vol. 17. Leiden: University Press, 57.
8. Veldman JE, Kaiserling E. In: Carr I, Daems WT, eds. The Reticuloendothelial System. Vol. I. New York, London: Plenum Press, 1980; 381.
9. Van Unnik JAM. The application of the metalophil method for the demonstration of histiocytes. *J Pathol* **144:** 233–239.
10. Yam LT, Ly CI, Crosby WH. Cytochemical identification of monocytes and granulocytes. *Am J Clin Path* 1971; **55:** 283.
11. Richter MN. Generalized reticular cell sarcoma of lymph nodes associated with lymphatic leukemia. *Amer J Path* 1928; **4:** 285.
12. Galton DAG, Goldman JM, Wiltshaw E, Catovsky D, Henry K, Goldenberg GJ. Prolymphocytic leukaemia. *Brit J Hemat* 1974; **27:** 7.
13. Lennert K, Mohri N. Histopathology and diagnosis of non-Hodgkin's lymphomas. In: Lennert K, ed. Malignant Lymphomas Other Than Hodgkin's Disease. Berlin, Heidelberg, New York: Springer Verlag, 1978; 302–409.
14. Stein H. The immunologic and immunochemical basis for the Kiel classification. In: Lennert K, ed. Malignant Lymphomas Other Than Hodgkin's Disease. Berlin, Heidelberg, New York: Springer Verlag, 1978; 651.
15. Curran RC, Jones EL. Non-Hodgkin's lymphomas: an immuno-histochemical and histological study. *J Pathol* 1979; **129:** 179.
16. Kaiserling E. Ultrastructure of non-Hodgkins lymphomas. In: Lennert K, ed. Malignant Lymphomas Other Than Hodgkin's Disease. Berlin, Heidelberg, New York: Springer Verlag, 1978; 473–522.
17. Mollo F, Monga G, Stramignioni A. Dark reticular cells in human lymphadenitis and lymphomas. *Virch Arch B* 1969; **3:** 117.
18. Bennett MH, Farrer-Brown G, Henry Kristin, Jeliffe AM. Classification of non-Hodgkin's lymphomas. *Lancet* 1974; **ii:** 405.
19. Curran RC, Gregory J, Jones EL. The distribution of immunoblobulins and other plasma proteins in human reactive lymph nodes. *J Pathol* 1982; **136:** 307.
20. Rademakers LHPM, Peters JPJ, Van Unnik JAM. Histiocytic and dendritic reticulum cells in follicular structures of follicular lymphoma and reactive hyperplasia. A quantitative electron microscopical analysis. *Virchows Archiv (Cell Pathol)* 1983; **44:** 85–98.
21. Lennert K, Stein H. The germinal centre: morphology, histo-chemistry and immunohistology. In: Goes M, Christophers E, eds. Lymphoproliferative Disease of the Skin. Berlin, Heidelberg, New York: Springer Verlag, 1982; 3–15.
22. Dick FR, Parks W, O'Conoor M. Transformation of nodular lymphoma to an immunoblastic IgM producing tumor. *Am J Clin Pathol* 1977; **68:** 611.
23. Le Tourneau A, Andouin J, Capron F, Diebold J. Lymphomes malins folliculaires centroblastiques-centrocytiques associés à un lymphome malin lymphoplasmacytaire. *Ann Pathol* 1981; **1:** 59.
24. Stein H, Tollesdorf G. In: Stacher A, Höcker P, eds. Lymphknoten Tumoren-Pathophysiologie, Klinik und Therapie. München-Wien-Baltimore: Urban and Schwarzenberg, 1979; 108.
25. Foucar K, McKenna RW, Frizzera G, Brunning R. Bone marrow and blood involvement by lymphoma in relationship to the Lukes–Collins classification. *Cancer* 1982; **49:** 888.
26. Mann RB, Jaffe ES, Braylan RC, Nanba K, Frank MM, Ziegler JL, Berard CW. Non-endemic Burkitt's lymphoma: a B-cell tumor related to germinal centers. *New Engl J Med* 1976; **295:** 685.
27. Rilke F, Pilotti S, Carbone A, Lombardi L. Morphology of lymphatic cells and of their derived tumours. *J Clin Pathol* 1978; **31:** 1009.

JOURNAL OF PATHOLOGY, VOL. **144**: 253–256 (1984)

PARANODAL TUMOUR IN BREAST CANCER: EXTRANODAL EXTENSION VERSUS VASCULAR SPREAD

F. HARTVEIT

Department of Pathology, The Gade Institute, The University, Bergen, Norway

Received 27 April 1984
Accepted 29 May 1984

SUMMARY

A detailed histological study of the axillary nodes from 98 breast carcinoma patients, in which 5 and 10 year follow-up data was available, has been undertaken. The presence of tumour cells in efferent vessels appears to be the only factor which is a marker of poor prognosis. Contrary to previous reports the direct infiltration of tumour cells through the nodal capsule into perinodal fat and connective tissue is of no prognostic significance. Distinction between site and type of tumour growth within nodes is thus essential for prognostic evaluation.

KEY WORDS—Breast cancer, extranodal extension, paranodal vascular spread.

INTRODUCTION

In the clinical evaluation of breast cancer patients the presence of enlarged and fixed lymph nodes in the axilla is uniformly accepted as a sign of advanced disease. It is probably this that has led to the ready acceptance of the histological finding of tumour infiltration in the paranodal fat as an indicator of poor prognosis.[1] Even so, as the present work shows, the finding should not be judged uncritically. Care is needed in its interpretation, and particular attention should be paid to the principles involved before an opinion is given.

This paper relates the findings in the paranodal tissues to the 5 and 10 year survival data for 98 node-positive patients with infiltrating breast carcinoma.

MATERIAL AND METHODS

The series of 115 consecutive node-positive cases of primary infiltrating breast carcinoma was first described in 1979.[2] All had been considered operable and treated by modified radical mastectomy with axillary node dissection. These specimens had been formalin-fixed and blocks taken from the nodes most obviously involved macroscpically. When one slide per node was reviewed tumour deposits were found in 269 of the 412 nodes investigated. Charts were drawn following projection of the slides and the position of the deposits marked. They were recorded as in the cortex, the medulla, or in the paranodal fatty tissue (subdivided into the efferent hilar area and the remaining afferent area, see Fig. 1). The presence of tumour cells in the afferent and/or efferent nodal vessels was noted separately.

In 14 cases no node was available in which the efferent hilar area could be identified. These cases were excluded, as were a further three dying of an unrelated cause within 10 years of operation. The present series thus consists of 98 cases, 49 of whom had died within 5 years of operation, 71 within 10 years. The follow-up data was supplied by the Norwegian Cancer Registry.

In 24 of the 98 cases four or more nodes were tumour-bearing. A mean ($\pm$ s.d.) of $2{\cdot}5 \pm 1{\cdot}7$ tumour-bearing and $1{\cdot}3 \pm 1{\cdot}6$ non-tumour-bearing nodes was available per case. In all but one case

Addressee for correspondence: Professor F. Hartveit, Department of Pathology, N 5016 Haukeland Hospital, Bergen, Norway.

0022–3417/84/120253–04$01.00

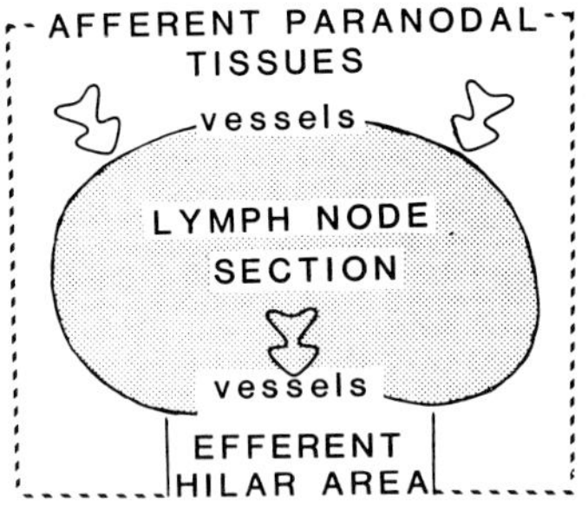

Fig. 1—Diagram of a lymph node section through the hilar area and the node's longest axis. Note: the afferent lymphatic vessels enter the node on its convex side; the efferent exit from the hilar area

tumour was present in both cortex and medulla in at least one node per axillary specimen.

The presence of a factor in at least one node in the axilla is used here to characterize the case. For example a case with tumour cells in an efferent vessel of one node only is termed positive for that factor. Further quantitation was not attempted due to the method of selection of the material.

The χ^2 test (1 df) was used to evaluate the survival differences between the groups at 5 and 10 years after operation.

RESULTS

Extranodal extension was present in 22 cases with four or more tumour-bearing nodes and absent in two. It was present in 47 of those with less than four tumour-bearing nodes and absent from 27. This difference is statistically significant ($\chi^2 = 6{\cdot}9$ $p < 0{\cdot}01$).

Table I relates the number of cases dead/alive at 5 and 10 years after operation to the presence/absence of extranodal extension in the two groups. Irrespective of presence/absence of extranodal extension those with four or more tumour-bearing nodes were at a prognostic disadvantage at both 5 and 10 years after operation, the difference at both times being highly significant statistically. As the great majority of these cases also showed extranodal extension, the presence/absence of the latter gave little further information. In those with under four tumour-bearing nodes the difference was not statistically significant at either 5 or 10 years.

The presence/absence of *paranodal tumour* and its site was related to the site of the intranodal deposits in 250 tumour-bearing axillary nodes (19 were excluded as the efferent area was not defined). None was recorded in the 143 non-tumour-bearing nodes examined.

Paranodal tumour was present in 62 per cent of the tumour-bearing nodes (Table II). Tumour in the afferent area (A or Av) was found in combination with tumour in the cortex (6·8 per cent), or cortex plus medulla (14·8 per cent), while deposits in the medulla alone were associated with tumour in the efferent area (Ev, E or E+Ev, 6+2+6=5·8 per cent). The latter combinations were found in 40·4 per cent of the nodes. The presence of tumour in the efferent vessels is not necessarily accompanied by tumour infiltration in the hilar (E) fat. Those with Ev and tumour in the medulla alone may be examples of retrograde spread.

The *site* of the paranodal tumour is related to the *proportion surviving* at 5 and 10 years after operation in Fig. 2. The two upper factors, tumour infiltrating the tissues (extranodal extension), and tumour in the efferent paranodal tissue only, did not give significant differences. Tumour cells in the efferent vessels (bottom factor) gave the greatest discrimination at 5 and 10 years ($p < 0{\cdot}0005$ for both). The weak significance at 5 years in the two other groups is dependent on the inclusion of cases with tumour cells in the efferent vessels. This is clear when the cases with tumour cells in the afferent vessels are further analysed. Of those with tumour cells in both afferent and efferent vessels 14 out of 15 were dead by 5 years, compared with three of 10 with tumour in the afferent vessels only (χ^2 with Yate's correction $= 8{\cdot}3$ $p < 0{\cdot}005$).

Table I—Extranodal extension of axillary metastases in breast cancer relative to the number of tumour-bearing nodes and survival 5 and 10 years after operation

Time post-op.	Tumour-bearing nodes	Extranodal extension +/−	No. of patients Dead	No. of patients Alive	Difference (χ^2)
5 years	4 or more	+	17	5	
		−	2	0	
		All	19	5	
	Under 4	+	20	27	All: $p < 0{\cdot}001$
		−	10	17	(10·8)
		All	30	44	
10 years	4 or more	+	21	1	
		−	2	0	
		All	23	1	
	Under 4	+	31	16	All: $p < 0{\cdot}005$
		−	17	10	(8·7)
		All	48	26	

Table II—The absence/presence and site of paranodal tumour related to the site of the intranodal tumour deposits in 250 tumour-bearing axillary nodes from 98 breast cancer patients

Paranodal tumour	Tumour deposits in nodal Cortex	Cortex + medulla	Medulla	Nodes All	%
None	18	74	3	95	38·0
Av	5	8	–		
Av + E	1	3	–	17	6·8
A	–	2	–		
A + E	–	12	–		
A + Ev	–	3	–		
A + E + Av	–	1	–		
A + E + Ev	–	5	–	37	14·8
A + E + Av + Ev	–	1	–		
A + Av + Ev	–	2	–		
E + Av + Ev	–	8	–		
Av + Ev	–	3	–		
Ev	2	16	6	24	
E	2	23	2	27	40·4
E + Ev	2	42	6	50	
All with pn tumour	12	129	14	155	62·0
Total	30	203	17	250	100·0

A: afferent; Av: afferent vessels; E: efferent; Ev: efferent vessels.

DISCUSSION

Extranodal extension of axillary metastases in breast cancer is considered a valuable prognostic discriminant for short-term treatment failure.[1] The present work shows that the prognostic information gained from study of tumour deposits around these nodes (paranodal tumour growth) is dependent on the presence/absence of tumour cells in the efferent nodal vessels, and that the presence of tumour infiltration, i.e. extranodal extension, by itself, is of no prognostic interest.

The definition of extranodal extension in the work quoted does not cover the paranodal vessels, or mention the possibility of finding tumour cells in them. The present study makes this distinction, and further defines the site involved as the afferent paranodal or efferent hilar area. The methods used are otherwise similar to those in Fisher *et al.*'s study,[1] and the material too is probably comparable, although fewer nodes were recovered per patient. Extranodal extension, for example, was seen more often in cases with four or more tumour-bearing nodes, than in those with fewer.

Here the similarity ends. Although cases with four or more tumour-bearing nodes were at a clear prognostic disadvantage no further distinction was gained on dividing the two groups into those with/without extranodal extention. Thus, although such extension is found more often when more tumour-bearing nodes are available per case, it does not give further prognostic discrimination.

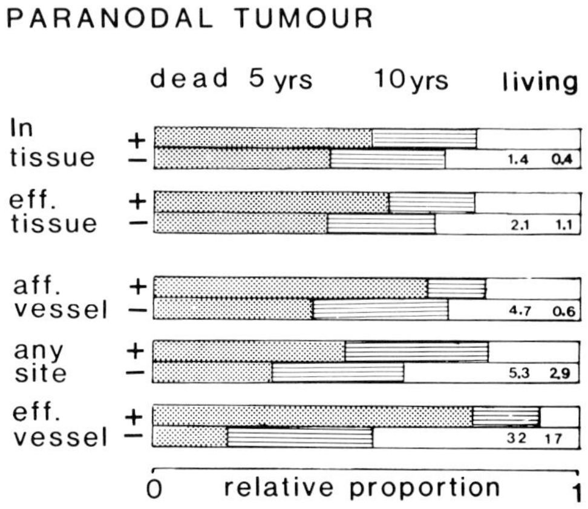

Fig. 2—The proportion of patients surviving at 5 and 10 years after operation for breast carcinoma related to the presence of paranodal tumour in different sites. (The figures in the lower right hand column for each factor are the χ^2 values for the survival difference at 5 and 10 years)

However, the presence of paranodal tumour (i.e. Fig. 2, any site) irrespective of the number of tumour-bearing nodes, gave weak prognostic discrimination at 5 years ($\chi^2 = 5{\cdot}3$). The presence/absence of tumour cells in the afferent vessels gave much the same result. Further analysis showed that the difference was dependent on the simultaneous presence of tumour cells in the efferent vessels in many of these cases, the latter being a major prognostic factor at 5 and 10 years. Tumour cells in the tissues alone gave no prognostic discrimination. On this basis it is tempting to suggest that Fisher *et al.*'s series,[1] in which there was 46·8 per cent treatment failure at 22 months follow-up in the group with extranodal tumour compared to 29·5 per cent in the group with metastases confined to the nodes, may also have included cases with tumour cells in the efferent vessels, as well as pure extranodal extension.

Understanding of the dynamics of nodal tumour growth is essential to the interpretation of the nodal histology in these cases. As tumour cells enter the nodes by the afferent vessels such a finding will not worsen prognosis in node-positive cases. On the other hand the finding of tumour cells in the efferent vessels, usually secondary to extensive tumour growth in the nodal cortex and medulla, suggests that tertiary spread may have occurred. It thus marks a later stage in nodal tumour growth than the mere presence of intranodal deposits. Extranodal extension is also, by definition, subsequent to intranodal growth, but its presence is not of prognostic significance.

There is a basic biological distinction here. Local infiltrative growth around regional deposits does not reflect the extent of distant metastatic spread. In contrast, the presence of an embolic growth form heralds the terminal phase of the disease. Thus, the more prone a tumour is to the embolic growth form the worse the prognosis, irrespective of the extent of local infiltrative growth.

ACKNOWLEDGEMENT

This work was supported by the Norwegian Cancer Society.

REFERENCES

1. Fisher ER, Gregorio RM, Redmond C, Kim WS, Fisher B. Pathological findings from the National Surgical Breast Project (Protocol No. 4) III. The significance of extranodal extension of axillary metastases. *Am J Clin Pathol* 1976; **65:** 439.
2. Hartveit F. Paranodal vascular spread in breast cancer with axillary node involvement. *J Pathol* 1979; **127:** 111.

JOURNAL OF PATHOLOGY, VOL. **144**: 257–267 (1984)

ISCHAEMIC CHANGES IN HUMAN MESENTERIC LYMPH NODES

N. J. MAHY AND J. D. DAVIES

University Department of Pathology, Bristol Royal Infirmary, Bristol, U.K.

Received 17 May 1984
Accepted 24 June 1984

SUMMARY

Lymph node lesions attributable to ischaemia are described in the mesenteric nodes from 10 patients with volvulus of the small and large bowel. Frank infarction, the microanatomy of which differs from that seen in superficial lymph nodes, is one of the nodal lesions evoked by ischaemia. Two others in the form of lymphocyte depletion and capsular hypervascularity also appear to result from vascular occlusion. These three lesions were also found in nodes associated with 'primary' venous and arterial infarction of the bowel mucosa, but not in non-vascular diseases of the small bowel or colon. The enhanced frequency of infarction in volvulus with mucosal necrosis, as opposed to cases with 'primary' vascular thromboses suggest that ischaemic lymph node changes are more frequent when several sets of vessels are occluded. Distension of lymph hode sinuses, erythrocyte extravasation, and dilatation of small intranodal vessels were not restricted to vascular cases, and appear to be less specific reactions to ischaemia. The range of ischaemia-induced reactions is wider than has hitherto been recognized in human lymph nodes.

KEY WORDS—Lymph nodes, ischaemia, mesentery, lymphocyte depletion, infarction, capsular hypervascularity.

INTRODUCTION

Spontaneous sub-total infarction of non-neoplastic superficial lymph nodes, apparently due to occlusion of hilar veins, was first described in man in 1972.[1] Experimental vascular occlusion in rabbits, dogs and rats had produced similar lesions.[2,3] Although several small series of cases of spontaneous infarction of human non-neoplastic lymph nodes have since been described,[4–6] there has been no consideration of ischaemic nodal lesions which fall short of sub-total necrosis.

Volvulus of the bowel may result in bowel ischaemia as a result of torsion and consequent occlusion of the mesenteric vessels.[7] Casual observation that this process may also be associated with the infarction of mesenteric lymph nodes led us to examine the mesenteric lymph nodes in a series of cases of bowel volvulus, and 'primary' venous and arterial infarction of the bowel. We wish to describe the range of lymph node changes which appear to be attributable to ischaemia in mesenteric lymph nodes. Our findings indicate that both infarction and lesser ischaemic lesions of lymph nodes are more common than is generally appreciated.

MATERIALS AND METHODS

Cases of large and small bowel volvulus were sought in the clinical and histopathological Disease Index files of the Bristol Royal Infirmary for the period January 1975 to June 1983. The cases were then examined after retrieval from the stored sections and paraffin blocks in the University Department of Pathology. After elimination of those cases in which lymph nodal sections were lacking, a total of 10 cases of volvulus was available for study (six from the small bowel; four of the sigmoid colon): see Table I. For comparison, 20 cases of small bowel ulceration (four cases of Crohn's disease, 15 cases of ischaemia due to 'primary' vascular thrombosis, 11 of which involved superior mesenteric arteries

Addressee for correspondence: J. D. Davies, University Department of Pathology, Level 9, Phase 1, Bristol Royal Infirmary, Bristol BS2 8HW, U.K.

0022–3417/84/120257–11$01.10

Table I—Summary of cases of volvulus and their mesenteric lymph node changes

Case no.	Sex	Age (years)	Bowel affected	Mucosal infarct	Nodal infarct	Lymphoid depletion	Capsular vascularity	Sinus distension	RBC extravasation	Vascular dilatation
1	Male	70	Sigmoid	–	–	–	+	+	+	–
2	Male	39	Sigmoid	+	+	+	–	–	+	+
3	Male	48	Sigmoid	–	–	+	–	+	+	+
4	Male	65	Sigmoid	–	–	–	–	+	+	+
5	Female	68	Small	+	–	+	–	–	–	–
6	Male	61	Small	+	+	+	–	–	+	–
7	Female	68	Small	+	+	+	–	–	+	+
8	Female	85	Small	+	+	+	–	+	+	–
9	Male	50	Small	+	+	+	+	+	–	–
10	Female	73	Small	+	–	+	+	+	+	–

and four the veins, one case of post-irradiation enteritis) and 14 cases of sigmoid colonic disease (colonic carcinoma (5), Crohn's disease (3), ulcerative colitis (2), post-irradiation colitis (1) and diverticulitis (3)) in which mesenteric or mesocolonic lymph nodes were available were also examined. The stored haematoxylin and eosin stained sections of the bowel wall and mesenteric or mesocolonic tissue were reviewed. In selected instances paraffin blocks were recut and the sections stained by Gordon and Sweets' reticulin method, Masson's trichrome, and Weigert's and Congo 'blue'[8] methods for elastic fibres. Assessment of the changes in the lymph nodes was made independently by two observers, initially without knowledge of the associated bowel pathology.

RESULTS

The mesenteric and bowel wall tissues from the cases of volvulus were all engorged. The veins, which were clearly distinguishable from arteries in the elastic-stained preparations, were dilated and contained focal or widespread thrombosis in all cases. Additionally, arterial thrombosis was found in four of the 10 cases of volvulus. Dilated thin walled vessels, which contained a fibrinous coagulum and appeared to be lymphatic channels, were also present. Seven volvulus cases showed frank necrosis of the mucosa (all six small bowels; one of four sigmoid colons). In every case there was an acute inflammatory exudate in the mesenteric and subserosal tissues.

The histological appearances of the non-volvulus comparison cases, on review, were typical of their initial diagnoses (listed in the Material and Methods section). Mucosal necrosis was present in all the cases of primary venous and arterial infarction. Reactive acute inflammation was also present in the serosal and mesenteric tissue but, in general, was less pronounced than in the volvulus cases.

Six main changes were found in the lymph nodes in the mesenteries of the small bowel and sigmoid colon (Table II). The morphology and distribution of these changes in the volvulus and comparison cases are described below.

Lymph node infarction

Frank necrosis of lymph nodes was found in six cases. Five cases were found in the volvulus group

Table II—Lymph node changes in cases of volvulus, 'primary' vascular and non-vascular bowel disease

Condition	Nodal infarct	Lymphoid depletion	Capsular vascularity	Sinus distension	RBC extravasation	Vascular dilatation	Total of cases
Volvulus: mucosal necrosis	4	7	2	3	5	2	7
Volvulus: no mucosal necrosis	0	1	1	3	3	2	3
'Primary' venous infarction	0	2	1	3	2	1	4
'Primary' arterial infarction	1	3	2	4	2	3	11
Non-vascular disease: colon	0	0	0	8	3	3	14
Non-vascular disease: small bowel	0	0	0	3	0	1	5

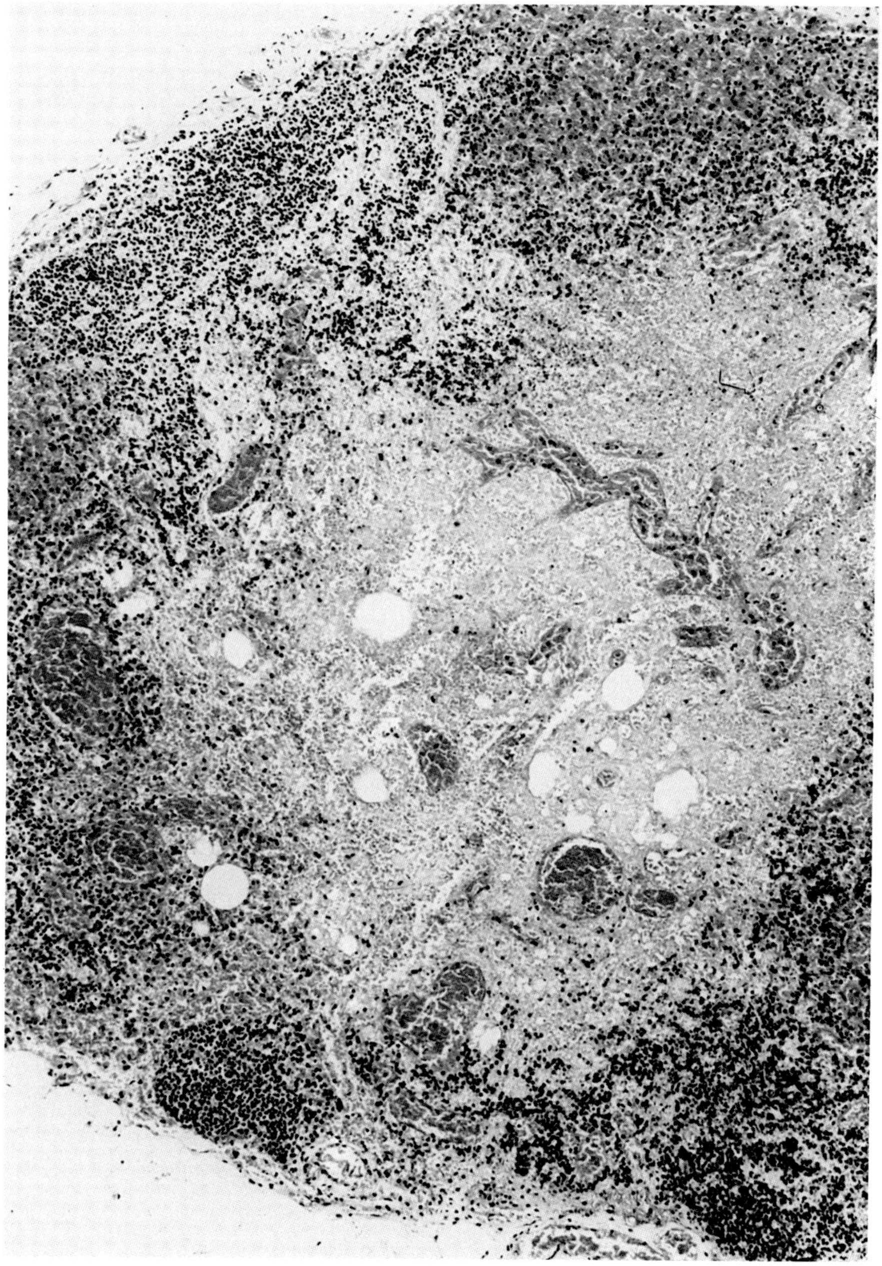

Fig. 1—(a) Infarction of central part of mesenteric lymph node, with survival of subcapsular lymphoid tissue. Pale central necrosis. Haematoxylin and eosin, × 100

(Table I), and one occurred in association with an arterial infarct of the small bowel. All four cases of volvulus with arterial thrombosis exhibited infarction of the mesenteric lymph nodes. Lymph node infarction was restricted to cases also showing necrosis of the bowel mucosa (five of the seven volvulus cases with mucosal infarction). None of the three cases of volvulus lacking mucosal infarction showed lymph nodal infarction, nor was nodal infarction found in the non-vascular colonic and small bowel lesions. The infarction of the lymph nodes ranged from sub-total necrosis to involve-

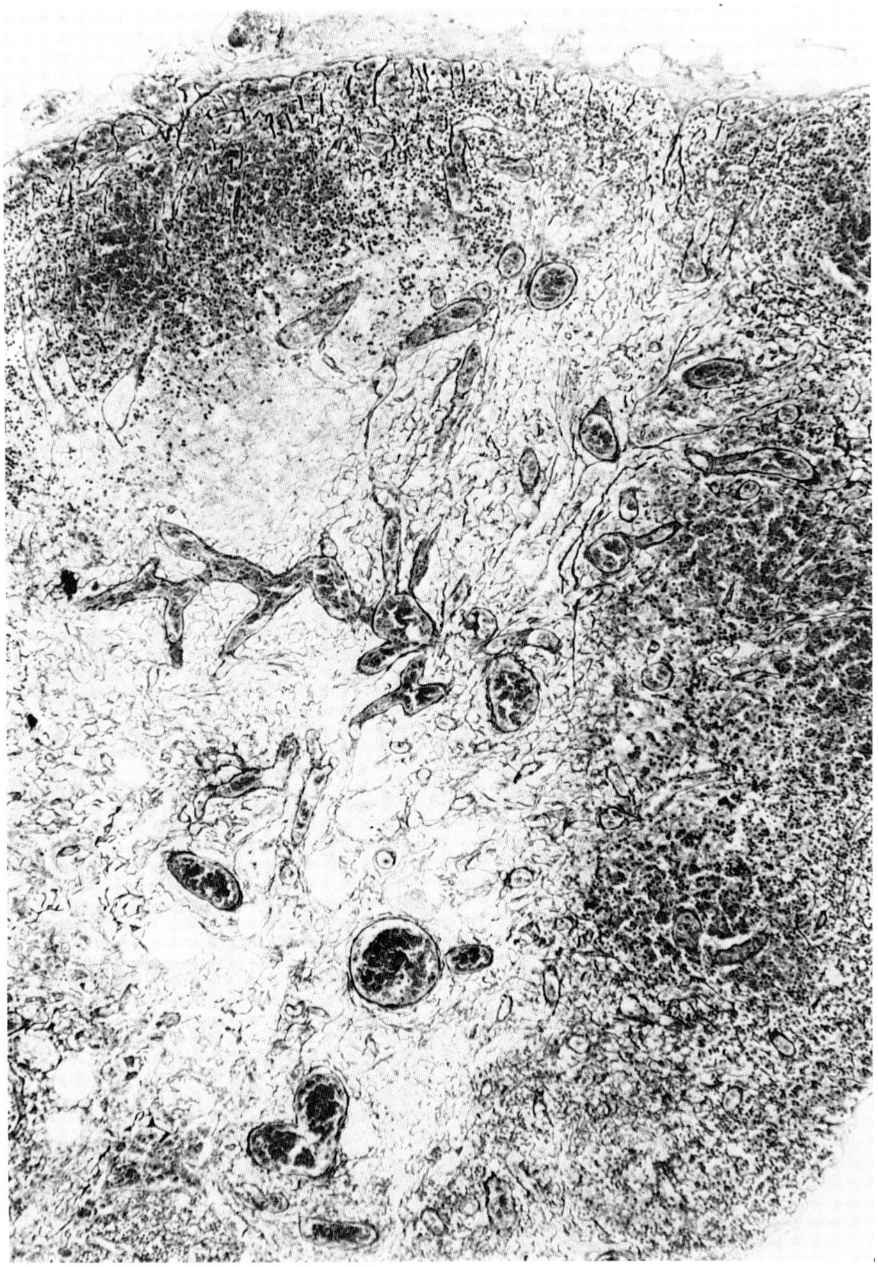

Fig. 1—(b) Infarction of central part of mesenteric lymph node, with survival of subcapsular lymphoid tissue. Structural preservation in central infarct, same node at deeper level. Gordon & Sweets' reticulin, × 100

ment only of the central part of the nodes (Fig. 1a, b). In contrast to the extensive relatively unselective necrosis of superficial (i.e. axillary of inguinal[9]) lymph nodes,[1,5] there was often a tendency to sparing of the deep peritrabecular lymphoid tissue (Fig. 2) in the mesenteric nodes. The nodal necrosis was visible as amorphous weakly eosinophilic material in the core of the lymph nodes. Reticulin staining showed the original connective tissue framework to be well preserved in the infarcted areas and Masson's trichrome gave a clearer impression of the ghost cells in the necrotic tissue

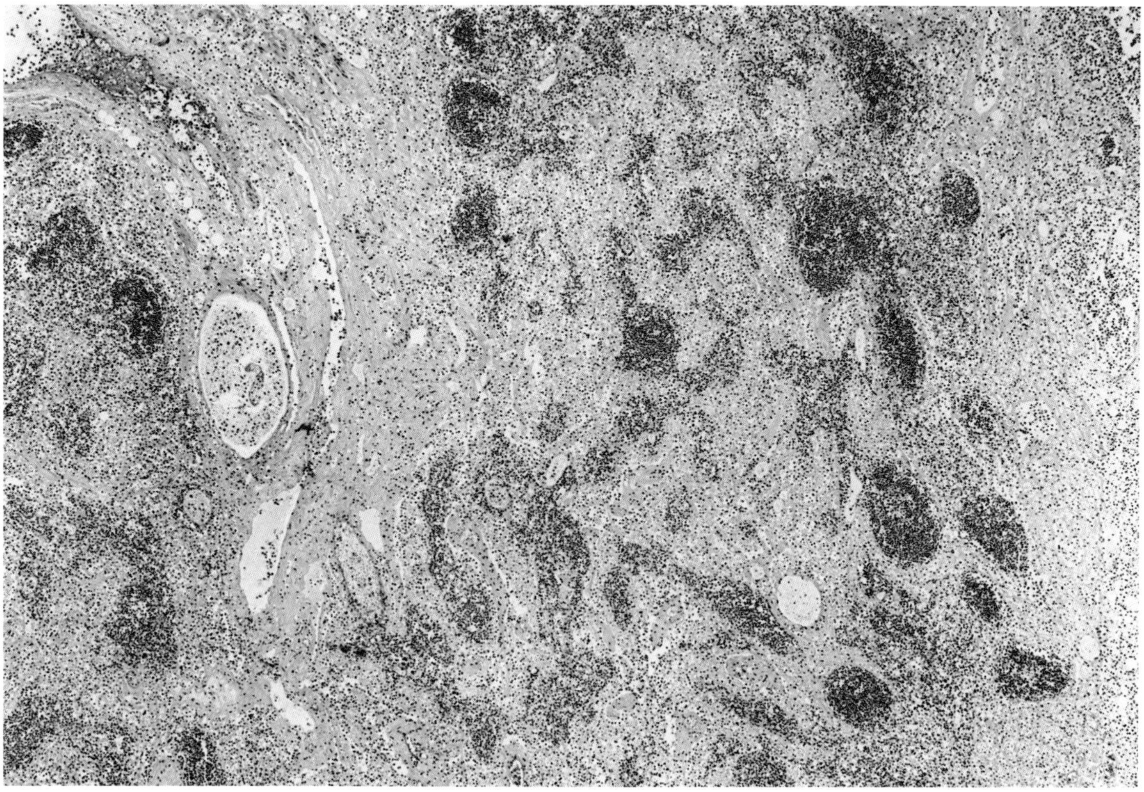

Fig. 2—Mesenteric lymph-node infarction with sparing of lymphoid tissue in trabecular areas (dark staining). Haematoxylin and eosin, ×40

than did haematoxylin and eosin preparations.

Lymphoid depletion

Lymphoid depletion was restricted to the cases of vascular bowel disease. Eight of the 10 cases of volvulus showed lymphoid depletion, and two of four 'primary' venous and three of 11 'primary' arterial bowel infarction cases displayed this change in the lymph nodes. The two cases of volvulus with mucosal necrosis lacking nodal infarction both exhibited lymphoid depletion in the mesenteric lymph nodes. Lymphoid depletion was characterized by a marked reduction in density of small nucleated lymphocytes in the intersinusoidal pulp of the lymph nodes (Fig. 3). The cellularity of the intervening sinuses appeared to be unaffected.

Capsular hypervascularity

A marked increase in the vascular content of the capsule and the adjacent perinodal tissue was found in six cases. Three were cases of volvulus (two with musosal necrosis; one lacking mucosal necrosis); one was found in association with 'primary' venous infarction and two with arterial infarction. The vessels in the nodal capsule and perinodal tissue were markedly distended and prominent on low-power microscopy (Fig. 4). The vessels affected were all thin-walled, and appeared to be both small veins and lymphatic channels in the nodal capsule (Fig. 5). The underlying lymph nodes were free of infarction but most displayed lymphoid depletion.

Distension of lymph node sinuses

Sinus distension was not limited to cases of volvulus or bowel ischaemia. Conspicuous dilation of the lymph node sinuses was found in six of the ten cases of volvulus, three of four venous bowel infarcts, four of 11 cases of arterial infaction of small bowel, eight of 14 and three of five cases of

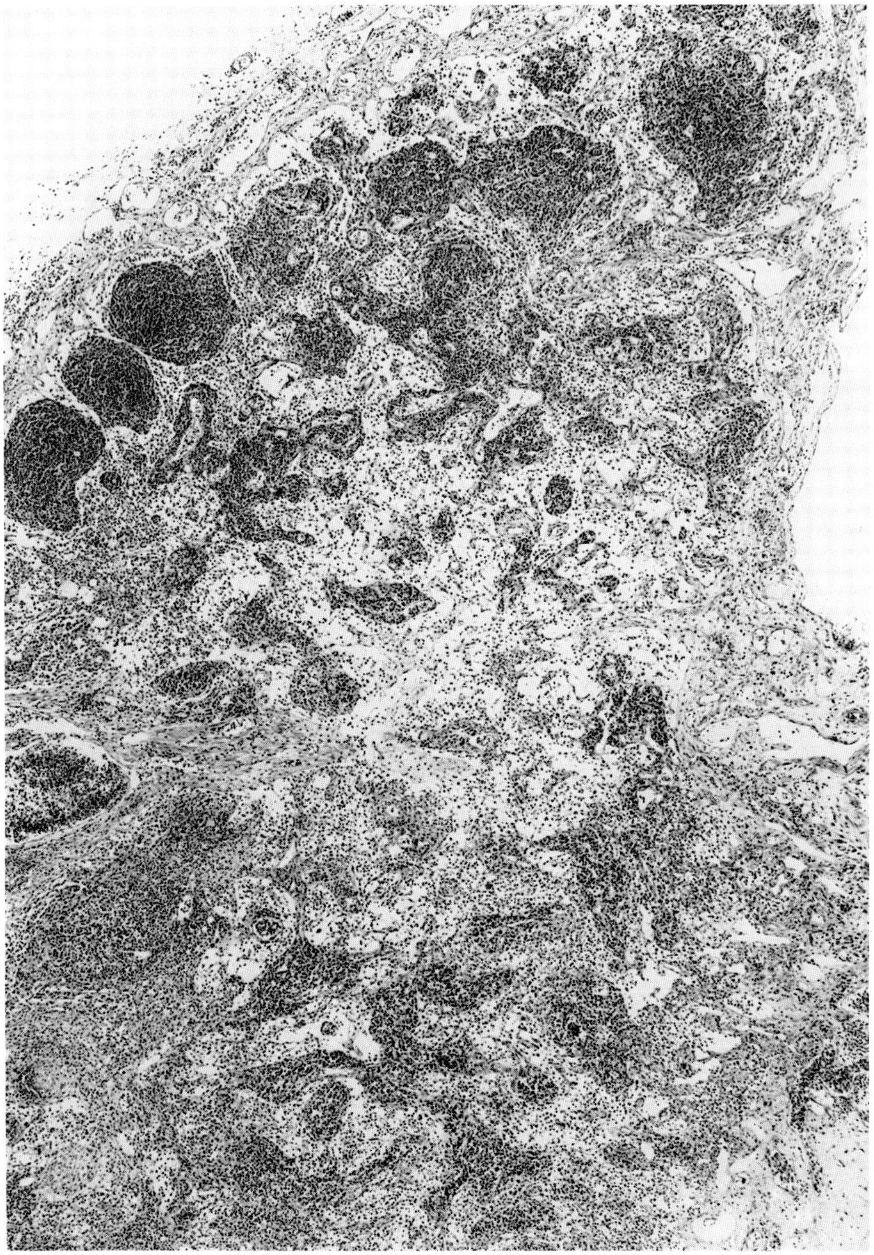

Fig. 3—Reduction of lymphocytic content of lymphoid trabeculae in lower part of mesenteric lymph node. Haematoxylin and eosin, × 35

non-vascular disease involving, respectively, the sigmoid colon and the small bowel. All lesions in this category showed expansion of some sinusoids to at least three or four times their normal diameter (Fig. 6). This dilatation was accompanied by the presence of cells and a coagulable fluid in the sinuses.

Nodal extravasation of erythrocytes

Extravasation of erythrocytes in the nodal pulp

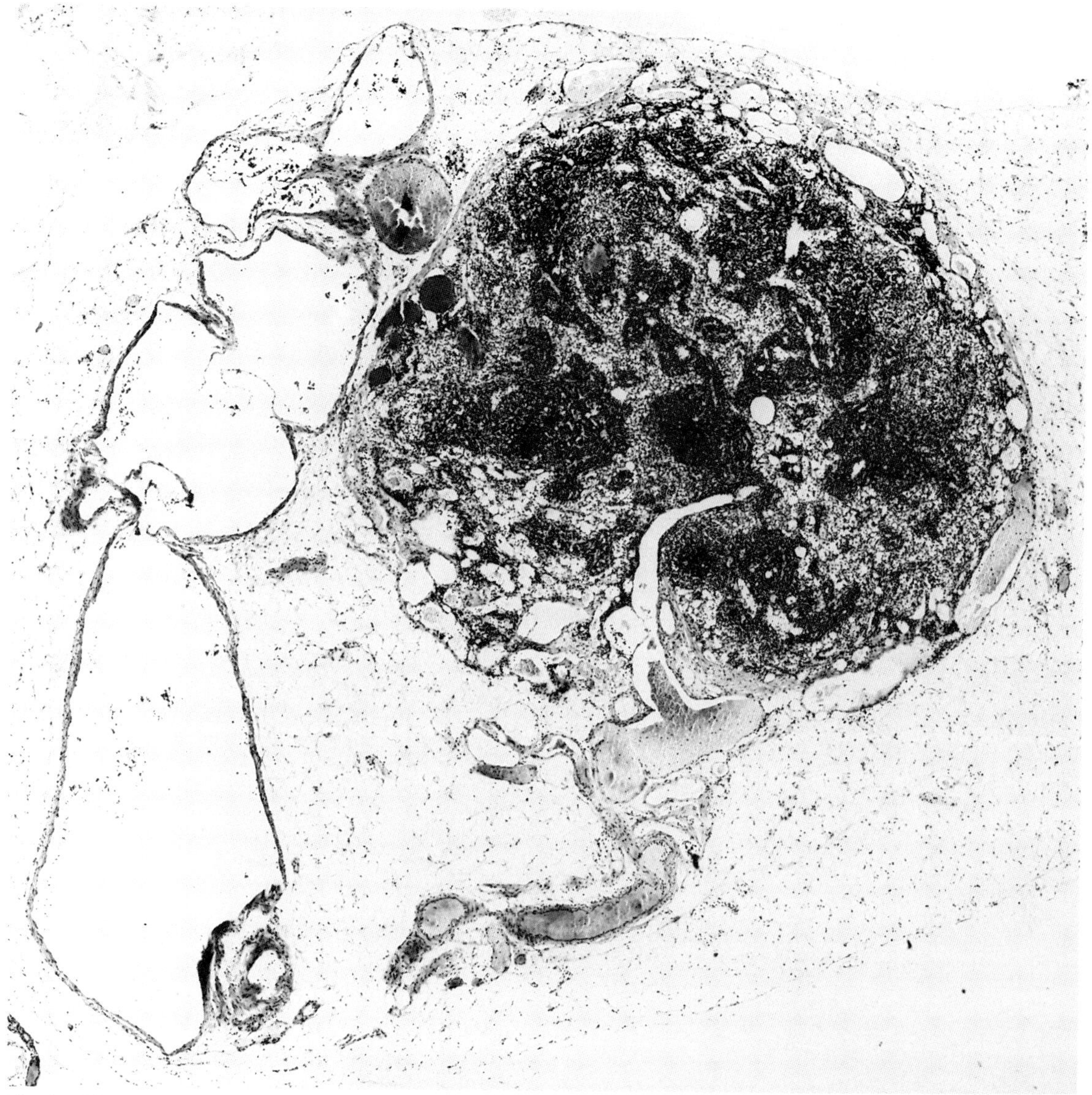

Fig. 4—Dilated veins and lymphatic vessels in perinodal and capsular tissue of mesenteric lymph node of small-bowel volvulus. Haematoxylin and eosin, ×29

(Fig. 7), sinuses or into the perinodal connective tissue was found in eight of 10 volvulus cases, four of 15 primary vascular bowel infarctions and in three of nineteen non-vascular small and large bowel lesions. It was found more commonly in association with volvulus (80 per cent) than in non-vascular cases (16 per cent): see Table II. 'Primary' venous infarction was more frequently (50 per cent) associated with red cell extravasation than was arterial infarction.

Generalized nodal vasodilatation

This was seen a little more frequently in cases of small bowel or colonic volvulus, where it was present in four of 10 cases (40 per cent) than in 'primary' vascular disease (four of 15 cases: 27 per cent) or in non-vascular small bowel and colonic disease (four of 19 cases: 21 per cent). The morphology of these lesions, as described earlier,[10] was that of vasodilation of small veins in all parts of the lymph

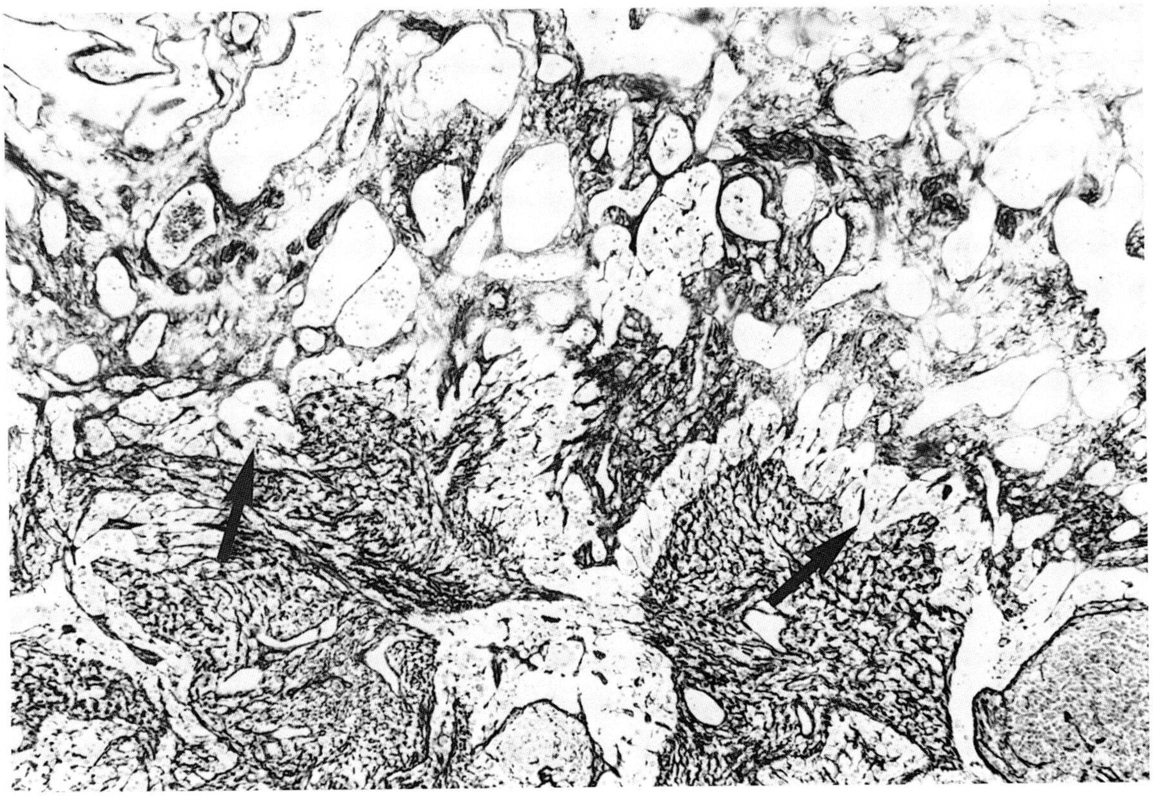

Fig. 5—Numerous dilated venous and lymphatic vessels present in capsule of mesenteric lymph node. The vertically striated marginal sinus (arrowed) passes through lower centre of field. Gordon & Sweets' reticulin, × 90

nodes and in the perinodal connective tissue.

DISCUSSION

'Spontaneous' infarction of superficial lymph nodes is usually held to be due to thrombosis of hilar veins.[1,11,12] Such infarction is rare, only being found once in 12000–20000 surgical biopsies.[13] Possibly on account of the rarity of this type of nodal infarction detailed injection studies are lacking, and lymph nodal necrosis due to identifiable extranodal vascular lesions is limited to infrequent reports of polyarteritis nodosum,[14,15] embolic atheroma,[16] and traumatic phlebothrombosis.[17] By comparison the ischaemic nodal lesions in our series are associated with more generalized vascular lesions. They are also potentially capable of further investigation by means of vascular injection.[18]

Volvulus of the intestine may involve the small bowel or the colon, the sigmoid region being the most frequently affected. With sufficient mesenteric rotation the blood and lymphatic vessels may be occluded to produce ischaemia of the bowel wall.[7] Initially the veins are obstructed, but in time arterial occlusion may ensue.[19] In view of their thin-walled character, it seems likely that mesenteric lymphatic channels will also be involved relatively early in established volvulus.

Infarction of mesenteric lymph nodes has not to our knowledge been reported in volvulus of the intestine. Indeed we are unaware of any formal accounts of lymph nodal infarction associated with ischaemia of adjacent organs supplied by the same blood vessels. However, intestinal volvulus appears to be a good model for gaining some insight into the lymph nodal reactions which result from vascular occlusion.

Three lesions in the mesenteric lymph nodes occurred only in ischaemic bowel groups, namely, frank infarction, lymphoid depletion and capsular hypervascularity. All three were found as often or more frequently in cases of volvulus than in simple

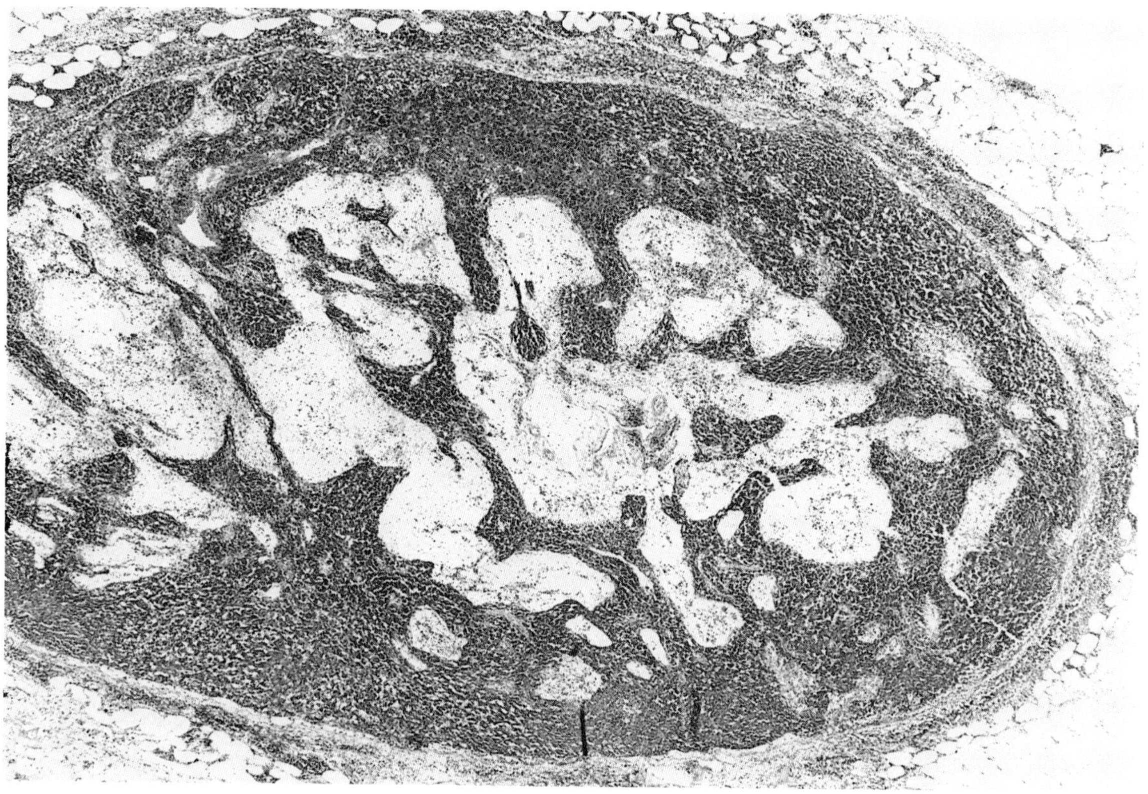

Fig. 6—Gross distension of central nodal sinuses in colonic volvulus. Haematoxylin and eosin, × 30

'primary' arterial infarction of the bowel. Frank infarction of lymph nodes was not seen in the groups without mucosal necrosis. Such observations suggest that these three nodal lesions are of ischaemic origin, that involvement of more than one set of blood vessels carries an enhanced liability of nodal ischaemia, and that the severity of the nodal lesions is related to the degree of ischaemia, which in extreme form evokes mucosal damage in the bowel wall. Similar conclusions have been reached about experimental lymph nodal ischaemia[2,20] in a variety of animals. Hitherto such graded effects have not been described in man. Clearly, however, it is not possible on our evidence to suggest that even these three nodal lesions, by themselves, are diagnostic of ischaemia in the absence of vascular abnormality. Nodal necrosis, lymphoid depletion and capsular hypervascularity may occur, respectively, in nodal neoplasms,[21] chronic disease,[22] and in inflammation.[13,23] Nonetheless, in the present series of mesenteric vascular occlusive lesions, these nodal changes do seem attributable to ischaemia and were not seen in non-vascular diseases of the bowel.

The other three lymph nodal abnormalities, sinus distension, erythrocyte extravasation and vasodilatation are much less specific. Whilst sinus distension is a feature of established lymph nodal infarction,[1,5] venous congestion[24] and erythrocyte extravasation would be anticipated in the presence of ischaemic and damaged blood vessels. However such changes are not confined to nodal ischaemia.[10] Dilatation of small intranodal vessels appears to be no more common in ischaemia than in other bowel conditions. In fact, it appears to be a positive response of the vessels to inflammation.[10] Our conclusion is that these latter three lesions, whilst seen in the mesenteric nodes of vascular lesions of the bowel, are probably non-specific reactions to a variety of stimuli.

The morphology of the infarcts in mesenteric lymph nodes differs from that seen in most superficial lymph nodes. In the latter only a small subcapsular rind of apparently viable tissue persists.[1,12]

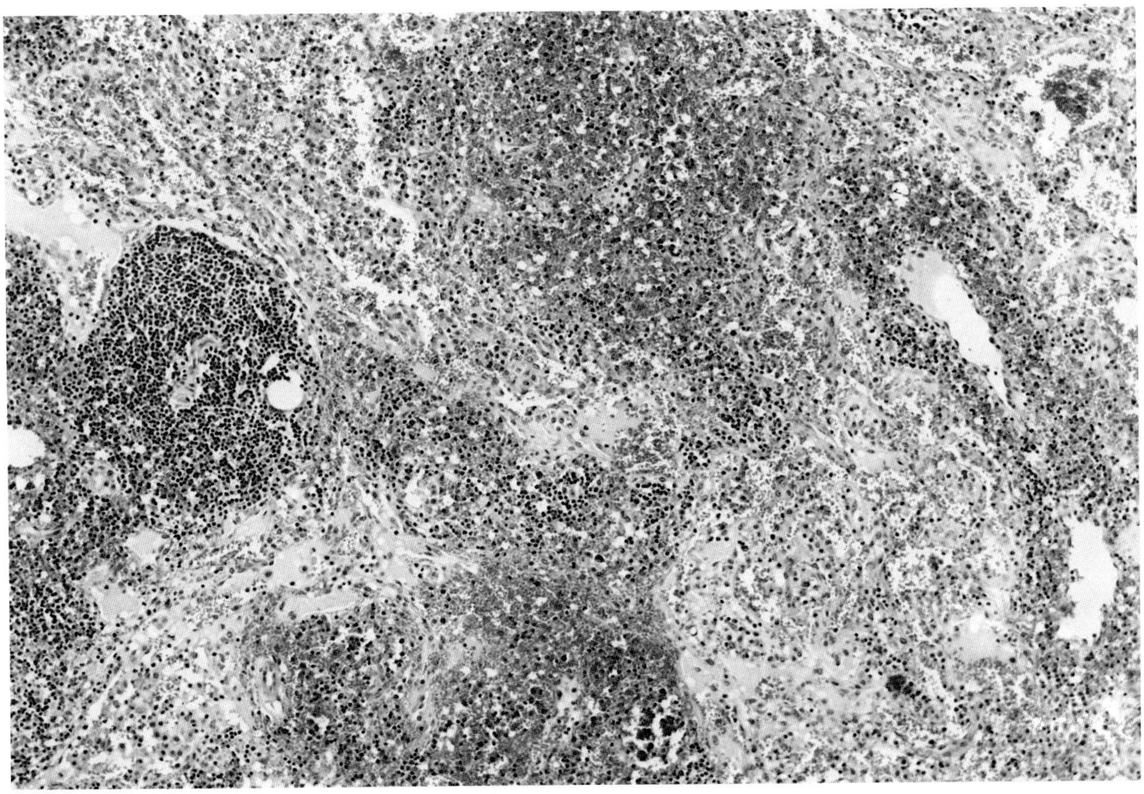

Fig. 7—Erythrocyte extravasation in white pulp of mesenteric lymph node (right part of field). Red cells present in necrosis (top) and around intranodal vessel on right. Right side of node displays lymphoid depletion, as compared with relatively normal trabeculae on left and centre. Haematoxylin and eosin, × 100

In mesenteric lymph nodes the necrosis may be as widespread as in superficial nodes, but is more often either central, or, when it extends to the superficial cortex, there may be zones of surviving lymphoid cells around the nodal trabeculae. These differences are likely to relate to the more complex structure of deep lymph nodes[25] in which cortex and paracortex are admixed. In consequence of this structure, the blood supply of deep lymph nodes appears to differ from superficial nodes[18] in possessing a more pronounced capsular and trabecular vascularity. As a result of these vascular differences the microanatomical distribution of the infarction in the mesenteric lymph nodes tends to be more centrally situated, with the survival of lymphoid tissue adjacent to the trabeculae.

Finally, our findings suggest that frank lymph nodal infarction and other lesser ischaemic lesions are more common than is supposed. Although lymph nodal infarction may herald malignant lymphoma,[21,26,27] such an ominous significance seems unlikely in cases where there is a demonstrable antecedant vascular cause of the infarction.

ACKNOWLEDGEMENTS

We are grateful to present and past surgical colleagues at the Bristol Royal Infirmary for access to clinical details of patients under their care. We are also indebted to Mr C. C. Jeal for help with the photomicrography, and to Mrs M. R. Lake for secretarial assistance. We are particularly pleased to acknowledge the opportunity to have reviewed published material from Professor J. Diebold, University of Paris (Ref. 23).

REFERENCES

1. Davies JD, Stansfeld AG. Spontaneous infarction of superficial lymph nodes. *J Clin Pathol* 1972; **25:** 689–696.

2. Osogoe B, Courtice FC. The effects of occlusion of the blood supply to the popliteal lymph node and on the histology of the node. *Austral J Exp Biol Med Sci* 1968; **46:** 515–524.
3. Tilak SP, Howard JM. Regeneration and autotransplantation of lymph nodes. *Ann Surg* 1965; **161:** 441–446.
4. Benisch BM, Howard RG. Lymph-node infarction in two young men. *Am J Clin Pathol* 1975; **63:** 818–823.
5. Schwarts A, Horáček J, Štěrba K. Infarkt mízni uzliny neznáme etiologie *Cas Lék čes* 1976; **115:** 524–526
6. Elie H, Joubert B, Mandard J-C. Infarctus ischémique spontané massif d'un ganglion cervical. *Ann Path (Paris)* 1982; **2:** 240–242.
7. Morson BC. The alimentary tract: 6. In: Wright GP, Symmers W StC, eds. Systemic Pathology. London: Longmans, Green, Vol 1. 1966: 522.
8. Davies JD, Young EW. Congo blue: a rapid stain for elastic fibres. *J Clin Pathol* 1982; **35:** 789–791.
9. Denz FA. Age changes in lymph nodes. *J Pathol Bact* 1947; **59:** 575–591.
10. Lott MF, Davies JD. Lymph node hypervascularity: haemangiomatoids and pan-nodal vasodilatation. *J Pathol* 1983; **140:** 209–219.
11. Robb Smith AHT, Taylor CR. Lymph Node Biopsy: A Diagnostic Atlas. London: Miller–Heyden, 1981; 222.
12. Ioachim HL. Lymph Node Biopsy. Philadelphia: Lippincott, 1982; 161–163.
13. Davies JD. Vascular disturbances. In: Stansfeld AG, ed. Lymph Node Biopsy Interpretation. Edinburgh: Churchill Livingstone, in press.
14. Lennert K. Lymphknoten: Diagnostik in Schnitt und Ausstrich. Berlin: Springer-Verlag, 1961; 379–380.
15. Symmers W StC. The lymphoreticular system. In: Symmers W StC, ed. Systemic Pathology. 2nd edn. Vol. 2. Edinburgh: Churchill-Livingstone, 1978; 504–891.
16. Shah KH, Kisilevsky R. Infarction of lymph nodes: a cause of palisading macrophage reaction mimicking necrotising granulomas. *Human Pathol* 1978; **9:** 597–599.
17. Davies JD, Webb AJ. Segmental lymph-node infarction following fine-needle aspiration. *J Clin Pathol* 1982; **35:** 855–857.
18. Semeraro D, Davies JD. The arterial supply of human lymph nodes. *Bristol Med-Chi J* 1984; **99:** 31.
19. Sutcliffe MML. Volvulus of the sigmoid colon. *Br J Surg* 1968; **55:** 903–910.
20. Steinmann G, Főldi E, Főldi M, Racz P, Lennert K. Morphologic findings in lymph nodes after occlusion of their efferent lymphatic vessels and veins. *Lab Invest* 1982; **47:** 43–50.
21. Cleary KR, Osborne BM, Butler JJ. Lymph node infarction fore-shadowing malignant lymphoma. *Am J Surg Pathol* 1982; **6:** 435–442.
22. Tsakraklides V, Tsakraklides E, Good RA. An autopsy study of human axillary lymph node histology. *Am J Pathol* 1975; **78:** 7–22.
23. Diebold J, Tulliez M, Bernadow A, Andouin J, Tricot G, Reynes M, Bilski-Pasquier G. Angio-follicular and plasmacytic polyadenopathy: a pseudotumorous syndrome with dysimmunity. *J Clin Pathol* 1980; **33:** 1068–1076.
24. Klishevich BA. Peculiarities of changes in paths of lymph circulation within lymph nodes in chronic circulatory insufficiency. (In Russian.) *Arkh Anat Hist Embr (Leningrad)* 1970; **54:** 56–63.
25. Bélisle C, Sainte-Marie G. Topography of the deep cortex of the lymph nodes of various mammalian species. *Anat Rec* 1981; **201:** 553–561.
26. Ballas M, Sanchez M, Lee J-H, Czepiel SJ, Kashani M. Syndrome of the infarcted lymph node. *Lab Invest* 1982; **46:** 7A.
27. Schmid U, Maurer R. Lymphknoteninfarkte. *Schweiz med Wschr* 1983; **113:** 755–756.

JOURNAL OF PATHOLOGY, VOL. **144**: 269–273 (1984)

FOCAL LYMPHOCYTIC THYROIDITIS IN SOUTHAMPTON

J. D. MITCHELL AND N. KIRKHAM
Department of Pathology, Faculty of Medicine, University of Southampton, Southampton, U.K.

AND

DAVID MACHIN
Department of Community Medicine and Medical Statistics, Faculty of Medicine, University of Southampton, Southampton, U.K.

Received 2 July 1984
Accepted 13 July 1984

SUMMARY

The presence of focal collections of lymphocytes within the thyroid gland has been associated with autoimmune thyroiditis. In a prospective study 197 thyroid glands were examined from post mortems performed in two Southampton hospitals over a 12 month period. The mean thyroid mass was 19·5 g in women and 22·2 g in men. Varying degrees of focal lymphocytic thyroiditis were present in 54 per cent of women and 24 per cent of men. Morphometry showed that on average less than 4 per cent of the gland was infiltrated by lymphocytes. There was no significant relationship with age. A possible association between focal lymphocytic thryoiditis and circulating thyroid autoantibodies has been shown.

KEY WORDS—Lymphocytes, thyroid gland, thyroiditis.

INTRODUCTION

The occurrence of microscopic foci of lymphocytes in grossly normal thyroid glands was first described by Simmonds[1] and has been examined previously in several studies.

Goudie *et al.*[2] found some degree of focal lymphocytic thyroiditis in 22 per cent of 77 post mortems. Williams and Doniach[3] reported a prevalence of 45 per cent in females and 19 per cent in males of the 612 adult thyroids studied and Weaver *et al.*[4] found thyroiditis in 18 per cent of males and 36 per cent of females (mean 22 per cent) in a study of 400 post mortems. Harris *et al.*[5] reported a lower prevalence of 3·3 per cent of 274 males and 13·8 per cent of 210 female Jamaican adults at post mortem.

These studies varied in their sampling of the thyroid. Williams and Doniach[3] give no mention of how many blocks they examined from each gland, whilst Weaver *et al.*[4] used a maximum of four. Despite this limitation a variation in the prevalence of focal lymphocytic thyroiditis has been shown. The results of a prospective study are reported in which post mortem thyroids from unselected clinically euthyroid Southampton residents were examined in detail for the presence of thyroiditis. In a proportion of cases we also looked for circulating thyroglobulin and microsomal antibodies.

MATERIALS AND METHODS

Thyroid glands were obtained from 197 unselected post mortems carried out on white adults between October 1982 and September 1983 in the two major teaching hospitals in Southampton. The clinical notes were consulted for details of the patient's age, sex and previously recognized thyroid disease.

The glands were removed intact, fixed in 10 per cent neutral buffered formol saline and cleaned of

Addressee for correspondence: N. Kirkham, Pathology Laboratory, Royal Sussex County Hospital, Brighton BN2 5BF, U.K.

0022–3417/84/120269–05$01.00

any non-thyroidal tissue. The total weight was measured on a Sartorious electric balance accurate to 0·01 g.

Each thyroid was sliced coronally into 3–4 mm thick sections. Alternate sections were processed for histology except in large glands where no more than 12 blocks were selected. The paraffin-embedded sections were stained with haematoxylin and eosin and systematically examined for focal lymphocytic thyroiditis, using the criteria of Williams and Doniach,[3] which was graded on a three point scale. Grade 1—small foci present on one or two blocks; Grade 2—small foci present on all or most blocks; Grade 3—large foci present on all or most blocks.

Computerized area analysis was employed on selected slides of all thyroids classified into grades 2 and 3. Each slide was projected onto the graphics tablet of an Apple II microcomputer at a magnification of ×10 using a Micro Promar projecting microscope (Leitz). One random point was selected on each slide by marking the slide with an ink dot. The four adjacent fields above, below and on either side of this point were then projected and the area of thyroid in each field and the area of each field occupied by lymphoid aggregates was outlined using the graphics light pen and calculated by the computer. The percentage area of each slide occupied by lymphocytic foci was then calculated. From this the percentage of the volume of the thyroid occupied by lymphocytic infiltrations was calculated by application of the Law of Deless.

Antibody studies

Circulating thyroid antibody levels were determined from the sera of 58 unselected clinically euthyroid patients, all of whom had been dead for less than 72 h. Antibodies to thyroglobulin and thyroid microsomal antigens were measured using the Thymune-T haemagglutination kit (Wellcome Diagnostics, Dartford)[6] for thyroglobulin antibodies and immunofluorescent technique for thyroid microsomal antibodies.[7]

Statistical methods

The influence of subject age, sex and grade of thyroiditis on the weight of the thyroid was examined by a multiple regression model which includes the effects of age, sex and grade. The model can be expressed for an individual of a given age as $W_{ij}=\eta+\eta^S_i+\eta^G_j+b$ (AGE) where W_{ij} is the thyroid weight corresponding to age i and grade j $i=0, 1, j=0, \ldots, 3$, η is a constant η^S_0 is the effect for males, η^S_1 for females, η^G_0 is the main effect for those with no thyroiditis, similar definitions hold for η^G_1, η^G_2, η^G_3, finally b is the multiple regression coefficient for age.

Each subject can be regarded as having thyroiditis (grades 1, 2 or 3), or not having it, with a certain probability p which depends on their age, sex and the weight of their thyroid. One method of modelling such a situation is by means of the multiple logistic model

$$\log\left(\frac{p}{1-p}\right)=c_0+c_1\,(\text{age})+c_2\,(\text{sex})+c_3\,(\text{weight})$$

where age and weight are the individual values for a particular subject and sex takes the value 0 or 1 depending on whether the subject is male or female. The c_0, c_1, c_2 and c_3 are numerical constants called logistic coefficients. $\text{Log}\left(\frac{p}{1-p}\right)$ is called the log odds of getting thyroiditis of any grade. The c_i values are estimated by means of the statistical computer package GENSTAT.[8]

RESULTS

Table I shows the mean thyroid weight and age of subjects classified by thyroid grade and sex. The thyroid appears somewhat heavier in the males and increases in weight with age (Fig. 1). Weight

Table I—Thyroid weight and age of subject by grade and sex. Number of subjects in parenthesis

Grade		Male	Female	Mean
Absent	Weight	22·7	20·1	21·0
	Age	62·5	68·6	64·5
		(81)	(41)	(122)
1	Weight	23·6	19·2	21·9
	Age	67·1	76·5	70·7
		(13)	(8)	(21)
2	Weight	17·0	17·9	17·6
	Age	55·3	68·4	63·4
		(8)	(13)	(21)
3	Weight	19·0	19·5	19·5
	Age	60·6	70·5	69·0
		(15)	(28)	(33)
All grades	Weight	22·2	19·5	21·0
	Age	62·4	69·9	65·8
		(107)	(90)	(197)

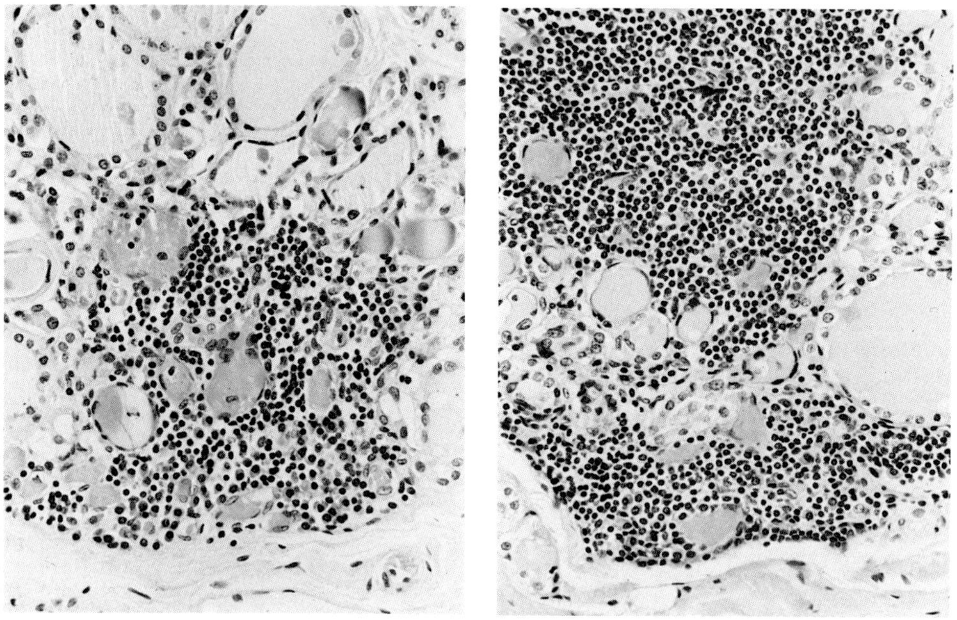

(a) (b)

Fig. 1—(a) Sparse lymphocytic infiltration seen in grades 1 and 2 thyroiditis. (b) Heavy lymphocytic infiltration of grade 3 thyroiditis

appears unaffected by grade or thyroiditis.

Formal statistical analysis summarized in Table II using selective multiple regression suggests that both sex and age are determinants of thyroid weight but weight appears uninfluenced by thyroiditis grade.

Table III shows the results of the logistic

Table II—Multiple regression for thyroid weight

Model	Variable			Regression coefficient	S.E.	t-value
	Constant term		η	14·006		
Full	Sex	Male	η_0^S	0		
		Female	η_1^S	−3·161	1·996	−1·58
	Grade	Absent	η_0^G	0		
		1	η_1^G	−0·560	2·993	−0·19
		2	η_2^G	−3·202	3·034	−1·06
		3	η_3^G	−1·343	2·670	−0·50
	Age	(years)	b	0·137	0·048	286
	Constant term		η'	13·483		
	Sex	Male	$\eta_0^{S'}$	0		
		Female	$\eta_1^{S'}$	−3·740	1·830	−2·04
	Age (years)		b′	0·140	0·048	2·94

regression analysis. Each variable has a logistic coefficient and its standard error was used to obtain t-values. Only sex has a significant t-value ($P<0{\cdot}001$) and is the only significant contribution to a patient's probability of having thyroiditis. The odds of a female having thyroiditis as compared to a male are given by exponentiating the logistic coefficient for sex of Table III (b), thus $e^{1{\cdot}1363}=3{\cdot}1$ which implies that women have approximately three times the risk as men.

Morphometry

The results of the analysis of 47 thyroids with grades 2 and 3 thyroiditis are shown in Table IV. There is considerable variation in the volume of gland occupied by lymphocytes, but even in Grade 3 thyroiditis the mean is only 3·58 per cent. In only six cases was the degree of infiltration greater than 5 per cent.

Antibody studies

Of the 54 cases tested, the majority were negative (Table V). However, 6/10 cases with grade 3 thyroiditis had positive microsomal antibodies. In a further 15 cases a full autoimmune profile had been performed in life. Of six cases with histological grade 3 thyroiditis, two had positive antibodies.

Table III—Multiple logistic model for presence of thyroiditis

Variable	Scale		Logistic coefficient (c_i)	S.E.	*t*-value
(a) Full model					
	Constant term	c_0	−1·186		
Age	(Years)	c_1	0·004	0·008	0·53
Sex	(0 = male 1 = female)	c_2	1·258	0·317	3·98
Thyroid weight	(g)	c_3	−0·010	0·013	0·83
(b) Reduced model					
Model excluding age and weight					
	Constant	c'_0	1·3145		
Sex	(0 = male, 1 = female)	c'_2	−1·1363	0·309	4·26

DISCUSSION

In this sample the thyroid glands from Southampton were similar in size to those found by Fukunaga and Yatani[9] in Japan, Canada and Columbia. It would seem that 20 g is approximately the normal human thyroid weight. Male subjects show a larger mean thyroid mass than the females, which may be due to their larger body size.

There was a clear increase in thyroid mass with age in females whilst it remained constant in males. This increase in female gland size reflects both an increased incidence of pathological englargement of the gland and an increased frequency of large but histologically normal glands.

Table IV

Grade of thyroiditis	No. of thyroids	Mean vol. % lymphocytes (S.D.)	Range (min 0·1%)
2	26	0·41 (0·37)	<0·1– 1·35
3	21	6·45 (8·65)	1·1–33·0
Total	47	3·58 (6·92)	<0·1–33·0

Table V

Thyroiditis	Microsomal antibodies Absent	Present
Absent	32	0
Grade 1	7	0
Grade 2	4	1
Grade 3	4	6
Total	47	7

The age and sex distribution in this study is similar to that found previously by Williams and Doniach[3] and Weaver *et al.*[4] in studies of predominantly white populations although different to that of Harris *et al.*[5] conducted on a female black population in Jamaica.

With respect to thyroiditis, the overall prevalence of 0·38 (95 per cent confidence limits 0·31–0·45) is higher than that previously reported. This is almost certainly because the whole thyroid was available for histological examination. Increased sampling has allowed us to detect small numbers of lymphocytic foci which would not have been found as readily in smaller samples of the gland. However, grades 1 and 2 thyroiditis do not seem to be associated with autoantibodies. Grade 3 thyroiditis, characterized by large lymphoid aggregates in more than two blocks of thyroid, is associated with microsomal autoantibodies. Thus when surgical thyroidectomy specimens are examined, a minimum of three tissue blocks should be examined. If grade 3 thyroiditis is present, then the patients may be found to have autoantibodies.

REFERENCES

1. Simmonds M. Uber lymphatische herde in der Schilddrüse. *Virchow's Arch Pathol Anat* 1913; **211:** 73–89.
2. Goudie RB, Anderson JR, Gray KG. Complement fixing antithyroid antibodies in hospital patients with asymptomatic thyroid lesions. *J Path Bact* 1959; **77:** 389–400.
3. Williams ED, Doniach I. The post-mortem incidence

of focal thyroiditis. *J Path Bact* 1962; **83:** 255–264.
4. Weaver DR, Doedhar SD, Hazard JB. A characterization of focal lymphocytic thyroiditis. *Cleve Clin Q* 1966; **33:** 59–72.
5. Harris M, Summerell JM, Swan AV. The prevalence of focal thyroiditis in Jamaican adults. *J Pathol* 1973; **110:** 309–318.
6. Cayzer I, Chalmers SR, Doniach D, Swana G. An evaluation of two new haemagglutination tests for the rapid diagnosis of autoimmune thyroid diseases. *J Clin Pathol* 1978; **31:** 1147–1151.
7. Doniach D. Thyroid autoimmune disease. *J Clin Pathol* 1967; **20:** 385–390.
8. Alvey N, Galwey N, Lane P. An Introduction to GENSTAT. London: Academic Press, 1982; 152.
9. Fukunaga FH, Yatani R. Geographic pathology of occult thyroid carcinomas. *Cancer* 1975; **36:** 1095–1099.

JOURNAL OF PATHOLOGY, VOL. **144**: 275–280 (1984)

HISTOGENESIS OF ADENOMATOID TUMOUR ASSOCIATED TO PSEUDOFIBROMATOUS PERIORCHITIS IN AN INFANT WITH HYDROCELE

M. NISTAL

Department of Morphology, School of Medicine, Autonomous University, Madrid, Spain, and Department of Pathology, La Paz Hospital, Madrid, Spain

R. PANIAGUA

Department of Cytology and Histology, Faculty of Biology, University of Salamanca, Salamanca, Spain

ELENA FUENTES

Department of Pathology, La Paz Hospital, Madrid, Spain

AND

J. REGADERA

Department of Morphology, School of Medicine, Autonomous University, Madrid, Spain

Received 9 April 1984
Accepted 17 July 1984

SUMMARY

An 18-month-old infant with recurrent congenital hydrocele presented with a mass in the caput epididymis. The tumour and several fragments of the tunica vaginalis were removed and studied by light and electron microscopy. The tumour showed the characteristic histological pattern of an adenomatoid tumour of mesothelial origin. The histological appearance of the tunica vaginalis was not uniform; some areas resembled the adenomatoid tumour to the epididymis, others exhibited histological and ultrastructural features of a haemangioma, whilst elsewhere, the two patterns were intermingled. Finally, areas of pseudofibromatous periorchitis with vascular proliferation and slit-like structures lined by mesothelial cells were recognized. These features suggest that the adenomatoid tumour originated from a localized reactive process with inflammation and vascular proliferation enclosing occasional slit-like structures originating from the mesothelial lining of the tunica vaginalis. Subsequent regression of vascular proliferation and inflammatory infiltration and continued mesothelial proliferation would give rise to the typical mesothelial pattern of adenomatoid tumour.

KEY WORDS—Adenomatoid tumour, pseudofibromatous periorchitis, hydrocele, haemangioma, mesothelial cell, endothelial cell.

INTRODUCTION

Paratesticular structures such as the tunica vaginalis testis, the epididymis and the spermatic cord, may often be involved in reactive processes like pseudofibromatous periorchitis (fibrous pseudotumour)[1–5] and tumours such as the adenomatoid tumour.[6–9] These two lesions have been reported many times but never associated. In the literature, only one case is reported in which both lesions were seen in the same patient within the space of a few months.[4] The present report concerns the association of pseudofibromatous periorchitis and adenomatoid tumour in an infant with recur-

Addressee for correspondence: Professor Dr Manuel Nistal, Departamento de Morfología, Facultad de Medicina, Universidad Autónoma, C/ Arzobispo Morcillo, 4; Madrid 28029, Spain.

0022–3417/84/120275–06$01.00

rent congenital hydrocele. Histological examination suggests a possible histogenesis of adenomatoid tumour.

METHODS

The patient, an 18-month-old infant, presented with recurrent right-sided congenital hydrocele which had required surgical intervention on two occasions. Surgical exploration showed a mass in the caput epididymis which was removed (Fig. 1). The tumour was a firm grey-white nodule measuring 1 cm on its longest axis. Slicing disclosed a whitish homogeneous cut surface. Several fragments of the tunica vaginalis testis, which appeared irregularly thickened, up to 1 cm in width, were also removed. They were white nodular and of moderately hard consistency.

The specimens were processed for both light and electron microscopy. For light microscopy they were fixed in formalin, dehydrated, embedded in paraffin wax and stained with haematoxylin and eosin, alcian blue (pH 1), periodic-acid–Schiff, Masson trichrome and Van Gieson stains. For electron microscopy, small fragments of fresh material were fixed in Karnovsky fixative (4 h), post-fixed in 1 per cent phosphate-buffered osmium tetroxide (2 h), dehydrated in ethanol and embedded in Epon-812. Sections (1 μm thick) were stained with toluidine blue. The ultrathin sections were double-stained with uranyl acetate and lead citrate and examined with a Philips-300 electron microscope.

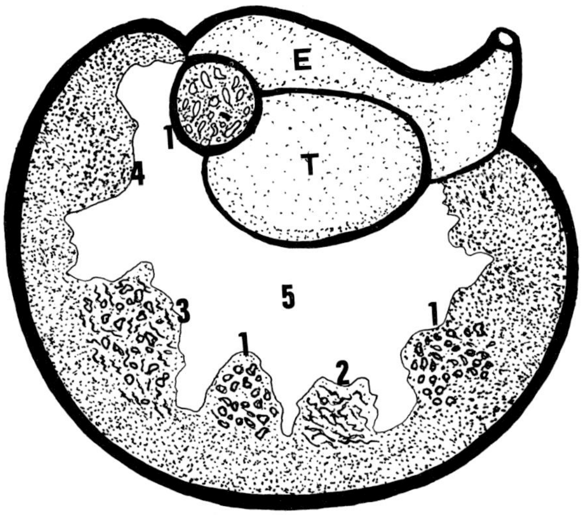

Fig. 1—Distribution of the different lesions in the epididymis and tunica vaginalis. 1: adenomatoid tumour; 2: haemangioma-like lesion; 3: adenomatoid tumour and haemangioma-like lesion intermingled; 4: pseudofibromatous periorchitis; 5: hydrocele. T: testis; E: epididymis

RESULTS

Light microscopic examination of the epididymal tumour revealed a typical adenomatoid pattern consisting of an unencapsulated mass of neoplastic cells arranged in solid cords, tubules and gland-like structures (Fig. 2A). These formed anastomosing irregular channels which occasionally contained sloughed cells. The channels were lined by cuboidal or flattened cells and were supported by a stroma of fibrous connective tissue with scattered lymphocytes. Electron microscopic examination revealed that the tumour cells possessed the typical ultrastructural features of mesothelial cells (Fig. 2B). They rested on a basal lamina and exhibited well-developed junctional complexes, but were separated by intercellular canaliculi in other areas. The plasma membrane projected microvilli on both adluminal and canalicular surfaces. The cytoplasm showed irregular, scattered, short cisternae of rough endoplasmic reticulum and moderately abundant polysomes, a prominent Golgi complex with some secretory vesicles and round mitochondria. Cytoplasmic microfilaments were numerous. In addition to 60 Å diameter non-specific microfilaments, 100 Å diameter filament bundles were also observed which probably corresponded to mesothelial keratin.[10] The nuclei were round or ovoid with deep infoldings (Fig. 2C).

The histological pattern of the tunica vaginalis varied widely from one zone to another (Figs 3, 4). In some zones, the light and electron microsopic appearance was similar to that of the adenomatoid tumour (Fig. 3A). Other zones showed a histological pattern similar to haemangioma. They were composed of anastomosing slit-like channels or papillae lined by cuboidal or flattened cells with nuclear infoldings, more frequent and prominent than those of the adenomatoid tumour. Inflammatory infiltrates were more abundant. The ultrastructural appearance differed markedly from that of the adenomatoid tumour, being rather similar to that of endothelial cells (Fig. 3B). There were no microvilli but there were irregular cytoplasmic projections into the lumen. Pinocytotic vesicles were frequent. Junctional complexes were not developed. Only focal points of occlusion and small

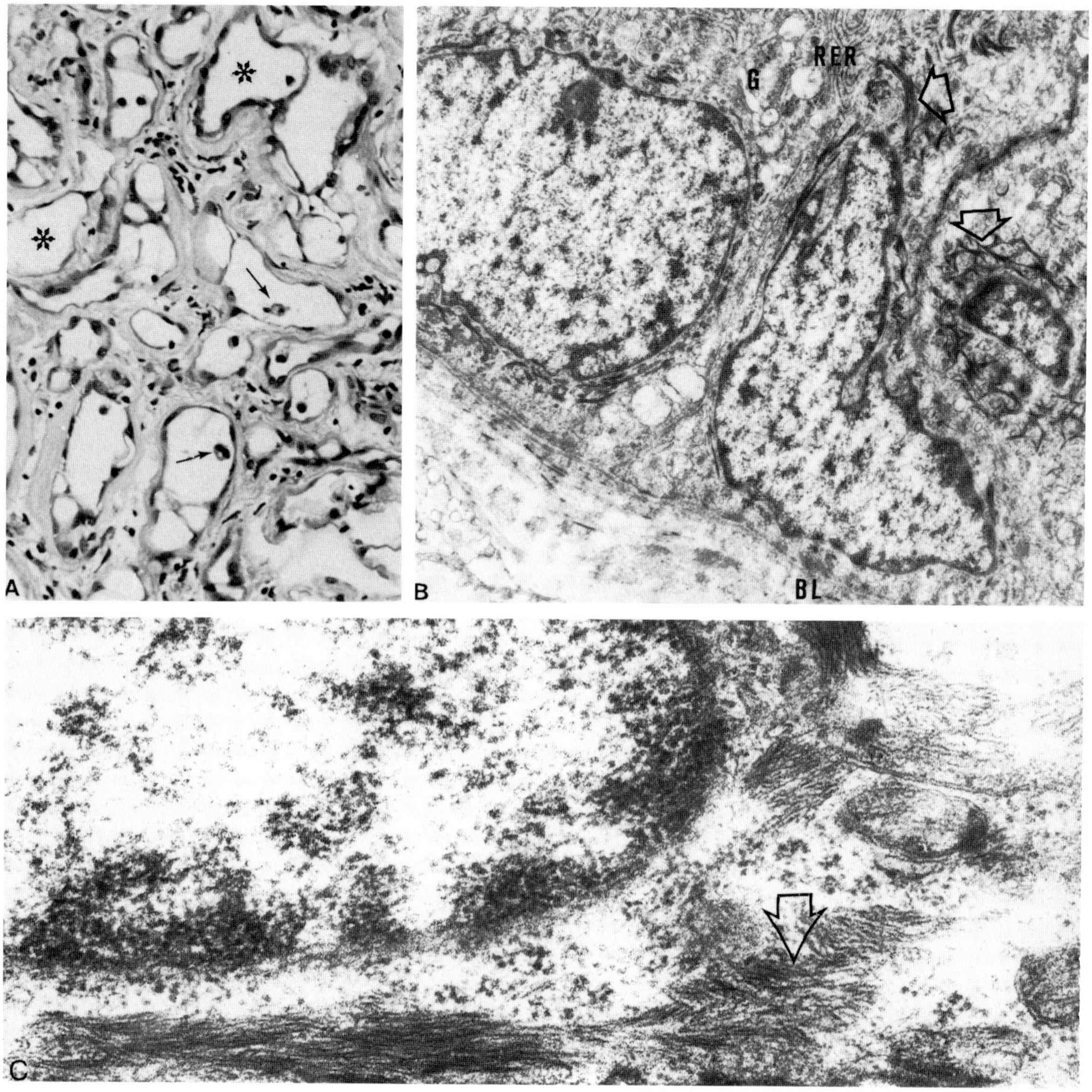

Fig. 2—Adenomatoid tumour in the caput epididymis. (A) Gland-like structures (asterisks) lined by cuboidal or flattened cells. Some sloughed cells (arrows) are also seen. H & E, ×238. (B) Mesothelial cells lining the adenomatoid tumour channels. Mesothelial keratin filaments (arrows) are seen. RER: rough endoplasmic reticulum; G: Golgi complex; BL: basal lamina, ×3325. (C) Higher magnification of keratin filament bundles (arrow), ×15675

desmosomes were observed. Mesothelial keratin filaments were absent, although 60 Å microfilaments were present. In addition, these cells contained specific endothelial granules (Weibel-Palade bodies) (Fig. 3C) and were resting on a multilayered basal lamina (Fig. 3B).

Other zones of the tunica vaginalis showed adenomatoid and vascular patterns intermingled.

In some areas the tunica vaginalis presented the characteristic features of pseudofibromatous periorchitis (Fig. 4A). They mainly consisted of fibrous connective tissue proliferation with irregularly arranged collagen fibre bundles which frequently surrounded blood vessels with thickened walls. The fibrous connective tissue occasionally contained slit-like structures (Figs 4A, B); some of

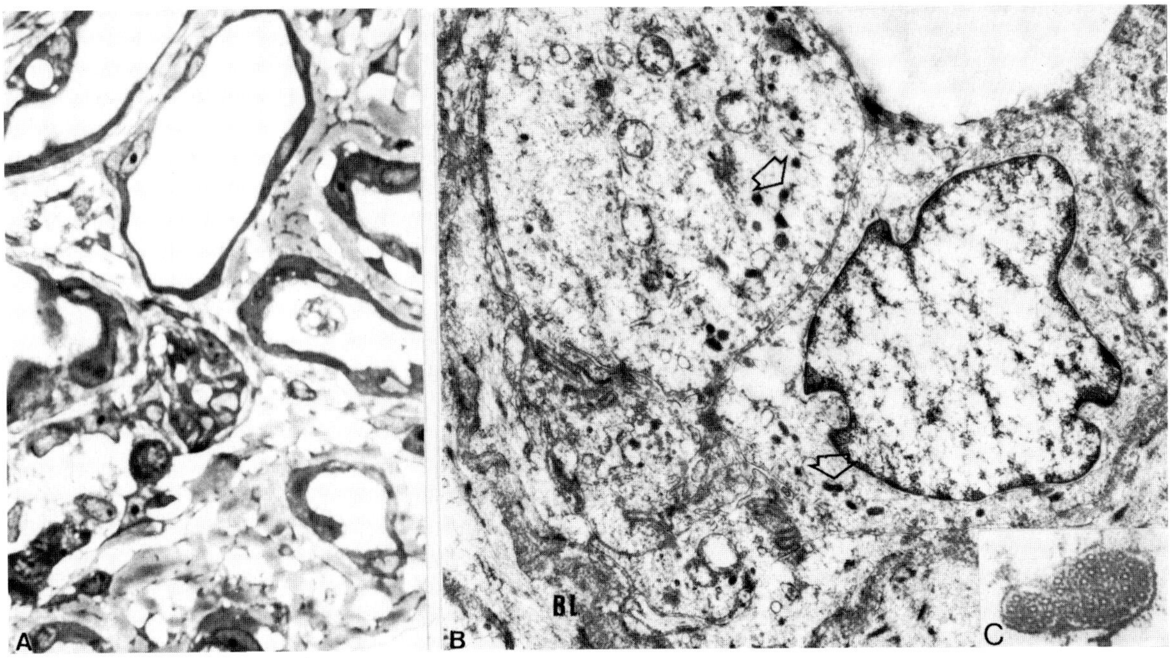

Fig. 3—Tunica vaginalis (A) Histological pattern similar to adenomatoid tumour. Toluidine blue, × 760. (B) Endothelial-like cells lining channels of the haemangioma-like lesion. The basal lamina (BL) displays several layers. Endothelial granules (arrows) are seen, × 3325. (C) Higher magnification of a specific endothelial granule in an endothelial-like cell, × 71 250

them were lined by mesothelial cells in continuity with the mesothelial lining of the tunica vaginalis, whilst others were lined by endothelial-like cells, as revealed by electron microscopy. In addition, there were mast cells and chronic inflammatory infiltrates.

The mesothelial lining of the tunica vaginalis exhibited generalized hyperplasia, displaying a papillary pattern (Fig. 4B). Mesothelial cell metaplasia towards either mucous-secreting cells or squamous cells was observed in areas with abundant inflammatory cell infiltration.

DISCUSSION

The histogenesis of adenomatoid tumours of the genital tract is still controversial. It has been suggested that they are derived from vascular endothelium,[11,12] mesonephros[13,14] or Müllerian epithelium[15–17] but more recently, a mesothelial origin of this tumour is supported.[6–9,18–21] Davy and Tang[22] have suggested that adenomatoid tumours be designated mesothelial or angiomatous on electron microscopic appearance.

The present case shows two different intermingled lesions in addition to hydrocele. The first lesion is similar to that previously reported under the terms 'nonspecific peritesticular fibrosis',[2] 'fibromatous periorchitis'[23] and 'fibromatous pseudotumour'.[3,4] The second lesion is a benign entity with a characteristic light microscopic appearance, designated as adenomatoid tumour. In some areas of the tunica vaginalis, the lesion exhibited ultrastructural features of both normal and neoplastic mesothelial cells.[24,25] Elsewhere, the tumour cells showed ultrastructural features similar to those of haemangioma,[26] suggesting the endothelial nature of these cells. In addition, the pseudofibromatous periorchitis contained slit-like structures lined by either mesothelial or endothelial cells. These features suggest a new hypothesis for adenomatoid tumour origin which combines the theories that are currently accepted.

We believe that the adenomatoid tumour is the end result of a localized reactive process with inflammatory cell infiltration and intense vascular proliferation. The slit-like structures, lined by mesothelial cells, arise from invaginations of mesothelial lining of the tunica vaginalis. If the tumour is observed at this stage, the histological pattern would be similar to that of haemangioma,

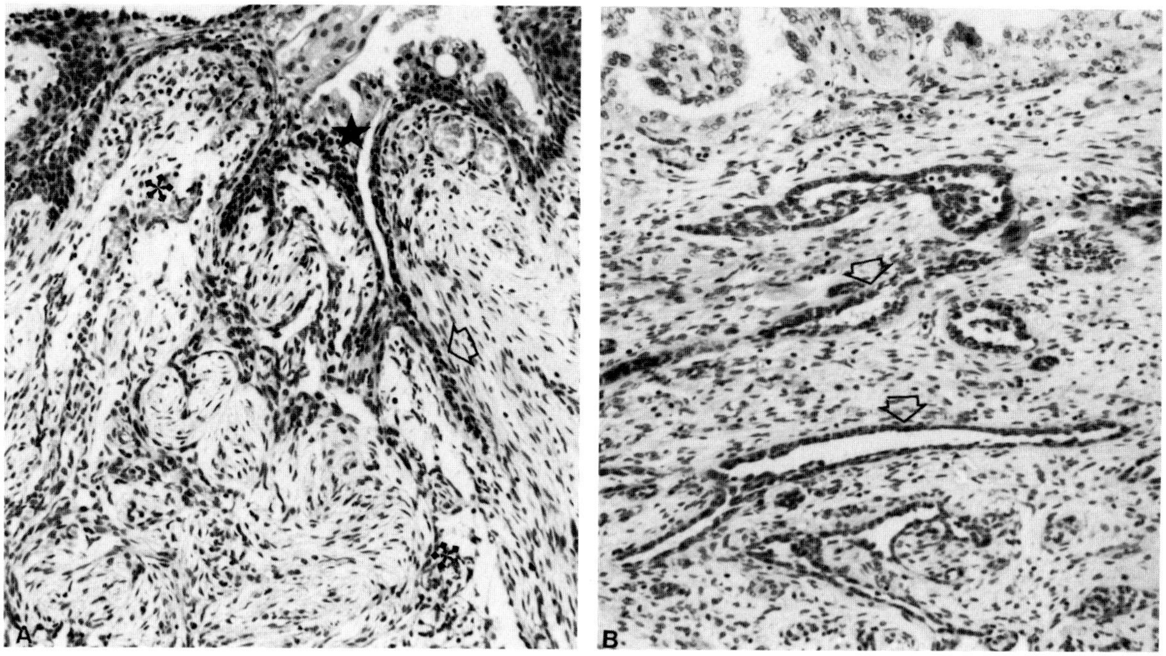

Fig. 4—Pseudofibromatous periorchitis in the tunica vaginalis. (A) Pseudofibromatous periorchitis with vascular proliferation (asterisk), inflammatory infiltrates, and slit-like structures (arrow) in continuity with the hyperplastic mesothelial lining (star). H&E, × 119. (B) Proliferation of slit-like structures (arrows) subjacent to the hyperplastic mesothelial lining. H&E, × 119

except for the presence of mesothelial-lined slit-like structures. Later, the connective tissue stroma, blood vessels and inflammatory infiltrate regress, and the mesothelium proliferates, giving rise to the typical mesothelial pattern of adenomatoid tumour.

ACKNOWLEDGEMENTS

This work was partially supported by a grant from the 'Fondo de Investigaciones Sanitarias de la Seguridad Social', Madrid, Spain. The authors thank Professor Dr Félix Contreras (Chairman of the Department of Pathology, La Paz Hospital, Madrid) for his help and for providing clinical material.

REFERENCES

1. Strom GW. Pseudotumor of testicular tunic. *J Urol* 1977; **118:** 340–341.
2. Honoré LH. Nonspecific peritesticular fibrosis manifested as testicular enlargement. Clinicopathological study of nine cases. *Arch Surg* 1978; **113:** 814–816.
3. Gilchrist KW, Benson RC. Multifocal fibrous pseudotumor of testicular tunics. Possible clinical dilemma. *Urology* 1979; **14:** 285–287.
4. Sarlis I, Yakomakis S, Rebelakos AG. Fibrous pseudotumor of the scrotum. *J Urol* 1980; **124:** 742–743.
5. Harris CJ, Das S, Vogt PJ. Fibrous hamartoma of infancy in the scrotum. *J Urol* 1982; **127:** 781–782.
6. Marcus JB, Lynn JA. Ultrastructural comparison of an adenomatoid tumor, lymphangioma, hemangioma and mesothelioma. *Cancer* 1970; **25:** 171–175.
7. MacKay B, Bennington JL, Skoglund RW. The adenomatoid tumor—fine structural evidence for a mesothelial origin. *Cancer* 1971; **37:** 109–115.
8. Nistal M, Contreras F, Paniagua R. Adenomatoid tumour of the epididymis: histochemical and ultrastructural study of 2 cases. *Brit J Urol* 1978; **50:** 121–125.
9. Söderström KO. Origin of adenomatoid tumor and epididymal duct cells. *Cancer* 1982; **49:** 2349–2357.
10. Wu YJ, Parker LM, Binder NE, *et al.* The mesothelial keratins: a new family of cytoskeletal proteins identified in cultured mesothelial cells and non-keratinizing opithelia. *Cell* 1982; **31:** 693–703.
11. Leighton AP. Lymphangioma of the fallopian tube. *Am J Obstet Gynecol* 1912; **65:** 573–581.
12. Sanes S, Warner R. Primary lymphangioma of the fallopian tube. *Am J Obstet Gynecol* 1939; **37:** 317–321.

13. Sakaguchi Y. Ueber das Adenomyon des Nebenhodens. *Frankfurt Z Pathol* 1916; **18:** 379–387.
14. Teilum G. Histogenesis and classification of mesonephric tumors of the female and male genital system and relationship to benign so-called adenomatoid tumors (mesotheliomas); comparative histological study. *Acta Pathol Microbiol Scand* 1954; **34:** 431–481.
15. Efskind J. Primary tumors of the fallopian tubes with report of 3 cases. *Acta Pathol Microbiol Scand* 1952; **30:** 384–394.
16. Sundarasivarao D. The Müllerian vestiges and benign epithelial tumors of epididymis. *J Pathol Bacteriol* 1953; **66:** 417–432.
17. Jackson JR. The histogenesis of the adenomatoid tumor of the genital tract. *Cancer* 1958; **11:** 337–350.
18. Broth G, Bullock WK, Morrow J. Epididymal tumors: report of 15 new cases including review of literature. Histochemical study of the so-called adenomatoid tumor. *J Urol* 1968; **100:** 530–536.
19. Salazar H, Kanbour A, Burgess F. Ultrastructure and observations on the histogenesis of mesotheliomas—'adenomatoid tumors' of the female genital tract. *Cancer* 1972; **29:** 141–151.
20. Ferenczy A, Fenoglio J, Richart RM. Observations on benign mesothelioma of the genital tract (adenomatoid tumor). *Cancer* 1972; **30:** 244–260.
21. Taxy JB, Battifora H, Oyasu R. Adenomatoid tumors: a light microscopic, histochemical and ultrastructural study. *Cancer* 1974; **34:** 306–316.
22. Davy CJ, Tang CK. Are all adenomatoid tumors adenomatoid mesotheliomas? *Hum Pathol* 1981; **12:** 360–369.
23. Grossman A, Gibson J, Stansfeld AG, Besser GM. Pituitary and testicular fibrosis in association with retroperitoneal fibrosis. *Clin Endocrinol* 1980; **12:** 371–374.
24. Efrati P, Nir E. Morphological and cytochemical investigations of human mesothelial cells from pleural and peritoneal effusions: a light and electron microscopy study. *Isr J Med Sci* 1976; **12:** 662–672.
25. Suzuki Y, Churg J, Kannerstein M. Ultrastructure of human malignant diffuse mesothelioma. *Am J Pathol* 1976; **85:** 241–262.
26. Rosai J, Gold J, Landy R. The histiocytoid hemangiomas. A unifying concept embracing several previously described entities of skin, soft tissue, large vessels, bone, and heart. *Hum Pathol* 1979; **10:** 707–730.

JOURNAL OF PATHOLOGY, VOL. **144**: 281–294 (1984)

CELL SURFACE CHARACTERIZATION OF THE HUMAN OSTEOCLAST: PHENOTYPIC RELATIONSHIP TO OTHER BONE MARROW-DERIVED CELL TYPES

M. A. HORTON, E. F. RIMMER AND D. LEWIS

Department of Haematology, St. Bartholomew's Hospital, London, U.K.

J. A. S. PRINGLE

Department of Morbid Anatomy, Institute of Orthopaedics,
The Royal National Orthopaedic Hospital, Stanmore, Middlesex, U.K.

AND

K. FULLER AND T. J. CHAMBERS

Department of Histopathology, St. Bartholomew's Hospital, London, U.K.

Received 28 April 1984
Accepted 4 June 1984

SUMMARY

Among the differentiated progeny of stem cells transplantable by bone marrow are osteoclasts, the multinucleate cells which are the major agents of bone resorption. Although the osteoclast is well characterized from a structural and functional standpoint, its development and origin are still far from clear. We have used monoclonal antibodies to investigate the interrelationship between osteoclasts and other haemopoietic cells in man. We have analysed the distribution of 19 granulocyte–monocyte antigens in eight reactivity clusters on the non-neoplastic osteoclasts present within nine osteoclastomas (syn. giant cell tumours of bone) and a single example of aneurysmal bone cyst. We found that osteoclasts are antigenically effete, failing to express granulocyte–monocyte, common leucocyte or other haemopoietic determinants; the only monocyte antigens detected on osteoclasts are My-7 and two closely related specificities, MCS.2 and DüHL60.4, which are also expressed by tissues outside the haemopoietic system. Our findings, taken together with recent transplantation studies, cast further doubt on the view that osteoclasts are specialized bone-resorbing macrophage-derived giant cells, and support a hypothesis that they are the end product of fusion of a hitherto unidentified circulating mononuclear cell type, the preosteoclast, which constitutes a cell lineage separate from those originating from the conventional multipotential haemopoietic stem cell, although still of bone marrow origin.

KEY WORDS—Osteoclasts, macrophage antigens, monoclonal antibodies, giant cell tumour.

INTRODUCTION

Osteoclasts are multinucleate giant cells with the property of mediating bone resorption[1,2]—although much is known about the structure and function of osteoclasts, their origin and development has been controversial. They were originally considered to be derived from a single osteoprogenitor stem cell, in common with the osteoblast, the bone-forming cell; however, a variety of experiments have demonstrated conclusively that the osteoclast arises from a bone marrow stem cell reaching the bone surface via a blood-borne mononuclear precursor,[1–3] in contrast to the osteoblast which develops from local skeletal mesenchyme.[4] Three major lines of evidence have

M.A.H. is a Wellcome Trust Senior Research Fellow in Clinical Science. This work was supported in part by grants from the Wellcome Trust, The Arthritis and Rheumatism Council, Cancer Research Campaign (M.A.H.), the Joint Research Board of St. Bartholomew's Hospital and the North East Thames Regional Health Authority (T.J.C.).

Addressee for correspondence: Dr M. A. Horton, Haemopoiesis Research Group, Department of Haematology, St. Bartholomew's Hospital, London EC1A 7BE, U.K.

0022–3417/84/120281–14$01.40

been provided in quail-chick limb grafting,[5,6] parabiosis[7] and transplantation experiments.[8,9] Definitive evidence came from the demonstration that grafts of compatible normal bone marrow cells cure osteopetrosis by substitution of the qualitatively defective osteoclasts with normal ones.[3,8,9]

Since osteoclasts are known to be formed by cell fusion,[1,2] and not by asymmetrical nuclear–cytoplasmic division, they have been generally considered to be a specialized skeletal form of phagocytic giant cell, derived from mononuclear macrophages in an analogous fashion to the formation of the inflammatory polykaryon.[10] However, although they have a number of properties in common, there are a number of important differences between osteoclasts and mononuclear phagocytes[1,2,10]—one of the most critical is the absence of calcitonin responsiveness in macrophages, a functional hallmark of osteoclasts.[11] Further evidence against a macrophage origin for osteoclasts comes from two studies. We have previously investigated the cell membrane phenotype of osteoclasts isolated from newborn rat and mouse bone and found that they fail to express Ia or granulocyte–monocyte surface antigens.[12] Secondly, work by Loutit and Nisbet[3] on radiation chimeras in osteopetrotic mice has demonstrated the existence of distinct stem cells for haemopoietic cell, including macrophage, and osteoclast formation.

Osteoclasts have been difficult to study in man, compared with rodents and birds, where procedures for isolation of osteoclasts from bone have been developed.[11] To circumvent this problem we have utilized tissues other than bone in which osteoclasts accumulate, namely oateoclastomas (syn. giant cell tumour of bone) and aneurysmal bone cyst. Although it has been argued[10,13,14] that the multinucleate giant cells of osteoclastomas are macrophage-derived, or possibly of neoplastic origin, more recent evidence has accrued to show that they exhibit a number of features in common with osteoclasts, many of which are unique to the specialized activities of bone resorption.[13,14] Hence, we have used these tumours as a convenient source of human osteoclasts for phenotypic studies and compared them with osteoclasts in aneurysmal bone cyst where there is no controversy over their origin. Thus, in this paper we present data on the cell surface phenotype of human osteoclastoma and aneurysmal bone cyst osteoclasts in an attempt to clarify the relationship between osteoclasts and other haemopoietic cell types, in particular of the macrophage cell lineage.

MATERIALS AND METHODS

Tissue specimens

Tissue from eight primary osteoclastomas (giant cell tumour of bone) and one metastatic lesion (total nine samples) were obtained at the time of surgical removal. The histopathological diagnosis was made by one of us (J.A.S.P.) according to standard diagnostic criteria.[15]

Tissue from a single patient with an aneurysmal bone cyst, which contains large numbers of osteoclasts in the septae, was also obtained.

Processing of tissue

Material was obtained at the time of the operation and stored in sterile tissue culture medium (20 mM HEPES buffered Medium 199) (Flow Laboratories Ltd, Irvine, Scotland) on ice and processed within between 1 and 5 h. Necrotic and haemorrhagic areas of tissue were dissected and a sample of the remainder was teased in medium and examined microscopically in order to check that ample osteoclasts were present. Two types of preparation were used for the cell surface phenotyping reported in this paper. First, tissue imprints were made by lightly dabbing 0·5 cm cubes of tumour on 6 mm multispot glass microscope slides (C. A. Hendley (Essex) Ltd., Loughton, Essex, U.K.); again, these were checked microscopically for the presence of adequate numbers of osteoclasts, air dried for 30 min, fixed in fresh acetone for 10 min, dried and then stored at −20°C before use (within 1 month). Second, samples of tumour or aneurysmal bone cyst were snap frozen and stored in liquid nitrogen in OCT embedding medium (Emscope Laboratories Ltd., Ashford, Kent, U.K.) until use; subsequently 5–8 μm frozen sections were prepared, air dried for 30 min, fixed in fresh acetone for 10 min, dried and stored at −20°C before use (within 1 month).

Characterization of osteoclastoma-derived giant cells as genuine osteoclasts

The cell suspensions from these osteoclastomas and from the aneurysmal bone cyst were also settled onto plastic substrates or slices of human femoral cortical bone for assessment of the calcitonin-responsiveness and bone resorptive capacity of the giant cells. The methods used will be described in detail (Pringle and Chambers, in preparation) but were essentially those described for rodent[11] and rabbit[16] osteoclasts.

Table I—Summary of phenotypic differences between osteoclasts, osteoclastoma giant cells, macrophages and inflammatory polykaryons

Cell type	Calcitonin responsiveness (inhibition of motility)	Fc receptors	Bone resorption (SEM)	Acid phosphatase
Macrophage	−	+	−	+
Inflammatory polykaryon	−	+	−	+
Osteoclast (rodent, rabbit)	+	−	+	+
Aneurysmal bone cyst osteoclast	+	−	+	+
Osteoclastoma giant cell	+	−	+	+

Antibodies

The mouse monoclonal antibodies to human haemopoietic cell surface antigens used in this study formed part of the granulocyte-monocyte specific panel of antibodies of the First International Workshop on Human Leukocyte Differentiation Antigens,[17] unless stated otherwise. As part of the workshop various antigenic 'clusters' were differentiated one from another which defined differing patterns of reactivity against circulating and tissue-fixed granulocytes and monocytes and their bone marrow precursors. The cluster designations, the names of the antibodies used from each cluster and their distribution on granulocytes and monocytes are summarized as part of Table III. Monoclonal antibodies reacting with other haemopoietic cell lineages and with common leucocyte determinants (Hle-1, T29/33, A3/D8) are summarized in Table II; these were purchased commercially or provided by their respective authors—2A1, Hle-1 (Dr P. Beverley); W6/32, CA2 (Dr W. Bodmer); R6A, R10 (Dr P. Edwards); My-7 (Dr J. Griffin).

All antibodies were provided as ascites, which was diluted to a predetermined optimal concentration before use.

Immunofluorescence techniques

Immunofluorescence analysis was performed on tumour imprints and frozen sections of osteoclastomas and the aneurysal bone cyst by an indirect technique. The stored imprints or sections were brought to room temperature, rehydrated for 10 min in Dulbecco's phosphate buffered saline containing 5 per cent fetal calf serum (PBS–FCS), excess medium wiped off and 50 μl of medium (negative control) or primary antibody applied for 30 min at room temperature in a humidified cham-

Table II—Cell surface antigens of human osteoclasts

Antigenic marker	Antibody	Osteoclast reactivity*: Osteoclastoma osteoclasts (three cases)	Osteoclast reactivity*: Aneurysmal bone cyst osteoclasts (one case)
HLA-A,B,C	2A1, W6/32	+++	+++
DrW(Ia)	CA2, I2	−	−
Common leucocyte†	Hle-1, T29/33, A3/D8	−	−
Widespread haemopoietic distribution	RFB1, OKT10, 5F1	−	nd
B lymphoid	SIg, CIg, J5	−	nd
T lymphoid	OKT6, 9.6, S33, WT1	−	nd
NK	Leu 7	−	nd
Erythroid	R6A, R10	−	nd
Megakaryocytic	AN51	−	nd

nd, Not determined.
* Assessed by indirect immunofluorescence on tissue imprints and frozen sections.
† Examined in all nine osteoclastomas and one aneurysmal bone cyst.

Table III—Absence of monclonal antibody defined granulocyte—monocyte antigens on human osteoclasts: osteoclastoma giant cells compared with aneurysmal bone cyst

Antigenic determinant	Antibodies used	Tissue distribution	Osteoclast reactivity: Osteoclastoma osteoclasts* (nine cases)	Osteoclast reactivity: Aneurysmal bone cyst osteoclasts* (one case)
HLA-A.B.C.	2A1, W6/32	Widespread. Positive control	+++	+++
DrW (Ia)	CA2, I2	Monocytes etc.	–	–
Granulocyte/monocyte†				
Cluster 11	FMC 10, 11, 12, 13	Most granulocytes, subpopulation of monocytes	–	–
Cluster 11a	TG1, IG10, G2	Most granulocytes, subpopulation of monocytes	–	–
Cluster 12	20.2	Large subpopulations of both granulocytes and monocytes	–	–
Cluster 13	My-7, MCS.2, DüHL60.4	Large subpopulations of both granulocytes and monocytes	+++	+++
Cluster 14	MO2, My4, 20.3	Most monocytes, subpopulation of granulocytes	–	–
Cluster 15	MO1, OKM1, M522	Large subpopulations of both granulocytes and monocytes	–	–
D5‡	—	Small subpopulations of both granulocytes and monocytes	–	–
My8‡	—	Large subpopulations of granulocytes and monocytes	–	–

* Assessed by indirect immunofluorescence on tissue imprints and frozen sections.

† Monoclonal antibody defined specificities arranged by their working groupings (First International Workshop on Human Leucocyte Differentiation Antigens[17]) according to their pattern of reactivity.

‡ Single specificities not assigned workshop grouping, but distinct from those in †.

ber. They were then washed in PBS–FCS for 30 min, excess medium removed and 50 μl optimally diluted, FITC conjugated goat anti-mouse immunoglobulin reagent added (GAM–Ig–FITC) (Coulter Immunology, Hialeah, Florida, U.S.A., 1/40 final concentration). After a further 30 min incubation, the slides were washed for a minimum of 60 min in PBS–FCS before mounting in PBS–glycerol and reading with a Zeiss epifluorescence microscope.

Controls and interpretation

Controls were included in all immunofluorescence tests to facilitate the interpretation of the reactions. Thus, the presence of a cell surface antigen was assessed by comparing the binding of a particular antibody to osteoclasts in the imprints or tissue sections with that of a negative (medium alone, i.e. the absence of primary antibody) and positive controls (antibody to common HLA–A,B,C determinants—2A1 or W6/32). The level of autofluorescence, in the absence of GAM–Ig–FITC, was also checked. Hence, the results given in Tables II and III are assigned as positive (+++ ; binding equivalent to positive control) or negative (−). Appropriate reactivity of the antibodies with inflammatory blood cells (monocytes, granulocytes and occasional lymphocytes), which were invariably present within the osteoclastomas and in the aneurysmal bone cyst, and the absence of reactivity with the tumour stromal cells, also served as internal controls for the assessment of the cell surface phenotype of osteoclasts.

RESULTS

Tissue morphology: osteoclastoma and aneurysmal bone cyst

The morphological appearance of the osteoclasts in the osteoclastoma tumour tissue and aneurysmal bone cyst used in this study is illustrated in stained sections (Fig. 1) and phase micrographs (Fig. 4a, 5a). The histopathological features of all nine tumours were typical of osteoclastoma (giant cell tumour of bone)[15] showing prominent, acid phosphatase positive (data not shown), multinucleate giant cells (osteoclasts) embedded in a mesh of elongate mononuclear stromal cells and intercellular ground substance, with a variable degree of infiltration with inflammatory cells (macrophages and occasional granulocytes and lymphocytes). The morphology of the aneurysmal bone cyst was also typical of that lesion. As can be seen, there are numerous multinucleate osteoclasts (marked (O)) (Figs. 4, 5) clearly identifiable in both tissues and easily separable from the stromal cells or inflammatory mononuclear cells infiltrating the lesions (Figs 1, 4).

Osteoclast properties exhibited by osteoclasts derived from osteoclastomas (giant cell tumour of bone) and aneurysmal bone cyst

We found that the giant cells obtained from osteoclastomas and from the aneurysmal bone cyst exhibited two properties which we have found to be characteristic of, and apparently specific for,

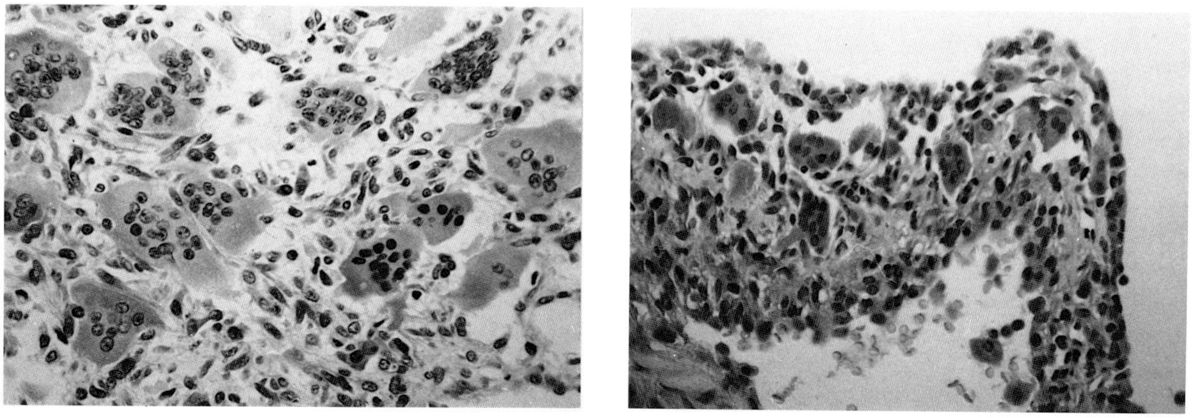

(a) (b)

Fig. 1—Haematoxylin and eosin stained section of an osteoclastoma tumour (a) and aneurysmal bone cyst (b) showing multinucleate osteoclasts and characteristic morphology of the lesions, × 155

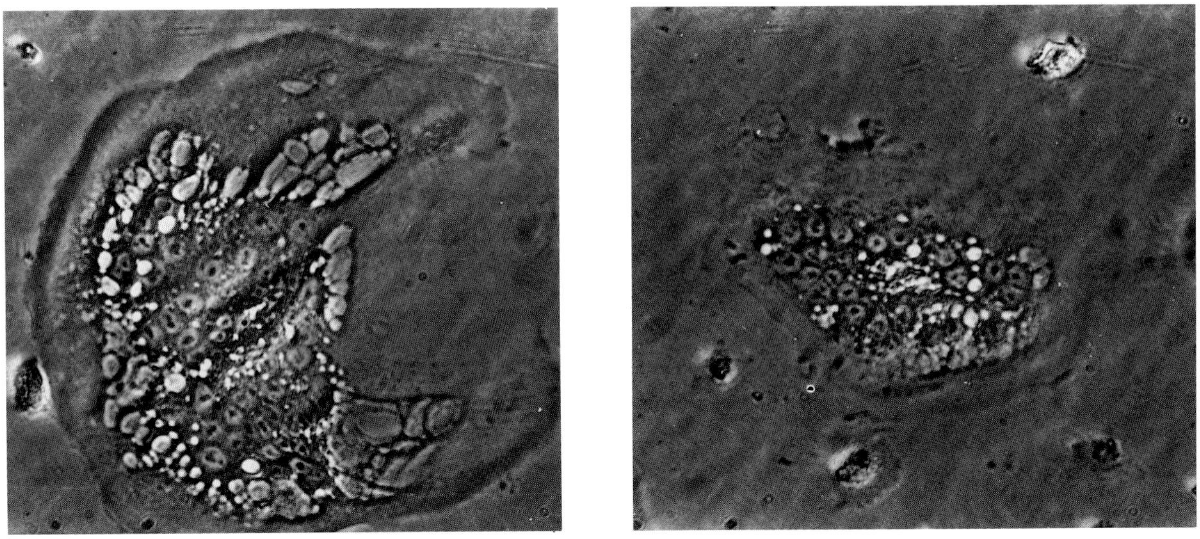

(a) (b)

Fig. 2—(a) Giant cell from osteoclastoma tumour incubated in control medium. The lobulated, smooth-contoured, phase-dense peripheral pseudopods are of an appearance which corresponds to active pseudopodial motility in time-lapse video observations. (b) Giant cell after 30 min incubation in salmon calcitonin (1 ng/ml) shows the phase-lucent, irregular periphery of an immotile cell. a and b, phase contrast, ×390

osteoclasts: the induction of cytoplasmic quiescence by calcitonin (Fig. 2) and the ability to resorb bone (Fig. 3) (results to be described in detail elsewhere). We have found that cells of the mononuclear phagocyte series, whether mononuclear or multinucleate, are both unresponsive to calcitonin and also incapable of bone resorption, measured in the scanning electron microscope as excavation of the surface of bone slices (see Table I and Refs 11, 16, 18).

The cell surface phenotype of osteoclastoma osteoclasts

Initially, we examined the cell surface phenotype of osteoclasts from 3 osteoclastomas with a number of monoclonal antibodies detecting cell surface antigens of haemopoietic cells. As the origin of the osteoclast is in dispute, but appears to be of bone marrow origin, antibodies specific for a wide range of different haemopoietic cell lineages were used in preliminary experiments. The results are shown in Table II; no evidence was found for expression of lymphoid, erythroid or megakaryocytic markers by osteoclasts. Low numbers of lymphocytes and a variable infiltration with monocytes and granulocytes was identifiable using lymphoid or common leucocyte specific antibodies. It should also be noted that the mononuclear neoplastic stromal cells only expressed HLA class I antigens and not DrW or haemopoietic cell restricted antigens.

Osteoclasts fail to express common leucocyte determinants

A number of cell surface antigens expressed on all nucleated cells of haemopoietic stem cell origin, but not other cell types, have been described. We examined the binding of three such antibodies (Hle-1, T29/33, A3/D8) to osteoclasts in all nine osteoclastomas, both as tumour imprints and in frozen sections, and in the aneurysmal bone cyst (see Table II and Fig. 4d). Although high background binding of these antibodies to the intercellular ground substance in three of the tumours made the interpretation of imprint, versus frozen section, results difficult, osteoclasts failed to express three monoclonal antibody defined common leucocyte antigens. The implication of such findings is discussed in detail later.

Absence of granulocyte–monocyte differentiation antigens on human osteoclasts

It has been suggested that osteoclasts might be a specialized form of mononuclear phagocyte-

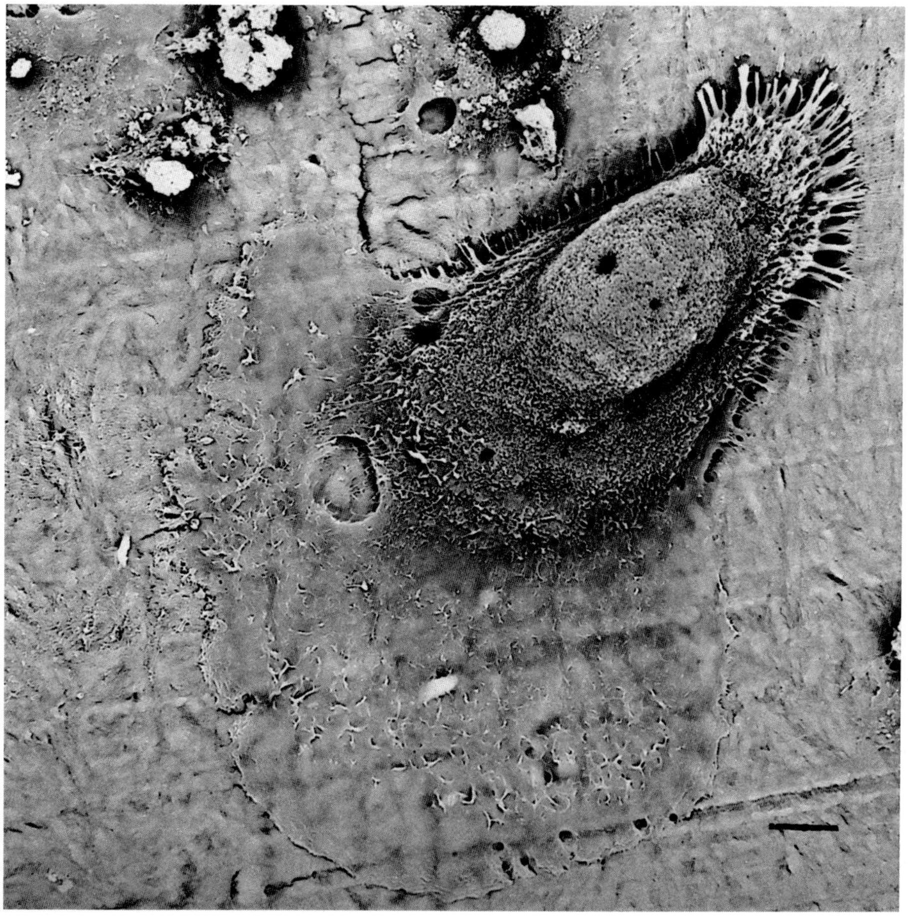

Fig. 3—(a) Scanning electron micrograph (backscatter electron image) of an osteoclastoma osteoclast shortly after sedimentation onto cortical bone surface showing characteristic morphological features—large size, complex structure and prominent microvilli over the central portion of the cell. Bar represents 10 μm

derived giant cell, a view based largely upon the analogy between fusion of macrophages to form polykaryons and the possibility of a similar mechanism operating for the formation of the multinucleate giant cell of bone, the osteoclast. For this reason, we examined the expression by osteoclasts of a wide range of antigens found on monocytes (and granulocytes)—the results are summarized in Table III and illustrated in Figs. 4 and 5 and are the same for both osteoclastoma and aneurysmal bone cyst osteoclasts. DrW(Ia) and granulocyte–monocyte antigens from seven of eight antigenically distinct reactivity clusters, defined in a recent international workshop,[17] are clearly absent from osteoclasts (but are present on the monocytes and/or granulocytes in the same lesions). One group of antigens (cluster 13), exemplified by the antibody My-7,[19] are uniformly and strongly expressed by osteoclasts in both sets of tissues (Figs. 4b, 4c, 5b). Moreover, preliminary observations suggest that, in some tumours containing a proportion of small osteoclasts with low nuclearity, there may be an increased expression of My-7 on the larger, more fully mature, osteoclasts; thus this antigen possibly represents an osteoclast, but not osteoclast-specific, differentiation antigen. As My-7 is expressed on some non-haemopoietic cells in addition to monocytes, for example umbilical cord vascular endothelium,[17] then the demonstration of this antigen on osteoclasts must be viewed with some caution as evidence for an origin in common with monocytes.

Monocytes and granulocytes within the tumour and cyst tissue reacted appropriately with the dif-

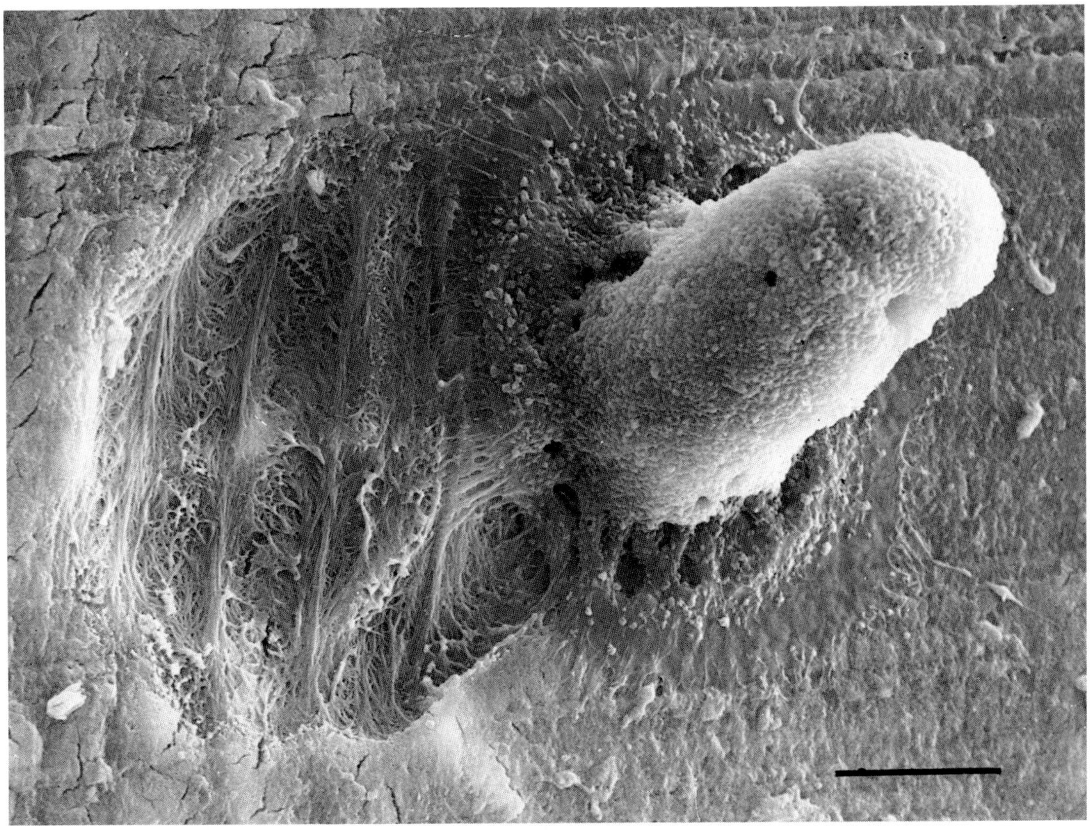

Fig. 3(b) Scanning electron micrograph (secondary electron image) of an osteoclastoma osteoclast, incubated for 16 h on bone surface, adjacent to resorption pit. These pits are never seen in the absence of added osteoclasts. Bar represents 10 μm

ferent granulocyte–monocyte specific antibodies; stromal cells consistently failed to bind all but the HLA positive control antibodies.

DISCUSSION

In this study we have investigated the cell lineage relationship between human osteoclasts and other bone marrow-derived cell types, in particular to the monocyte–macrophage cell lineage, using a series of monoclonal antibodies with defined specificities to haemopoietic cells (see Tables II and III). Human osteoclasts have been particularly difficult to study due to the lack of suitable procedures for isolating this numerically sparse cell type from normal bone—for this reason we have used an alternative tissue source, namely giant cell tumour and aneurysmal bone cyst osteoclasts.

Several conventionally applied criteria used for the identification of osteoclasts (see Table I) are fulfilled by the multinucleate giant cells characteristic of osteoclastomas (giant cell tumours of bone), which are also abundant in the cyst wall of the aneurysmal bone cyst. Furthermore, these features also clearly distinguish the cell type analysed in this study from the monocyte–macrophage derived inflammatory giant cell (Table I).

The morphological appearance[14,20] of giant cells at both light and ultrastructural level in both tissues is characteristic of the osteoclast; moreover the presence of a well-defined clear zone and plasma membrane ruffled border, together with the active bone resorption which is occasionally seen *in vivo*, support the osteoclastic nature of these cells. Osteoclastoma-derived giant cells share other properties found in osteoclasts of rodent and human bone—for example, the absence of Fc and C3 receptors,[21–23] histochemical profile[14,21] and low phagocytic potential *in vitro*.[21,22,24] We found that

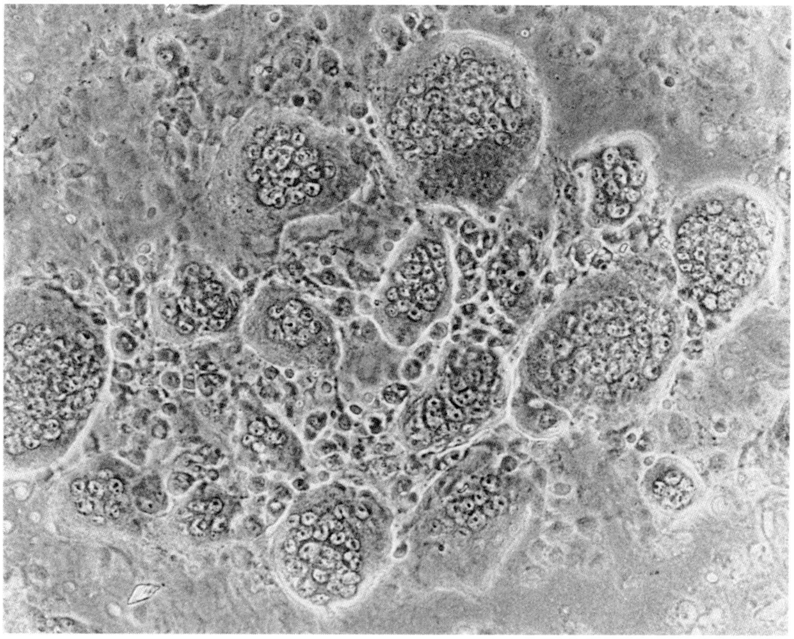

Fig. 4—(a) Tissue imprint of osteoclasts within an osteoclastoma tumour. Phase contrast micrograph with osteoclasts clearly visible, identified by their multinuclearity and granular cytoplasm, × 148

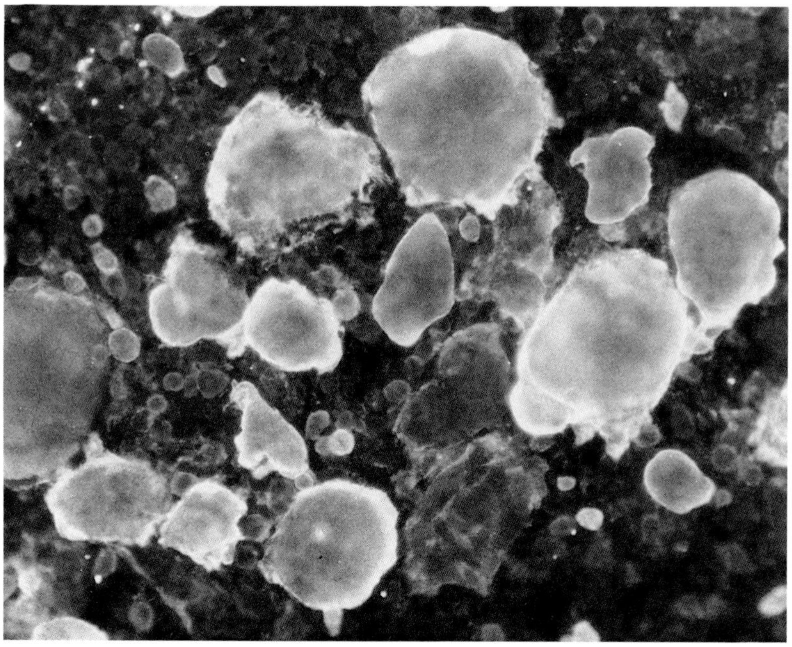

Fig. 4—(b) Tissue imprint of osteoclasts within an osteoclastoma tumour. Fluorescence micrograph using My-7 monoclonal antibody. Osteoclasts and macrophages are positive, whereas stromal cells are negative, × 148

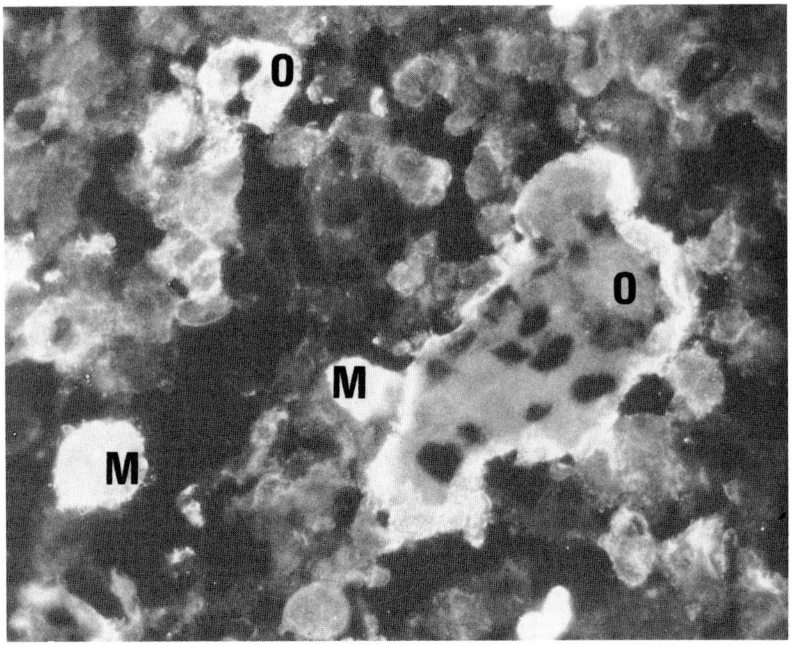

Fig. 4—(c) Frozen section of osteoclasts within an osteoclastoma tumour. Fluorescence micrograph using My-7 monoclonal antibody. Osteoclasts (O) and macrophages (M) are positive, whereas stromal cells are negative, × 390

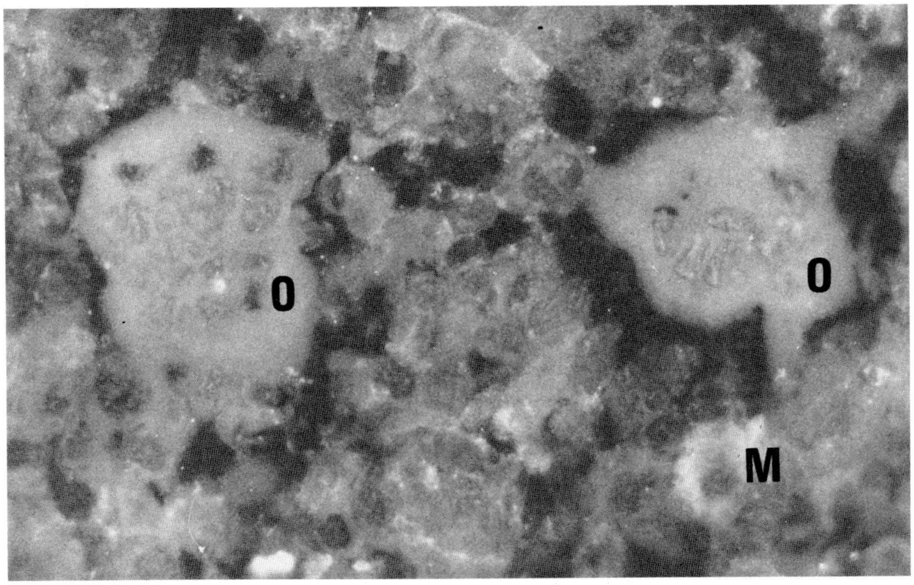

Fig 4—(d) Frozen section of osteoclasts within an osteoclastoma tumour. Fluorescence micrograph using Hle-1 monoclonal antibody. Osteoclasts (O) and stromal cells are negative whereas a single macrophage (M) is positive, × 390

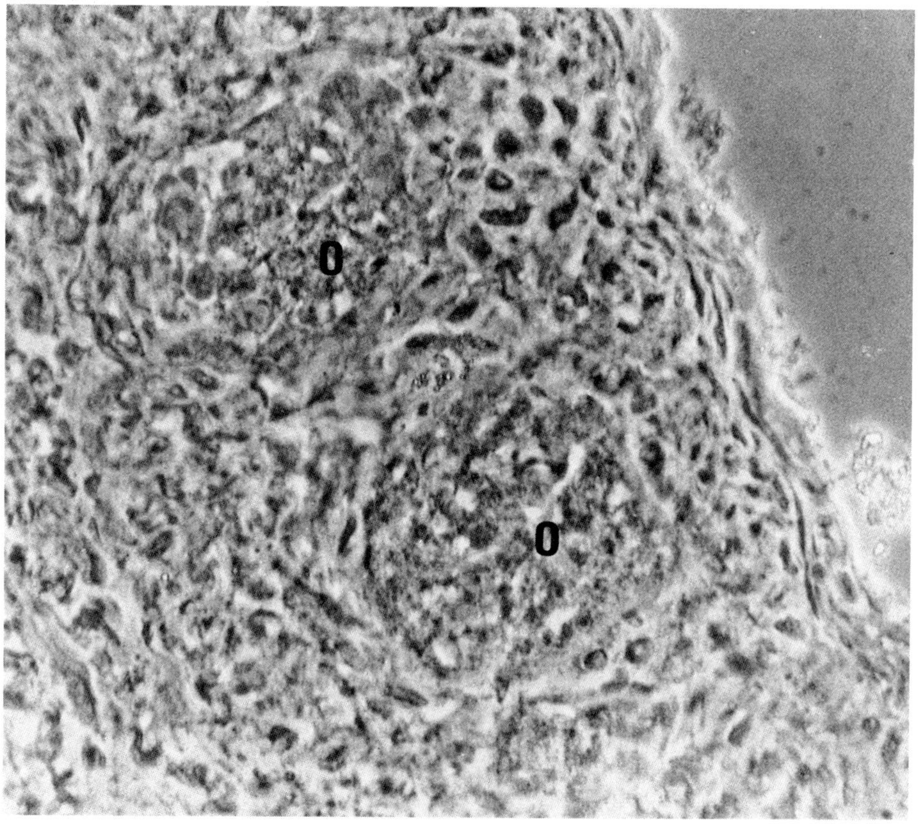

Fig. 5—(a) Phase contrast micrograph of a frozen section of osteoclasts in an aneurysmal bone cyst. Two osteoclasts (O) can be seen, × 390

the osteoclastoma giant cells used in the present communication undergo characteristic shape changes in response to calcitonin and resorb bone *in vitro* (Figs 2, 3) (Pringle and Chambers, in preparation) in a similar way to rabbit osteoclasts isolated from bone,[16] activities which macrophages and inflammatory polykaryons fail to exhibit.[11,18]

Taken together, these features serve not only to distinguish the giant cells of osteoclastomas from macrophages but also provide strong and convincing evidence that (a) the tumour-derived giant cells are osteoclasts and (b) that they are not phenotypically or functionally altered as part of a neoplastic process. Furthermore, we have also studied osteoclasts from an example of an aneurysmal bone cyst and found similar results by both functional and phenotypic criteria. As these latter cells are present in a non-neoplastic lesion, about which there is no controversy over their origin, we believe that it is valid to extend data derived from this study to the phenotype of osteoclasts in the normal environment of bone.

We have found that osteoclastoma and aneurysmal bone cyst osteoclasts fail to express markers characteristic of haemopoietic cell types (see Tables II and III and Figs. 4, 5). In particular, we would draw attention to the lack of expression of DrW and 16 of 19 monoclonal antibody defined monocyte–granulocyte determinants from eight antigenic clusters[17] (Table III); common leucocyte antigens, molecules expressed on all of the progeny of the multipotential haemopoietic stem cell, are also absent. These findings are in accord with our previous results for osteoclasts isolated from newborn rat and mouse bone.[12]

Two previous studies have analysed the macrophage characteristics of osteoclastoma giant cells.[21,24] Wood *et al.*[21] demonstrated the lack of cell surface Fc and C3 receptors found on monocytes, tissue macrophages and inflammatory polykaryons and also showed that osteoclastoma giant cells were poorly phagocytic and lacked non-

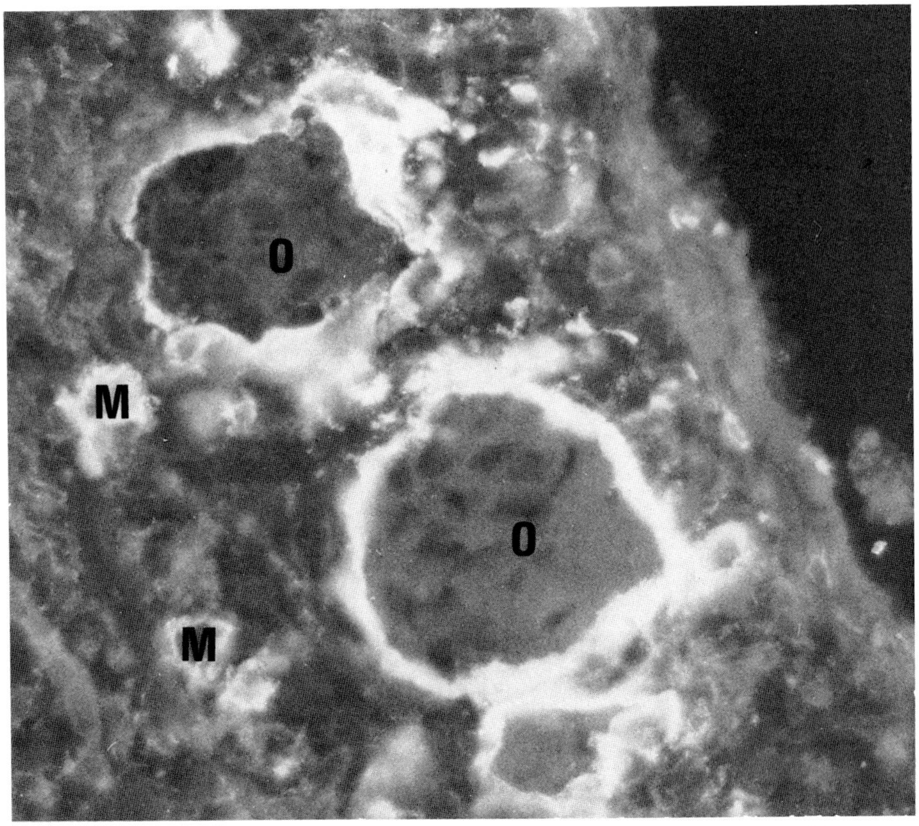

Fig. 5—(b) Fluorescence micrograph of a frozen section of osteoclasts in an aneurysmal bone cyst. The osteoclasts and at least two macrophages (M) are positive with My-7 monoclonal antibody, ×390

specific esterase activity, found in abundance in mononuclear phagocytes. From these studies they concluded that it was unlikely that osteoclastoma giant cells were macrophage derived—their conclusions are further supported by the fact that osteoclasts *in vivo* or freshly isolated from bone[1,2] also showed these differences from macrophages.

In a recent study by Burmester *et al.*,[24] the distribution on osteoclastoma giant cells of a series of monocyte–macrophage specific cell surface antigens was reported. The giant cells were found to be heterogeneous and either antigenically effete (Fc receptor$^-$, DrW(Ia)$^-$ and monocyte antigen$^-$) or Ia positive but, with one exception (MϕU50), not expressing surface antigens found on conventional circulating monocytes or tissue-fixed macrophages. In our series we found a consistent expression of a single antigenically related group of surface markers, including My-7,[17,19] on osteoclastoma osteoclasts; it is unclear how this specificity relates to the MϕU50 antigen, as we were unable to test both reagents in parallel. As My-7 is also found on cell types other than the monocytic lineage and outside the haemopoietic system,[17] and the full distribution of MϕU50 is not known, it cannot yet be ascertained whether expression of My-7 or MϕU50 is relevant to the question of whether or not osteoclasts come from monocytes. The reason for the finding of DrW on some giant cells in Burmester's study,[24] but its total absence in our cases (and in rodent newborn bone osteoclasts[12]) is also unclear. The class II major histocompatibility is known to consist of a series of biochemically related but antigenically distinct gene products[25] and it is possible that the difference between these results may be explained by differences in the antigenic specificity recognized by the monoclonal antibodies used.

Our findings on the surface antigenic profile of human osteoclasts allow us to conclude that they are quite unlike other bone marrow derived cell types; the absence of monocyte restricted surface antigens on osteoclasts, taken with other published data, makes it unlikely that there is a direct relationship between osteoclasts and the mononuclear phagocyte system. Moreover, the absence of common leucocyte antigens on human (and rodent[12]) osteoclasts strongly suggests that they arise by terminal differentiation of a bone marrow cell lineage distinct from the multipotential haemopoietic stem cell which gives rise to conventional blood cells; this view is supported by recent transplantation studies[3] which demonstrate that osteoclasts and macrophages arise from different stem cells.

However, in the type of phenotypic study reported herein, we cannot totally exclude that either (a) the mononuclear precursors of osteoclasts separate and diverge from the multipotential stem cell at a very early development stage or (b) that osteoclasts represent a highly specialized, terminally differentiated monocyte-derived cell type which has altered to such an extent in the local environment of bone that all the features of its precursor cell are lost. Conclusive proof against these possibilities will depend upon the isolation of mononuclear osteoclast precursors, capable of fusion *in vitro* to form functional multinucleate cells, and the demonstration that they are phenotypically distinct from circulating monocytes. Clearly one approach will be to make monoclonal antibodies to antigens unique to multinucleate osteoclasts, and hence their mononuclear precursors, which will enable them to be isolated and thus investigated.

NOTE ADDED IN PROOF

Since this paper was submitted we have examined a further 140 monoclonal antibodies to myeloid cells (some reactive with tissue macrophages) and found all but two to be negative on osteoclastoma osteoclasts.

ACKNOWLEDGEMENTS

We would like to thank the following orthopaedic surgeons for kindly allowing us access to surgical specimens and without whose cooperation this study would not have been possible: Mr S. D. Wilson, Mr H. B. S. Kemp, Royal National Orthopaedic Hospital, Stanmore; Mr Rodney Sneath, Royal Orthopaedic Hospital, Birmingham; Mr J. Hobbs and Dr A. MacFarlane, Kingsmill Hospital, Nottingham; Mr P. Stiles, Royal Surrey County Hospital, Guildford, U.K. We also thank Dr M. B. Wilkinson, Department of Biomedical Engineering, Institute of Orthopaedics for the scanning electron microscope pictures.

REFERENCES

1. Chambers TJ. The cellular basis of bone resorption. *Clin Orthop Rel Res* 1980; **151:** 283–293.
2. Marks SC. The origin of osteoclasts: evidence, clinical implications and investigative challenges of an extra-skeletal source. *J Oral Pathol* 1983; **12:** 226–256.
3. Loutit JF, Nisbet NW. The origin of the osteoclast. *Immunobiology* 1982; **161:** 193–203.
4. Vaughan J. Osteogenesis and haematopoiesis. *Lancet* 1981; **ii:** 133–135.
5. Kahn AJ, Simmons DJ. Investigations of cell lineage in bone using a chimaera of chick and quail embryonic tissue. *Nature* 1975; **258:** 325–327.
6. Jotereau FV, Le Douarin NM. The developmental relationship between osteocytes and osteoclasts, a study using quail-chick nuclear marker in endochrondral ossification. *Develop Biol* 1978; **63:** 253–265.
7. Göthlin G, Ericsson JLE. On the histogenesis of cells in fracture callus. Electron microscopic autoradiographic observations in parabiotic rats and studies on labelled monocytes. *Virchows Arch Cell Pathol* 1973; **12:** 318–329.
8. Walker DG. Control of bone resorption by hemopoietic tissue. The induction and reversal of congenital osteopetrosis in mice through use of bone marrow and splenic transplants. *J Exp Med* 1975; **142:** 651–663.
9. Ash P, Loutit JF, Townsend KMS. Osteoclasts derived from haemopoietic stem cells. *Nature* 1980; **283:** 669–670.
10. Chambers TJ. Multinucleate giant cells. *J Pathol* 1978; **126:** 125–148.
11. Chambers TJ, Magnus CJ. Calcitonin alters behaviour of isolated osteoclasts. *J Pathol* 1982; **136:** 27–39.
12. Horton MA, Rimmer EF, Moore A, Chambers TJ. On the origin of the osteoclast: the cell surface phenotype of rodent osteoclasts. *Calc Tissue Int*, in press.
13. Stewart MJ. Observations on myeloid sarcoma, with an analysis of 50 cases. *Lancet* 1914; **ii:** 1236–1242.
14. Schajowicz F. Giant cell tumour of bone (osteoclastoma): a pathological and histochemical study. *J Bone Jt Surg* 1961; **43A:** 1–29.
15. Jaffe HL, Lichtenstein L, Portis RB. Giant cell tumor of bone. Its pathological appearance, grading, supposed variants and treatment. *Arch Pathol* 1940; **30:** 993–1031.
16. Chambers TJ, Revell PA, Fuller K, Athanasou NA. Resorption of bone by isolated rabbit osteoclasts. *J Cell Sci* 1984; **66:** 383–399.
17. Bernard A, Boumsell L, Dausset J, Milstein C, Schlossman SF. (eds). Human Leucocyte Differentiation Antigens Detected by Monoclonal Antibodies. Heidelberg: Springer-Verlag, 1984.

18. Chambers TJ, Horton MA. Failure of cells of the mononuclear phagocyte series to resorb bone. *Calc Tissue Int*, in press.
19. Griffin JD, Ritz J, Nadler LM, Schlossman SF. Expression of myeloid differentiation antigens on normal and malignant myeloid cells. *J Clin Invest* 1981; **68:** 932–941.
20. Göthlin G, Ericsson JLE. The osteoclast. Review of ultrastructure, origin and structure–function relationship. *Clin Orthop Rel Res* 1976; **120:** 201–231.
21. Wood GW, Nett JR, Gollahon KA, Gourley WK. Macrophages in giant cell tumours of bone. *J Pathol* 1978; **125:** 53–58
22. Chambers TJ. Phagocytosis and trypsin-resistant glass adhesion by osteoclasts in culture. *J Pathol* 1979; **127:** 55–59.
23. Hogg N, Shapiro IM, Jones SJ, Slusarenko M, Boyde A. Lack of Fc receptors on osteoclasts. *Cell Tissue Res* 1980; **212:** 509–516.
24. Burmester GR, Winchester RJ, Dimitriu-Bona A, Klein M, Steiner G, Sissons HA. Delineation of four cell types comprising the giant cell tumor of bone: expression of Ia and monocyte–macrophage lineage antigens. *J Clin Invest* 1983; **71:** 1633–1648.
25. Steinmetz M, Minard K, Horvarth S, McNicholas J, Srelinger J, Wake C, Long E, Mach B, Hood L. A molecular map of the immune response region from the major histocompatibility complex of the mouse. *Nature* 1982; **300:** 35–42.

JOURNAL OF PATHOLOGY, VOL. **144**: 295–296 (1984)

LETTER TO THE EDITOR

OSTEOCLASTS: PUTATIVE, SURROGATE AND AUTHENTIC

We share the enthusiasm of your editorial for osteoclasts, and would like to take this opportunity to add some comments of our own and to clarify our views concerning the relationship between osteoclasts and cells of the mononuclear phagocyte series.

Despite its central position in bone pathobiology, the osteoclast is a poorly understood cell. Until recently[1] it was completely unavailable for study outside bone, and even now can be extracted only in very small numbers, too few for the liking of biochemists, difficult to separate from other bone cells and in a non-proliferative state. For these reasons there is intense current interest in the origin of the osteoclast: the precursors and their progeny might represent an alternative source of osteoclasts.

The confidence with which results, derived from the use of such surrogates, can be extrapolated to the pathobiology, of osteoclastic bone resorption, depends heavily upon the degree to which such cells share ontogenetic and phenotypic similarities with osteoclasts. Osteoclasts are undoubtedly derived from a haemopoietic stem cell, and the morphologically similar cells of the mononuclear phagocyte series are candidates as osteoclast precursors. How close is this relationship? To answer this we have compared hormonal responsiveness, bone-resorptive potential and antigenic markers of osteoclasts (which we define as multinucleate cells disaggregated from normal bone) and mononuclear phagocytes.

We have found[1] that exquisitely low concentrations of calcitonin regularly induce a dramatic behavioural change in osteoclasts, a response we have never observed in any cell of the mononuclear phagocyte lineage, including polykaryons, at any concentration. This difference does not mean that osteoclasts do not develop from mononuclear phagocytes, but does mean that mononuclear phagocytes, lacking this response, cannot be used as reliable osteoclast surrogates.

Excavation of bone, the primary function of osteoclasts, has never been demonstrated by osteoclast surrogates. Although mononuclear phagocytes release calcium and hydroxyproline from devitalized bone *in vitro* we have found[2] that monocytes, macrophages, monocytic cell lines and macrophage polykaryons, even in the presence of agents currently considered to enhance osteoclastic differentiation in these cells, are without perceptible effect on slices of bone in which osteoclasts, under identical conditions, rapidly induce deep excavations.[3] This suggests that there may be a fundamental biological difference between osteoclasts and mononuclear phagocytes.

We have also been struck by the degree of dissimilarity between the cell surface phenotypes of osteoclasts and mononuclear phagocytes. Using osteoclasts disaggregated from mouse, rat[4] and fetal human[5] long bones all macrophage-specific markers (My7 is not macrophage-specific), although present on macrophage polykaryons, were absent from osteoclasts. Furthermore, common leucocyte antigens, present on all nucleated derivatives of the haemopoietic stem cell, shared by red cell, platelet, lymphoid, granulocytic and monocytic cell lineages from the most primitive to the terminally differentiated, are absent from osteoclasts. If osteoclasts differentiate from mononuclear phagocytes this represents a degree of phenotypic divergence unprecedented amongs haemopoietic cells. The alternative is separation of osteoclasts from other haemopoietic cells at a very early stage, a possibility favoured by bone marrow transplantation experiments which suggest a separate haemopoietic stem cell for osteoclasts.[6] In either case, such phenotypic dissimilarity makes mononuclear phagocytes unpromising osteoclast surrogates.

With these phenotypic and functional distinctions between osteoclasts and mononuclear phagocytes in mind we assessed the nature of the polykaryons in giant cell tumours. The giant cells, like osteoclasts and unlike mono- and multinucleated macrophages, excavate bone, and demonstrate the behavioural change in the presence of calcitonin which appears characteristic of osteoclasts. Antigenically the giant cells were effete for mononuclear phagocyte and other haemopoietic cell antigens: as your editorial mentions, if the giant cells were macrophage polykaryons, even if the giant cells are the neoplastic component, we would have expected retention of at least a few markers, especially since these are in general so well conserved on haemopoietic neoplasms; the markers therefore also support an identity of these cells as osteoclasts.

Opinion is growing that the polykaryons in these lesions are a reactive, immigrant population, not derived from the neoplastic cell but attracted by it into the lesion. Our results thus indicate the osteoclastic nature of giant cell tumour polykaryons, emphasize the phenotypic and functional distinctions between osteoclasts and mononuclear phagocytes, and suggest that the giant cells in these lesions represent a source of a cell type otherwise for practical purposes unavailable from adult man.

J. J. CHAMBERS
Senior Lecturer in Histopathology
St Bartholomew's Hospital
London EC1
U.K.

M. A. HORTON
Wellcome Senior Research Fellow
St Bartholomew's Hospital
London EC1
U.K.

REFERENCES

1. Chambers TJ, Magnus CJ. Calcitonin alters behaviour of isolated osteoclasts. *J Pathol* 1982; **136:** 27–39.
2. Chambers TJ, Horton MA. Failure of cells of the mononuclear phagocyte series to resorb bone. *Calc Tissue International*, in press.
3. Chambers TJ, Revell PA, Fuller K, Athanasou NA. Resorption of bone by isolated rabbit osteoclasts. *J Cell Science* 1984; **66:** 383–399.
4. Horton MA, Rimmer EF, Moore A, Chambers TJ. On the origin of the osteoclast: the cell surface phenotype of rodent osteoclasts. *Calc Tiss International*, in press.
5. Horton MA, Pringle JAS, Chambers TJ. Cell surface phentotype of human foetal osteoclasts. Submitted.
6. Loutit JF, Nisbet NW. The origin of the osteoclast. *Immunobiology* 1982; **161:** 193–203.

BOOK REVIEWS

Precancer. Edited by J. J. DeCosse. Vol. 2, No. 3 of Cancer Surveys. Published for the Imperial Cancer Research Fund by Oxford University Press, Oxford. 1983. Price: £14.00.

This book is about the cell and tissue lesions which are associated with and may lead to subsequent development of cancer. Although the morphological features of these lesions are usually described in words and sometimes with pictures, the bulk of the text assumes a basic histopathological understanding and concentrates on analysis of the strength of the associations with subsequent cancer, and on the possible mechanisms whereby progression may occur from pre-cancerous lesions to full-blown malignancy. Like many little books that attempt great things, this book has some defects. Cancer scientists without a histopathological background—for whom perhaps, the book is primarily intended—may find it heavy going, as some important definitions are confuscated (for example 'dysplasia refers to an intraepithelial change whose maturation is altered'). Some chapters are disappointing, where they are little more than compilations of statistical associations. Others have omissions which reflect personal bias (for example Lagios' failure to mention radial scars in the breast). Nonetheless, this is an admirable book on an important subject. It brings together many hard facts and enough speculation on human pre-cancer to counter some misconceptions and encourage new ideas. The panel of authors are recognized authorities and present an up-to-date picture of our understanding of pre-cancer in the human cervix uteri, breast, mouth, lung, stomach, colorectum and bladder. The book finishes with a well-written account on multi-stage carcinogenesis in animals, with some reference to recent work on oncogenes. Diagnostic histopathologists, experimentalists, cytologists and teachers of pathology should all find the book of value.

A. H. Wyllie
University of Edinburgh

The Healing and Scarring of Atheroma. Edited by Moshe Wolman. Advances in Experimental Medicine and Biology, Volume 168. Plenum Press, New York, 1984. No. of pages: 622. Price: $32.50. ISBN: 0 306 41514 3.

This book is a compilation of seven papers from the 1981 meeting of the World Congress of Pathology and is intended to address the question, can atherosclerosis be prevented, halted or reversed? The title is intriguing and suggests a tissue orientated approach likely to be of interest to histopathologists. Indeed, the first chapter attempts to describe atherosclerosis in terms of 'normal pathological principles'. However, rather than drawing fresh insights from analogies with examples of chronic inflammation in other tissues, such as the potential reversibility of hepatic fibrosis, a more narrow attitude is adopted. 'The proliferation of smooth muscle in atherosclerosis is, thus, attributed to a variant of a basic pathological mechanism, and does not require a more complex mechanism, such as the action of a somatotropin, mitogen or mutagen.' Thus, are the exciting new areas, such as platelet derived growth factor, monoclonality of plaques, etc., summarily dismissed.

The chapters on such topics as macrophage enzyme activity, ultrastructural features and hormonal effects on experimental atherosclerosis are written in a particularly loose and rambling style which makes for hard reading. Conclusions are not clearly summarized. There are no sections of discussion between the speakers at the conference. A recurrent difficulty is the failure of several authors to consider whether fibrosis should be regarded as 'healing', being part of regression, or 'scarring', being part of progression. From analogy with the healing wound, why not both, if arterial endothelium is repeatedly disturbed? The later chapters do tackle such problems and are written in a Crisper and more convincing style. A book then, to irritate the specialist, perhaps with some benefit, and not for the general reader.

W. D. Thompson
University of Aberdeen

Cardiac Pathology, An Integrated Text and Colour Atlas. Anton E. Becker and Robert H. Anderson. Churchill Livingstone, Edinburgh; Gower Medical Publishing, London, 1984. Price: £48.00. ISBN: 0 443 03114 2 (Churchill Livingstone); 0 906923 10 7 (Gower Medical Publishing).

This long and extensively illustrated work is indeed a combination of a colour atlas and a textbook of cardiac pathology. It is as an atlas that it scores most highly for the illustrations are really magnificent and almost faultless. Many complex conditions are lucidly illustrated, often with an adjacent black and white pen drawing to highlight different pathological features. The general pathologist will find the earlier chapters of this book the most useful. Chapter 3, 'Acquired conditions primarily affecting myocardial contractility' includes excellent sections on the pathology of coronary artery bypass grafting, myocarditis and unusual myocardial diseases. Equally useful are the sections in chapter 4 on pathological changes involving prosthetic valves and the short chapter 6 on injuries produced during cardiac catheterization and pacemaker insertion.

Both authors are international authorities on the anatomy and pathology of congenital heart disease. It is, perhaps, for this reason that eight of the 16 chapters deal with malformations of the heart, great arteries and conducting system. The first of these is the most valuable for the non-expert as it describes briefly and clearly the criteria that should be used for the identification of different anatomical chambers. Subsequent sections describe individual anomalies in ever increasing detail. Again the illustrations are excellent and line drawings highlight the important features of many of the photographs. These chapters are not for the faint hearted! Pediatric pathologists and cardiac surgeons will find them fascinating but I doubt that any general pathologists would read these chapters systematically.

Departments of cardiac surgery and pediatric pathology will obviously need and use this book extensively. The heavy bias toward pediatric pathology will probably make most pathologists think twice before dipping into their pockets for £48.00.

P. J. GALLAGHER
Southampton General Hospital

Proteases Potential Role in Health and Disease. Edited by WALTER H. HORL and AUGUST HEIDLAND. Advances in Experimental Medicine and Biology, Volume 167. Plenum Press, New York, 1983. No of pages: 591. Price $85.00. ISBN 0 306 41167 9.

This volume represents a camera-ready compilation of papers presented at the symposium 'Proteases: Potential Role in Health and Disease' which was held in Würzburg (FRG), 17–20 October 1982. There are 51 contributions, of which some are reviews, but most are scientific communications. Papers are arranged into sections primarily concerned with the physiology and pathophysiology of proteases and their inhibitors, proteases and hormones, proteases in kidney and gastrointestinal tract, proteases and blood, proteases and lung, proteases and arthritis, hypercatabolism, pancreatitis, proteases and muscle function. It is rather a parochial collection of papers, with almost all originating from West German laboratories. All the papers are written in English, although with scattered grammatical and spelling errors. My judgement would be that this compilation would be of use in those laboratories actively engaged in connective tissue protease research.

T. S. CHAMBERS
St. Bartholomew's Hospital
London

International Medical Reviews in Haematology. Vol 1. Leukaemias. Edited by JOHN M. GOLDMAN and HARVEY D. PRIESLER. Butterworth, London, 1984. No. of pages: xi + 372. Price: ISBN: 0 407 02336 4.

This, the first volume on a haematological subject in the series of International Medical Reviews published by Butterworths, amply fulfils what it sets out to do. It fills the gap between the textbook descriptions of the leukaemias and the comprehensive monograph. It is recommended as a stimulating update in a field where the data base of information from research is expanding rapidly and the busy clinician cannot hope to keep pace.

Inevitably in a multi-author compendium there is a certain amount of repetition but this is kept to a minimum and the slightly differing versions given by haematologists from opposite sides of the Atlantic make for added interest. Each main variety of leukaemia is allocated one descriptive chapter and one on treatment. In addition, there are excellent resumées on retroviruses in leukaemia, cytotoxic drugs, bone marrow transplantation and supportive care. Thus, in one volume we have an authoritative and comprehensive review covering both theoretical aspects and management of the disease. Generally, the chapters are clearly laid out with aptly chosen tables. If one had to select just one for special comment it would be the delightfully lucid account of the treatment of chronic lymphocytic leukaemia by Professor Galton. This will certainly be of practical use to the clinical haematologist in deciding whether treatment is appropriate, when it should be commenced and what should be the aims of treatment.

For anyone regretting lack of detail there are, on average, 134 references for each chapter, many of which are up to date. For the curious some historical reports are cited which throw light on the way in which treatments have developed. I would recommend this book to clinicians and laboratory haematologists who wish to keep abreast of changes in the field. It augurs well for future numbers in this series by Butterworths.

D. S. GILLETT
Kings College Hospital
London

Practical Aspiration Cytology. DAVID MELCHER, JOHN LINEHAN and RUSSELL SMITH. Churchill Livingstone, New York, 1984. No. of pages iii + 230. Price: £25.00. ISBN: 0 443 02633 5.

Though long established in a few centres, the diagnosis of tumours by aspiration cytology has only recently been started in many British hospitals. Some applications are still of debatable value (thyroid and parotid), while others are undeniably of practical importance (confirmation of metastatic deposits). The present book, with simple explanations and clear photographs, succeeds well as an introduction to the subject. Besides the three editors who deal with the breast, prostate, lymph nodes and a few other sites, there are chapters by A. John Webb on the thyroid and salivary glands, by Chandra Grubb on the lungs and abdominal organs, and a chapter (curiously out of place in this context) by Ken Chippendale on the technique of identification of B and T lymphocytes by E-rosettes and immunofluorescence of cells in suspension.

Of the two commonly used fixation and staining techniques, Webb shows Romanowsky-stained cells only, as does Melcher for breast and lymph nodes, while the other sites are illustrated from Papanicolaou smears in addition.

Because smears contain subtler information than histological sections, one might expect that aspirates would need to be interpreted by a higher-powered type of pathologist. Why then should a book on this subject be aimed at non-medical readers? Judging by the brief glossary this even extends to people who did no science at school, else it would not feature 'hormone', 'mitosis', 'DNA', and 'pH'. Clearly, the intention is to involve all grades of staff in the diagnostic process. The rising tide of needle aspiration cytology should force us to take a new look at the roles of pathologist, MLSO and 'screener'.

I will not carp at certain anomalies and over-simplifications in this book. There are some actual mistakes, for instance an excellent photograph of starch grains is called 'talc' both in the text and the caption; and the statement, contradicted elsewhere, that lymphoblasts are 'only seen with certainty in the rare mediastinal malignant lymphoma of the young adult'. Latin or Greek expressions tend to be wrong, e.g. a large corpora amylacea, a criteria, the bursa of fabricus.

There are other new or nearly new books on the same subject—for instance those of Kline, Frable, and Linsk and Franzén. The present one is certainly the simplest, clearest and quickest to read. Its relatively large pictures are the easiest to find and use and will make this book a valuable one for the novice. It also contains wise advice about the principles of reporting.

What we need now is a heavy-weight textbook of histopathology which will include histochemistry and cytology with every section.

A. I. SPRIGGS
The Churchill Hospital
Oxford

JOURNAL OF PATHOLOGY, VOL. **144**: 300 (1984)

ANNOUNCEMENT

POSTGRADUATE COURSE IN GYNECOLOGIC AND OBSTETRIC PATHOLOGY

22–26 April 1985

The Departments of Pathology, Massachusetts General Hospital, and Brigham and Women's Hospital, Harvard Medical School will present a postgraduate course in Gynecologic and Obstetric Pathology under the direction of Drs Robert E. Scully, Robert H. Young and Shirley G. Driscoll. This course is designed for pathologists and obstetrician–gynecologists at resident and practitioner levels. It will provide an in-depth review of gynecologic and obstetric pathology with emphasis on morphologic diagnostic features and clinicopathologic correlation including management. Special attention will be paid to recent advances and newly recognized entities. Instruction will be primarily by lecture, but will also include case presentations and discussion periods. Each participant will receive a comprehensive course syllabus. The course has Category I accreditation for 35 h CME credit by the American Medical Association and 35 cognates, formal learning, by the American College of Obstetricians and Gynecologists. The fee for the course is $475.00.

Further information from: Department of Continuing Education, Harvard Medical School, 25 Shattuck Street, Boston, MA 02115, U.S.A. Telephone 617 732 1526.

JOURNAL OF PATHOLOGY, VOL. **144**: vii–viii (1984)

KEY WORD INDEX

Acute hepatitis, 213
Adenoma of breast, 15
Adenomatoid tumour, 275
Adrenal glands, 1
Alveolar macrophages, 149
Aminonucleoside, 45
Amiodarone lung toxicity, 73
Angiofollicular lymph node hyperplasia, 131
Atypical fibroxanthoma, 189

Basement membrane, 35
Breast, 15
Breast cancer, 109, 253
Breast carcinoma, 101

Capsular hypervascularity, 257
CCK, 171
Chemotactic tripeptide, 201
Chronic gastritis, 171

Dendritic histiocytes, 241
Dendritic reticulum cells, 233
Desmoplastic malignant melanoma, 189
Ductal adenoma, 15

Endocrine cells, 171
Endothelial cells, 201, 213, 275
Enteroglucagon, 171
Enzyme-histochemistry, 131
Extranodal extension, 253

Ferritin, 45
Fibronectin, 35
Fibrosis, 149
Fluorescent probes, 201
Focal glomerular sclerosis, 45
Fucose, 109

Gastrin, 171
Giant cell tumour, 281
GIP, 171
Glomerulonephritis, 45
Glomerulus, 179
Granulocyte adherence, 201

Haemangioma, 275
Histiocytes, 233
Histomorphometry, 163
Hodgkin's disease, 227, 233
Hydrocele, 275

Idiopathic myeloid metaplasia, 163
Immunohistochemistry, 131, 189
Infarction, 257
Inflammatory mediator, 25
Intestinal metaplasia, 171
Iron–dextran, 179
Ischaemia, 257

Juxtaglomerular cells, 1

Laminin, 35
Laryngeal carcinomas, 35
Lectin histochemistry, 101
Lectins, 109
Lipid pneumonia, 73
Lung development, 89
Lung injury, 149
Lymph nodes, 257
Lymphocyte depletion, 257
Lymphocytes, 269

Macrophage antigens, 281
Malignant lymphomas, 233, 241
Membrane dynamics, 201
Mesangium, 45, 179
Mesentery, 257
Mesothelial cell, 275
Metalophil histiocytes, 241
Metalophil method, 233
Monoclonal antibodies, 281
Mouse lungs, 89

Nicotine toxicity, 89

Oral lesions, 119
Osteoclasts, 281

Paf-acether, 25
Paraffin sections, 119
Paranodal vascular spread, 253
Particulate matter, 119

Peritoneal macrophages, 81
Pigmented villondular synovitis, 57
Platelet activating factor, 25
Precancerous lesions, 171
Psoriatic arthritis, 57
Pulmonary histocytosis, 73

Radiation mouse chimaeras, 81
Rat, 179
Reed–Sternberg cells, 227
Reticulum cells, 227

Pseudofibromatous periorchitis, 275

Sclerotic bone, 163
Secretin, 171
Sheep, 1
Silica, 149
Somatostatin, 171
Spindle-cell squamous carcinoma, 189

Thyroid gland, 269
Thyroiditis, 269
Toxaemia of pregnancy, 1
Tumour heterogeneity, 101
Type IV collagen, 35
Type V collagen, 35

Ultrastructure, 213

Vascular permeability, 25

XES, 119

AUTHOR INDEX

Adamson, I.Y.R., 149
Aparicio, S. R., 179
Archer, C. B., 25
Archer-Harvey, J. M., 57
Azzopardi, J. G., 15, 189

Bardadin, K. A., 213
Bellon, G., 35
Bowden, D. H., 149
Broustet, A., 163

Cam, Y., 35
Carlei, F., 171
Cattell, V., 45
Caulet, T., 35
Ceccarelli, C., 189
Chambers, T. J., 281
Chen, M.-F., 89
Coghlan, J.P., 1
Coindre, J. M., 163
Corrin, B., 73
Costa-Jussà, F. R., 73
Covotta, A., 171
Cristofolini, M., 189
Crocker, J., 131
Crocker, P. R., 119
Curran, R. C., 131

Davies, J. D., 257
Davison, A. M., 179
De Mascarel, A., 163
Dewar, A., 25
De Weger, R. A., 241

Eusebi, V., 189
Fuentes, E., 275
Fuller, K., 281

Goode, N. P., 179
Goussot, J. F., 163
Gowland, G., 179
Gregory, J., 131
Grounds, M. D., 81
Guibarra, M., 131

Hartveit, F., 253
Henderson, D. W., 57
Hill, P. A., 1
Horton, M. A., 281

Kirkham, N., 269
Kirkpatrick, C. J., 201

Jacobs, J. M., 73
Jones, E. L., 131, 227

Lee, G., 119
Legros, M., 35
Levison, D. A., 119
Lewis, D., 281
Lezoche, E., 171

MacDonald, D. M., 25
Machin, D., 269
Mahy, N.J., 257
Malchiodi-Albedi, F., 171
Melcion, C., 45
Melzner, I., 201
Mingazzini, P., 171
Mitchell, J. D., 269
Morley, J., 25
Murch, A. R., 81

Nistal, M., 275

Page, C. P., 25
Paniagua, R., 275
Papadimitriou, J. M., 57, 81
Paul, W., 25
Piscioli, F., 189
Polak, J. M., 171
Poulin, G., 35
Pringle, J. A. S., 281
Pytlinska, M., 35

Regadera, J., 275
Reiffers, J., 163
Rimmer, E. F., 281
Ryan, G. B., 1
Rozenbilds, M. A. M., 57

Salm, R., 15
Scheuer, P. J., 213
Schraufnagel, D. E., 89
Scoggins, B. A., 1
Shepherd, N. A., 119
Shires, M., 179
Smith, A. P., 119
Smith, J., 45
Speranza, V., 171

Van Unnik, J. A. M., 233, 241

Walker, R. A., 101, 109
Wang, N.-S., 89

Yao, Y.-T., 89